Gynaecology: Evidence-Based Algorithms

COMPANION VOLUME:
Obstetrics: Evidence-Based Algorithms,
Jyotsna Pundir and Arri Coomarasamy
(ISBN 9781107618930)

Gynaecology: Evidence-Based Algorithms

Jyotsna Pundir

*Sub-Speciality Fellow in Reproductive Medicine and Surgery,
St Bartholomew's Hospital, London, UK*

Arri Coomarasamy

*Professor of Gynaecology, School of Clinical and Experimental Medicine,
College of Medical and Dental Sciences, University of Birmingham,
and Birmingham Women's Hospital Foundation Trust, Birmingham, UK*

CAMBRIDGE
UNIVERSITY PRESS

CAMBRIDGE
UNIVERSITY PRESS

University Printing House, Cambridge CB2 8BS, United Kingdom

Cambridge University Press is part of the University of Cambridge.

It furthers the University's mission by disseminating knowledge in the pursuit of education, learning and research at the highest international levels of excellence.

www.cambridge.org
Information on this title: www.cambridge.org/9781107480698

First printed 2016
3rd printing 2017

Printed in the United Kingdom by Print on Demand, World Wide

A catalogue record for this publication is available from the British Library

Library of Congress Cataloguing in Publication data

Pundir, Jyotsna, author.
Gynaecology : evidence-based algorithms / Jyotsna Pundir, Arri Coomarasamy.
    p. ; cm.
Includes bibliographical references and index.
ISBN 978-1-107-48069-8 (Paperback)
I. Coomarasamy, Arri, author.   II. Title.
[DNLM: 1. Genital Diseases, Female–diagnosis.   2. Genital Diseases, Female–therapy.
3. Algorithms.   4. Decision Support Techniques. WQ 140]
RG101
618.1–dc23   2015006508

ISBN 978-1-107-48069-8 Paperback

"To my mother for everything I am today, to my husband and two lovely boys for their patience and endless support, to my brothers and in-laws for their faith and encouragement, and finally to my father for his wisdom." Jyotsna

"Dedicated to the memory of Poongo Aunty, who treaded the earth ever so gently." Arri

We would like to acknowledge Dr Justin Chu MBChB MRCOG, Academic Clinical Lecturer, Obstetrics and Gynaecology, College of Medical and Dental Sciences, University of Birmingham; and Helen Williams BSc (Hons), Research Associate, Institute of Metabolism and Systems Research, College of Medical & Dental Sciences, University of Birmingham for their help and time with editing the chapters.

TABLE OF CONTENTS

SECTION 7: Sexual and reproductive health, sexually transmitted infection, and vaginal infection

SECTION 8: Contraception

PREFACE

Evidence-based medicine is the conscientious, explicit, and judicious use of current best evidence in making decisions about the care of individual patients. With the evolution of evidence-based medicine, and the explosion of medical literature, there has been a continuous stream of guidelines published in obstetrics and gynaecology. These guidelines, designed to provide systematically developed recommendations, assist clinicians and patients in making decisions about appropriate treatment for specific conditions. They also provide crucial information for candidates preparing for the Member of the Royal College of Obstetricians and Gynaecologists (MRCOG) examination. Our attempt is to bring together the essential information contained in these guidelines in these comprehensive books. Where guidelines do not exist, we have relied on available evidence and accepted norms of practice. The information is presented in flowcharts, representing a step-by-step method of solving a clinical problem.

As our books are a revision guide for MRCOG candidates, we have focused primarily on RCOG and other UK national guidelines. However, many chapters contain a 'Guideline Comparator' box carrying information from other important international guidelines, thus providing an international perspective. Several chapters also contain a 'what not to do' box, which should act as a source of rich debate! Our desire is that these books act as an essential tool for clinicians and examination candidates. However, they should not replace a close study of the guidelines themselves.

Jyotsna Pundir and Arri Coomarasamy

ABBREVIATIONS LIST

A1C – haemoglobin A1 C
AAP – American Academy of Paediatricians
AC – abdominal circumference
ACA – anticardiolipin antibodies
ACE – angiotensin-converting enzyme
ACOG – American Congress of Obstetricians
ACS – acute chest syndrome
ACTH – adrenocorticotropic hormone
AED – antiepileptic drug
AFI – amniotic fluid index
AFP – α-feto protein
AFV – amniotic fluid volume
AH – abdominal hysterectomy
AIDS – acquired immune deficiency syndrome
AIS – androgen insensitivity syndrome
AJCC – American Joint Committee on Cancer
ALO – actionmyces-like organism
ALPP – abdominal leak point pressure
AM – abdominal myomectomy
AMH – antimüllerian hormone
AMS – antenatal magnesium sulphate
ANC – antenatal care
ANCS – antenatal corticosteroids
anti-D Ig – anti-D immunoglobulin
anti-HT – antihypertensive
AP – anteroposterior
APA – antiphospholipid antibodies
APH – antepartum haemorrhage
APS – antiphospholipid syndrome
ARBs – angiotensin II receptor blockers
ARDS – adult respiratory distress syndrome
ART – assisted reproductive techniques
ASA – anti-sperm antibodies
ASAP – as soon as possible
ASC – abdominal sacrocolpopexy
ASRM – American Society of Reproductive Medicine
ATD – anti-thyroid treatment
AUA – American Urological Association
BASHH – British Association for Sexual Health and HIV
BD – twice a day (*bis in die*)
BEP – bleomycin, etoposide, cisplatin
BF – breastfeeding
BG – blood glucose
BMD – bone mass/mineral density
BMI – body mass index
BP – blood pressure

BPP – biophysical profile
BSO – bilateral salpingo-oopherectomy
BT – brachytherapy blood transfusion
BV – bacterial vaginosis
CAH – congenital adrenal hyperplasia
CAIS – complete androgen insensitivity syndrome
CBAVD – congenital bilateral absence of vas deferens
CBT – cognitive behavioural therapy
CC – clomiphene citrate
CDC – Centers for Disease Control and Prevention
CEE – conjugated equine oestrogens
CEMD – confidential enquiries into maternal death
CF – cystic fibrosis
cGIN – cervical glandular intra-epithelial neoplasia
CHC – combined hormonal contraception
CHD – congenital heart disease
ChT – chemotherapy
CIN – cervical intra-epithelial neoplasia
CKS – Clinical Knowledge Summaries
CLPP – cough leak point pressure
CMP – cardiomyopathy
COC – combined oral contraceptive pills
CPA – cyproterone acetate
CPP – chronic pelvic pain central precocious puberty
CPR – clinical pregnancy rate cardiopulmonary resuscitation
CRL – crown–rump length
CRP – C-reactive protein
CRS – congenital rubella syndrome
CS – Caesarean section
CSF – cerebrospinal fluid
CT – computerized tomography
CTG – cardiotocography
CTP – combined transdermal patch
CTPA – computed tomography pulmonary angiogram
Cu-IUD – copper-bearing intrauterine device
CVR – combined vaginal ring
CVS – chorionic villus sampling
CVST – cerebral venous sinus thrombosis
Cx – circumflex
D&E – dilatation and evacuation
DA – dopamine agonist
DBP – diastolic blood pressure
DCDA – dichorionic diamniotic

DDAVP – trade name for desmopressin acetate
DEXA – dual-emission X-ray absorptiometry
DHEA – dehydroepiandrosterone
DHT – dihydro-testosterone
DI – donor insemination
DIC – disseminated intravascular coagulopathy
DM – diabetes mellitus
DMPA – depot medroxyprogesterone acetate
DNA – deoxyribonucleic acid
DO – detruser overactivity
DR – detection rate
DSD – disorders of sexual development
DV – domestic violence
DVT – deep vein thrombosis
E2 – oestradiol
EA – endometrial ablation
EBW – estimated birth weight
EC – emergency contraception
ECG – electrocardiograph
EE – ethinyl oestradiol
EEG – electroencephalograph
EFM – electronic fetal monitoring
EFW – estimated fetal weight
EIA/ELISA – enzyme immunoassay
EIN – endometrial intra-epithelial neoplasia
ELITT – endometrial laser intrauterine thermal therapy
EMA-CO – etoposide, methotrexate, dactinomycin, vincristine, and cyclophosphamide
EMAS – European Menopause and Andropause Society
EMG – electromyography
EMI – endometrial–myometrial interface
EPAU – early pregnancy assessment unit
ER – extended release
ERCS – elective repeat Caesarean section
ERPC – evacuation of retained products of conception
ESCP – Endocrine Society clinical practice guidelines
ESGE – European Society for Gynaecological Endoscopy
ESHRE – European Society of Human Reproduction and Embryology
ESR – erythrocyte sedimentation rate
ET – endometrial thickness/embryo transfer

EUA – examination under anaesthesia
FAS – fetal alcohol syndrome
FASD – fetal alcohol spectrum disorder
FBC – full blood count
FBG – fasting blood glucose
FBS – fetal blood sampling
FFA – free fatty acids
FFTS – feto-fetal transfusion syndrome
FGR – fetal growth restriction
FHR – fetal heart rate
FIGO – International Federation of Gynecology and Obstetrics
FISH – fluorescence *in situ* hybridization
FM – fetal movements/full mutation
FMH – feto-maternal haemorrhage
FMR – fragile-X mental retardation
FMU – fetal medicine unit
FNAC – fine-needle aspiration cytology
FPA – Family Planning Association
FPG – fasting plasma glucose
FPR – false positive rate
FSH – follicle stimulating hormone
fT4 – free T4
fT3 – free T3
FTA-abs – fluorescent treponemal antibody-absorbed
FVL – factor V Leiden
FVS – fetal vericella syndrome
FXS – fragile-X syndrome
FXT – fragile-X testing
FXTAS – fragile-X tremor ataxia syndrome
GA – general anaesthesia
GCT – germ cell ovarian tumour
GDM – gestational diabetes mellitus
GDPP – gonadotrophin-dependent precocious puberty
GH – growth hormone
GI – gastrointestinal
GIFT – intra-Fallopian gamete transfer
GIPP – gonadotrophin-independent precocious puberty
GLN – groin lymph node
GND – groin node dissection
GnRH – gonadotrophin releasing hormone
GnRHa – GnRH agonist
GTD – gestational trophoblastic disease
GTN – gestational trophoblastic neoplasia
GTT – glucose tolerance test
GUD – genital ulcerative desease
GUM – genitourinary medicine
HAART – highly active anti-retroviral therapy
HC – hormonal contraception
hCG – human chorionic gonadotrophin
HCP – healthcare professional
HES – hydroxyethyl starch
HERS – Heart and Oestrogen– Progestogen Replacement Study

HFEA – Human Fertilisation and Embryology Authority
HFI – hormone free interval
HG – hyperemesis gravidarum
HIE – hypoxic ischaemic encephalopathy
HIFU – high-intensity focused ultrasound
HIT – heparin-induced thrombocytopenia
HIV – human immunodeficiency virus
HLA – human leucocyte antigen
HMB – heavy menstrual bleeding
hMG – human menopausal gonadotrophins
HNPCC – hereditary non-polyposis colonic cancer
HOMA-IR – Homeostasis Model Assessment – insulin resistant
HOS – hypo-osmotic swelling test
HPA – health protection agency
HPV – human papilloma virus
HRT – hormone replacement therapy
HSG – hysterosalpingogram
HSV – herpes simplex virus
HT – hypertension
HTA – hydrothermal ablation/health technology assessment
HVS – high vaginal swabs
Hx – history
IADPSG – International Association of Diabetes and Pregnancy Study Groups
IBS – irritable bowel syndrome
IC – interstitial cystitis
ICS – International Continence Society
ICSI – intra-cytoplasmic sperm injection
ICU – intensive care unit
ID – iodine deficiency
IDDM – insulin-dependent DM
IFG – impaired fasting glycaemia
Ig – immunoglobulin
IgA – immunoglobulin A
IgG – immunoglobulin G
IgM – immunoglobulin M
IGT – impaired glucose tolerance
IHD – ischaemic heart disease
IM – intramuscular/intramural
IMB – inter-menstrual bleeding
IOL – induction of labour
IOTA – International Ovarian Tumor Analysis Group
IR – immediate release
IU – international unit
IUCD – intrauterine contraceptive device
IUD – intrauterine device/ intrauterine deaths
IUFD – intrauterine fetal death
IUGR – intrauterine growth restriction
IUI – intrauterine insemination
IUP – intrauterine pregnancy
IUS – intrauterine system
IUT – intrauterine transfusion
IV – intravenous

IVF – in vitro fertilization
IVH – intraventricular haemorrhage
JZ – junctional zone
KCl – potassium chloride
LA – local anaesthesia
LAC – lupus anticoagulant
LAM – lactational amenorrhoea method
LARC – long-acting reversible contraception
LAVH – laparoscopic assisted vaginal hysterectomy
LB – live births
LBC – liquid-based cytology
LBR – live birth rate
LBW – low-birth weight
LFT – liver function test
LGV – lymphogranuloma venerum
LH – leutinizing hormone/laparoscopic hysterectomy
LLETZ – large loop excision of the transition zone
LLP – low-lying placenta
LM – laparoscopic myomectomy
LMP – last menstrual period
LMWH – low molecular-weight heparin
LN – lymph node
LND – lymph node dissection
LNG – levonorgestrel
LNG-IUS – levonorgestrel-releasing intrauterine system
LOD – laparoscopic ovarian drilling/ diathermy
LR – likelihood ratio
LR– – negative test result
LR+ – positive test result
LUNA – laparoscopic uterosacral nerve ablation
LVSI – lymphovascular space involvement
MCA – middle cerebral artery
MCDA – monochorionic diamniotic
MCH – mean cell haemoglobin
MCHC – mean cell haemoglobin concentration
MCMA – monochorionic monoamniotic
MCV – mean cell volume
MDT – multi-disciplinary team
MEA – microwave endometrial ablation
MI – myocardial infarction
MIS – müllerian inhibitory substance
MOH – massive obstetric haemorrhage
MP – multiple pregnancy
MPA – medroxyprogesterone acetate
MRC – Medical Research Council
MRI – magnetic resonance imaging
MSL – meconium-stained liquor
MSM – men who have sex with men
MSU – midstream urine
MTX – methotrexate

MUCP – maximum urethral closure pressure

MUI – mixed urinary incontinence

MVP – maximum vertical pocket

MWS – The Million Women Study

Mx – management

N – normal

NAATs – nucleic acid amplification tests

NCRI – National Cancer Research Institute

NCSP – National Cervical Screening Programme

Nd-YAG – neodymium-YAG

NEC – necrotizing enterocolitis

NET – norethisterone

NET-EN – norethisterone enantate

NGU – non-gonococcal urethritis

NICE – National Institute of Clinical Excellence

NICU – neonatal intensive care units

NIFH – non-immune hydrops fetalis

NK – natural killer

NND – neonatal deaths

NNT – number needed to treat

NPV – negative predictive value

NSAID – nonsteroidal anti-inflammatory

NT – nuchal translucency

NTD – neural tube defect

OAB – overactive bladder

OC – obstetric cholestasis

OCD – obsessive compulsive disorder

OCP – oral contraceptive pill

OGTT – oral glucose tolerance test

OH – overt hypothyroidism

OHSS – ovarian hyperstimulation syndrome

OI – ovulation induction

ONTDs – open neural tube defects

ORS – ovarian remnant syndrome

OVD – operative vaginal delivery

PAIS – partial androgen insensitivity syndrome

PAPP-A – pregnancy-associated plasma protein A

PBC – platinum-based compound

PBT – platinum-based therapy

PCB – post-coital bleeding

PCO – polycystic ovarian

PCOS – polycystic ovarian syndrome

PCP – Pneumocystis carinii pneumonia

PCR – polymerase chain reaction

PCT – progesterone challenge test

PE – pulmonary embolism

PESA – percutaneous epididymal aspiration

PET – positron emission tomography/ pre-eclamptic toxaemia

PFM – pelvic floor muscles

PFMT – pelvic floor muscle training

PGD – preimplantation genetic diagnosis

PID – pelvic inflammatory disease

PLDH – pegylated liposomal doxorubicin hydrochloride

PLN – pelvic lymph node

PMB – postmenopausal bleeding

PME – postmortem examination

PMS – premenstrual syndrome

PMW – post-menopausal women

PNM – perinatal mortality

PNMR – perinatal mortality rate

POC – products of conception/ progestogen-only contraceptives

POD – pouch of Douglas

POEC – progestogen-only emergency contraception

POF – premature ovarian failure

POI – premature ovarian insufficiency

POIC – progestogen-only injectable contraception

POIM – progestogen-only implant

POP – progestogen-only pill

POP-Q – pelvic organ prolapse quantification

POPSE – post-exposure prophylaxis following sexual exposure

POSDIs – progestogen-only subdermal implants

PP – postprandial/precocious puberty

PPH – post-partum haemorrhage

PPROM – premature preterm rupture of membranes

PPV – positive predictive value

PRL – prolactin

PROM – premature rupture of membranes

PSN – presacral neurectomy

PSTT – placental site trophoblastic tumour

PTB – preterm birth

PTD – preterm delivery

PTL – preterm labour

PUL – pregnancy of unknown location

QOL – quality of life

RAADP – routine antenatal anti-D prophylaxis

RAT – radical abdominal trachelectomy

RBC – red blood cell

RBG – random blood glucose

RCOG – Royal College of Obstetricians and Gynaecologists

RCT – randomized controlled trial

RDS – respiratory distress syndrome

RFM – reduced fetal movements

RhD – rhesus D

RM – recurrent miscarriage

RMI – risk of malignancy index

ROS – residual ovary syndrome reactive oxygen species

RPG – random plasma glucose

RPL – recurrent pregnancy loss

RPOC – retained products of conception

RPR – rapid plasma reagin

RR – relative risk

RT – radiotherapy

RVT – radical vaginal trachelectomy

SA – semen analysis

SANS – Stoller afferent nerve stimulator

SB – stillbirth

SBP – systolic blood pressure

SC – subcutaneous

SCC – squamous cell carcinoma

SCD – sickle-cell disease

SCH – subclinical hypothyroidism

SCST – sex cord stromal tumour

SET – single embryo transfer

SGA – small for gestational age

SHBG – sex hormone-binding globulin

SLE – systemic lupus erythematosus

SM – submucosal

SMM – surgical management of miscarriage

SNS – sacral nerve stimulation

SNRI – selective noradrenaline reuptake inhibitor

SOGC – Society of Obstetricians and Gynaecologists of Canada

SPTB – spontaneous preterm birth

SR – systematic review

SRL – systematic retroperitoneal lymphadenectomy

SS – subserosal

SSC – secondary sexual characteristic

SSF – sacrospinous fixation

SSR – surgical sperm retrieval

SSRI – selective serotonin reuptake inhibitor

SSRIs – selective serotonin reuptake inhibitors

STH – subtotal hysterectomy

STI – sexually transmitted infection

STL – second-trimester loss

SUI – stress urinary incontinence

T4 – thyroxine

TAH – total abdominal hysterectomy

TAS – trans absominal scan

TBG – T4-binding globulin

TCRE – transcervical resection of endometrium

TDS – three times a day (ter die sumendus)

TEDS – thromboembolic deterrent stockings

TENS – transcutaneous nerve stimulation

TESA – testicular sperm aspiration

TESE – testicular sperm extraction

TFTs – thyroid function tests

TH – total hysterectomy

TLH – total laparoscopic hysterectomy

TOC – test of cure

TOP – termination of pregnancy

TORCH – Toxoplasma gondii, other viruses, rubella, cytomegalovirus, herpes simplex

TP – thromboprophylaxis

TPHA – Treponema pallidum haemagglutination assay

TPPA – Treponema pallidum particle agglutination assay

TRUS – transrectal ultrasound

TSAb – thyroid stimulating antibodies

TSH – thyroid stimulating hormone

TTN – transient tachypnoea of newborn

TV – Trichomonas vaginalis/transvaginal

TVS – transvaginal scan

TVT – tension-free vaginal tape

TXA – trenaxemic acid

UAD – uterine artery Doppler

UAE – uterine artery embolization

UDA – urodynamic assessment

uE3 – unconjugated oestradiol

UI – urinary incontinence/unexplained infertility

UKCTOCS – United Kingdom Collaborative Trial of Ovarian Cancer Screening

UKFOCSS – United Kingdom Familial Ovarian Cancer Screening Study

UKMEC – United Kingdom Medical Eligibility Criteria

UKOSS – United Kingdom Obstetric Surveillance System

UmAD – umbilical artery Doppler

UOP – urine output

UPA – ulipristal acetate

uPCR – urinary protein:creatinine ratio

UPSI – unprotected sexual intercourse

USCL – ultrasound cervical length

USO – unilateral salpingo-oopherectomy

USS – ultrasound scan

UTI – urinary tract infection

UUI – urge urinary incontinence

VaIN – vaginal intra-epithelial neoplasia

VDRL – venereal disease research laboratory

VH – vaginal hysterectomy

VIN – vulval intraepithelial neoplasia

VLPP – Valsalva leak point pressure

VMS – vasomotor menopausal symptoms

V/Q – ventilation–perfusion lung scan

VTE – venous thromboembolism

VVC – vulvovaginal candidiasis

VZIG – Varicella zoster immunoglobulin

VZV – Varicella zoster virus

WHI – Women's Health Initiative

WHO – World Health Organization

WLE – wide local excision

WWE – woman with epilepsy

ZIFT – intra-Fallopian zygote transfer

CHAPTER 1 Early pregnancy bleeding and miscarriage

Spontaneous loss of a pregnancy before 24 weeks' gestation.

Background and prevalence

- Miscarriage in early pregnancies occurs in 10–20% of pregnancies.
- Biochemical miscarriage – by measuring β-hCG at a stage when the woman is unaware that she is pregnant, up to 30% of pregnancies are found to miscarry.
- Approximately 50% of women with bleeding in early pregnancy have a miscarriage.
- Miscarriage risk is reduced in women with continuing pregnancy-associated vomiting.
- Most non-recurrent miscarriages are caused by abnormalities in the embryo; e.g., chromosomal abnormalities, genetic abnormalities, defects in the development of the placenta or embryo.
- The risk of miscarriage increases with increasing maternal age:
  * 10% in women aged < 30 years.
  * 15–20% in women aged 35–39 years.
  * > 50% in women aged > 45 years.
- Risk of miscarriage reduces with increasing gestational age, with up to 75% of miscarriages occurring before 12 weeks' gestation.

Clinical features

- Period of amenorrhoea/positive pregnancy test.
- Pain and/or bleeding.
- **Threatened miscarriage** – scanty vaginal bleeding, varying from a brownish discharge to bright red bleeding. Lower abdominal cramping pain or lower backache usually develops after the onset of bleeding. Tenderness of the abdomen or pelvis may be present. **Cervical os is closed.**
- Inevitable miscarriage – same symptoms as threatened miscarriage but more severe. **Internal cervical os is open** or pregnancy tissue may be found to be coming through the os.
- **Complete miscarriage** – resolving symptoms and signs of a miscarriage.
- **Delayed miscarriage** – may present with resolving symptoms of pregnancy in women with no pain or bleeding. Fetal heartbeat is undetectable and the uterus may be small for dates. May be found incidentally during a routine ultrasound assessment of pregnancy.

Risks or complications

- Psychological complications – grief, anxiety, or depression. Risk of more intense or longer-lasting distress if the woman has:
  * Strongly desired the pregnancy.
  * Waited a long time to conceive.
  * History of miscarriage or other pregnancy.
  * Miscarriage later in the pregnancy.
  * Limited social support.
  * History of difficulty coping with distressing situations.

Be aware of the psychological sequelae associated with pregnancy loss and provide support, follow-up, and access to formal counselling when necessary.

Differential diagnosis – bleeding in early pregnancy

DDx

Extrauterine causes

- Urethral bleeding.
- Cervical ectropion.
- Cervical polyps.
- Gynaecological cancers.

Uterine causes

- Ectopic pregnancy:
  * Cardiovascular shock.
  * Fainting.
  * Shoulder-tip pain.
  * Abdominal pain.
  * Abdominal tenderness on examination.
  * Cervical tenderness.
- Molar pregnancy:
  * Absent fetal heart sounds.
  * Heavy and prolonged bleeding.
  * Symptoms of pregnancy are exaggerated.
  * Uterus is large for dates.
  * Vesicles may be passed vaginally.
- **Intrauterine pregnancy.**

Clinical

Inevitable – when bleeding is associated with an open cervix. However, pregnancy may continue successfully in women diagnosed to have an open cervix; therefore, aim for expectant management.
Threatened – vaginal bleeding and/or pain with viable pregnancy and closed cervix.
Incomplete – when all the pregnancy tissue has not been expelled from the uterus and bleeding may or may not be present.
Complete – when all the pregnancy tissue has been expelled and bleeding has stopped.
Delayed/missed miscarriage/anembryonic pregnancy/early fetal demise – when the pregnancy has failed but there is no bleeding, and pregnancy tissues have not been expelled.

Ultrasound-based

Pregnancy of unknown location – no identifiable pregnancy on scan, with positive hCG.
Fetal loss – previous CRL measurement with subsequent loss of fetal heart activity.
Empty sac – gestational sac with absent or minimal structures.
Biochemical pregnancy loss – pregnancy not located on the scan.
Delayed/missed miscarriage/anembryonic pregnancy/early fetal demise.

Gestational age

Early miscarriage – the spontaneous loss of a pregnancy before 12 weeks' gestation.
Late miscarriage – loss of fetal heart activity after 12 completed weeks.

Investigations

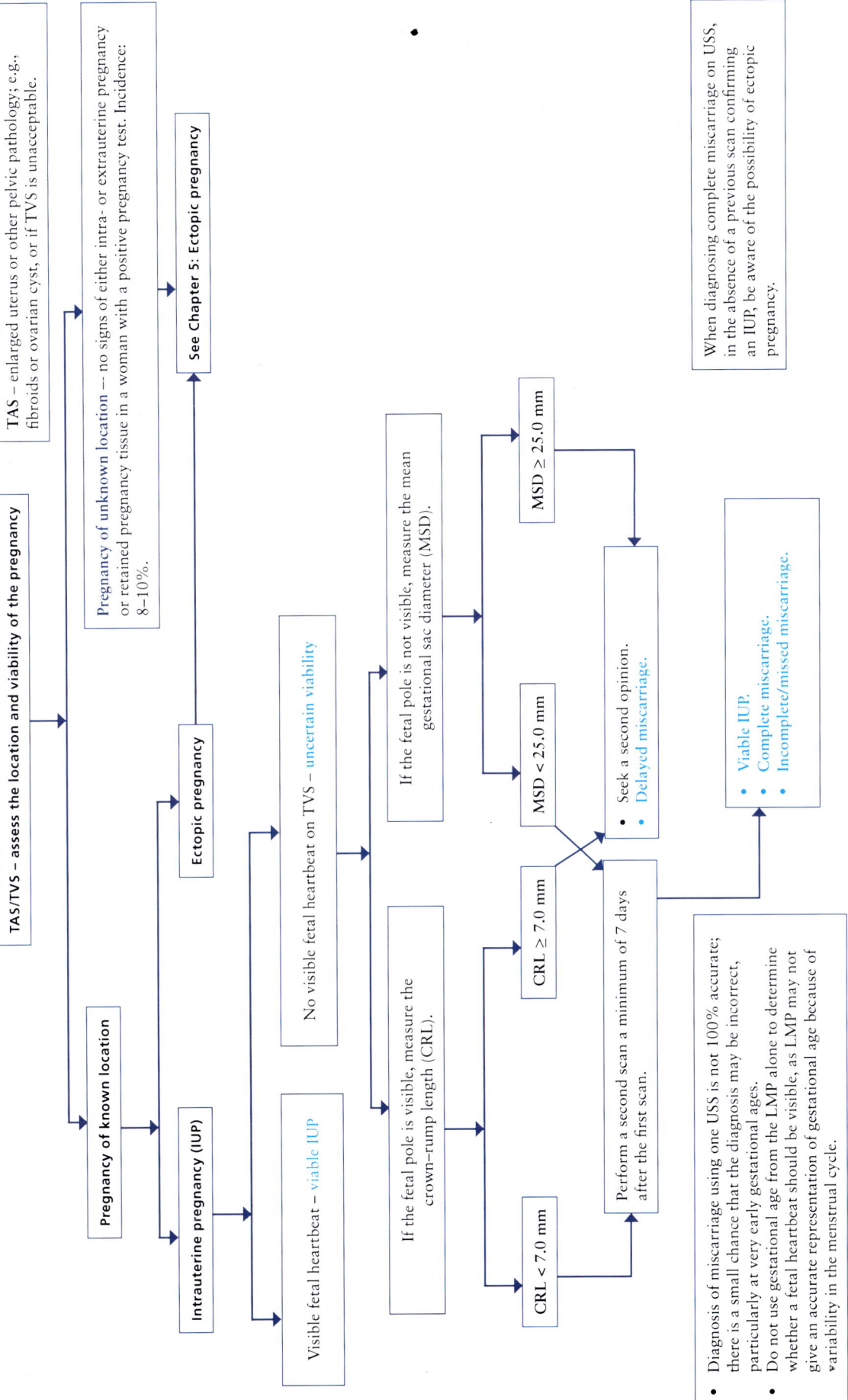

TAS/TVS – assess the location and viability of the pregnancy

TAS – enlarged uterus or other pelvic pathology; e.g., fibroids or ovarian cyst, or if TVS is unacceptable.

Pregnancy of unknown location -- no signs of either intra- or extrauterine pregnancy or retained pregnancy tissue in a woman with a positive pregnancy test. Incidence: 8–10%.

See Chapter 5: Ectopic pregnancy

Pregnancy of known location

Intrauterine pregnancy (IUP)

Ectopic pregnancy

Visible fetal heartbeat – viable IUP

No visible fetal heartbeat on TVS – uncertain viability

If the fetal pole is visible, measure the crown–rump length (CRL).

If the fetal pole is not visible, measure the mean gestational sac diameter (MSD).

CRL < 7.0 mm

CRL ≥ 7.0 mm

MSD < 25.0 mm

MSD ≥ 25.0 mm

Perform a second scan a minimum of 7 days after the first scan.

- Seek a second opinion.
- Delayed miscarriage.

- Viable IUP.
- Complete miscarriage.
- Incomplete/missed miscarriage.

When diagnosing complete miscarriage on USS, in the absence of a previous scan confirming an IUP, be aware of the possibility of ectopic pregnancy.

- Diagnosis of miscarriage using one USS is not 100% accurate; there is a small chance that the diagnosis may be incorrect, particularly at very early gestational ages.
- Do not use gestational age from the LMP alone to determine whether a fetal heartbeat should be visible, as LMP may not give an accurate representation of gestational age because of variability in the menstrual cycle.

℞ **Management**

Outpatient – refer women with a threatened or suspected incomplete/delayed miscarriage to an early pregnancy assessment unit (EPAU) for confirmation of the diagnosis.
Inpatient – refer women with severe pain or bleeding, or who are shocked for **immediate admission to hospital.**

General measures

- Threatened miscarriage (vaginal bleeding and a confirmed viable IUP):
  * If her bleeding gets worse, or persists beyond 14 days, return for further assessment.
  * If the bleeding stops, start or continue routine ANC.
- Medical/expectant management – can be offered only in units where women can access 24-hour telephone advice and emergency admission, if required. Protocols with selection criteria, therapeutic regimens, and arrangements for follow-up should be in place.
- Encourage patient choice – associated with positive quality-of-life outcomes.
- Screen for infections – including Chlamydia trachomatis, in women undergoing SMM.
- Histology of the tissue obtained at the time of miscarriage to confirm pregnancy and to exclude ectopic pregnancy or unsuspected GTD.
- NICE – anti-D rhesus prophylaxis at a dose of 250 IU (50 µg) to all rhesus-negative women who have a surgical procedure to manage an ectopic pregnancy or a miscarriage.
- NICE – do not offer anti-D rhesus prophylaxis to women who:
  * Receive solely medical management for an ectopic pregnancy or miscarriage.
  * Have a threatened miscarriage.
  * Have a complete miscarriage.
  * Have a pregnancy of unknown location.

Service provision

Early pregnancy loss accounts for over 50,000 admissions in the UK annually.
Outpatient EPAU service – hospital admission can be avoided in 40% of women, with a further 20% requiring a shorter hospital stay.
NICE – EPAU services should be:

- Available – 7 days a week.
- Accessibility – direct access for GPs and selected patient groups. EPAU should accept self-referrals from women who have had a recurrent miscarriage or a previous ectopic or molar pregnancy. All other women with pain and/or bleeding should be assessed by an HCP (GP, A&E doctor, midwife, or nurse) before referral.
- Appropriate setting – ideally sited in a dedicated area.
- Appropriate staff – HCPs competent to diagnose and care for women with pain and/or bleeding in early pregnancy, trained in sensitive communication and breaking bad news.
- Diagnostic and therapeutic algorithms.
- USS equipment and staff appropriately trained.
- Laboratory facilities – rhesus antibody testing, serial β-hCG with results available within 24 hours, progesterone estimation (NICE – only β-hCG).
- Standardized information leaflets, referral, and discharge letters, with clear plans for follow-up.
- Access to formal counselling.
- Ensure that a system is in place to enable women referred to their local EPAU to attend within 24 hours if the clinical situation warrants this.

Management options

Rx Largely based on the woman's preference, unless there are clinical indications for surgical intervention.

First-line option – expectant management (NICE)

A management approach in which treatment is not administered, with the aim of seeing whether the condition will resolve naturally.

NICE – use expectant management for 7–14 days as the first-line management strategy for women with a confirmed diagnosis of miscarriage.

- **Advantages:**
  * Avoids hospitalization and risks of surgery.
  * Reduction in clinical pelvic infection rates.
- **Risks** – Symptoms may take several weeks to resolve and, sometimes, surgical intervention is required for failed cases.
- Most women will need no further treatment.
- Provide oral and written information about what to expect throughout the process, advice on pain relief, where and when to get help in an emergency, and further treatment options.

- **Factors that affect the success rates:**
  * Type of miscarriage (delayed or incomplete).
  * Duration of follow-up.
  * Serum progesterone levels.
- Highly effective in incomplete miscarriage.
- Success rates for delayed miscarriage for expectant *vs* surgical management are 28% and 81% and for incomplete miscarriage, the rates are 94% and 99%.
- **Retained pregnancy tissue** – genuine retained pregnancy tissue is less likely to be confirmed histologically when USS shows heterogenous shadows with a maximum AP diameter of ≤ 15 mm. These could include some cases of incomplete miscarriage but are best managed conservatively as there is a trend towards a lower complication rate compared with surgical management.

Success rates

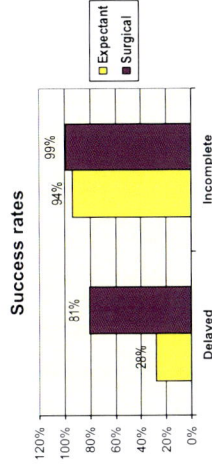

- Resolution of bleeding and pain during 7–14 days suggests complete miscarriage. Advise a urine pregnancy test after 3 weeks.
  * Negative – complete miscarriage.
  * Positive – return for individualized care.

- If after the period of 7–14 days the bleeding and pain:
  * Have not started (miscarriage has not begun).
  * Are persisting and/or increasing (incomplete miscarriage).
- Repeat scan.
- Further treatment options – continued expectant, medical, or surgical management.

- If the woman opts for continued expectant management, review at a minimum of 14 days after the first follow-up appointment.

Failed expectant management or Expectant management not acceptable

Medical or surgical management

Explore management options other than expectant management if:

- Woman is at increased risk of haemorrhage (late first trimester).
- History of adverse and/or traumatic experience associated with pregnancy (stillbirth, miscarriage, or antepartum haemorrhage).
- Increased risk from the effects of haemorrhage (coagulopathies or is unable to have a blood transfusion).
- There is evidence of infection.

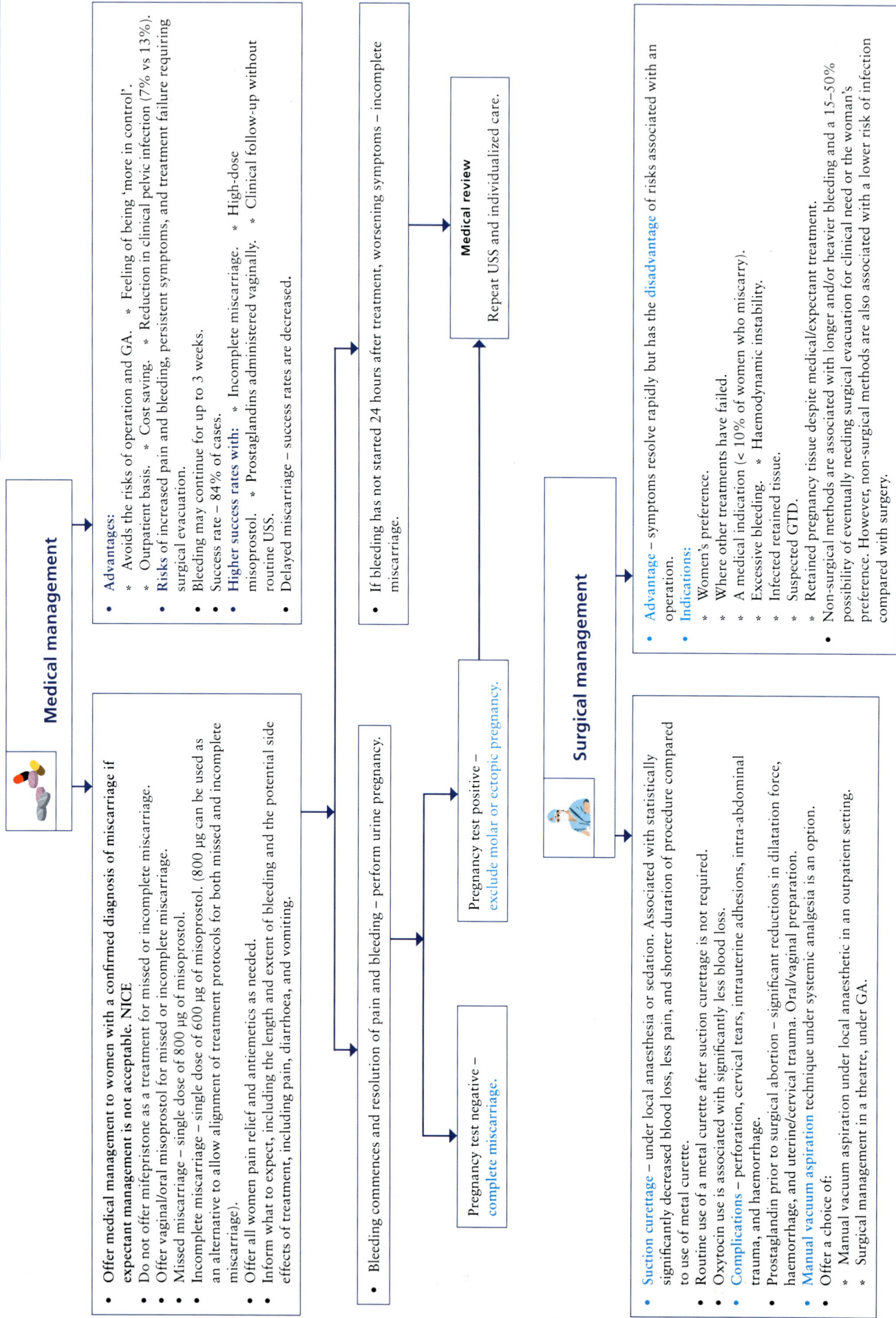

Medical management

- **Offer medical management to women with a confirmed diagnosis of miscarriage if expectant management is not acceptable. NICE**
- Do not offer mifepristone as a treatment for missed or incomplete miscarriage.
- Offer vaginal/oral misoprostol for missed or incomplete miscarriage.
- Missed miscarriage – single dose of 800 μg of misoprostol.
- Incomplete miscarriage – single dose of 600 μg of misoprostol. (800 μg can be used as an alternative to allow alignment of treatment protocols for both missed and incomplete miscarriage).
- Offer all women pain relief and antiemetics as needed.
- Inform what to expect, including the length and extent of bleeding and the potential side effects of treatment, including pain, diarrhoea, and vomiting.

- **Advantages:**
  - * Avoids the risks of operation and GA. * Feeling of being 'more in control'.
  - * Outpatient basis. * Cost saving. * Reduction in clinical pelvic infection (7% vs 13%).
- **Risks** of increased pain and bleeding, persistent symptoms, and treatment failure requiring surgical evacuation.
- Bleeding may continue for up to 3 weeks.
- Success rate – 84% of cases.
- **Higher success rates with:** * Incomplete miscarriage. * High-dose misoprostol. * Prostaglandins administered vaginally. * Clinical follow-up without routine USS.
- Delayed miscarriage – success rates are decreased.

- Bleeding commences and resolution of pain and bleeding – perform urine pregnancy.

Pregnancy test positive – exclude molar or ectopic pregnancy.

Pregnancy test negative – complete miscarriage.

- If bleeding has not started 24 hours after treatment, worsening symptoms – incomplete miscarriage.

Medical review

Repeat USS and individualized care.

Surgical management

- **Suction curettage** – under local anaesthesia or sedation. Associated with statistically significantly decreased blood loss, less pain, and shorter duration of procedure compared to use of metal curette.
- Routine use of a metal curette after suction curettage is not required.
- Oxytocin use is associated with significantly less blood loss.
- **Complications** – perforation, cervical tears, intrauterine adhesions, intra-abdominal trauma, and haemorrhage.
- Prostaglandin prior to surgical abortion – significant reductions in dilatation force, haemorrhage, and uterine/cervical trauma. Oral/vaginal preparation.
- **Manual vacuum aspiration** technique under systemic analgesia is an option.
- Offer a choice of:
  - * Manual vacuum aspiration under local anaesthetic in an outpatient setting.
  - * Surgical management in a theatre, under GA.

- **Advantage** – symptoms resolve rapidly but has the **disadvantage** of risks associated with an operation.
- **Indications:**
  - * Women's preference.
  - * Where other treatments have failed.
  - * A medical indication (< 10% of women who miscarry).
  - * Excessive bleeding. * Haemodynamic instability.
  - * Infected retained tissue.
  - * Suspected GTD.
  - * Retained pregnancy tissue despite medical/expectant treatment.
- Non-surgical methods are associated with longer and/or heavier bleeding and a 15–50% possibility of eventually needing surgical evacuation for clinical need or the woman's preference. However, non-surgical methods are also associated with a lower risk of infection compared with surgery.

Follow-up

- Assess woman's psychological wellbeing and offer counselling, if appropriate. Grief, anxiety, and depression are common following miscarriage. Grief following miscarriage is comparable in nature, intensity, and duration to grief reactions in people suffering other types of major loss. Distress is commonly at its worst 4–6 weeks after a miscarriage and may last 6–12 months.
- Menstruation can be expected to resume within 4–8 weeks of the miscarriage, but may take several cycles to re-establish a regular pattern.
- For women who wish to become pregnant – they can do so as soon as they feel psychologically and physically ready.
- Offer pre-conception advice.
- For women who do not wish to become pregnant – advise on contraception immediately after the miscarriage.

Consent – surgical evacuation of the uterus for early pregnancy loss

(Surgical management of miscarriage)

Discuss

- Explain – removal of early pregnancy tissue from the uterus, usually with suction. Cervix may need to be dilated to allow empty.ng of the uterine contents.
- Intended benefit – to treat an incomplete or delayed miscarriage, or retained placental tissue.
- Discuss alternative treatment options: medical and expectant management, particularly for women without an intact sac. If tissue is sent for histology, the reasons (to exclude ectopic or molar pregnancy) should be explained.
- Form of anaesthesia.

- **Serious risks:**
  * Serious morbidity – 2.1% with a mortality of 0.5/100,000.
  * Uterine perforation – up to 5/1000.
  * Significant trauma to the cervix (rare).
  * No substantiated evidence of any impact on future fertility.
- **Frequent risks:**
  * Bleeding that lasts for up to 2 weeks is very common but blood transfusion is uncommon (1.2/1000).
  * Need for repeat surgical evacuation – up to 5/100.
  * Localized pelvic infection – 3/100 women.

Extra procedures

- That may become necessary – laparoscopy or laparotomy to diagnose and/or repair organ injury, e.g., uterine trauma, perforation.

Risks	
Very common	1/1 to 1/10.
Common	1/10 to 1/100.
Uncommon	1/100 to 1/1000.
Rare	1/1000 to 1/10,000.

Guideline comparator

- Anti-D immunoglobulin (RCOG) - non-sensitized rhesus (Rh)-negative women should receive it in cases of:
  * Ectopic pregnancy.
  * All miscarriages > 12 weeks of gestation (including threatened).
  * All miscarriages where the uterus is evacuated (medically or surgically).
  * It should only be given for threatened miscarriage under 12 weeks gestation, when bleeding is heavy or associated with pain.
  * It should be given in any case where there is clinical doubt.

What not to do

- Routine antibiotic prophylaxis prior to surgical uterine evacuation.
- Anti-D in spontaneous miscarriages < 12 weeks of gestation.
- Mifepristone as a treatment for missed or incomplete miscarriage.
- Routine use of a metal curette after suction curettage.
- NICE – anti-D rhesus prophylaxis to women who:
  * Receive solely medical management for an ectopic pregnancy or miscarriage.
  * Have a threatened miscarriage or a complete miscarriage.
  * Have a pregnancy of unknown location.

1. *Ectopic Pregnancy and Miscarriage: Diagnosis and Initial Management in Early Pregnancy of Ectopic Pregnancy and Miscarriage. NICE Clinical Guidelines, 2012.*
2. *The Management of Early Pregnancy Loss. RCOG Green-top Guideline No. 25, October 2006.*
3. *Clinical Knowledge Summaries. http://www.cks.nhs.uk/miscarriage.*
4. *Surgical Evacuation of the Uterus for Early Pregnancy Loss. RCOG Consent Advice No. 10, June 2010.*

CHAPTER 1 Early pregnancy bleeding and miscarriage

CHAPTER 2 Care of patients requesting termination of pregnancy

Prevalence and incidence

- About one third of women have a TOP by the age of 45 years in the UK.
- Most commonly performed gynaecological procedure in the UK, with around 200,000 terminations performed annually in England and Wales and around 11,500 in Scotland.
- Over 98% of TOPs in the UK are undertaken because of the risk to the mental or physical health of the woman or her children. Remaining done for fetal abnormality.

History

- Take detailed history to identify those who require more support in decision making (such as psychiatric history, poor social support, or evidence of coercion).
- Assess risk for STIs and screening for Chlamydia.

Investigations

- Haemoglobin.
- ABO and rhesus blood groups.
- Screening for red cell antibodies.
- HIV, hepatitis B and C, and haemoglobinopathies – indicated in the light of clinical features, individual risk factors, or local prevalence.
- Cervical smear.
- USS – not essential prerequisite in all cases. Undertake where gestation is in doubt or extrauterine pregnancy is suspected.

Prevention of infective complications

- **Ideally, test for lower genital tract organisms with treatment of positive cases.**
- **Minimum – antibiotic prophylaxis.**
- Regimens for peri-TOP prophylaxis:
  * Metronidazole, 1 g rectally at the time of TOP plus doxycycline, 100 mg orally BD for 7 days, commencing on the day of abortion.
  * Metronidazole, 1 g rectally at the time of TOP plus azithromycin, 1 g orally on the day of TOP.
  * Metronidazole, 1 g rectally or 800 mg orally, prior to or at the time of TOP for women tested negative for Chlamydia.

Service provision

- The earlier in the pregnancy a TOP is performed, the lower the risk of complications.
- Service arrangements should be such that:
  * Referral to abortion services should be made within 2 days.
  * Assessment appointment should be within 5 days of referral.
  * Offer abortion procedure within 5 working days of decision to proceed.
  * Total time from seeing the abortion provider to the procedure should not exceed 10 working days.
- Care pathways for additional support – access to social services and access to services for women with special needs.
- Information and support for those who consider but do not proceed.
- Maintain confidentiality.
- May be managed on a day-case basis.
- Inpatient beds must be available for women who are unsuitable for day case (up to 5%).
- Should be cared for separately from other gynaecological patients.
- Second-trimester TOP – must be cared for by experienced midwife or nurse.

Information to women

- Adapt national information to reflect local circumstances.
- Possible complications:
  * Haemorrhage requiring blood transfusion – 1/1000 in early gestation increasing to 4/1000 in gestation beyond 20 weeks.
  * Uterine perforation 1–4/1000.
  * Uterine rupture (mid-trimester medical TOP) < 1/1000.
  * Cervical trauma – no greater than 1/100.
  * Failed abortion – < 1/100 (surgical = 2.3/1000; medical =1–14/1000).
  * Need for further intervention (surgical intervention following medical termination or repeat evacuation following surgical termination) – < 5%.
  * Post-abortion infection – 10%.
- No proven associations between induced abortion and subsequent ectopic pregnancy, placenta praevia, or infertility.
- May be associated with a small increase in the risk of subsequent PTD, which increases with number of abortions.
- Termination regimens containing misoprostol are not licensed. Inform women if a prescribed treatment is unlicensed.

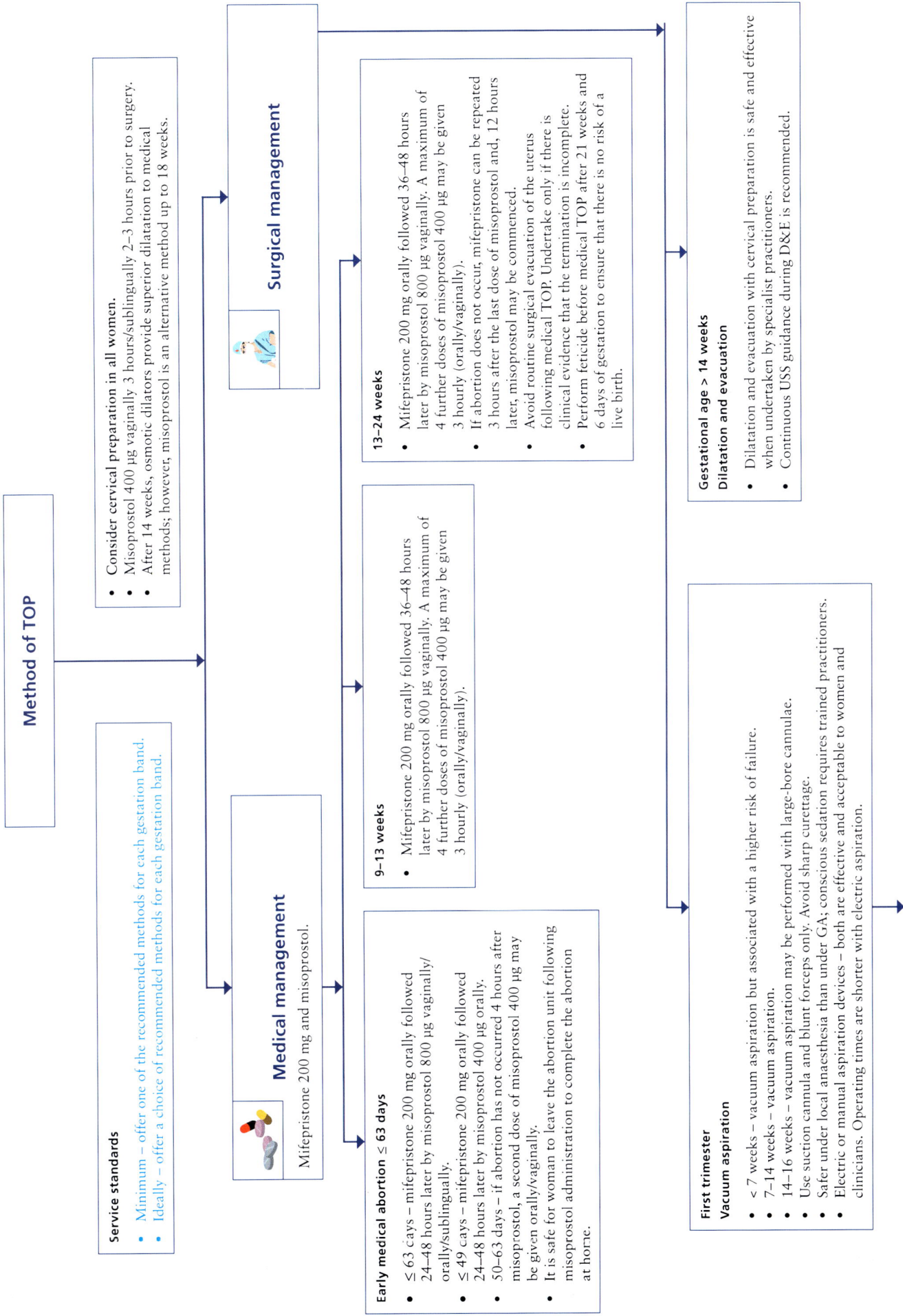

Method of TOP

Service standards

- Minimum – offer one of the recommended methods for each gestation band.
- Ideally – offer a choice of recommended methods for each gestation band.

Medical management

Mifepristone 200 mg and misoprostol.

Early medical abortion ≤ 63 days

- ≤ 63 days – mifepristone 200 mg orally followed 24–48 hours later by misoprostol 800 µg vaginally/orally/sublingually.
- ≤ 49 days – mifepristone 200 mg orally followed 24–48 hours later by misoprostol 400 µg orally.
- 50–63 days – if abortion has not occurred 4 hours after misoprostol, a second dose of misoprostol 400 µg may be given orally/vaginally.
- It is safe for woman to leave the abortion unit following misoprostol administration to complete the abortion at home.

9–13 weeks

- Mifepristone 200 mg orally followed 36–48 hours later by misoprostol 800 µg vaginally. A maximum of 4 further doses of misoprostol 400 µg may be given 3 hourly (orally/vaginally).

13–24 weeks

- Mifepristone 200 mg orally followed 36–48 hours later by misoprostol 800 µg vaginally. A maximum of 4 further doses of misoprostol 400 µg may be given 3 hourly (orally/vaginally).
- If abortion does not occur, mifepristone can be repeated 3 hours after the last dose of misoprostol and, 12 hours later, misoprostol may be commenced.
- Avoid routine surgical evacuation of the uterus following medical TOP. Undertake only if there is clinical evidence that the termination is incomplete.
- Perform feticide before medical TOP after 21 weeks and 6 days of gestation to ensure that there is no risk of a live birth.

Surgical management

- Consider cervical preparation in all women.
- Misoprostol 400 µg vaginally 3 hours/sublingually 2–3 hours prior to surgery.
- After 14 weeks, osmotic dilators provide superior dilatation to medical methods; however, misoprostol is an alternative method up to 18 weeks.

First trimester
Vacuum aspiration

- < 7 weeks – vacuum aspiration but associated with a higher risk of failure.
- 7–14 weeks – vacuum aspiration.
- 14–16 weeks – vacuum aspiration may be performed with large-bore cannulae.
- Use suction cannula and blunt forceps only. Avoid sharp curettage.
- Safer under local anaesthesia than under GA; conscious sedation requires trained practitioners.
- Electric or manual aspiration devices – both are effective and acceptable to women and clinicians. Operating times are shorter with electric aspiration.

Gestational age > 14 weeks
Dilatation and evacuation

- Dilatation and evacuation with cervical preparation is safe and effective when undertaken by specialist practitioners.
- Continuous USS guidance during D&E is recommended.

Aftercare

- Analgesia.
- Routine histopathological examination of tissue is unnecessary.
- Rhesus prophylaxis.
- Written account of the warning symptoms.
- 24-hour telephone helpline.
- Urgent clinical assessment and emergency admission when necessary.
- Discharge letter that includes sufficient information.

Follow-up

- No need for routine follow-up if successful abortion has been confirmed at the time of the procedure.
- Women having medical TOP, in whom successful abortion has not been confirmed at the time of the procedure – offer follow-up to exclude continuation of pregnancy.
- Routine follow-up if woman wishes.
- Refer for further counselling if necessary.
- Do not scan routinely to screen women for incomplete abortion. Decide to evacuate the uterus following incomplete abortion based on clinical signs and symptoms and not on USS appearance.
- Contraception – discuss, offer, and initiate.
- IUCD can be inserted immediately following a first- or second-trimester TOP.
- Sterilization can be safely performed at the time of TOP. However, combined procedures are associated with higher rates of failure and of regret on the part of the woman.

Method of termination of pregnancy based on gestational age

Gestation in weeks

| 5 | 6 | 7 | 8 | 9 | 10 | 11 | 12 | 13 | 14 | 15 | 16 | 17 | 18 | 19 | 20 | 21 | 22 | 23 | 24 |

Medical termination with mifepristone and prostaglandin

Prostaglandin
Single dose < 49 days
Two doses 50–63 days

Prostaglandins – multiple doses

Surgical termination of pregnancy

Suction aspiration

Strict protocols

Suction termination

Suction termination

Experienced surgeon

Dilatation and evacuation

Experienced surgeon

Mifepristone

- **Mechanism** – anti-progesterone. It works by blocking the effects of progesterone.
- **Indications:**
  - * Medical TOP.
  - * Induction of labour in cases of IUD.
- **Dose** – 200 mg tablets. Used in combination with prostaglandins such as misoprostol.
- **Side effects** – diarrhoea, nausea, uterine contractions or cramps, vomiting, vaginal bleeding, infection, stomach cramps.
- Uncommon: hypersensitivity reactions, lowered blood pressure, skin rash or rashes, fever, general feeling of being unwell, headaches, rupture of the uterus, skin problems, toxic epidermal necrolysis, urticaria, vasovagal reaction such as hot flushes, dizziness or chills, toxic shock syndrome.

Misoprostol

- **Mechanism** – a synthetic prostaglandin E1 analogue that causes cervical softening and dilatation and uterine contractions.
- **Indications:**
  - * Medication TOP.
  - * Medical management of miscarriage.
  - * Induction of labour in cases of intrauterine death.
  - * Cervical ripening before surgical procedures – first-trimester surgical abortion, second-trimester D&E, hysteroscopy.
  - * Treatment of postpartum haemorrhage.
  - * Cervical ripening and induction of labour for a viable fetus.
  - * To treat or prevent stomach and duodenal ulcers.
- **Doses** – 200–800 μg oral, vaginal, sublingual, buccal, or rectal.
- **Side effects** – nausea, vomiting, diarrhoea, fever, and chills.
- Termination regimens containing misoprostol are not licensed; women should be informed if a prescribed treatment is unlicensed.
- Misoprostol's advantages over other synthetic prostaglandin analogues are its low cost, long shelf life, lack of need for refrigeration, and worldwide availability.

What not to do

- Routine crossmatch.
- Routine USS.
- Routine surgical evacuation of the uterus following medical TOP.
- Surgical evacuation – routine use of oxytocin/ergometrine for prophylaxis; sharp curettage.
- Routine USS to screen women for incomplete abortion.

1. *The Care of Women Requesting Induced Abortion.* RCOG Evidence-Based Clinical Guideline No. 7, 2011.

CHAPTER 3 Recurrent first-trimester (≥ 3) and second-trimester (≥ 1) miscarriage

Definition and prevalence

- First-trimester recurrent miscarriage (RM) – loss of 3 or more consecutive pregnancies.
- 1–2% of second-trimester pregnancies miscarry before 24 weeks of gestation.
- Approximately 15% of all clinical pregnancies end in pregnancy loss, with 3 or more losses affecting 1–2% of women of reproductive age and 2 or more losses affecting around 5% of women.

History

- **Obstetric history** – risk increases after each successive pregnancy loss, reaching approximately 40% after 3 consecutive pregnancy losses.
- **Details of previous losses** – gestational age, scan confirmation of fetal pole, painless or painful loss especially in second trimester loss.
- **Past history** – diabetes or thyroid disorders, congenital or acquired thrombophilias.
- **Heavy alcohol consumption** is toxic to the embryo and the fetus. Even moderate consumption of ≥ 5 units per week may increase the risk of sporadic miscarriage.
- **Occupational history** – working with or using video display terminals does not increase the risk of miscarriage. The evidence on the effect of anaesthetic gases for theatre workers is conflicting.
- **Maternal smoking and caffeine** – associated with an increased risk of spontaneous miscarriage in a dose-dependent manner. However, current evidence is insufficient to confirm this association.

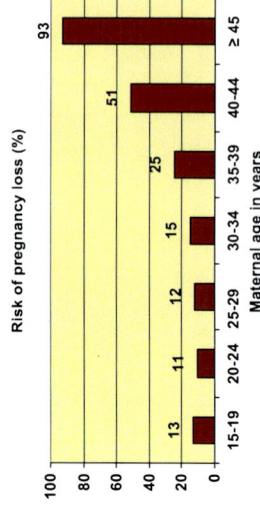

Risk factors

- Cause of recurrent pregnancy loss (RPL) remains unknown in the majority of women.
- **Maternal and paternal age** – risk of miscarriage is highest among couples where the woman is > 35 years of age and the man > 40 years of age.
  * Maternal age – advancing maternal age is associated with a decline in both the number and quality of the remaining oocytes.
  * The age-related risk of miscarriage – see graph.
- Advanced paternal age is also a risk factor for miscarriage.
- **BMI** – obesity increases the risk of both sporadic and RPL.

Risk of pregnancy loss (%)

Maternal age in years	Risk
15-19	13
20-24	11
25-29	12
30-34	15
35-39	25
40-44	51
≥ 45	93

Investigations and recommendations

Antiphospholipid antibodies (LAC/ACA)

- Screen women with first-trimester RPL and women with one or more second-trimester miscarriage before pregnancy.
- Two positive tests at least 6 weeks apart for either LAC or ACA of IgG and/or IgM class in medium or high titre are necessary for diagnosis.

Uterine anomalies

- Offer pelvic USS for women with first-trimester RPL and women with one or more second-trimester miscarriages.
- 2D USS and/or HSG can be used as an initial screening test.
- Combined hysteroscopy and laparoscopy and possibly 3D USS should be used for definitive diagnosis.
- Value of MRI scanning remains undetermined.

Cervical weakness

- Women with a history of second-trimester miscarriage and suspected cervical weakness who have not undergone a history-indicated cerclage may be offered serial cervical sonographic surveillance.

Genetic factors

- Perform cytogenetic analysis of the products of conception on third and subsequent miscarriage.
- Perform parental peripheral blood karyotyping of both partners in couples with RPL where testing of products of conception reports an unbalanced structural chromosomal abnormality.
- Current data suggest that routine karyotyping of couples with RPL cannot be justified owing to the cost. Selective parental karyotyping may be more appropriate when an unbalanced chromosome abnormality is identified in the products of conception.

Inherited thrombophilic defects

- Screen women with second-trimester miscarriage for inherited thrombophilias including factor V Leiden, factor II (prothrombin) gene mutation, and protein S.

Risk factors

Antiphospholipid syndrome (APS)

- **APA are present in 15% of women with RPL.**
- **APS** – antiphospholipid antibodies (APA) + adverse pregnancy outcome or vascular thrombosis.
- **APA** – lupus anticoagulant (LAC), anticardiolipin antibodies (ACA), and anti-B2 glycoprotein-I antibodies.
- **Adverse pregnancy outcomes:**
  * ≥ 3 consecutive miscarriages < 10 weeks of gestation.
  * ≥ 1 morphologically normal fetal loss > 10 weeks.
  * ≥ 1 PTB < 34 weeks owing to placental disease.
- Mechanisms – inhibition of trophoblastic function and differentiation, activation of complement pathways at the maternal–fetal interface resulting in a local inflammatory response and in later pregnancy, thrombosis of the uteroplacental vasculature.
- LBR with no medical intervention is as low as 10%.

Genetic

- **Parental structural chromosomal anomaly** – 2–5% of couples. Most commonly a balanced reciprocal or Robertsonian translocation.
  * Carriers are phenotypically normal, but their pregnancies are at increased risk of miscarriage and may result in a live birth with multiple congenital anomalies.
  * Risk of miscarriage is influenced by the size and genetic content of the rearranged chromosomal segments.
- **Embryonic chromosomal abnormalities** – account for 30–57% of further miscarriages. Risk increases with advancing maternal age.

Endocrine factors

- **Diabetes and thyroid disorders** – women with uncontrolled diabetes in the first trimester are at risk of miscarriage. Well-controlled diabetes mellitus and treated thyroid dysfunction are not risk factors for RPL.
- **Anti-thyroid antibodies** – women with RPL are no more likely than women without RPL to have circulating thyroid antibodies.
- **PCOS** – possible increased risk of miscarriage but the exact mechanism remains unclear. The increased risk is attributed to insulin resistance, hyperinsulinaemia, and hyperandrogenaemia. The prevalence of insulin resistance is increased in women with RPL compared with fertile controls.
  * Polycystic ovarian morphology, elevated LH levels, or elevated serum testosterone levels do not predict an increased risk of future pregnancy loss.
  * Elevated free androgen index appears to be a prognostic factor for a subsequent miscarriage in women with RPL.

Immune factors

- No evidence to support the hypothesis of **human leucocyte antigen (HLA)** incompatibility between couples.
- **Natural killer (NK) cells** – peripheral blood NK cells are phenotypically and functionally different from uterine NK cells. No evidence that altered peripheral blood NK cells are related to RPL.

Anatomical factors

- **Congenital uterine malformations** – risk of RPL is unclear and the association is debatable. Prevalence of uterine anomalies in RPL – 2–38%. Prevalence is higher in women with second-trimester miscarriages compared with women who suffer first-trimester miscarriages.
- **Cervical weakness** – recognized cause of second-trimester miscarriage. The true incidence is unknown, as the diagnosis is essentially clinical, based on a history of second-trimester miscarriage preceded by spontaneous rupture of membranes or painless cervical dilatation.

Infective agents

- Any severe infection that leads to bacteraemia or viraemia can cause sporadic miscarriage.
- **TORCH** – for an infective agent to be implicated in the aetiology of RPL, it must be capable of persisting in the genital tract and avoiding detection, or must cause insufficient symptoms to disturb the woman. Toxoplasmosis, rubella, cytomegalovirus, herpes, and *Listeria* infections do not fulfil these criteria.
- **Bacterial vaginosis:**
  * BV in the first trimester has been reported as a risk factor for second-trimester miscarriage and PTD, but the evidence for an association with first-trimester miscarriage is inconsistent.
  * Treatment of BV with oral clindamycin early in the second trimester significantly reduces the incidence of second-trimester miscarriage and PTD.
  * No published data to assess the role of antibiotic therapy in women with a previous second-trimester miscarriage.

Inherited thrombophilic defects

- Activated protein C resistance (factor V Leiden mutation), deficiencies of protein C/S and antithrombin III, hyperhomocysteinaemia, and prothrombin gene mutation.
- Possible cause of RPL and late pregnancy complications owing to thrombosis of the uteroplacental circulation.
- Association between inherited thrombophilias and fetal loss varies according to type of thrombophilia.
- Association between thrombophilia and late pregnancy loss has been consistently stronger than for early pregnancy loss.

- **Male factor** – increasing evidence suggests that abnormal integrity (intactness) of sperm DNA may affect embryo development and possibly increase miscarriage risk. However, these data are still very preliminary, and it is not known how often sperm defects contribute to RPL. (ASRM)

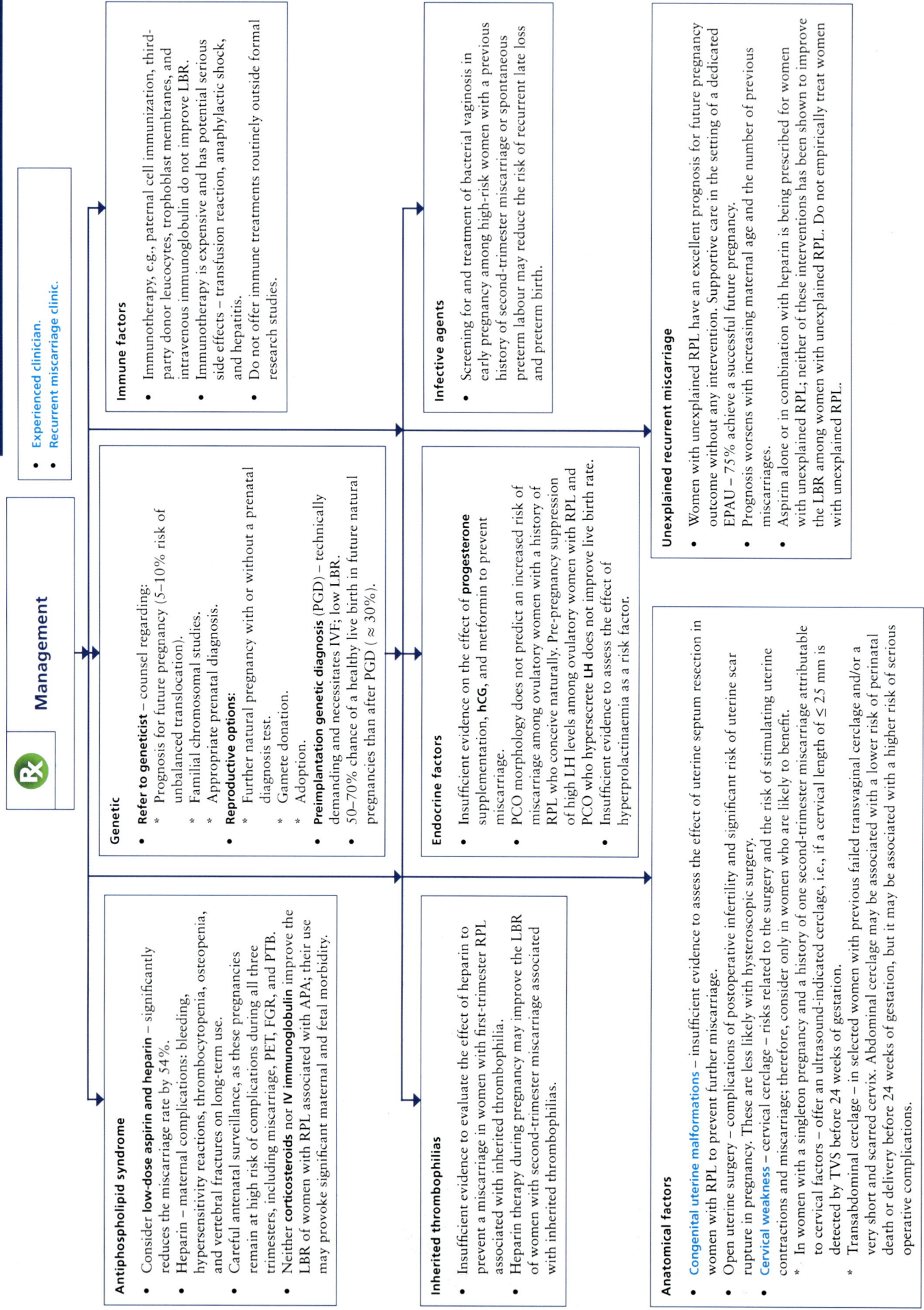

℞ Management

- Experienced clinician.
- Recurrent miscarriage clinic.

Immune factors

- Immunotherapy, e.g., paternal cell immunization, third-party donor leucocytes, trophoblast membranes, and intravenous immunoglobulin do not improve LBR.
- Immunotherapy is expensive and has potential serious side effects – transfusion reaction, anaphylactic shock, and hepatitis.
- Do not offer immune treatments routinely outside formal research studies.

Infective agents

- Screening for and treatment of bacterial vaginosis in early pregnancy among high-risk women with a previous history of second-trimester miscarriage or spontaneous preterm labour may reduce the risk of recurrent late loss and preterm birth.

Unexplained recurrent miscarriage

- Women with unexplained RPL have an excellent prognosis for future pregnancy outcome without any intervention. Supportive care in the setting of a dedicated EPAU – 75% achieve a successful future pregnancy.
- Prognosis worsens with increasing maternal age and the number of previous miscarriages.
- Aspirin alone or in combination with heparin is being prescribed for women with unexplained RPL; neither of these interventions has been shown to improve the LBR among women with unexplained RPL. Do not empirically treat women with unexplained RPL.

Genetic

- **Refer to geneticist** – counsel regarding:
  * Prognosis for future pregnancy (5–10% risk of unbalanced translocation).
  * Familial chromosomal studies.
  * Appropriate prenatal diagnosis.
- **Reproductive options:**
  * Further natural pregnancy with or without a prenatal diagnosis test.
  * Gamete donation.
  * Adoption.
- **Preimplantation genetic diagnosis** (PGD) – technically demanding and necessitates IVF; low LBR. 50–70% chance of a healthy live birth in future natural pregnancies than after PGD ($\approx$ 30%).

Endocrine factors

- Insufficient evidence on the effect of **progesterone** supplementation, **hCG**, and metformin to prevent miscarriage.
- PCO morphology does not predict an increased risk of miscarriage among ovulatory women with a history of RPL who conceive naturally. Pre-pregnancy suppression of high LH levels among ovulatory women with RPL and PCO who hypersecrete **LH** does not improve live birth rate.
- Insufficient evidence to assess the effect of hyperprolactinaemia as a risk factor.

Antiphospholipid syndrome

- Consider **low-dose aspirin and heparin** – significantly reduces the miscarriage rate by 54%.
- Heparin – maternal complications: bleeding, hypersensitivity reactions, thrombocytopenia, osteopenia, and vertebral fractures on long-term use.
- Careful antenatal surveillance, as these pregnancies remain at high risk of complications during all three trimesters, including miscarriage, PET, FGR, and PTB.
- Neither **corticosteroids** nor **IV immunoglobulin** improve the LBR of women with RPL associated with APA; their use may provoke significant maternal and fetal morbidity.

Inherited thrombophilias

- Insufficient evidence to evaluate the effect of heparin to prevent a miscarriage in women with first-trimester RPL associated with inherited thrombophilia.
- Heparin therapy during pregnancy may improve the LBR of women with second-trimester miscarriage associated with inherited thrombophilias.

Anatomical factors

- **Congenital uterine malformations** – insufficient evidence to assess the effect of uterine septum resection in women with RPL to prevent further miscarriage.
- Open uterine surgery – complications of postoperative infertility and significant risk of uterine scar rupture in pregnancy. These are less likely with hysteroscopic surgery.
- **Cervical weakness** – cervical cerclage – risks related to the surgery and the risk of stimulating uterine contractions and miscarriage; therefore, consider only in women who are likely to benefit.
  * In women with a singleton pregnancy and a history of one second-trimester miscarriage attributable to cervical factors – offer an ultrasound-indicated cerclage, i.e., if a cervical length of $\leq$ 25 mm is detected by TVS before 24 weeks of gestation.
  * Transabdominal cerclage – in selected women with previous failed transvaginal cerclage and/or a very short and scarred cervix. Abdominal cerclage may be associated with a lower risk of perinatal death or delivery before 24 weeks of gestation, but it may be associated with a higher risk of serious operative complications.

Tests not recommended

- MRI for uterine anomalies – value of MRI remains undetermined.
- Routine karyotyping of couples with RPL cannot be justified owing to the cost.
- Human leucocyte antigens – maternal leucocytotoxic antibodies or maternal blocking antibodies.
- Cervical weakness – no satisfactory objective test that can identify women with cervical weakness in the non-pregnant state; the diagnosis is essentially a clinical one.
- Blood NK cells – testing for peripheral blood NK cells as a surrogate marker of the events at the maternal–fetal interface is inappropriate.
- Cytokines – routine cytokine tests outside research context.
- TORCH screening.
- Antithyroid antibodies – routine screening for thyroid antibodies.
- Screening for occult diabetes and thyroid (GTT, TFT) in asymptomatic women.

Management not recommended

- Corticosteroids and IV immunoglobulins in APA.
- Uterine septum resection, hCG, metformin, and progesterone supplementation.
- Prepregnancy suppression of high LH levels among ovulatory women with RPL and polycystic ovaries who hypersecrete LH.
- Heparin to prevent a miscarriage associated with inherited thrombophilia.
- Aspirin alone or in combination with heparin for women with unexplained RPL.
- Use of empirical treatment in women with unexplained RPL.

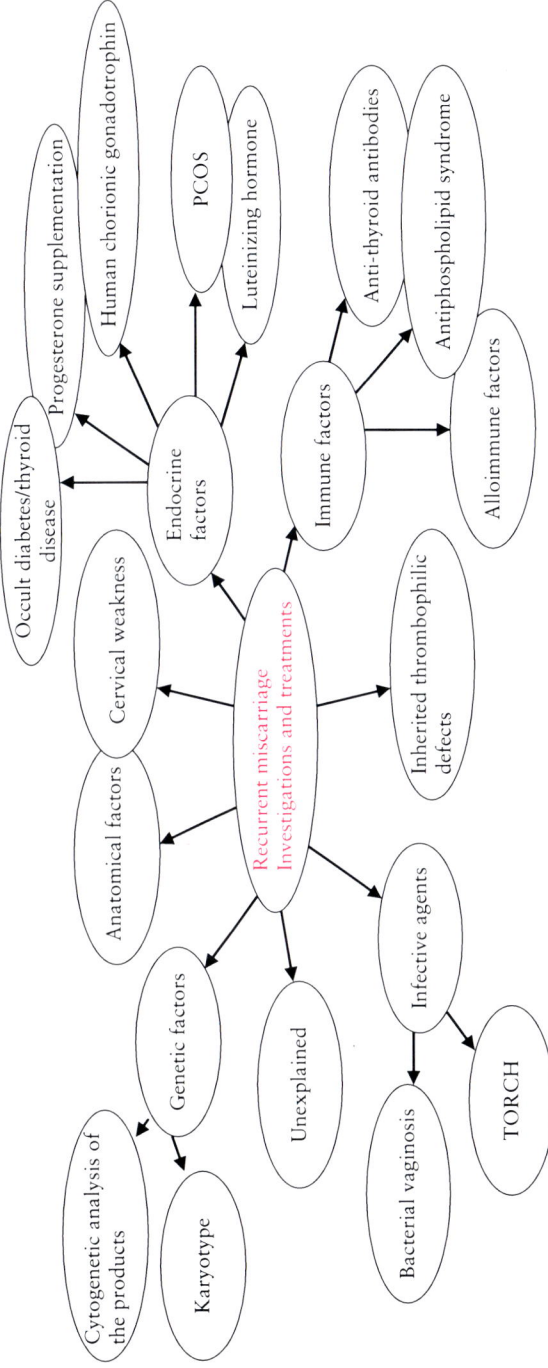

1. *The Use of Antithrombotics in the Prevention of Recurrent Pregnancy Loss*. RCOG Scientific Advisory Committee Opinion Paper 26, June 2011.
2. *The Investigation and Treatment of Couples with Recurrent First-trimester and Second-trimester Miscarriage*. RCOG Green-top Guideline No. 17, April 2011.
3. *Recurrent Pregnancy Loss*. ASRM Patient's Fact Sheet, 2008.

CHAPTER 3   Recurrent first-trimester (≥ 3) and second-trimester (≥ 1) miscarriage

CHAPTER 4 Gestational trophoblastic disease and neoplasia

- **GTD** – group of disorders ranging from complete and partial molar pregnancy to the malignant conditions of invasive mole, choriocarcinoma, and placental site trophoblastic tumour (PSTT). 1/714 live births. Higher incidence in Asian women. • **GTN** – any evidence of persistence of GTD, most commonly defined as a persistent elevation of β-hCG. Persistent GTN may develop after a molar pregnancy, a non-molar pregnancy, or a live birth.

  - **Complete moles:**
    - * Diploid and androgenetic – usually due to duplication of the haploid sperm following fertilization of an 'empty' ovum (75–80%).
    - * Some due to dispermic fertilization of an 'empty' ovum (20–25%).
    - * No evidence of fetal tissue.
  - **Partial moles:**
    - * Triploid – two sets of paternal haploid genes and one set of maternal haploid genes (90%) due to dispermic fertilization of an ovum.
    - * Tetraploid or mosaic conceptions – 10%.
    - * Usually evidence of fetal tissue or fetal RBCs.

History

- Majority present with symptoms of early pregnancy failure – irregular vaginal bleeding, hyperemesis.
- Presentation with early severe PET, abdominal distension due to theca lutein cysts and hyperthyroidism is rare.
- Very rarely – acute respiratory failure or neurological symptoms such as seizures due to metastatic disease.

Examination – excessive uterine enlargement

Investigations

- Urine pregnancy test.
- Serum hCG levels greater than two multiples of the median may help.
- USS is helpful in making a diagnosis but the definitive diagnosis is by histopathology of pregnancy tissues.

  - **Early complete molar pregnancy:**
    - * Commonly associated with the USS diagnosis of delayed miscarriage or anembryonic pregnancy.
  - **Partial molar pregnancy:**
    - * USS has limited value in detecting as it is more complex. Finding of multiple soft markers, including both cystic spaces in the placenta and a ratio of transverse to AP dimension of the gestation sac of > 1.5 is required for a reliable diagnosis. (RCOG)

Management – evacuation

- Suction evacuation is the method of choice.
- Experienced surgeon to manage excessive vaginal bleeding.
- Preparation of the cervix immediately before evacuation is safe.
- Avoid prolonged cervical preparation, particularly with prostaglandins, to reduce the risk of embolization of trophoblastic cells.
- Use of oxytocic infusion before completion of the evacuation is not recommended.
- Where possible, commence oxytocic infusion only once evacuation is completed.

  - **Complete molar pregnancies:**
    - * Suction curettage is the method of choice of evacuation.
    - * Avoid medical termination if possible.
    - * Anti-D is not required in complete molar pregnancies because of poor vascularization of the chorionic villi and absence of the anti-D antigen.
  - **Partial molar pregnancies:**
    - * Suction curettage is the method of choice except when the size of the fetal parts deters the use of suction curettage, when medical evacuation can be used.
    - * Anti-D to Rh-negative women.

  - Evidence – data with mifepristone and misoprostol are limited – avoid, as it increases the sensitivity of the uterus to prostaglandins.

Persisting symptoms such as vaginal bleeding after initial evacuation

- hCG, USS.
- Consult with the trophoblastic screening centre before repeat surgical intervention.
- **Routine repeat evacuation is not warranted.**

Histological examination

- Perform histological examination of all pregnancy tissues obtained after evacuation (medical or surgical).
- There is no need to routinely send pregnancy tissues for histological examination following TOP, provided that fetal parts have been identified on prior USS.
- Ploidy status and immunohistochemistry staining for P57 may help in distinguishing partial from complete moles.

Monitoring/follow-up

- Register women with trophoblastic screening centre for follow-up.
- If hCG has reverted to normal within 56 days of the pregnancy, follow-up for 6 months from the date of evacuation.
- If hCG has not reverted to normal within 56 days of the pregnancy, follow-up for 6 months from normalization of the hCG level.

Risk of recurrence

- Risk of a further molar pregnancy is low (1/80).
- > 98% of women who become pregnant following a molar pregnancy will not have a further mole or be at increased risk of obstetric complications.
- If a further molar pregnancy does occur, in 68–80% of cases it will be of the same histological type.
- After the conclusion of any further pregnancy, at any gestation and outcome, advise women to notify the trophoblastic screening centre. Urine or blood hCG levels are measured 6–8 weeks after the end of the pregnancy to exclude disease recurrence.

Contraception

- Advise women not to conceive until the hCG level has been normal for 6 months.
- Advise women who undergo chemotherapy not to conceive for one year after completion of treatment.
- Advise women to use barrier methods of contraception until hCG levels revert to normal.
- COC pill and HRT are safe to use after hCG levels have reverted to normal.
- There is no evidence on whether single-agent progestogens have any effect on GTN.
- COC pill, if taken while hCG levels are raised – there is a potential increased risk of developing GTN.
- Do not use IUCD until hCG levels are normal, to reduce the risk of uterine perforation.
- Small potential risk of use of emergency hormonal contraception, in women with raised hCG levels, outweighs the potential risk of a pregnancy.

Twin pregnancy with one viable fetus and the other a molar pregnancy

- Refer to regional fetal medicine unit and the trophoblastic screening centre.
- Consider prenatal invasive testing for fetal karyotype in cases:
  * Where it is unclear if the pregnancy is a complete mole with a coexisting normal twin or a partial mole.
  * Of abnormal placenta, such as suspected mesenchymal hyperplasia of the placenta.

- Increased risk of PNM and morbidity – approximately 25% chance of a live birth along with increased risk of early fetal loss (40%) and premature delivery (36%).
- Incidence of PET is variable: 4–20%.
- Outcome for GTD:
  * No increased risk of developing GTN after such a twin pregnancy.
  * Pregnancy outcome after chemotherapy is unaffected.

Persistent GTN

- Persistent vaginal bleeding after a pregnancy event is the most common presenting symptom.
- Symptoms from metastatic disease, such as dyspnoea or abnormal neurology, occur very rarely.

A urine pregnancy test to exclude persistent GTN
Urgent referral to specialist centre

Placental site trophoblastic tumour is recognized as a variant of GTN. It may be treated with surgery as it is less sensitive to chemotherapy.

FIGO staging

The need for chemotherapy following:
- A complete mole is 15%.
- A partial mole is 0.5 %.

Scoring six or less (low risk).
- * IM methotrexate (MTX).
- * Resistance to MTX – use combined dactinomycin and etoposide.

Scoring seven or more (high risk).
- * Combination chemotherapy – IV etoposide, methotrexate, dactinomycin, vincristine, and cyclophosphamide (EMA-CO).

- Continue treatment in all cases, until the hCG level has returned to normal and then for a further 6 weeks.
- Prognosis for women with GTN after non-molar pregnancy may be worse (21% mortality after a live birth, 6% after a non-molar miscarriage) and, in part, is due to delay in diagnosis.
- Women who receive chemotherapy are likely to have an earlier menopause.
- Women who require multi-agent chemotherapy (including etoposide) may be at increased risk of developing secondary cancers.

What not to do

- There is a theoretical concern over the routine use of potent oxytocic agents owing to the potential to embolize and disseminate trophoblastic tissue. Therefore:
  - * Avoid prolonged cervical preparation, particularly with prostaglandins.
  - * Do not use oxytocic infusion prior to completion of the evacuation.
- Avoid medical termination, if possible.
- In complete molar pregnancies, anti-D is not required because of poor vascularization of the chorionic villi and absence of the anti-D antigen.
- Routine repeat evacuation is not warranted.
- Advise women not to conceive until the hCG level has been normal for 6 months.
- Advise women who undergo chemotherapy, not to conceive for one year after completion of treatment.
- Avoid COC while hCG levels are raised.
- Do not use intrauterine contraceptive devices until hCG levels are normal.

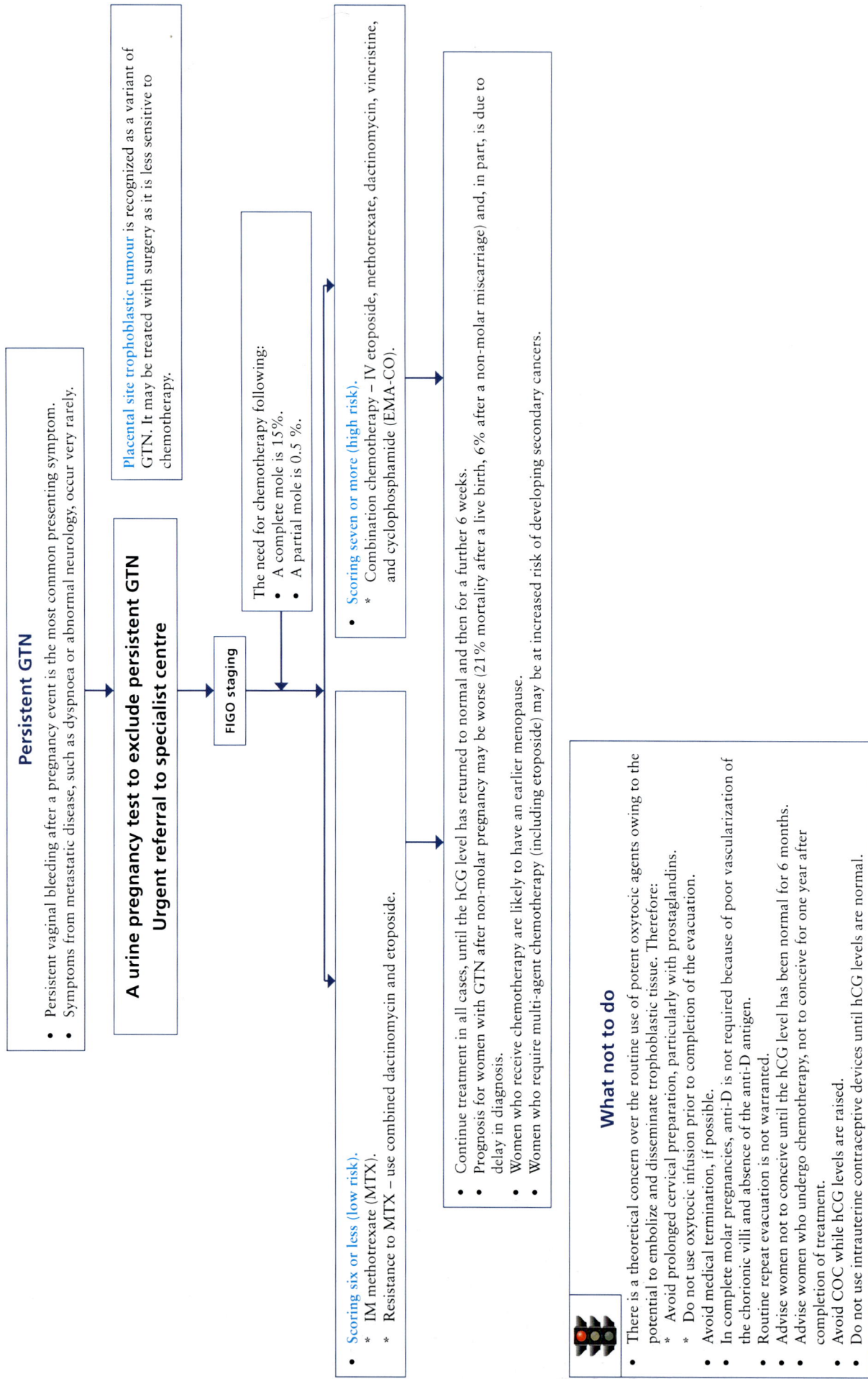

1. *The Management of Gestational Trophoblastic Disease.* RCOG Green-top Guideline No. 38, February 2010.
2. *Gestational Trophoblastic Disease.* SOGC Clinical Practice Guidelines No. 114, May 2002.

Pregnancy outside the uterine cavity

Prevalence and incidence

- Incidence (static in recent years) – 1% of pregnancies.
- Maternal mortality of 0.2/1000 estimated ectopic pregnancies.
- Sites – tubal (98%); others – abdomen, ovary, cervix, caesarean section scar.
- Heterotopic pregnancy – combination of both an IUP and an extrauterine pregnancy; occurs in 1/4000 natural pregnancies and in about 1/100 pregnancies following assisted reproduction.

History

- Amenorrhoea. Women may appear not to have missed a menstrual period, as vaginal bleeding may occur at the time of the expected period.
- Pain or bleeding between 5 and 14 weeks' gestation.
- Lower abdominal or pelvic pain – mild to severe; often unilateral.
- Vaginal bleeding – usually intermittent, bright or dark red, rarely exceeds the normal menstrual flow.
- Beware of uncommon symptoms – fainting or dizziness, breast tenderness, gastrointestinal symptoms (vomiting or diarrhoea), shoulder-tip pain (referred pain due to peritoneal irritation), urinary symptoms, passage of tissue, rectal pressure or pain on defecation.
- Asymptomatic – found incidentally on an early pregnancy scan.

Examination

- General examination – cardiovascular shock in cases of ruptured ectopic.
- Abdominal examination – tenderness, rebound tenderness, guarding, rigidity, or distension.
- Vaginal examination – cervical and/or adnexal tenderness.
- Common signs – pelvic, adnexal, and abdominal tenderness.
- Other signs – cervical motion tenderness, rebound tenderness or peritoneal signs, pallor, abdominal distension, enlarged uterus, tachycardia (> 100 beats per minute) or hypotension (< 100/60 mmHg), shock or collapse, orthostatic hypotension.
- Advise not to perform a pelvic examination if a tubal rupture is suspected, as it is usually difficult and information gained is limited because of generalized haemoperitoneum and pain. It could cause total rupture of the ectopic pregnancy and it may delay management.

Risk factors

- Conditions that damage the fallopian tube, impair its ability to transport gametes or embryos, and predispose to faulty implantation.
- Risk factors for ectopic pregnancy:
  * Prior pelvic or abdominal surgery.
  * History of an STI, previous elective TOP, history of infertility, history of PID, previous ectopic pregnancy, or history of IUCD.
  * Prior tubal surgery or endometriosis.
  * About a third of women have no known risk factors.

Risks or complications

- Tubal rupture (time of rupture depends on the site of implantation and usually occurs after 6 weeks) – intra-abdominal bleeding, shock.
- Death is rare but the leading cause of pregnancy-related death in the first trimester.
- Tubal infertility.
- Psychological – grief, anxiety, or depression. Distress is commonly at its worst 4–6 weeks after pregnancy loss and may last 6–12 months.

Prognosis if untreated

- Spontaneous tubal miscarriage – occurs in about 50% of ectopic pregnancies and the woman may have no symptoms. Some spontaneous tubal abortions may bleed, but the bleeding is self-limiting.
- Ruptured ectopic – intra-abdominal bleeding, shock, death.
- Chronic ectopic pregnancy.

Differential diagnosis

DDx

- Pain or bleeding in early pregnancy.

Pregnancy-related
- Miscarriage.
- Molar pregnancy.
- Early intrauterine pregnancy.
- Ruptured corpus luteal cyst.
- Degeneration of a fibroid.

Non-pregnancy-related
- Cervicitis, cervical ectropion, or polyps.
- Vaginitis.
- Cancer of the cervix, vagina, or vulva.
- UTI, urethral bleeding, renal colic.
- Irritable bowel syndrome, haemorrhoids.
- Appendicitis. • PID.
- Torsion/degeneration of a fibroid.
- Ovarian cyst (torsion, rupture, or bleeding).
- Musculoskeletal pain. • Adhesions.

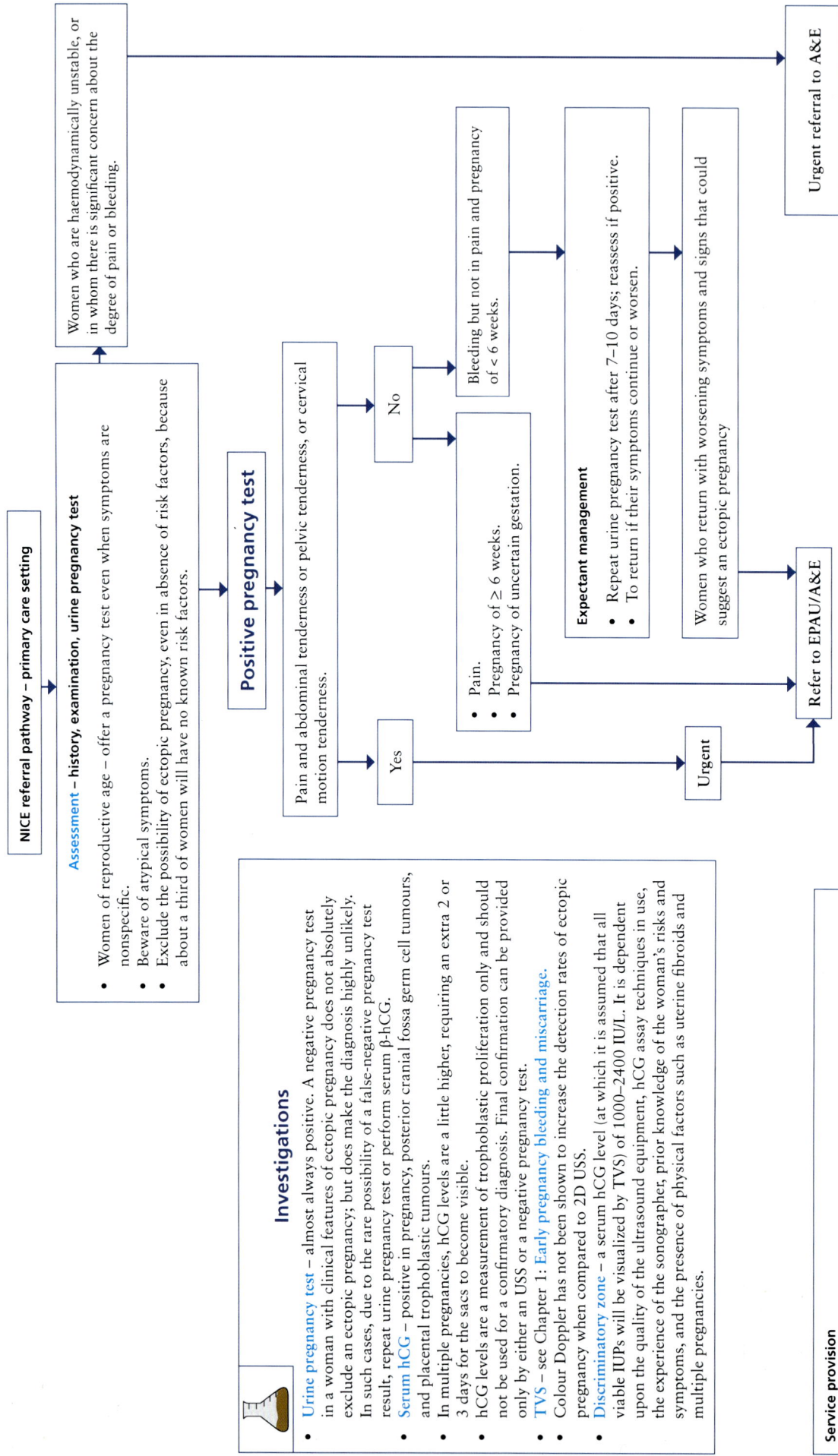

NICE referral pathway – primary care setting

Women who are haemodynamically unstable, or in whom there is significant concern about the degree of pain or bleeding.

Assessment – history, examination, urine pregnancy test

- Women of reproductive age – offer a pregnancy test even when symptoms are nonspecific.
- Beware of atypical symptoms.
- Exclude the possibility of ectopic pregnancy, even in absence of risk factors, because about a third of women will have no known risk factors.

Positive pregnancy test

Pain and abdominal tenderness or pelvic tenderness, or cervical motion tenderness.

Yes → **No**

- Pain.
- Pregnancy of ≥ 6 weeks.
- Pregnancy of uncertain gestation.

Bleeding but not in pain and pregnancy of < 6 weeks.

Expectant management

- Repeat urine pregnancy test after 7–10 days; reassess if positive.
- To return if their symptoms continue or worsen.

Women who return with worsening symptoms and signs that could suggest an ectopic pregnancy

Urgent

Refer to EPAU/A&E

Urgent referral to A&E

Investigations

- **Urine pregnancy test** – almost always positive. A negative pregnancy test in a woman with clinical features of ectopic pregnancy does not absolutely exclude an ectopic pregnancy; but does make the diagnosis highly unlikely. In such cases, due to the rare possibility of a false-negative pregnancy test result, repeat urine pregnancy test or perform serum β-hCG.
- **Serum hCG** – positive in pregnancy, posterior cranial fossa germ cell tumours, and placental trophoblastic tumours.
- In multiple pregnancies, hCG levels are a little higher, requiring an extra 2 or 3 days for the sacs to become visible.
- hCG levels are a measurement of trophoblastic proliferation only and should not be used for a confirmatory diagnosis. Final confirmation can be provided only by either an USS or a negative pregnancy test.
- **TVS** – see Chapter 1: Early pregnancy bleeding and miscarriage.
- Colour Doppler has not been shown to increase the detection rates of ectopic pregnancy when compared to 2D USS.
- **Discriminatory zone** – a serum hCG level (at which it is assumed that all viable IUPs will be visualized by TVS) of 1000–2400 IU/L. It is dependent upon the quality of the ultrasound equipment, hCG assay techniques in use, the experience of the sonographer, prior knowledge of the woman's risks and symptoms, and the presence of physical factors such as uterine fibroids and multiple pregnancies.

Service provision

- EPAU services – see Chapter 1: Early pregnancy bleeding and miscarriage.
- Offer counselling and provide clear information about the importance of the possible need for further treatment, adverse effects with the treatment, and compliance with follow-up.
- Offer anti-Dimmunoglobulin to non-sensitized women who are rhesus negative with a confirmed or suspected ectopic pregnancy.

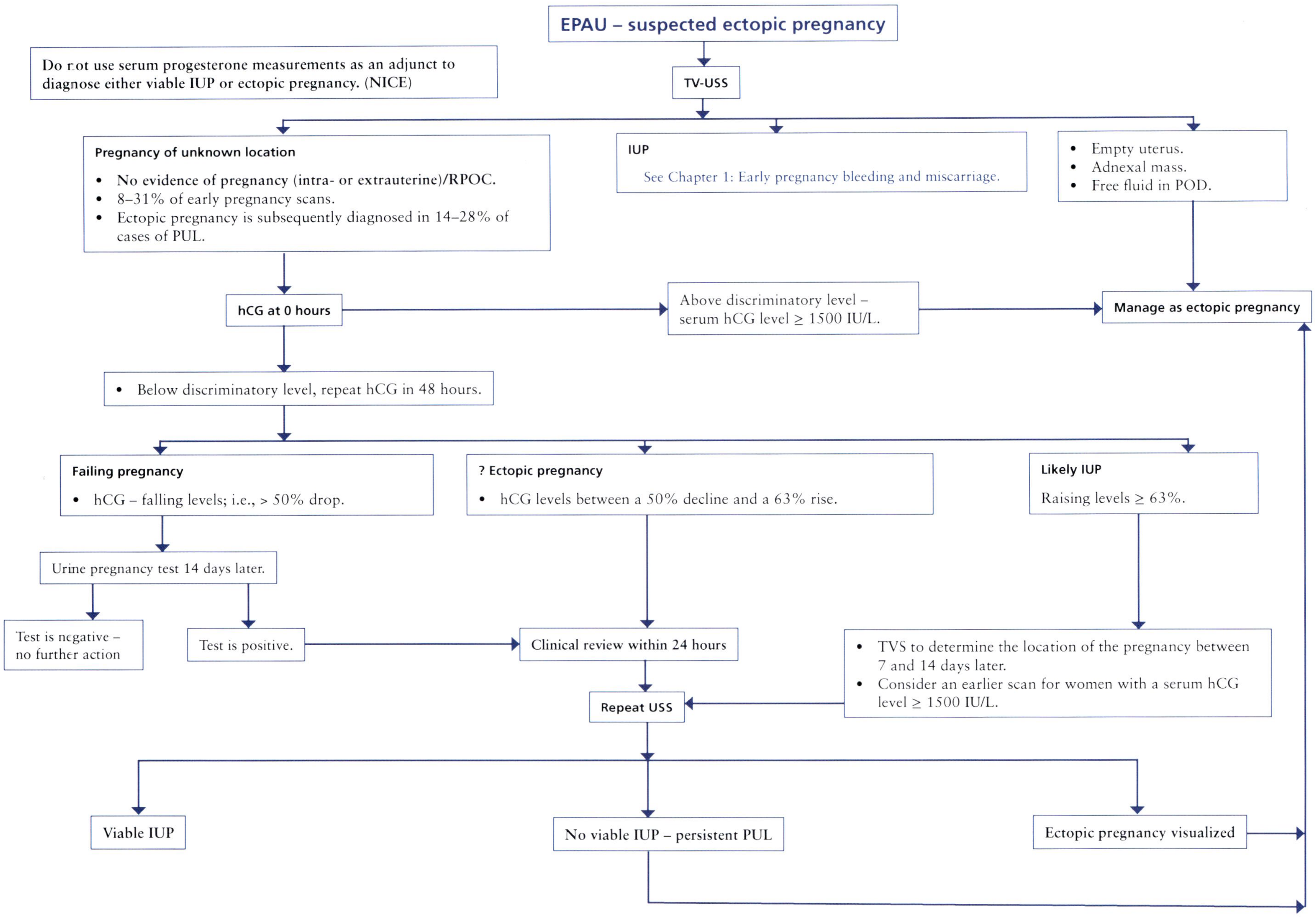

EPAU – suspected ectopic pregnancy

Do not use serum progesterone measurements as an adjunct to diagnose either viable IUP or ectopic pregnancy. (NICE)

TV-USS

Pregnancy of unknown location

- No evidence of pregnancy (intra- or extrauterine)/RPOC.
- 8–31% of early pregnancy scans.
- Ectopic pregnancy is subsequently diagnosed in 14–28% of cases of PUL.

IUP

See Chapter 1: Early pregnancy bleeding and miscarriage.

- Empty uterus.
- Adnexal mass.
- Free fluid in POD.

Manage as ectopic pregnancy

Above discriminatory level – serum hCG level ≥ 1500 IU/L.

hCG at 0 hours

- Below discriminatory level, repeat hCG in 48 hours.

Failing pregnancy

- hCG – falling levels; i.e., > 50% drop.

Urine pregnancy test 14 days later.

Test is positive.

Test is negative – no further action

? Ectopic pregnancy

- hCG levels between a 50% decline and a 63% rise.

Likely IUP

Raising levels ≥ 63%.

Clinical review within 24 hours

- TVS to determine the location of the pregnancy between 7 and 14 days later.
- Consider an earlier scan for women with a serum hCG level ≥ 1500 IU/L.

Repeat USS

No viable IUP – persistent PUL

Viable IUP

Ectopic pregnancy visualized

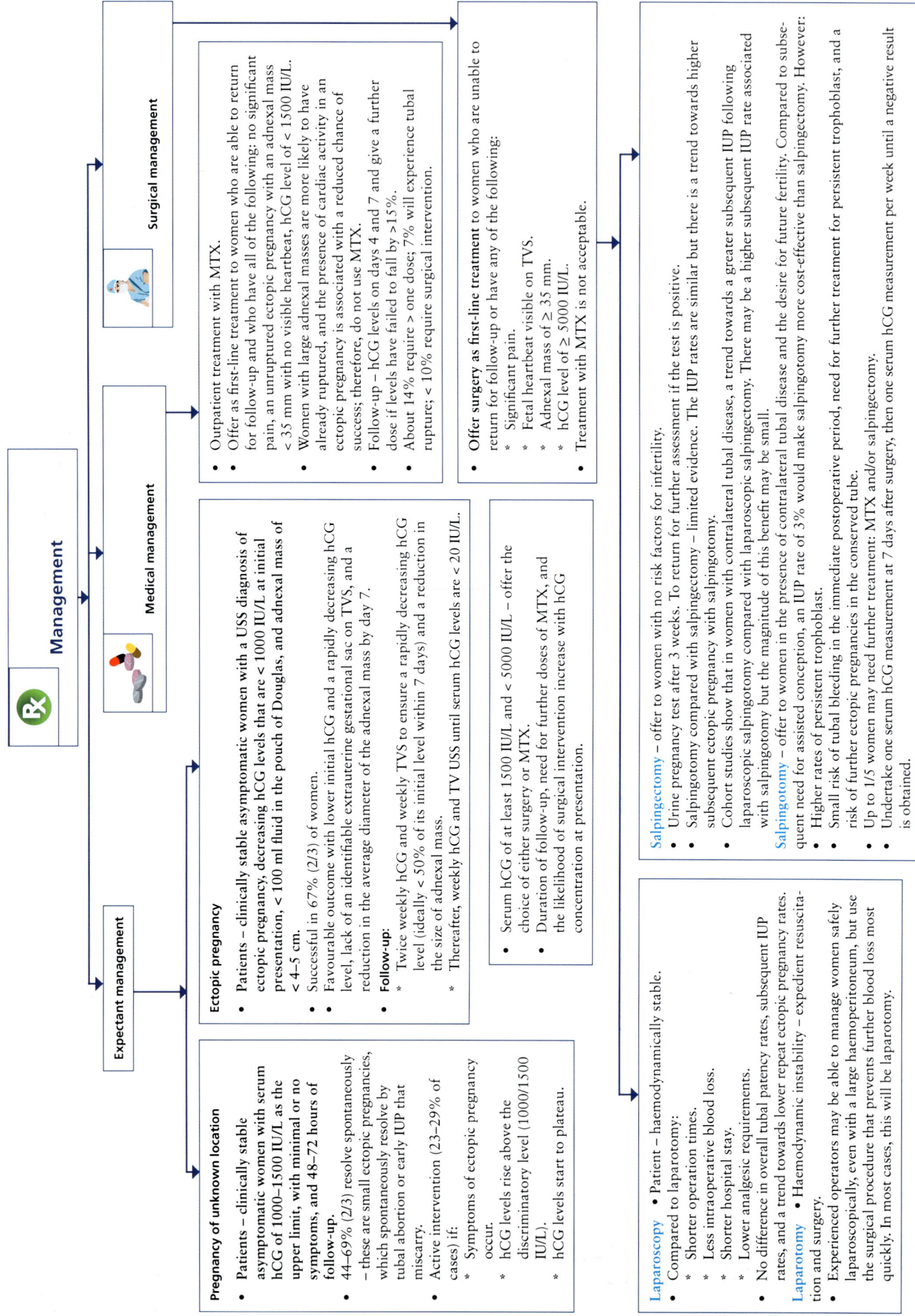

Management

- Expectant management
- Medical management
- Surgical management

Pregnancy of unknown location

- **Patients** – clinically stable asymptomatic women with serum hCG of 1000–1500 IU/L as the upper limit, with minimal or no symptoms, and 48–72 hours of follow-up.
- 44–69% (2/3) resolve spontaneously – these are small ectopic pregnancies, which spontaneously resolve by tubal abortion or early IUP that miscarry.
- Active intervention (23–29% of cases) if:
  * Symptoms of ectopic pregnancy occur.
  * hCG levels rise above the discriminatory level (1000/1500 IU/L).
  * hCG levels start to plateau.

Ectopic pregnancy

- **Patients** – clinically stable asymptomatic women with a USS diagnosis of ectopic pregnancy, decreasing hCG levels that are < 1000 IU/L at initial presentation, < 100 ml fluid in the pouch of Douglas, and adnexal mass of < 4–5 cm.
- Successful in 67% (2/3) of women.
- Favourable outcome with lower initial hCG and a rapidly decreasing hCG level, lack of an identifiable extrauterine gestational sac on TVS, and a reduction in the average diameter of the adnexal mass by day 7.
- **Follow-up:**
  * Twice weekly hCG and weekly TVS to ensure a rapidly decreasing hCG level (ideally < 50% of its initial level within 7 days) and a reduction in the size of adnexal mass.
  * Thereafter, weekly hCG and TV USS until serum hCG levels are < 20 IU/L.

- Serum hCG of at least 1500 IU/L and < 5000 IU/L – offer the choice of either surgery or MTX.
- Duration of follow-up, need for further doses of MTX, and the likelihood of surgical intervention increase with hCG concentration at presentation.

- Outpatient treatment with MTX.
- Offer as first-line treatment to women who are able to return for follow-up and who have all of the following: no significant pain, an unruptured ectopic pregnancy with an adnexal mass < 35 mm with no visible heartbeat, hCG level of < 1500 IU/L.
- Women with large adnexal masses are more likely to have already ruptured, and the presence of cardiac activity in an ectopic pregnancy is associated with a reduced chance of success; therefore, do not use MTX.
- Follow-up – hCG levels on days 4 and 7 and give a further dose if levels have failed to fall by >15%.
- About 14% require > one dose; 7% will experience tubal rupture; < 10% require surgical intervention.

- **Offer surgery as first-line treatment** to women who are unable to return for follow-up or have any of the following:
  * Significant pain.
  * Fetal heartbeat visible on TVS.
  * Adnexal mass of ≥ 35 mm.
  * hCG level of ≥ 5000 IU/L.
  * Treatment with MTX is not acceptable.

Laparoscopy • Patient – haemodynamically stable.
- Compared to laparotomy:
  * Shorter operation times.
  * Less intraoperative blood loss.
  * Shorter hospital stay.
  * Lower analgesic requirements.
- No difference in overall tubal patency rates, subsequent IUP rates, and a trend towards lower repeat ectopic pregnancy rates.
Laparotomy • Haemodynamic instability – expedient resuscitation and surgery.
- Experienced operators may be able to manage women safely laparoscopically, even with a large haemoperitoneum, but use the surgical procedure that prevents further blood loss most quickly. In most cases, this will be laparotomy.

Salpingectomy – offer to women with no risk factors for infertility.
- Urine pregnancy test after 3 weeks. To return for further assessment if the test is positive.
- Salpingotomy compared with salpingectomy – limited evidence. The IUP rates are similar but there is a trend towards higher subsequent ectopic pregnancy with salpingotomy.
- Cohort studies show that in women with contralateral tubal disease, a trend towards a greater subsequent IUP following laparoscopic salpingotomy compared with laparoscopic salpingectomy. There may be a higher subsequent IUP rate associated with salpingotomy but the magnitude of this benefit may be small.
Salpingotomy – offer to women in the presence of contralateral tubal disease and the desire for future fertility. Compared to subsequent need for assisted conception, an IUP rate of 3% would make salpingotomy more cost-effective than salpingectomy. However:
- Higher rates of persistent trophoblast.
- Small risk of tubal bleeding in the immediate postoperative period, need for further treatment for persistent trophoblast, and a risk of further ectopic pregnancies in the conserved tube.
- Up to 1/5 women may need further treatment: MTX and/or salpingectomy.
- Undertake one serum hCG measurement at 7 days after surgery, then one serum hCG measurement per week until a negative result is obtained.

Follow-up

- **Risk of recurrence** – 8–14%. 25% in women with ≥ 2 previous ectopic pregnancies.
- **Future fertility** – about 60% of women who have had an ectopic pregnancy are able to have a subsequent spontaneous IUP.
- Assess psychological wellbeing and offer counselling.
- **Future pregnancies** – patient should inform the GP as soon as she suspects she is pregnant, for an early USS at 6–7 weeks to establish the location and viability of the pregnancy.
- **Contraception** – history of ectopic pregnancy is not a contraindication to any form of hormonal contraception or IUD.
- Advise reliable contraception for 6 months post-treatment with MTX (teratogenic risk).

Persistent trophoblast

- Rate – 8.1–8.3% after laparoscopic salpingotomy and 3.9–4.1% after open salpingotomy.
- Increased risk in cases of high preoperative serum hCG levels (> 3000 IU/L), a rapid preoperative rise in serum hCG, and the presence of active tubal bleeding.
- Can present with delayed haemorrhage.
- Diagnosis – failure of serum hCG levels to fall as expected after initial treatment. MTX single dose, if levels fail to fall as expected.
- Prophylactic MTX at the time of laparoscopic salpingotomy – when compared with simple salpingotomy, there is a significant reduction in the rate of persistent trophoblast (1.9% vs 14%) has been reported.

Know your drug – methotrexate

- Mechanism – anti-metabolite and anti-folate; acts by inhibiting the metabolism of folic acid.
- Indications:
  * Ectopic pregnancy.
  * Gestational trophoblastic disease.
  * Cancers.
  * Autoimmune disease.
- Dose – a single IM injection (50 mg/m^2).
- Side effects – nearly 75% experience abdominal pain. Differentiating so-called 'separation pain' owing to a tubal abortion from pain because of tubal rupture can be difficult, and women may need to be admitted for observation and assessment.
- **Other side effects** – conjunctivitis, stomatitis, and gastrointestinal upset.
- **Advise** – to avoid sexual intercourse during treatment and to use reliable contraception for 3 months after MTX because of possible teratogenic risk.

What not to do

- Pelvic examination if a tubal rupture is suspected.
- Medical management in women with large adnexal masses and presence of cardiac activity in an ectopic pregnancy.
- Laparoscopy for haemodynamically unstable patient.
- Serum progesterone as an adjunct to diagnose either viable IUP or ectopic pregnancy.

Evidence round-up

Surgical management compared with medical management using systemic MTX:
- Meta-analysis:
  * No difference in success rate, in future pregnancy rates, and in recurrent ectopic pregnancy rates.
  * Resolution time is shorter, need for further intervention is lower, and hospital stay is longer with surgical management.

Laparoscopy vs laparotomy:
- Meta-analysis – no difference in the incidence of subsequent viable IUP, incidence of recurrent ectopic pregnancy, need for further surgery; however, the length of hospital stay is longer with laparotomy.
- Incidence of abdominal pain, intraoperative blood loss, and need for a blood transfusion is higher with laparotomy.

Salpingectomy vs salpingotomy:
- One study found that a subsequent live birth is significantly less likely with salpingectomy compared with salpingotomy. A further 7 studies did not find a statistically significant difference in a subsequent live birth between the two groups.
- For the recurrent ectopic pregnancy, there is a general trend that the incidence is lower with salpingectomy.
- **For women without any coexistent fertility factors, future reproductive potential is unlikely to be strongly affected by which mode of surgery is performed. However, for women with factors prognostic of infertility, the evidence suggest that salpingotomy is associated with a higher chance of a subsequent IUP.**

1. *Ectopic Pregnancy and Miscarriage: Diagnosis and Initial Management in Early Pregnancy of Ectopic Pregnancy and Miscarriage.* NICE Clinical Guidelines, 2012.
2. *The Management of Tubal Pregnancy.* RCOG Guideline No. 21, May 2004, reviewed 2010.
3. Sagili H, Mohamed K. Pregnancy of unknown location: an evidence-based approach to management. *The Obstetrician and Gynaecologist* 2008;10:224–230.

CHAPTER 6 Hyperemesis gravidarum (HG)

Background and prevalence

- Nausea and vomiting of pregnancy affects at least 50% of women in the first trimester of pregnancy. Symptoms usually begin between 5 and 6 weeks with peak severity around week 11, and in 90% of women these symptoms resolve by week 16.
- HG – persistent vomiting in pregnancy, which leads to weight loss of > 5% of pre-pregnancy weight with electrolyte imbalance and ketonuria. HG affects 1% of pregnant woman.
- Pathogenesis of HG is poorly understood and the aetiology is likely to be multifactorial.

Clinical features

- Severe and persistent nausea and vomiting leading to dehydration and weight loss.
- There may be ptyalism (inability to swallow saliva) and spitting.
- Signs of dehydration, tachycardia, and postural hypotension.

Differential diagnosis

- Urinary tract infection.
- Hepatitis.
- Appendicitis.
- Cholecystitis.
- Small bowel obstruction.
- Pancreatitis.
- Thyrotoxicosis, gestational thyrotoxicosis.
- Hyperparathyroidism.
- Diabetic ketoacidosis.
- Uraemia.
- Addison's disease.
- Iron supplementation.

Management

Dietary and lifestyle changes – no evidence to prove the effectiveness of dietary changes on relieving symptoms.

Non-pharmacological therapies

- Emotional support with frequent reassurance and encouragement.
- Psychotherapy, hypnotherapy, and behavioural therapy may be helpful.
- Ginger, alternative therapies, such as acupuncture and acupressure, may be beneficial.

Risks or complications

Maternal

- Weight loss and muscle wasting.
- Mallory–Weiss tears and haematemesis.
- Thiamine deficiency – Wernicke's encephalopathy – diplopia, abnormal ocular movements, ataxia, and confusion. IV glucose may precipitate it. Thiamine replacement may improve the symptoms but residual impairment is not uncommon.
- Korsakoff's psychosis – retrograde amnesia, impaired ability to learn, and confabulation. The recovery rate is only about 50%.
- Hyponatraemia – lethargy, seizures, respiratory arrest. Both severe hyponatraemia and its rapid reversal may precipitate central pontine myelinolysis – spastic quadraparesis, pseudobulbar palsy, and impaired consciousness.
- Other vitamin deficiencies – (cyanocobalamin and pyridoxine) can cause anaemia and peripheral neuropathy.
- Maternal death.

Fetal – lower birth weight; fetal death in severe Wernicke's encephalopathy.

Psychological impact

- Affects work and quality of life.
- Depression.
- Difficulties between partners.
- In some, the condition is so intolerable that they elect to have a termination of pregnancy.

Evidence round-up

- Systematic review – women with HG during pregnancy are more likely to have a baby with low birthweight and premature birth. There is no association with Apgar scores, congenital anomalies, or perinatal death.

Service provision – role of day-care units

- Advantages:
  * Women can be discharged within 24 hours of admission.
  * A study showed up to 88% patient satisfaction rate.
- Disadvantage:
  * Misuse of the services.

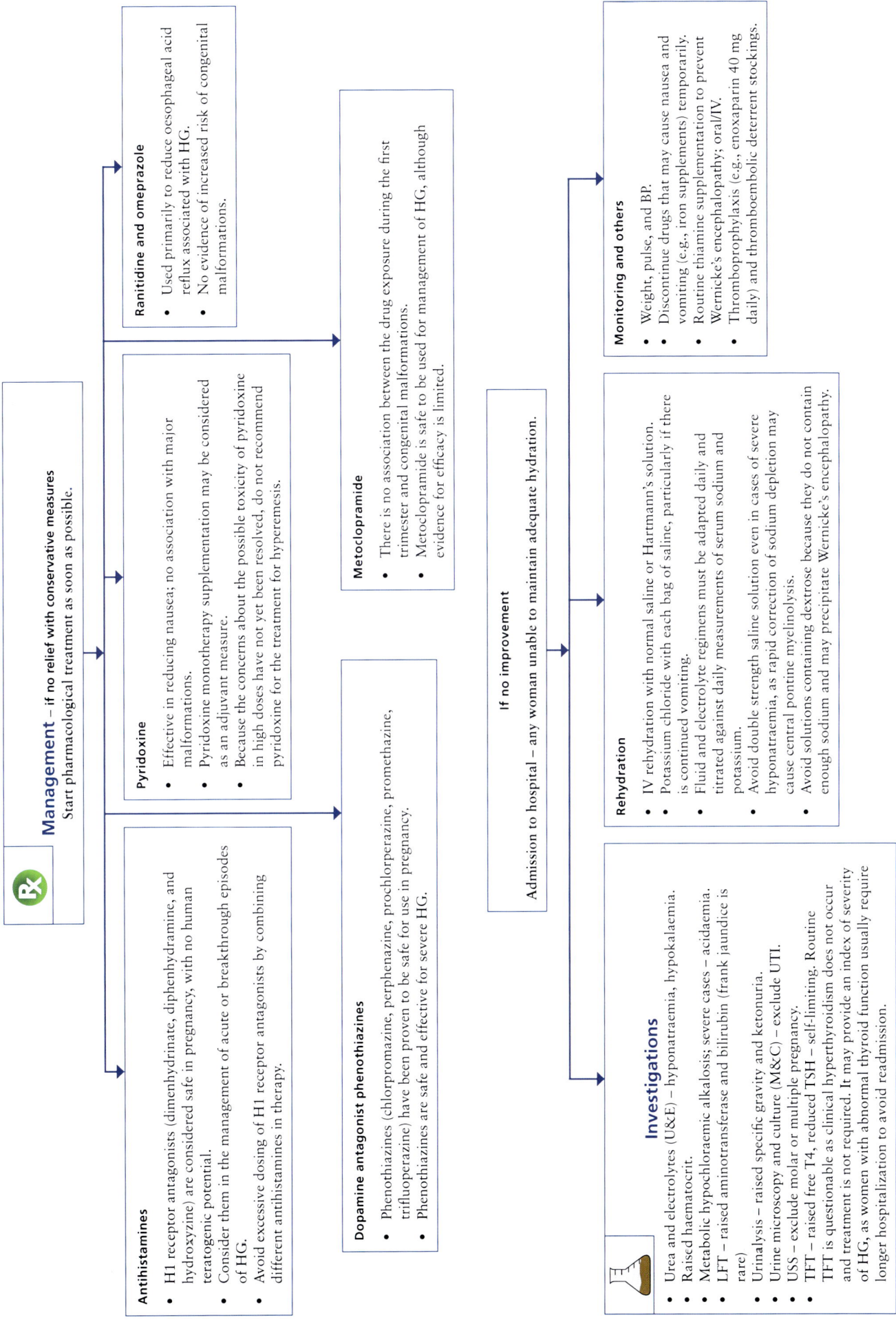

℞ Management – **if no relief with conservative measures**
Start pharmacological treatment as soon as possible.

Antihistamines
- H1 receptor antagonists (dimenhydrinate, diphenhydramine, and hydroxyzine) are considered safe in pregnancy, with no human teratogenic potential.
- Consider them in the management of acute or breakthrough episodes of HG.
- Avoid excessive dosing of H1 receptor antagonists by combining different antihistamines in therapy.

Ranitidine and omeprazole
- Used primarily to reduce oesophageal acid reflux associated with HG.
- No evidence of increased risk of congenital malformations.

Pyridoxine
- Effective in reducing nausea; no association with major malformations.
- Pyridoxine monotherapy supplementation may be considered as an adjuvant measure.
- Because the concerns about the possible toxicity of pyridoxine in high doses have not yet been resolved, do not recommend pyridoxine for the treatment for hyperemesis.

Dopamine antagonist phenothiazines
- Phenothiazines (chlorpromazine, perphenazine, prochlorperazine, promethazine, trifluoperazine) have been proven to be safe for use in pregnancy.
- Phenothiazines are safe and effective for severe HG.

Metoclopramide
- There is no association between the drug exposure during the first trimester and congenital malformations.
- Metoclopramide is safe to be used for management of HG, although evidence for efficacy is limited.

If no improvement
Admission to hospital – any woman unable to maintain adequate hydration.

Investigations
- Urea and electrolytes (U&E) – hyponatraemia, hypokalaemia.
- Raised haematocrit.
- Metabolic hypochloraemic alkalosis; severe cases – acidaemia.
- LFT – raised aminotransferase and bilirubin (frank jaundice is rare)
- Urinalysis – raised specific gravity and ketonuria.
- Urine microscopy and culture (M&C) – exclude UTI.
- USS – exclude molar or multiple pregnancy.
- TFT – raised free T4, reduced TSH – self-limiting. Routine TFT is questionable as clinical hyperthyroidism does not occur and treatment is not required. It may provide an index of severity of HG, as women with abnormal thyroid function usually require longer hospitalization to avoid readmission.

Rehydration
- IV rehydration with normal saline or Hartmann's solution.
- Potassium chloride with each bag of saline, particularly if there is continued vomiting.
- Fluid and electrolyte regimens must be adapted daily and titrated against daily measurements of serum sodium and potassium.
- Avoid double strength saline solution even in cases of severe hyponatraemia, as rapid correction of sodium depletion may cause central pontine myelinolysis.
- Avoid solutions containing dextrose because they do not contain enough sodium and may precipitate Wernicke's encephalopathy.

Monitoring and others
- Weight, pulse, and BP.
- Discontinue drugs that may cause nausea and vomiting (e.g., iron supplements) temporarily.
- Routine thiamine supplementation to prevent Wernicke's encephalopathy; oral/IV.
- Thromboprophylaxis (e.g., enoxaparin 40 mg daily) and thromboembolic deterrent stockings.

If no improvement

Refractory – severe hyperemesis gravidarum

If no improvement

Ondansetron

- The selective serotonin (5HT3) receptor antagonist ondansetron is effective in some women with HG.
- Limited evidence on effectiveness.
- It may be safe to use during the first trimester, but the data are scant.
- Because of its limited effectiveness, do not offer as first-line, until agents with established safety and effectiveness have been tried and have failed.

Corticosteroid therapy

- May produce a dramatic and rapid improvement; may need long-term therapy.
- Screening for the complications of steroid treatment in pregnancy, particularly UTI and GDM, is necessary.
- Recent case–control studies showed a small but significantly increased risk of oral clefting associated with first-trimester exposure.
- Data on effectiveness are weak. Although a few controlled studies showed some effectiveness, pooled results of those studies failed to show a reduction in the number of subsequent readmissions to hospital compared with controls.
- Until more data are available, use corticosteroids as the last line of therapy and only when maternal benefits outweigh fetal risk.
- Avoid corticosteroids during the first trimester because of possible increased risk of oral clefting, and restrict its use to refractory cases. (SOGC, ACOG)

Total parenteral nutrition

- Produces a rapid therapeutic effect.
- Recommended if optimal rehydration, antiemetic therapy, and a trial of corticosteroids and/or ondansetron have failed to result in improvement.
- Risks – metabolic and infectious complications – line sepsis, bacterial endocarditis, and pneumonia.
- Strict protocol with careful monitoring is essential.

What not to do

- Pyridoxine for the treatment for hyperemesis. (NICE)
- Double-strength saline solution.
- Solutions containing dextrose.
- Corticosteroids during the first trimester should be restricted to refractory cases because of possible increased risk of oral clefting. (SOGC, ACOG)

Evidence round up

Cochrane review, 2010 – acupressure, acustimulation, acupuncture, ginger, vitamin B6, and several antiemetic drugs:

- P6 acupressure, auricular acupressure, and acustimulation of the P6 point – limited evidence.
- Acupuncture – no significant benefit.
- Ginger products may be helpful, but the evidence of effectiveness is limited.
- Limited evidence to support the use of vitamin B6 and antiemetic drugs to relieve mild or moderate nausea and vomiting.
- Little information on maternal and fetal adverse outcomes on psychological, social, or economic outcomes.

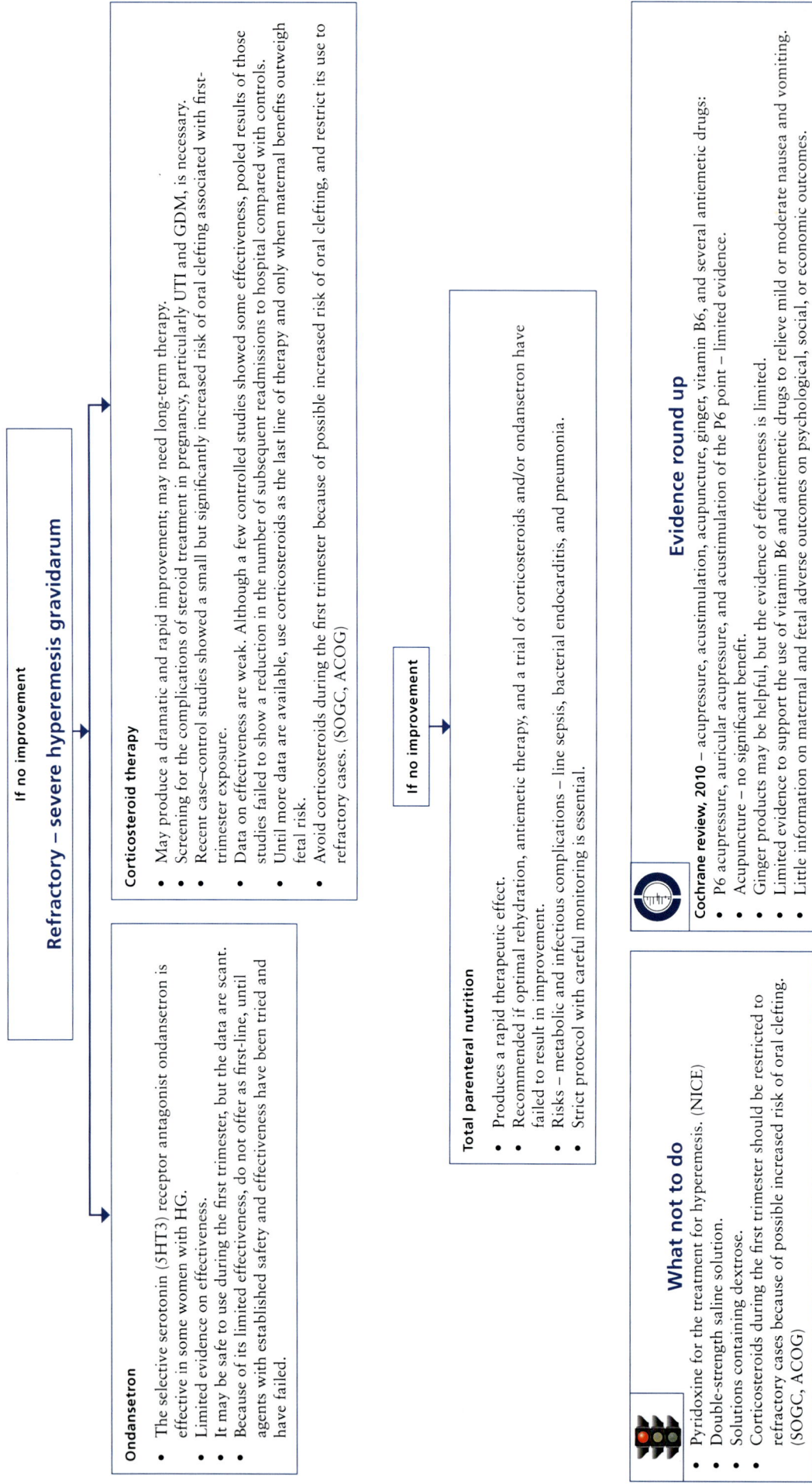

1. Gadsby R, Barnie-Adshead T. Severe nausea and vomiting of pregnancy: should it be treated with appropriate pharmacotherapy? *The Obstetrician and Gynaecologist* 2011;13:107–111.
2. Neill A-M, Nelson-Piercy C. Hyperemesis gravidarum. *The Obstetrician and Gynaecologist* 2003;5:204–207.
3. Alalade AO, Khan R, Dawlatly B. Day-case management of hyperemesis gravidarum: feasibility and clinical efficacy. *Journal of Obstetrics and Gynaecology* 2007;27(4):363–364.
4. Veenendaal MV, van Abeelen AF, Painter RC, van der Post JA, Roseboom TJ. Consequences of hyperemesis gravidarum for offspring: a systematic review and meta-analysis. *British Journal of Obstetrics and Gynaecology* 2011;118(11):1302–1313.
5. Matthews A, Dowswell T, Haas DM, Doyle M, O'Mathúna DP. Interventions for nausea and vomiting in early pregnancy. *Cochrane Database of Systematic Reviews* 2010;9:CD007575.

CHAPTER 7 Dysmenorrhoea

Prevalence and incidence

- The most common gynaecological symptom reported by women. It affects between 50% and 90% of menstruating women.
- It can lead to absence from school or work; 13–51% report having been absent and 5–14% report being frequently absent.

Risk factors

- Age – more pronounced in adolescents.
- Early menarche, heavy and increased duration of menstrual flow.
- Family history.
- Nulliparity.
- Smoking.
- More frequent life changes, fewer social supports, and stressful close relationships.
- Lower socioeconomic groups.
- Obesity, physical activity, and alcohol – controversial.

History

- To rule out secondary dysmenorrhoea and other causes of pelvic pain.
- Menstrual history – age at menarche, length and regularity of cycles, duration and amount of the bleeding, IMB, PCB.
- Length of time elapsed between menarche and beginning of dysmenorrhoea.
- Pain – type, location, radiation, associated symptoms, chronology of the onset of pain in relation to menstrual bleeding.
- Severity and duration of symptoms, the progression over time, and the degree of the patient's disability.
- Significant gastrointestinal symptoms or the presence of pelvic pain not related to the menstrual cycle.
- Rectal pain and bleeding.
- Sexual activity, dyspareunia, and contraception.
- Gynaecological history – STIs, pelvic infection, infertility.
- Pelvic/cervix surgery – cerclage, cryotherapy, or conization (cervical stenosis).
- Any family history of endometriosis.
- All types of therapy tried in the past.
- **Establish the impact of dysmenorrhoea on the woman's life.**

Examination

- To rule out the presence of any pelvic pathology.
- Abdominal examination – any mass, tenderness.
- Inspect – external genitalia to exclude an abnormality of the hymen.
- Pelvic examination – when history is suggestive of organic disease or when the patient does not respond to the conventional therapy.
- In the adolescent with a typical history of mild to moderate primary dysmenorrhoea, who has never been sexually active – pelvic examination is not necessary.

Investigations

- USS:
  * No evidence for the routine use of USS in the evaluation of primary dysmenorrhoea. May be helpful if there is any abnormality on examination, dysmenorrhoea refractory to first-line therapy, adolescents in whom a pelvic examination is not possible or unsatisfactory.
  * USS cannot detect subtle signs of organic diseases such as uterosacral ligament tenderness or nodules and cervical motion tenderness; therefore, will not replace a thorough bimanual examination.
- MRI – for adenomyosis, but this expensive test has limited clinical usefulness.
- Hysteroscopy and saline sonohysterography – for endometrial polyps and submucosal fibroids.
- Laparoscopy – a definite diagnosis of endometriosis, PID, or pelvic adhesions. Indicated when these pathologies are strongly suspected or when first-line therapy has failed.

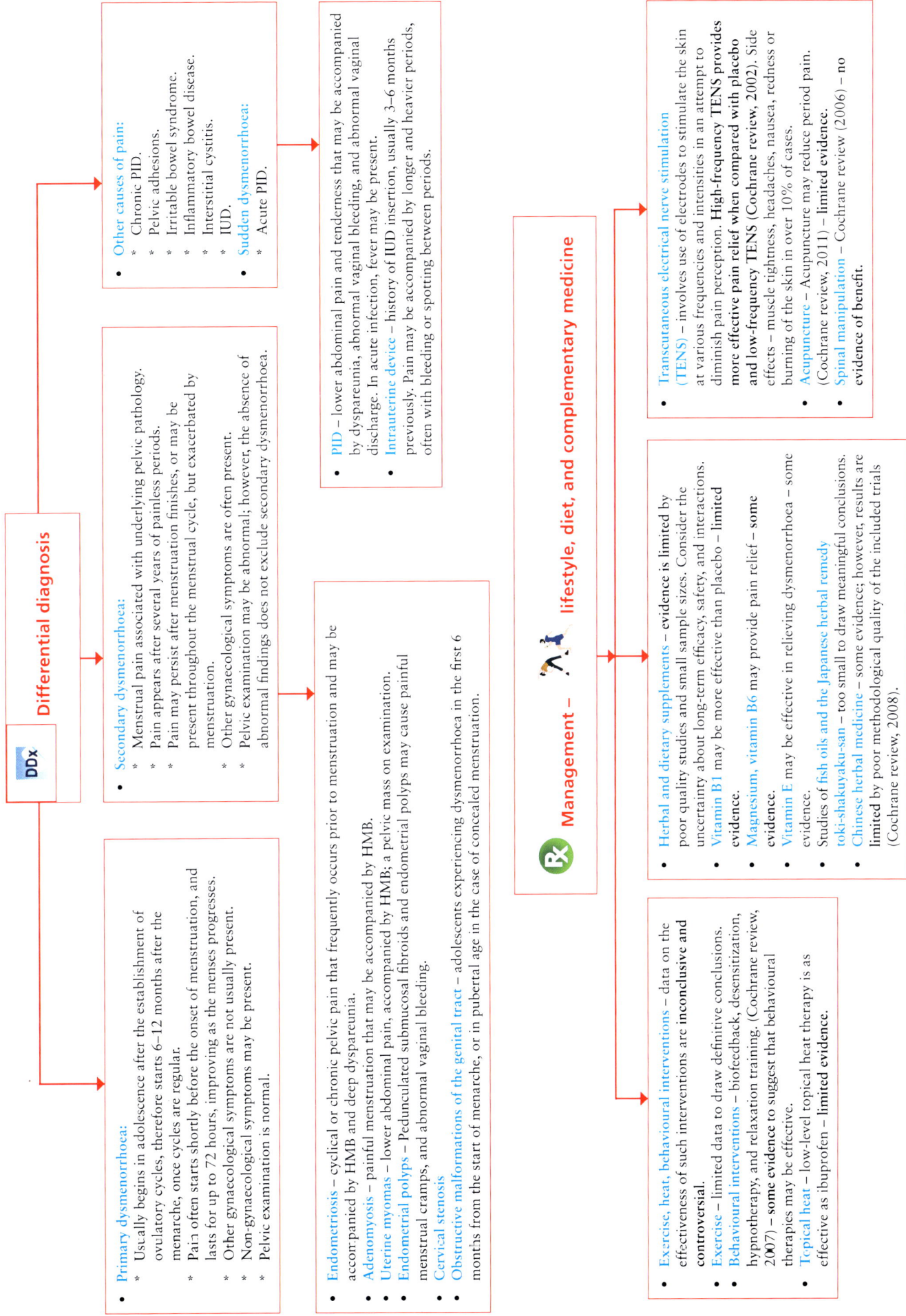

DDx Differential diagnosis

Primary dysmenorrhoea:
* Usually begins in adolescence after the establishment of ovulatory cycles, therefore starts 6–12 months after the menarche, once cycles are regular.
* Pain often starts shortly before the onset of menstruation, and lasts for up to 72 hours, improving as the menses progresses.
* Other gynaecological symptoms are not usually present.
* Non-gynaecological symptoms may be present.
* Pelvic examination is normal.

- Endometriosis – cyclical or chronic pelvic pain that frequently occurs prior to menstruation and may be accompanied by HMB and deep dyspareunia.
- Adenomyosis – painful menstruation that may be accompanied by HMB.
- Uterine myomas – lower abdominal pain, accompanied by HMB; a pelvic mass on examination.
- Endometrial polyps – Pedunculated submucosal fibroids and endometrial polyps may cause painful menstrual cramps, and abnormal vaginal bleeding.
- Cervical stenosis
- Obstructive malformations of the genital tract – adolescents experiencing dysmenorrhoea in the first 6 months from the start of menarche, or in pubertal age in the case of concealed menstruation.

Secondary dysmenorrhoea:
* Menstrual pain associated with underlying pelvic pathology.
  * Pain appears after several years of painless periods.
  * Pain may persist after menstruation finishes, or may be present throughout the menstrual cycle, but exacerbated by menstruation.
  * Other gynaecological symptoms are often present.
  * Pelvic examination may be abnormal; however, the absence of abnormal findings does not exclude secondary dysmenorrhoea.

- PID – lower abdominal pain and tenderness that may be accompanied by dyspareunia, abnormal vaginal bleeding, and abnormal vaginal discharge. In acute infection, fever may be present.
- Intrauterine device – history of IUD insertion, usually 3–6 months previously. Pain may be accompanied by longer and heavier periods, often with bleeding or spotting between periods.

Other causes of pain:
* Chronic PID.
* Pelvic adhesions.
* Irritable bowel syndrome.
* Inflammatory bowel disease.
* Interstitial cystitis.
* IUD.

Sudden dysmenorrhoea:
* Acute PID.

Rx Management – lifestyle, diet, and complementary medicine

- Exercise, heat, behavioural interventions – data on the effectiveness of such interventions are inconclusive and controversial.
- Exercise – limited data to draw definitive conclusions.
- Behavioural interventions – biofeedback, desensitization, hypnotherapy, and relaxation training. (Cochrane review, 2007) – some evidence to suggest that behavioural therapies may be effective.
- Topical heat – low-level topical heat therapy is as effective as ibuprofen – limited evidence.

- Herbal and dietary supplements – evidence is limited by poor quality studies and small sample sizes. Consider the uncertainty about long-term efficacy, safety, and interactions.
- Vitamin B1 may be more effective than placebo – limited evidence.
- Magnesium, vitamin B6 may provide pain relief – some evidence.
- Vitamin E may be effective in relieving dysmenorrhoea – some evidence.
- Studies of fish oils and the Japanese herbal remedy toki-shakuyaku-san – too small to draw meaningful conclusions.
- Chinese herbal medicine – some evidence; however, results are limited by poor methodological quality of the included trials (Cochrane review, 2008).

- Transcutaneous electrical nerve stimulation (TENS) – involves use of electrodes to stimulate the skin at various frequencies and intensities in an attempt to diminish pain perception. High-frequency TENS provides more effective pain relief when compared with placebo and low-frequency TENS (Cochrane review, 2002). Side effects – muscle tightness, headaches, nausea, redness or burning of the skin in over 10% of cases.
- Acupuncture – Acupuncture may reduce period pain. (Cochrane review, 2011) – limited evidence.
- Spinal manipulation – Cochrane review (2006) – no evidence of benefit.

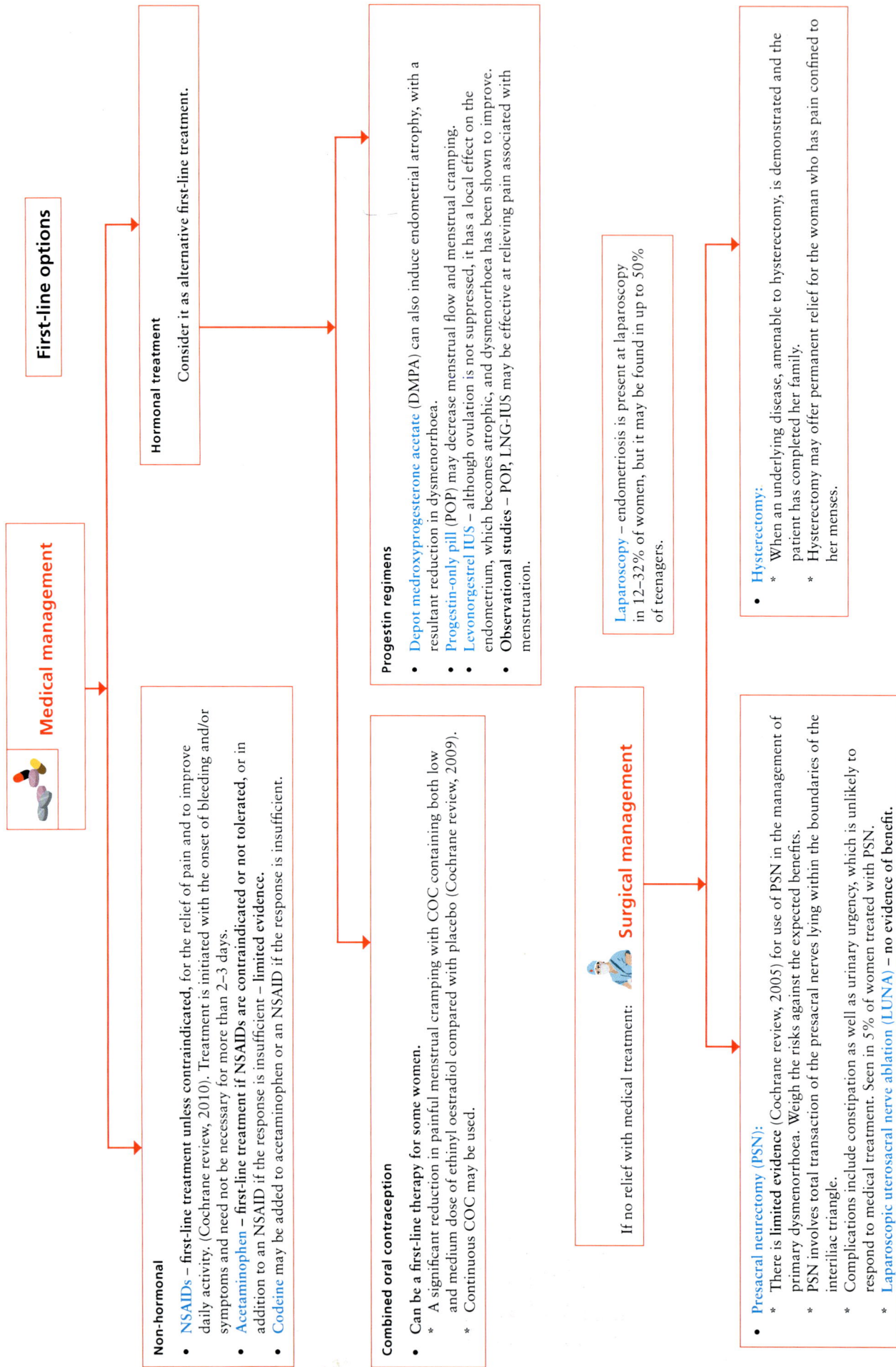

First-line options

Medical management

Non-hormonal

- NSAIDs – first-line treatment unless contraindicated, for the relief of pain and to improve daily activity. (Cochrane review, 2010). Treatment is initiated with the onset of bleeding and/or symptoms and need not be necessary for more than 2–3 days.
- Acetaminophen – first-line treatment if NSAIDs are contraindicated or not tolerated, or in addition to an NSAID if the response is insufficient – limited evidence.
- Codeine may be added to acetaminophen or an NSAID if the response is insufficient.

Combined oral contraception

- Can be a first-line therapy for some women.
  - A significant reduction in painful menstrual cramping with COC containing both low and medium dose of ethinyl oestradiol compared with placebo (Cochrane review, 2009).
  - Continuous COC may be used.

Hormonal treatment

Consider it as alternative first-line treatment.

Progestin regimens

- Depot medroxyprogesterone acetate (DMPA) can also induce endometrial atrophy, with a resultant reduction in dysmenorrhoea.
- Progestin-only pill (POP) may decrease menstrual flow and menstrual cramping.
- Levonorgestrel IUS – although ovulation is not suppressed, it has a local effect on the endometrium, which becomes atrophic, and dysmenorrhoea has been shown to improve.
- Observational studies – POP, LNG-IUS may be effective at relieving pain associated with menstruation.

Surgical management

If no relief with medical treatment:

- Presacral neurectomy (PSN):
  - There is limited evidence (Cochrane review, 2005) for use of PSN in the management of primary dysmenorrhoea. Weigh the risks against the expected benefits.
  - PSN involves total transaction of the presacral nerves lying within the boundaries of the interiliac triangle.
  - Complications include constipation as well as urinary urgency, which is unlikely to respond to medical treatment. Seen in 5% of women treated with PSN.
  - Laparoscopic uterosacral nerve ablation (LUNA) – no evidence of benefit.

- Laparoscopy – endometriosis is present at laparoscopy in 12–32% of women, but it may be found in up to 50% of teenagers.

- Hysterectomy:
  - When an underlying disease, amenable to hysterectomy, is demonstrated and the patient has completed her family.
  - Hysterectomy may offer permanent relief for the woman who has pain confined to her menses.

What not to do

- Spinal manipulation.
- Uterosacral ligament resection.

Know your drug – NSAIDS (mefenemic acid)

- **Mechanism** – inhibit the COX enzymes and production of prostaglandins.
- Indications:
  * Dysmenorrhoea (first-line drug).
  * HMB.
- **Typical dose** – 500 mg TDS.
- **Side effects** – indigestion, diarrhoea, headache, and drowsiness. Rare: worsening of asthma, peptic ulcers.
- Contraindications – asthma, peptic ulcers.

1. SOGC Clinical Practice Guideline No 169, December 2005.
2. Safe practical clinical answers – dysmenorrhoeas. Clinical Knowledge Summaries, nhs. uk, 2009.
3. Smith CA, Zhu X, He L. Acupuncture for primary dysmenorrhoea. *Cochrane Database Syst Rev* 2011;1:CD007854.
4. Marjoribanks J, Proctor M, Farquhar C, Derks RS. Nonsteroidal anti-inflammatory drugs for dysmenorrhoea. *Cochrane Database Syst Rev* 2010;1:CD001751.
5. Wong CL, Farquhar C, Roberts H, Proctor M. Oral contraceptive pill for primary dysmenorrhoea. *Cochrane Database Syst Rev* 2009;4:CD002120.
6. Zhu X, Proctor M, Bensoussan A, Wu E, Smith CA. Chinese herbal medicine for primary dysmenorrhoea. *Cochrane Database Syst Rev* 2008;2:CD005288.
7. Proctor ML, Murphy PA, Pattison HM, Suckling J, Farquhar CM. Behavioural interventions for primary and secondary dysmenorrhoea. *Cochrane Database Syst Rev* 2007;3:CD002248.
8. Proctor ML, Latthe PM, Farquhar CM, Khan KS, Johnson NP. Surgical interruption of pelvic nerve pathways for primary and secondary dysmenorrhoea. *Cochrane Database Syst Rev* 2005;4:CD001896.
9. Proctor ML, Hing W, Johnson TC, Murphy PA. Spinal manipulation for primary and secondary dysmenorrhoea. *Cochrane Database Syst Rev* 2006;3:CD002119.
10. Proctor ML, Smith CA, Farquhar CM, Stones RW. Transcutaneous electrical nerve stimulation and acupuncture for primary dysmenorrhoea. *Cochrane Database Syst Rev* 2002;1:CD002123

CHAPTER 8 Premenstrual syndrome

Background and definition

- A condition that manifests with distressing physical, behavioural, and psychological symptoms in the absence of organic or underlying psychiatric disease, which regularly recurs during the luteal phase of each menstrual cycle and disappears or significantly regresses by the end of menstruation.
- Mild – does not interfere with personal/social and professional life.
- Moderate – interferes with personal/social and professional life but still able to function and interact, although maybe suboptimally.
- Severe – unable to interact personally/socially/professionally; withdraws from social and professional activities.
- Precise aetiology is unknown but cyclical ovarian activity and the effect of oestradiol and progesterone on the neurotransmitters serotonin and γ aminobutyric acid (GABA) may be key factors.

History

- Psychological – mood swings, irritability, depression, and feeling out of control.
- Physical – breast tenderness, bloating, and headaches.
- Behavioural – reduced visuospatial and cognitive ability and an increase in accidents.
- Record symptoms prospectively, over two cycles, using a symptom diary.

Prevalence

- Prevalence of severe PMS – 3–30%.
- More prevalent in women who are:
  * obese.
  * perform less exercise and are of lower academic achievement.
- Less prevalent in women using hormonal contraception.

- Refer to a psychiatrist – women with marked underlying psychopathology as well as PMS.
- Refer to a gynaecologist – when simple measures fail and when the severity of the PMS justifies gynaecological intervention.
- Manage in an MDT – gynaecologist, psychiatrist, dietician, and counsellor.
- SSRIs prescription only by psychiatrists and doctors with a special interest.

Management

First-line options

Medical management

Selective serotonin reuptake inhibitors (SSRIs) – proven efficacy and safety (Cochrane review, 2009).
- Continuous or luteal phase (day 15–28) low-dose SSRIs.
- Abrupt withdrawal can result in withdrawal symptoms; withdraw gradually over a few weeks. Not necessary with low-dose luteal-phase SSRIs.
- Luteal-phase regimens with the newer agents such as citalopram and either luteal-phase or symptom-onset dosing with citalopram may produce resolution of symptoms where other SSRIs have failed.
- No data confirming the synergistic effects of SSRIs with ovulation suppression methods.

Combined new-generation pill – Yasmin, Cilest.
- Drospirenone plus ethenyl oestradiol 20 μg may help treat PMS (Cochrane review, 2009).
- Lower-dose Yasmin (Yaz – 20μg EE and 3 mg drospirenone) is effective; however, it is not yet available in the UK.
- Use the contraceptive pill continuously rather than cyclically.

Lifestyle measures

- Consider lifestyle adjustments such as improved self-care, low glycaemic index diet, stress reduction and exercise.
- Exercise – evidence from non-RCTs – some benefit.

Cognitive behavioural therapy (CBT)

- Consider routinely as a treatment option.
- Systematic review – low quality evidence from RCTs; CBT may have important beneficial effects in managing symptoms associated with PMS.

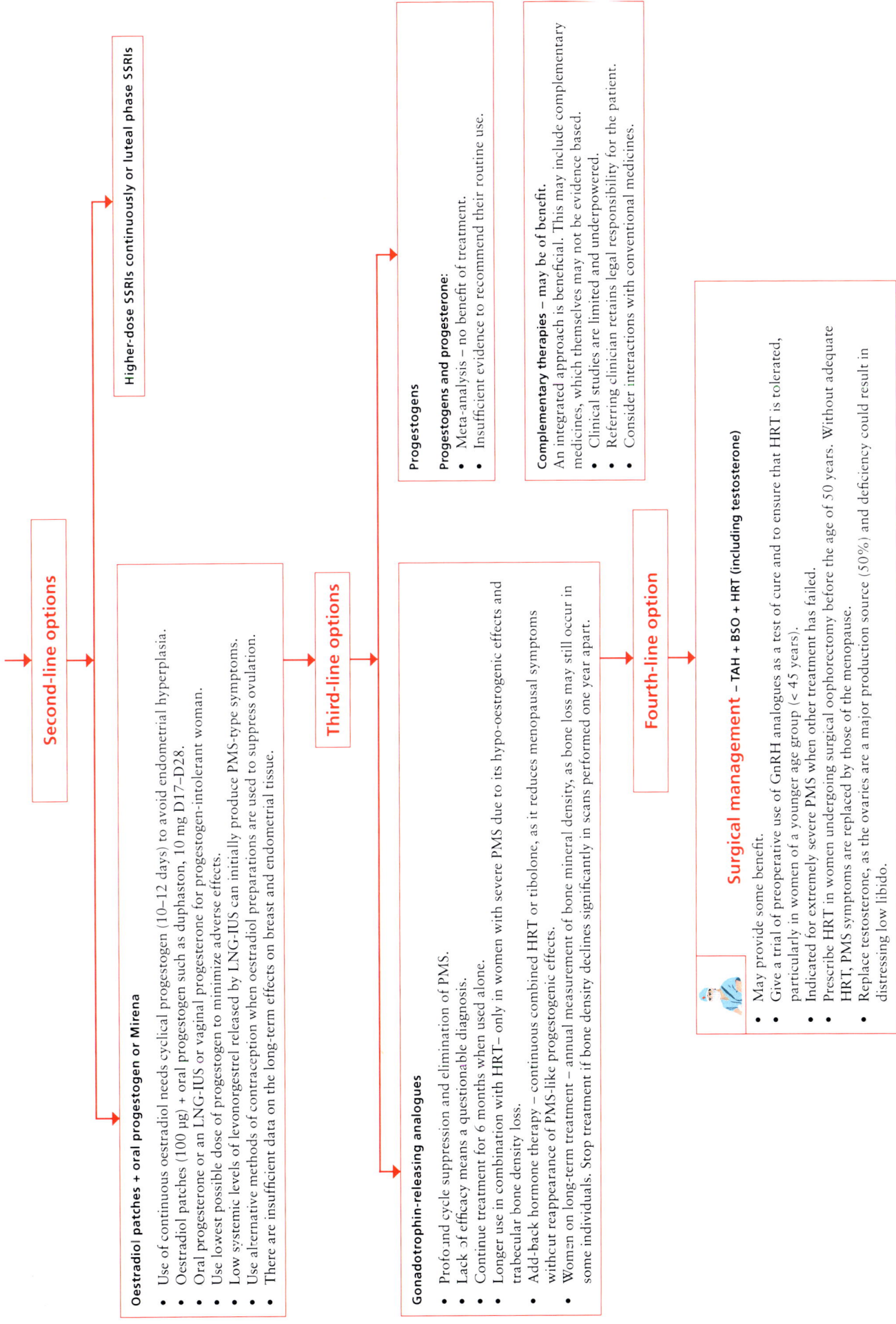

Higher-dose SSRIs continuously or luteal phase SSRIs

Second-line options

Oestradiol patches + oral progestogen or Mirena

- Use of continuous oestradiol needs cyclical progestogen (10–12 days) to avoid endometrial hyperplasia.
- Oestradiol patches (100 µg) + oral progestogen such as duphaston, 10 mg D17–D28.
- Oral progesterone or an LNG-IUS or vaginal progesterone for progestogen-intolerant woman.
- Use lowest possible dose of progestogen to minimize adverse effects.
- Low systemic levels of levonorgestrel released by LNG-IUS can initially produce PMS-type symptoms.
- Use alternative methods of contraception when oestradiol preparations are used to suppress ovulation.
- There are insufficient data on the long-term effects on breast and endometrial tissue.

Third-line options

Gonadotrophin-releasing analogues

- Profound cycle suppression and elimination of PMS.
- Lack of efficacy means a questionable diagnosis.
- Continue treatment for 6 months when used alone.
- Longer use in combination with HRT– only in women with severe PMS due to its hypo-oestrogenic effects and trabecular bone density loss.
- Add-back hormone therapy – continuous combined HRT or tibolone, as it reduces menopausal symptoms without reappearance of PMS-like progestogenic effects.
- Women on long-term treatment – annual measurement of bone mineral density, as bone loss may still occur in some individuals. Stop treatment if bone density declines significantly in scans performed one year apart.

Progestogens

Progestogens and progesterone:

- Meta-analysis – no benefit of treatment.
- Insufficient evidence to recommend their routine use.

Complementary therapies – may be of benefit.
An integrated approach is beneficial. This may include complementary medicines, which themselves may not be evidence based.

- Clinical studies are limited and underpowered.
- Referring clinician retains legal responsibility for the patient.
- Consider interactions with conventional medicines.

Fourth-line option

Surgical management – TAH + BSO + HRT (including testosterone)

- May provide some benefit.
- Give a trial of preoperative use of GnRH analogues as a test of cure and to ensure that HRT is tolerated, particularly in women of a younger age group (< 45 years).
- Indicated for extremely severe PMS when other treatment has failed.
- Prescribe HRT in women undergoing surgical oophorectomy before the age of 50 years. Without adequate HRT, PMS symptoms are replaced by those of the menopause.
- Replace testosterone, as the ovaries are a major production source (50%) and deficiency could result in distressing low libido.

Know your drug

What not to do

- Combine SSRIs with ovulation suppression methods.
- Progestogens and progesterone – routine use.
- Use of continuous oestradiol.
- GnRHa for more than 6 months.

SSRIs

- Mechanism – SSRIs increase the extracellular level of the neurotransmitter serotonin by inhibiting its reuptake into the presynaptic cell, increasing the level of serotonin in the synaptic cleft available to bind to the postsynaptic receptor; helps lift mood.
- Dose – smallest dose possible, generally TDS.
- Indications:
  * depression, anxiety disorder, obsessive compulsive disorder (OCD), panic disorder, serious phobias.
  * PMS.
- Side effects – nausea, insomnia, and reduction in libido and other sexual dysfunction. Withdrawal symptoms on abrupt withdrawal – GIT disturbances, headache, anxiety, dizziness, paraesthesia, sleep disturbances, fatigue, influenza-like symptoms, and sweating.

Yasmin – ethinyl oestradiol and drospirenone

- Mechanism – it has potent anti-mineralocorticoid properties, counteracts the oestrogen, and has mild anti-androgen activity.
- Indications:
  * Contraception.
  * PMS.
  * Hirsuitism.
  * Acne.
- Side effects – breast pain or tenderness, depressed mood, headaches, irregular bleeding, migraine, nausea, risk of thromboembolism, hyperkalaemia.

1. *Management of Premenstrual Syndrome*. RCOG Green-top Guideline No. 48, December 2007.
2. Lopez LM, Kaptein AA, Helmerhorst FM. Oral contraceptives containing drospirenone for premenstrual syndrome. *Cochrane Database Syst Rev* 2009;2:CD006586.
3. Brown J, O'Brien PM, Marjoribanks J, Wyatt K. Selective serotonin reuptake inhibitors for premenstrual syndrome. *Cochrane Database Syst Rev* 2009;2:CD001396.
4. Busse JW, Montori VM, Krasnik C, Patelis-Siotis I, Guyatt GH. Psychological intervention for premenstrual syndrome: a meta-analysis of randomized controlled trials. *Psychother Psychosom* 2009;78(1):615.
5. Clinical Knowledge Summaries. http://www.cks.nhs.uk/premenstrual_syndrome.

Background and definition

- Excessive menstrual blood loss that interferes with the woman's physical, emotional, social, and material QOL.
- An objectively measured blood loss of 60–80 ml or more per menstruation (average blood loss is 30–40 ml, and 90% of women have losses < 80 ml). Objective measurement is not practical in the clinical setting, and correlates poorly with a woman's subjective assessment of blood loss and its impact on QOL.

Prevalence and incidence

- About one third of women describe their periods as heavy.
- One in 20 women aged 30–49 years consult their GP each year for HMB.
- Menstrual disorders are the second most common gynaecological condition resulting in hospital referral and account for 12% of all gynaecological referrals.

Causes

- Unexplained (dysfunctional uterine bleeding) – 40–60%.
- Uterine and ovarian pathologies:
  * Uterine fibroids. * Adenomyosis. * PCOS.
  * Endometrial polyps. * Endometrial hyperplasia or carcinoma.
- Systemic diseases and disorders:
  * Coagulation disorders (e.g., von Willebrand disease).
  * Hypothyroidism. * Liver or renal disease.
- Iatrogenic causes: * Anticoagulant treatment. * Chemotherapy.
  * IUCD (blood loss may be increased by 40–50% over 6–12 months).

History

- Nature of the bleeding – age at menarche and details of menstrual cycle; length of cycle, the number of days of menstruation, length of heavy periods, previous periods.
- Symptoms that might suggest potential underlying causes – persistent IMB or PCB.
- Dyspareunia, dysmenorrhoea, pelvic pain and/or pressure symptoms, vaginal discharge.
- Impact on QOL and woman's ideas, concerns, expectations, and needs.
- Factors that may determine treatment options (such as presence of co-morbidity).
- Symptoms suggesting an underlying systemic disease, such as hypothyroidism or coagulation disorder (e.g., von Willebrand disease).
- Smear status, contraceptive history, fertility history, and future plans for a family.
- Family history of endometriosis and coagulation disorders.
- **Diagnose menorrhagia – when both the woman and clinician agree menstrual bleeding is heavy after a history.**

Examine and/or investigate if history suggests structural or histological abnormality.

Examination

- Required in women in whom:
  * Symptoms are suggestive of underlying abnormalities.
  * LNG-IUS is being considered.
  * Initial treatment has been ineffective.
- Vulva: examination – evidence of external bleeding and signs of infection.
- Speculum examination.
- Vaginal examination – uterine or adnexal enlargement or tenderness.
- Systemic signs of underlying disease – hirsutism, thyroid enlargement or nodularity, or changes in skin pigmentation, bruises, or petechiae (coagulation disorders).

Risks or complications

- Affects QOL by limiting normal activities, social life, and work.
- Woman's sex life may be negatively affected.
- Mood changes.
- Iron deficiency anaemia in about two thirds of women.

- If history suggests no structural or histological abnormality, the cause of menorrhagia is likely to be idiopathic with no obvious underlying pathology. In most cases, this will respond to symptomatic treatment.
- One can start medical treatment without carrying out an examination or other investigations at initial consultation in primary care, unless the treatment chosen is LNG-IUS.

Service provision

Refer to secondary care:

- HMB despite adequate trials of medical treatment.
- Women with fibroids that are palpable abdominally, or who have intra-cavity fibroids, and/or whose uterine length as measured at USS or hysteroscopy is > 12 cm.
- Urgently, if a suspicious mass is detected. Symptoms suggesting a possible malignancy – persistent IMB or PCB, vulval mass, or bleeding due to ulceration, features of cervical cancer.
- Woman who wishes to consider surgery.
- Woman who has iron deficiency anaemia that has failed to respond to treatment.

Advice and counselling

- Discuss the natural variability and range of menstrual blood loss.
- For some women, reassurance may be all that is required, and treatment may not be needed.
- If reassurance alone is not appropriate, discuss the different treatment option, effectiveness and acceptability of treatments, including adverse effects.
- Discuss the impact on fertility of any planned surgery or uterine artery embolization (UAE) may have, and if a potential treatment (hysterectomy or ablation) involves the loss of fertility.
- No specific lifestyle changes (e.g., diet or exercise) benefit menorrhagia.

Management

Rx

Medical management

- Where no structural or histological abnormality is present.
- For fibroids < 3 cm in diameter causing no distortion of the uterine cavity.

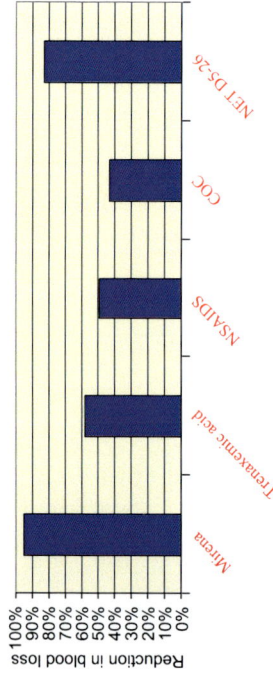

First-line medical option

- LNG-IUS if long-term (at least 12 months) use is anticipated. • Warn regarding changes in the bleeding pattern, particularly in the first few cycles and maybe lasting longer than 6 months, therefore advise to persevere for at least 6 cycles to see the benefits of the treatment.

Second-line medical options

- Trenaxemic acid (TXA) and NSAIDs – indicated:
  * If hormonal treatments are not acceptable to the woman.
  * If contraception is not desired.
  * Can be commenced as first-line drugs while investigations or definitive treatment is being organized.
- Ongoing use is recommended for as long as they are found to be beneficial.
- Use should be stopped if it does not improve symptoms within three menstrual cycles.
- When HMB coexists with dysmenorrhoea, NSAIDs should be preferred to TXA.
- COCs.

Third-line medical options

- Oral norethisterone (NET, 15 mg) daily from D5–26 of the menstrual cycle. Not an effective form of contraception. However, a dose that is effective in decreasing menstrual blood loss is also likely to inhibit ovulation, and so its use is not appropriate in women wishing to conceive.
- Depot medroxyprogesterone acetate (DMPA) is the recommended long-acting progestogen. Bleeding is likely to stop completely.
- Do not use oral progestogens given during the luteal phase only for the treatment of HMB.

Investigations

- Full blood count to rule out iron deficiency anaemia.
- Test for coagulation disorders in women who have had HMB since menarche and have personal or family history suggesting a coagulation disorder.
- Thyroid function test when other signs and symptoms of thyroid disease are present.
- Biopsy to exclude endometrial cancer or atypical hyperplasia if:
  * Women aged 45 years and over.   * Persistent IMB.   * Treatment failure or ineffective treatment.
- Opportunistic cervical screening if appropriate.
- Do not carry out a routine serum ferritin and female basal hormone tests.
- Imaging if: * Uterus is palpable abdominally.   * Vaginal examination reveals a pelvic mass of uncertain origin.   * Medical treatment fails.
- USS is the first-line diagnostic tool for identifying structural abnormalities.
- Perform hysteroscopy only when USS results are inconclusive; e.g., to determine the exact location of a fibroid or the exact nature of the abnormality.
- Do not use saline infusion sonography, MRI, or dilatation and curettage alone as a first-line diagnostic tool.

If initial treatment fails

- When a first medical treatment has proved ineffective, consider a second medical treatment. Typically, combine TXA with a NSAID or an NSAID with the COCs. There is no evidence on the effectiveness of combining treatments. Nevertheless, this is often done in practice and anecdotal evidence suggests that it can be beneficial.
- Refer for examination, investigations, and to consider surgical options.

Surgical management

Effectiveness of medical management of HMB

(Bar chart: Reduction in blood loss, y-axis 0%–100%. Categories: Mirena, Trenaxemic acid, NSAIDS, COC, NET D5–26)

Know your drugs

1. TXA

- Mechanism – anti-fibrinolytic.
- Indications – HMB.
- Typical dose – 500 mg TDS on bleeding days.
- Side effects – indigestion, diarrhoea, headaches.
- Contraindications – NSAIDs (mefenemic acid).
- See Chapter 7: Dysmenorrhoea.

2. COCs

- Mechanism – suppresses ovulation and endometrial proliferation, thereby decreasing menstrual fluid volume and prostaglandin secretion; regulates cycles.
- Indications:
  * HMB.
  * Dysmenorrhoea.
  * Contraceptive.
- Typical dose.
- Side effects – mood changes, headaches, nausea, fluid retention, breast tenderness, DVT, stroke, heart attacks.

3. GnRHa

- Mechanism – stops production of oestrogen and progesterone. In 89% of women, bleeding stops completely.
- Indications – could be considered prior to surgery or when all other treatment options for uterine fibroids, including surgery or UAE, are contraindicated.
- Typical dose – 3.6 mg implant every 4 weeks.
- Side effects – menopausal symptoms, vaginal dryness, osteoporosis, particularly trabecular bone, with longer than 6 months use.
- If this treatment is to be used for > 6 months or if adverse effects are experienced, then HRT 'add-back' therapy is recommended.

4. Progestogens

Oral norethisterone

- Mechanism – prevents proliferation of the endometrium.
- Indications – HMB.
- Typical dose for HMB – 15 mg daily from D5 to D26.
- Side effects – weight gain, bloating, breast tenderness, headaches, acne, depression.

LNG-IUS

- Mechanism – slowly releases progestogen locally and prevents proliferation of the endometrium.
- Indications:
  * HMB.
  * Contraceptive.
  * Endometriosis.
- Duration of effectiveness – 5 years.
- Side effects – irregular bleeding that may last for over 6 months; hormone-related problems such as breast tenderness, acne, or headaches (minor and transient), amenorrhoea, uterine perforation at the time of IUD insertion.

DMPA

- Mechanism – it is a long-acting progestogen. Works primarily by suppressing ovulation; prevents proliferation of the endometrium.
- Indications:
  * HMB.
  * Contraceptive.
- Typical dose – IM injection every 12 weeks.
- Side effects – weight gain, irregular bleeding, amenorrhoea, premenstrual-like syndrome, small loss of bone mineral density, largely recovered when treatment is discontinued.

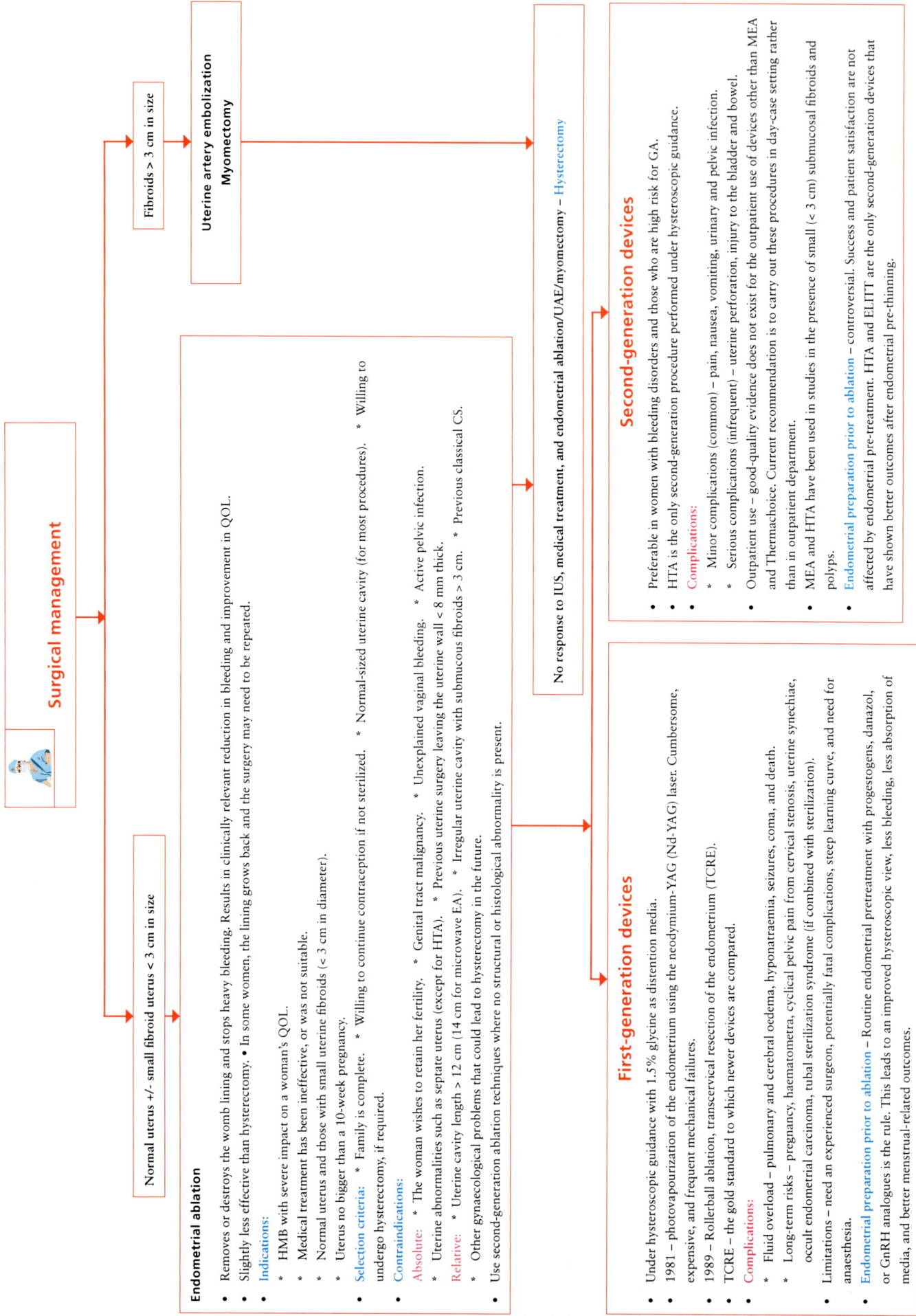

Surgical management

Normal uterus +/- small fibroid uterus < 3 cm in size

Endometrial ablation

- Removes or destroys the womb lining and stops heavy bleeding. Results in clinically relevant reduction in bleeding and improvement in QOL.
- Slightly less effective than hysterectomy. • In some women, the lining grows back and the surgery may need to be repeated.
- Indications:
  * HMB with severe impact on a woman's QOL.
  * Medical treatment has been ineffective, or was not suitable.
  * Normal uterus and those with small uterine fibroids (< 3 cm in diameter).
  * Uterus no bigger than a 10-week pregnancy.
- Selection criteria: * Family is complete. * Willing to continue contraception if not sterilized. * Normal-sized uterine cavity (for most procedures). * Willing to undergo hysterectomy, if required.
- Contraindications:
  Absolute: * The woman wishes to retain her fertility. * Genital tract malignancy. * Unexplained vaginal bleeding. * Active pelvic infection.
  Relative: * Uterine abnormalities such as septate uterus (except for HTA). * Previous uterine surgery leaving the uterine wall < 8 mm thick.
  * Uterine cavity length > 12 cm (14 cm for microwave EA). * Irregular uterine cavity with submucous fibroids > 3 cm. * Previous classical CS.
  * Other gynaecological problems that could lead to hysterectomy in the future.
- Use second-generation ablation techniques where no structural or histological abnormality is present.

Fibroids > 3 cm in size

Uterine artery embolization
Myomectomy

No response to IUS, medical treatment, and endometrial ablation/UAE/myomectomy – Hysterectomy

First-generation devices

- Under hysteroscopic guidance with 1.5% glycine as distention media.
- 1981 – photovapourization of the endometrium using the neodymium-YAG (Nd-YAG) laser. Cumbersome, expensive, and frequent mechanical failures.
- 1989 – Rollerball ablation, transcervical resection of the endometrium (TCRE).
- TCRE – the gold standard to which newer devices are compared.
- Complications:
  * Fluid overload – pulmonary and cerebral oedema, hyponatraemia, seizures, coma, and death.
  * Long-term risks – pregnancy, haematometra, cyclical pelvic pain from cervical stenosis, uterine synechiae, occult endometrial carcinoma, tubal sterilization syndrome (if combined with sterilization).
- Limitations – need an experienced surgeon, potentially fatal complications, steep learning curve, and need for anaesthesia.
- Endometrial preparation prior to ablation – Routine endometrial pretreatment with progestogens, danazol, or GnRH analogues is the rule. This leads to an improved hysteroscopic view, less bleeding, less absorption of media, and better menstrual-related outcomes.

Second-generation devices

- Preferable in women with bleeding disorders and those who are high risk for GA.
- HTA is the only second-generation procedure performed under hysteroscopic guidance.
- Complications:
  * Minor complications (common) – pain, nausea, vomiting, urinary and pelvic infection.
  * Serious complications (infrequent) – uterine perforation, injury to the bladder and bowel.
- Outpatient use – good-quality evidence does not exist for the outpatient use of devices other than MEA and Thermachoice. Current recommendation is to carry out these procedures in day-case setting rather than in outpatient department.
- MEA and HTA have been used in studies in the presence of small (< 3 cm) submucosal fibroids and polyps.
- Endometrial preparation prior to ablation – controversial. Success and patient satisfaction are not affected by endometrial pre-treatment. HTA and ELITT are the only second-generation devices that have shown better outcomes after endometrial pre-thinning.

	Mechanism of action	Limitations	Other information
Balloon thermal ablation	Hot fluid is circulated within the balloon positioned in the uterine cavity.	Not useful in large, irregular cavities or in the presence of polyps or fibroids.	• Cavaterm – balloon size can be adjusted to size of the uterine cavity. Depth of EA 6–8 mm. • Thermachoice – depth of EA – 4.5 mm. Associated with high level of nausea and uterine cramps, which limit its outpatient use. • Thermablate – EA to a depth of 4–5 mm. Good potential for outpatient use because of its narrow catheter and short application time.
NovaSure (impedance controlled bipolar radiofrequency EA)	Bipolar radiofrequency energy. Depth of EA is controlled by tissue impedance. The endometrium has low impedance, which is vaporized. On reaching the myometrium, the tissue impedance increases, resulting in automatic termination of ablation.	It cannot be reliably used if the uterine cavity is enlarged or irregular. Need to dilate the cervix to 8 mm. The blind nature of the procedure.	It can alert the operator to a perforated uterine wall prior to treatment using CO_2 gas. Complete EA in 90–120 seconds. Potentially ideal office-based procedure due to its short operating time, safety profile, and low pain scores.
Hydrothermal ablation (HTA)	Hot saline is instilled into the uterine cavity under direct hystero-scopic vision.	Significant pain, necessitates GA. Risk of vaginal, perineal, and thigh burns if fluid leaks from the cervix.	Can be used in women who have large or abnormally shaped uterine cavities, in presence of uterine septa, submucous fibroids, or polyps.
Microwave EA (MEA)	Microwave energy at a fixed frequency. Depth of EA is 5–6 mm and duration of treatment is 3 minutes.	Extremely bulky and cumbersome unit; large diameter of the probe, limiting its outpatient application.	Endometrial curettage prior to MEA is not recommended as it increases the risk of unrecognized uterine perforation and subsequent bowel damage.
Endometrial laser intrauterine thermal therapy (ELITT)	Laser beam undergoes diffusion, leading to uniform heating of the endometrium.	Cervix needs to be dilated to 7 mm and the procedure takes 7 minutes.	This device is not currently in widespread use and NICE has not yet produced guidance on its use.
Chemoablation	The most attractive form of EA. It involves instilling a chemical into the uterine cavity.	Remains investigational at present.	Trichloroacetic acid – amenorrhoea and patient satisfaction rates similar to second-generation EA.
Photodynamic therapy	A photosensitizing chemical is injected into the uterine cavity, followed by laser, which activates the chemical and results in EA.	Remains investigational at present.	
Cryotherapy	EA by freezing to –90°C. The depth of the ablation is up to 12 mm and the treatment can take 10–20 minutes.	Reports of pelvic abscesses. USS guidance needed; demands scanning skills and equipment.	It is thought that the low temperatures provide anaesthesia, leading to better outpatient tolerance of the device.

Evidence round-up

- **The MISTLETOE study:**
  * Complications associated with first-generation devices – total complication rate of 4.4%, including two directly related deaths.
  * Rollerball ablation was found to be safer than laser and TCRE.
- **Cochrane review** – equipment failure, nausea, vomiting, and uterine cramping are more common with the second-generation devices. The second-generation devices are less likely to be associated with fluid overload, uterine perforation, cervical laceration, and haematoma when compared with first-generation devices.

Surgical management continued – fibroids > 3 cm in size

Myomectomy

- Only potential fertility sparing surgical treatment option.

Know your procedure – myomectomy

Mechanism – fibroids are removed – reduce bleeding; fertility is potentially retained. Abdominal, vaginal, laparoscopic, and hysteroscopic – choice of route determined by the size, number, and position of the fibroids.

Indications – HMB, sub-fertility, pressure symptoms, dysmenorrhoea.

Pre-procedure – consider pre-treatment with a GnRHa for 3–4 months should be considered.

Side effects – adhesions (which may lead to pain and/or impaired fertility), need for additional surgery, recurrence of fibroids, perforation (hysteroscopic route), infection.

Its main disadvantage is that uterine fibroids can grow back, requiring further surgery.

Contraindications – medical co-morbidities.

Uterine artery embolization

- For women with large fibroids and HMB, and other significant symptoms such as dysmenorrhoea or pressure symptoms, one can recommend UAE as first-line treatment.

Know your procedure – UAE

Mechanism – blood supply to the fibroids is blocked and this causes them to shrink; it may reduce bleeding, fertility is potentially retained.

Pre-procedure – assess by USS or MRI (position, size, number, and vascularity of fibroids). If a woman is on GnRHa, stop it as soon as UAE is scheduled.

Side effects – persistent vaginal discharge, post-embolization syndrome (pain, nausea, vomiting, and fever), need for additional surgery, premature ovarian failure, particularly in women over 45 years old, puncture site haematoma.

Effectiveness – up to 85% improvement in HMB, mean fibroid volume decreases by 30–60%.

Contraindications: do not recommended for women who wish to retain their fertility because of inadequate safety data.

Evidence round-up – UAE

Systematic review, 2012:

- Symptomatic improvement – 78–90%, with a follow-up of up to 2 years.
- Major complications rate – 2.9%. There were no reported deaths.
- Rate of hysterectomy for resolution of a complication from UAE was 0.7%, and the rate of readmission was 2.7%.
- Other complications – leiomyoma tissue passage (4.7%), DVT or PE (0.2%), and permanent amenorrhoea (3.9%).
- Re-intervention rates (repeat UAE, myomectomy, hysterectomy) – 5.3%

Cochrane review, 2012:

- Satisfaction rate similar to hysterectomy and myomectomy.
- Advantage – shorter hospital stay and a quicker return to routine activities.
- Disadvantages – higher rate of minor short-term and long-term complications, more unscheduled readmissions, and an increased likelihood of requiring surgical intervention within 2–5 years.
- Very low level of evidence suggesting that myomectomy may be associated with better fertility outcomes than UAE, but more research is needed.
- No significant difference in ovarian failure rates at long-term follow-up.

No response to IUS, medical treatment, and endometrial ablation/UAE/myomectomy

Hysterectomy

- **Consider hysterectomy only when:**
  - Other treatment options have failed, are contraindicated, or are declined by the woman.
  - Large fibroids. * There is a wish for amenorrhoea.
  - Woman no longer wishes to retain her uterus and fertility.
- Discussion: sexual feelings, fertility impact, bladder function, need for further treatment, complications, the woman's expectations, alternative surgery, and psychological impact.
- Route – abdominal, vaginal, laparoscopic, robotic – consider complications and cost.
- Factors that may influence the route – uterine size, presence and size of uterine fibroids, mobility, accessibility, descent of uterus, extra uterine disease (adnexal pathology; endometriosis, adhesions/pathology obliterating pouch of Douglas), size and shape of vagina, need for concurrent surgery, surgical training and expertise, availability of technology/devices history of previous surgery.
- First-line vaginal, second-line abdominal. If morbid obesity or the need for BSO during vaginal hysterectomy, consider the laparoscopic approach.
- Discuss both the total and subtotal methods.
- The VALUE study – complications with hysterectomy – serious complication rate of 3%, mortality of 0.38/1000, long hospital stay and postoperative recovery.

Recommendations on oophorectomy (NICE):
- Refer women with a significant family history of breast or ovarian cancer for genetic counselling prior to a decision about oophorectomy.
- Take age into account, not only as a marker for cancer risk, but because of QOL issues such as long-term HRT use and loss of fertility.
- Women aged < 45 years considering hysterectomy for HMB with other symptoms that may be related to ovarian dysfunction (PMS) – give a trial of pharmaceutical ovarian suppression for at least 3 months to assess the need for oophorectomy.
- Disadvantages – menopausal symptoms and possible need for HRT.
  - Advantages:
  * Prevention of ovarian cancer and reduction in breast cancer.
  * Undertaking oophorectomy subsequently to hysterectomy can present technical problems.
  * Reduction in likelihood of residual ovary syndrome.
- Oophorectomy at the same time as hysterectomy is not recommended unless there is a family history of breast or ovarian cancer (refer for genetic counselling first) or the woman expressly requests it (after appropriate counselling).

Evidence round-up – route of hysterectomy

Cochrane review, 2009:
- The benefits of VH versus AH – speedier return to normal activities, fewer febrile episodes or unspecified infections, and shorter duration of hospital stay.
- The benefits of LH versus AH – speedier return to normal activities, lower intraoperative blood loss, smaller drop in haemoglobin, shorter hospital stay, and fewer wound or abdominal wall infections at the cost of more urinary tract (bladder or ureter) injuries (OR 2.4) and longer operation time.
- The benefits of LAVH versus TLH – fewer febrile episodes or unspecified infection and shorter operation time.
- No evidence of benefits of LH versus VH and the operation time as well as substantial bleeding are increased in LH.
- Because of equal or significantly better outcomes on all parameters, perform VH in preference to AH where possible. Where VH is not possible, LH may avoid the need for AH; however, the length of the surgery increases as the extent of the surgery performed laparoscopically increases.
- Experience with robotic assisted hysterectomy is limited. Very expensive.

Evidence round-up – BSO at the time of hysterectomy in postmenopausal women not at high risk for ovarian cancer

Systematic review, 2012:
- Arguments to support – prevention of ovarian cancer, ovarian benign disease, and chronic pelvic pain due to postoperative ovarian adhesions.
- Arguments against – effect on endocrine function, bone density, cardiovascular disease, and increased mortality.
  - < 65 years – the literature is clear and a BSO is recommended.
  - > 65 years – consider benefits and relative risks on an individual basis.

Evidence round-up – total (TH) versus subtotal hysterectomy (STH)

Cochrane review, 2012:
- No difference in the outcomes such as urinary, bowel, or sexual function either in the short or long term. No difference in other complications, recovery from surgery, alleviation of pre-surgery symptoms, or readmission rates between the two types of hysterectomy.
- Length of operation (difference of 11 minutes) and amount of blood lost during surgery (difference of 57 ml) are significantly reduced with STH. These differences are unlikely to constitute a clinical benefit.
- Postoperative fever and urinary retention are less likely and ongoing cyclical vaginal bleeding up to two years after surgery is more likely after STH.
- This review does not confirm the perception that STH offers improved outcomes for sexual, urinary, or bowel function when compared with TAH.

Consent – hysterectomy

Total/subtotal abdominal hysterectomy, preserve/remove normal ovaries.

Discuss

- Explain the procedure.
- Operation will leave her infertile.
- Potential impact of the operation on sexual function, bladder function, and psychology.
- Intended incision (midline or transverse).
- If the plan is for a total hysterectomy, occasionally it may be necessary to limit the operation to a subtotal hysterectomy for technical reasons.
- Potential for unexpected disease of the ovaries.
- If the ovaries are to be removed in a premenopausal woman, this would mean immediate surgical menopause, and discuss the long-term health implications.
- Intended benefits – while menstrual bleeding is guaranteed to be abolished, the effect on pelvic pain and premenstrual symptoms is not guaranteed.
- Alternative treatment options – discuss other treatments, such as vaginal hysterectomy, the LNG-IUS, endometrial ablation, and pharmacological therapies, together with the option of no treatment.
- Discuss total method and subtotal method.
- Removal of the ovaries – inform of the effect of this on the risk of ovarian and breast cancer.
- Form of anaesthesia.

Risks

Very common	1/1 to 1/10.
Common	1/10 to 1/100.
Uncommon	1/100 to 1/1000.
Rare	1/1000 to 1/10,000.
Very rare	Less than 1/10,000.

- Serious risks: 4/100.
  * Haemorrhage requiring blood transfusion – 23/1000.
  * Damage to the bladder and/or the ureter – 7/1000.
  * Return to theatre (bleeding/wound dehiscence) – 7/1000.
  * Venous thrombosis or pulmonary embolism – 4/1000.
  * Pelvic abscess/infection – 2/1000.
  * Damage to the bowel – 4/10,000.
  * Risk of death within 6 weeks – 32/10,0000. (Main causes of death are PE and cardiac disease.)
  * Long-term disturbance to bladder function (uncommon).

- Frequent risks:
  * Wound infection, pain, bruising, delayed wound healing, or keloid formation.
  * Numbness, tingling or burning sensation around the scar (self-limiting but could take weeks or months to resolve).
  * Frequency of micturition, UTI, ovarian failure.
  * Surgical and anaesthetic risks are increased with obesity.

Extra procedures

- Any extra procedures that may become necessary:
  * Blood transfusion.
  * Repair to bladder, bowel, or major blood vessel.
- Do not perform oophorectomy for unsuspected disease found at hysterectomy without consent. Inform all women undergoing hysterectomy that unexpected disease may be found in one or both ovaries and document their wishes (to remove this or leave alone).

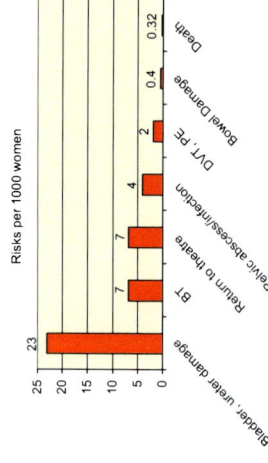

Risks per 1000 women

Bladder, ureter damage	23
Return to theatre	7
Pelvic abscess/infection	7
BT	7
DVT, PE	4
Bowel Damage	2
Death	0.4
	0.32

Evidence round-up – management strategies of HMB

The HTA systematic review (2011):

- Although hospital stay and time to resumption of normal activities are longer, more women are satisfied after hysterectomy than after first-generation EA.
- Indirect estimates suggest that hysterectomy is also preferable to second-generation EA in terms of patient satisfaction.
- Dissatisfaction rates are comparable between first- and second-generation EA techniques, although second-generation techniques are cheaper, quicker, and associated with faster recovery and fewer complications.
- The few data available suggest that Mirena is potentially cheaper and more effective than first-generation EA techniques, with rates of satisfaction that are similar to those of second-generation EA techniques.
- Owing to a paucity of trials, there is limited evidence to suggest that hysterectomy is preferable to Mirena.
- Hysterectomy is considered the most cost-effective strategy, but owing to its invasive nature and higher risk of complications, is considered a final option by gynaecological experts and consumers.

What not to do

- Measuring menstrual blood loss either directly (alkaline haematin) or indirectly ('pictorial blood loss assessment chart').
- Routine serum ferritin test and female hormones.
- Saline infusion sonography, dilatation and curettage alone, or MRI as a first-line diagnostic tool.
- No specific lifestyle changes (e.g., diet or exercise) benefit menorrhagia.
- Use of Danazol or Etamsylate for the treatment of HMB.
- Oral progestogens given during the luteal phase only for the treatment of HMB.
- Hysterectomy as a first-line treatment solely for HMB.
- Dilatation and curettage as a therapeutic treatment.
- Removal of healthy ovaries at the time of hysterectomy.

1. *Heavy Menstrual Bleeding*. NICE Clinical Guidelines 44, January 2007.
2. Clinical Knowledge Summaries – Menorrhagia. http://www.cks.nhs.uk/menorrhagia.
3. Justin W, Ibraheim M, Bagtharia S, Haloob R. Current minimal access techniques in the treatment of heavy menstrual bleeding. *The Obstetrician and Gynaecologist* 2007;9:223–232.
4. Bhattacharya S, Middleton LJ, Tsourapas A, et al. Hysterectomy, endometrial ablation and Mirena for heavy menstrual bleeding: a systematic review of clinical effectiveness and cost effectiveness analysis. *Health Technol Assess* 2011;15(19);DOI: 10.3310/hta15190.
5. Johnson N, Barlow D, Lethaby A, et al. Methods of hysterectomy: systematic review and meta-analysis of randomised controlled trials. *BMJ* 2005;330(7506):1478.
6. Ouldamer L, Marret H, Jacquet A, Denakpo J, Body G. Profits of post-menopausal ovarian conservation at the time of hysterectomy for benign disease: mirage or reality? *J Gynecol Obstet Biol Reprod (Paris)* 2012;S0368-2315(12)00337-7;DOI:10.1016/j.jgyn.2012.10.014.
7. Toor SS, Jaberi A, Macdonald DB, et al. Complication rates and effectiveness of uterine artery embolization in the treatment of symptomatic leiomyomas: a systematic review and meta-analysis.; *AJR Am J Roentgenol* 2012;199(5):1153–1163.
8. Lethaby A, Mukhopadhyay A, Naik R. Total versus subtotal hysterectomy for benign gynaecological conditions. *Cochrane Database Syst Rev* 2012;4:CD004993.
9. Gupta JK, Sinha A, Lumsden MA, Hickey M. Uterine artery embolization for symptomatic uterine fibroids. *Cochrane Database Syst Rev* 2012;5:CD005073
10. Nieboer TE, Johnson N, Lethaby A, et al. Surgical approach to hysterectomy for benign gynaecological disease. *Cochrane Database Syst Rev* 2009;3:CD003677.
11. *Choosing the Route of Hysterectomy for Benign Disease*. ACOG Committee Opinion Paper, 2009.
12. *Abdominal Hysterectomy for Benign Conditions*. RCOG Consent Advice No. 4, May 2009.

CHAPTER 10 Fibroids (leiomyoma)

Background and definition

- Benign tumours arising from the myometrium of the uterus.
- Subserosal (SS) fibroids develop near the outer serosal surface of the uterus and extend into the peritoneal cavity. Asymptomatic; may cause pressure symptoms.
- Intramural (IM) fibroids develop within the myometrium. May cause HMB, dysmenorrhoea.
- Submucosal (SM) fibroids develop near the endometrial surface of the uterus and extend into the uterine cavity. May cause HMB, pain, and subfertility.
- Pedunculated – attached to the myometrium by a pedicle. May cause torsion.

Prevalence and incidence

- Prevalence increases progressively from puberty until the menopause – 40–60% of women have fibroids by 35 years of age, which is increased to 70–80% by 49 years of age.
- Usually shrink after menopause as they are promoted and maintained by oestrogen and progestogen.
- Prevalence is higher in:
  * Black women – tend to occur at an earlier age, are larger, and more likely to be symptomatic.
  * Women with early onset of puberty.
  * Obese women – probably due to higher oestrogen levels.
- Risk is reduced by pregnancy and decreases with increasing number of pregnancies.

History

- Symptoms depend on the size, number, and location of the fibroids.
- Most common – heavy and prolonged bleeding.
- Abdominal swelling, pelvic or abdominal pain or discomfort.
- Dyspareunia.
- Pressure symptoms – constipation or urinary symptoms such as frequency or difficulty in voiding.
- Acute, severe abdominal or pelvic pain following torsion of a pedunculated fibroid or 'red degeneration'.
- Subfertility, miscarriage.

Examination

- Abdominal examination – mass arising from the pelvis, smooth/multi-nodular, firm, mobile from side-to-side.
- Pelvic examination – mass arising out of the pelvis, with an irregular knobbly shape, a firm or hard consistency, and can be moved slightly from side-to-side. Any movement of the abdominal mass moves the cervix.

Risks or issues

- Gynaecological:
  * HBM – anaemia, affects QOL.
  * Compression of ureters by large fibroids – hydronephrosis.
  * Torsion of pedunculated fibroid – acute pain.
  * Leiomyosarcoma – minimal risk.
- Fertility issues.
- Pregnancy complications:
  * First- and second-trimester miscarriage.
  * Higher rates of Caesarean delivery.
  * Preterm delivery.
  * Malpresentation, mechanical complications in labour.
  * PPH.
  * Acute pain requiring hospital admission (5–6%) – red degeneration of fibroid owing to avascular necrosis (when rapid growth of a fibroid, promoted by high levels of sex hormones, outgrows its blood supply).

Differential diagnosis

- Adenomyosis may be difficult to distinguish from multiple small fibroids and may coexist with them.
- Pregnancy.
- Benign causes of a pelvic mass: benign ovarian mass – hemorrhagic cyst, dermoid cyst, or endometrioma.
- Malignant causes of a pelvic mass: ovarian cancer, endometrial cancer, leiomyosarcoma.

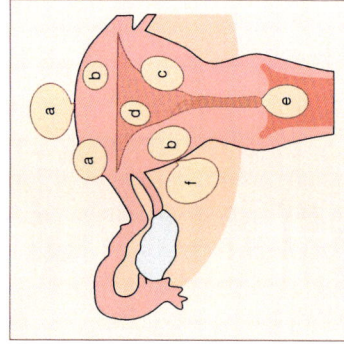

a=subserosal fibroids, b=intramural fibroids, c=submucosal fibroid, d=pedunculated, submucosal fibroid, e=fibroid in cervix, f=fibroid of the broad ligament.

Investigations

- USS, depending on the uterine size, a transabdominal or TVS (or both) to assess the location, number, and size of the fibroids.
- Saline or contrast sonography – use of saline as a contrast medium improves the accuracy of assessment of SM fibroids.
- 3D USS can locate fibroids accurately.
- MRI – provides information on exact location and size of fibroids for the interventional radiologist and is superior to conventional ultrasound.

Asymptomatic fibroids

- Refer for secondary care if:
  * Fibroids are palpable abdominally.   * Intra-cavity fibroids.
  * Uterine length on USS >12 cm.
- No need to monitor the size of asymptomatic fibroids.
- Do not advise hysterectomy for asymptomatic fibroids solely to improve detection of adnexal masses, to prevent impairment of renal function, or to rule out malignancy.

Management

Symptomatic fibroids

Surgical management

Medical management

Tends to give only short-term relief.

NSAIDS

- Effective in reducing dysmenorrhoea, but there are no studies that document improvement in women with dysmenorrhoea caused by fibroids.

Anti-progesterone agents

- Mifepristone acts at the level of the progesterone receptors, found in high concentration in fibroids.
- Reduction in fibroid volume of 26–74% (comparable to GnRHa, slower rate of recurrent growth after cessation of mifepristone treatment), amenorrhoea rates up to 90%, and stable bone mineral density.
- Side effects – endometrial hyperplasia without atypia (14–28%) and transient elevations in transaminase levels (4%) requiring LFT monitoring.
- May have a short-term role in the preoperative management of leiomyomas, but further research is necessary.

Contraceptive steroids

- Data is limited.
- COCs may control bleeding without stimulating further growth.
- Studies of progestin therapy – mixed results.
- While on COCs, monitor the fibroids and uterine size.

Aromatase inhibitors

- Aromatase inhibitors block ovarian and peripheral oestrogen production and decrease oestradiol levels.
- Fewer side effects than GnRHa, with the benefit of a rapid effect.
- Small studies showed reduction in leiomyoma size and symptoms.
- Further research is necessary.

GnRHa

- A 35–65% reduction in fibroid volume within 3 months.
- Preoperative in women with anaemia and to reduce the size of fibroids and blood loss during surgery.
- Systematic review – no significant difference in blood loss with preoperative GnRHa has been demonstrated.
- Add-back therapy. (See Chapter 12: Endometriosis.)
- A sequential regimen, in which a GnRHa is first used to achieve downregulation to which steroids are added after 1–3 months of therapy, gives maximal results. However, the addition of progestin add-back therapy results in an increase in mean uterine volume to 95% of baseline within 24 months.

LNG-IUS

- Small studies suggest that it may be effective for treatment of HMB.
- However, these women may have a higher rate of expulsion and vaginal spotting.

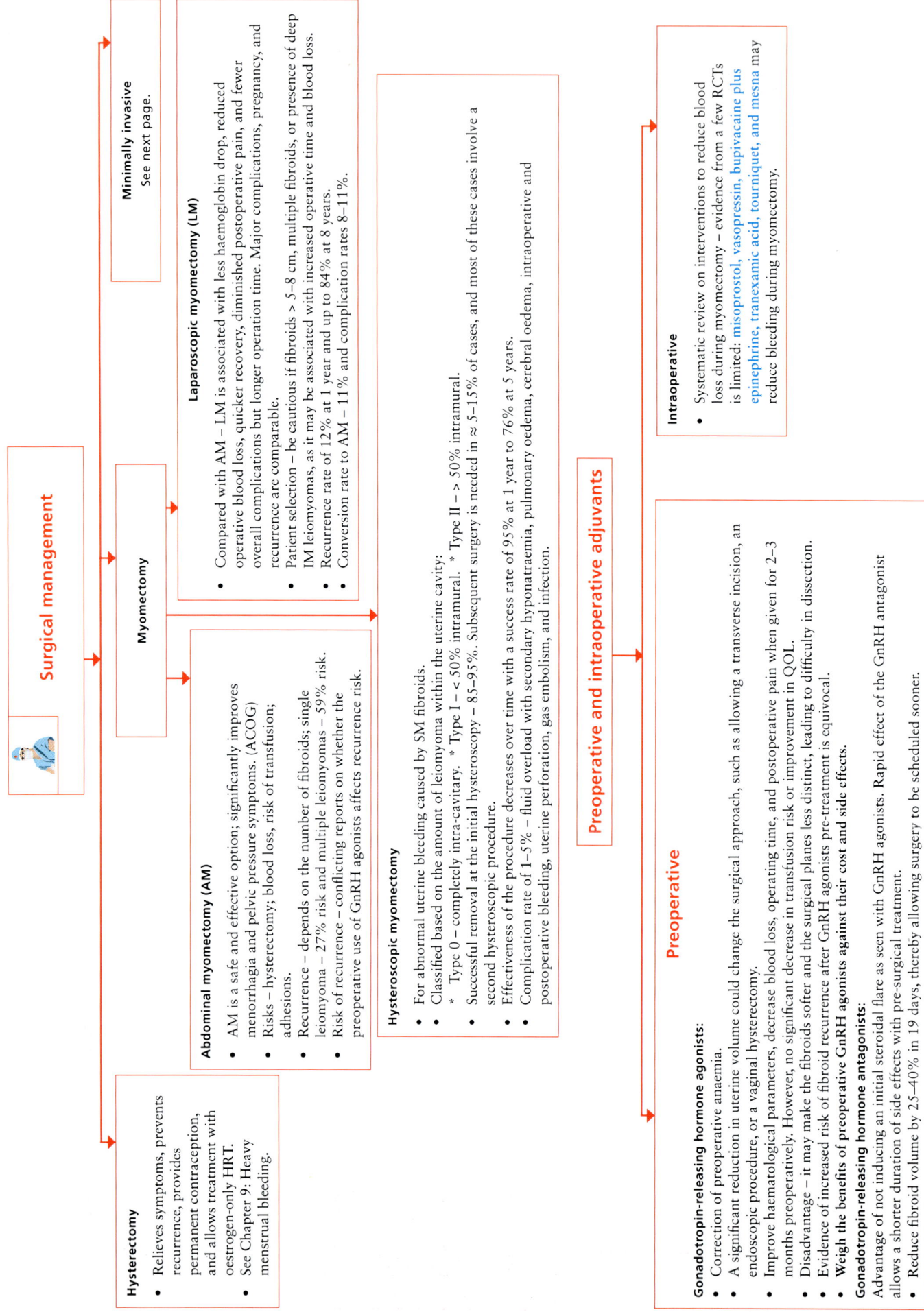

Surgical management

→ **Minimally invasive**
See next page.

→ **Hysterectomy**

- Relieves symptoms, prevents recurrence, provides permanent contraception, and allows treatment with oestrogen-only HRT. See Chapter 9: Heavy menstrual bleeding.

→ **Myomectomy**

Laparoscopic myomectomy (LM)

- Compared with AM – LM is associated with less haemoglobin drop, reduced operative blood loss, quicker recovery, diminished postoperative pain, and fewer overall complications but longer operation time. Major complications, pregnancy, and recurrence are comparable.
- Patient selection – be cautious if fibroids > 5–8 cm, multiple fibroids, or presence of deep IM leiomyomas, as it may be associated with increased operative time and blood loss.
- Recurrence rate of 12% at 1 year and up to 84% at 8 years.
- Conversion rate to AM – 11% and complication rates 8–11%.

Abdominal myomectomy (AM)

- AM is a safe and effective option; significantly improves menorrhagia and pelvic pressure symptoms. (ACOG)
- Risks – hysterectomy; blood loss, risk of transfusion; adhesions.
- Recurrence – depends on the number of fibroids; single leiomyoma – 27% risk and multiple leiomyomas – 59% risk.
- Risk of recurrence – conflicting reports on whether the preoperative use of GnRH agonists affects recurrence risk.

Hysteroscopic myomectomy

- For abnormal uterine bleeding caused by SM fibroids.
- Classified based on the amount of leiomyoma within the uterine cavity:
  * Type 0 – completely intra-cavitary. * Type I – < 50% intramural. * Type II – > 50% intramural.
- Successful removal at the initial hysteroscopy – 85–95%. Subsequent surgery is needed in ≈ 5–15% of cases, and most of these cases involve a second hysteroscopic procedure.
- Effectiveness of the procedure decreases over time with a success rate of 95% at 1 year to 76% at 5 years.
- Complication rate of 1–5% – fluid overload with secondary hyponatraemia, pulmonary oedema, cerebral oedema, intraoperative and postoperative bleeding, uterine perforation, gas embolism, and infection.

Preoperative and intraoperative adjuvants

Intraoperative

- Systematic review on interventions to reduce blood loss during myomectomy – evidence from a few RCTs is limited: misoprostol, vasopressin, bupivacaine plus epinephrine, tranexamic acid, tourniquet, and mesna may reduce bleeding during myomectomy.

Preoperative

Gonadotropin-releasing hormone agonists:
- Correction of preoperative anaemia.
- A significant reduction in uterine volume could change the surgical approach, such as allowing a transverse incision, an endoscopic procedure, or a vaginal hysterectomy.
- Improve haematological parameters, decrease blood loss, operating time, and postoperative pain when given for 2–3 months preoperatively. However, no significant decrease in transfusion risk or improvement in QOL.
- Disadvantage – it may make the fibroids softer and the surgical planes less distinct, leading to difficulty in dissection.
- Evidence of increased risk of fibroid recurrence after GnRH agonists pre-treatment is equivocal.
- **Weigh the benefits of preoperative GnRH agonists against their cost and side effects.**

Gonadotropin-releasing hormone antagonists:
Advantage of not inducing an initial steroidal flare as seen with GnRH agonists. Rapid effect of the GnRH antagonist allows a shorter duration of side effects with pre-surgical treatment.
- Reduce fibroid volume by 25–40% in 19 days, thereby allowing surgery to be scheduled sooner.

Minimally invasive procedures/myolysis

A number of energy sources and techniques have been used to induce necrosis in fibroids, including diathermy, laser ablation, and radiofrequency ablation. Good quality evidence is lacking on the effectiveness and safety of these techniques.

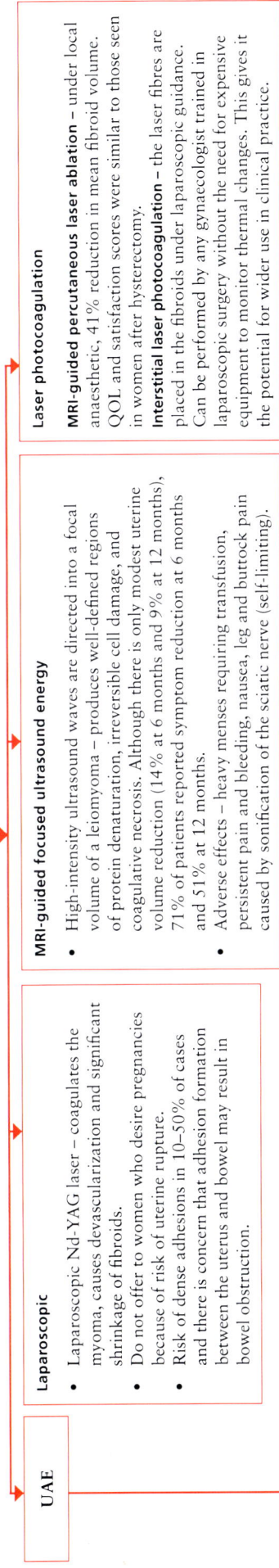

Laparoscopic

- Laparoscopic Nd-YAG laser – coagulates the myoma, causes devascularization and significant shrinkage of fibroids.
- Do not offer to women who desire pregnancies because of risk of uterine rupture.
- Risk of dense adhesions in 10–50% of cases and there is concern that adhesion formation between the uterus and bowel may result in bowel obstruction.

MRI-guided focused ultrasound energy

- High-intensity ultrasound waves are directed into a focal volume of a leiomyoma – produces well-defined regions of protein denaturation, irreversible cell damage, and coagulative necrosis. Although there is only modest uterine volume reduction (14% at 6 months and 9% at 12 months), 71% of patients reported symptom reduction at 6 months and 51% at 12 months.
- Adverse effects – heavy menses requiring transfusion, persistent pain and bleeding, nausea, leg and buttock pain caused by sonification of the sciatic nerve (self-limiting).

Laser photocoagulation

- **MRI-guided percutaneous laser ablation** – under local anaesthetic, 41% reduction in mean fibroid volume. QOL and satisfaction scores were similar to those seen in women after hysterectomy.
- **Interstitial laser photocoagulation** – the laser fibres are placed in the fibroids under laparoscopic guidance. Can be performed by any gynaecologist trained in laparoscopic surgery without the need for expensive equipment to monitor thermal changes. This gives it the potential for wider use in clinical practice.

Uterine artery embolization

Consider UAE for women with symptomatic fibroids as a treatment option. (NICE)

- Femoral artery is cannulated and an embolic agent is injected into the uterine arteries to impair the blood supply to the uterus and fibroids. This has a differential effect on fibroids (that have a higher blood supply than the surrounding myometrium).
- Fibroid shrinkage – 60% by the end of 6 months with further shrinkage up to one year.
- Indications:
  * Women with medical conditions that contraindicate surgery.
  * Women who are unwilling to have a blood transfusion.
  * Women who had previous unsuccessful surgery for fibroids.

Contraindications

- Absolute:
  * Current or recent infection of genital tract.
  * Patient refusing hysterectomy under any circumstances.
  * Doubtful diagnosis due to the clinical factors or inadequate imaging.
- Relative:
  * Narrow-stalked, pedunculated SS fibroids – might detach and cause significant complications.
  * Large fibroids – the outcome for smaller fibroids is better than for larger fibroids with similar complication rates. Large fibroid is not a contraindication. However, volume reduction might not be sufficient to satisfy patient's expectations.

UAE

- Do not give GnRHa within 2 months prior to the procedure.
- MDT – gynaecologist and interventional radiologist.
- MRI – superior to USS for diagnosing fibroids and adenomyosis. UAE in the presence of adenomyosis is less effective.
- Remove any IUD, if used, prior to the procedure.

Complications

- Immediate:
  * Groin haematoma, arterial thrombosis, dissection, and pseudo-aneurysm.
  * Non-target embolization – presence of ovarian-uterine anastomoses can compromise the ovary.
  * Early – post-embolization syndrome – pain, nausea, fever, flu-like symptoms with raised inflammatory markers and white cell count. Frequent and self-limiting. Manage with analgesics and anti-inflammatory drugs. Re-admission may be required in 3–5% of cases.
- Late:
  * Vaginal discharge (self-limiting) – 20–30%.
  * Persistent discharge with pain may be due to expulsion of fibroid.
  * Fibroid expulsion – 10%, more common with SM fibroids, may require hysteroscopic removal in 6% of cases.
  * Sexual dysfunction – 12% risk of changes in sexual function.
  * Infection (endometritis) – 0.5%. Rarely septicaemia and multi-organ failure. Emergency hysterectomy may be needed as life-saving surgery in 2–3%.
  * Need for further treatment (repeat UAE, exploration of uterine cavity, myomectomy, hysterectomy) in future – 25% if < 40 years; 10% if 40–50 years of age.
  * Amenorrhoea (POI) – 1.5–7%, but the majority of these patients are > 45 years old (25% risk in this age group).

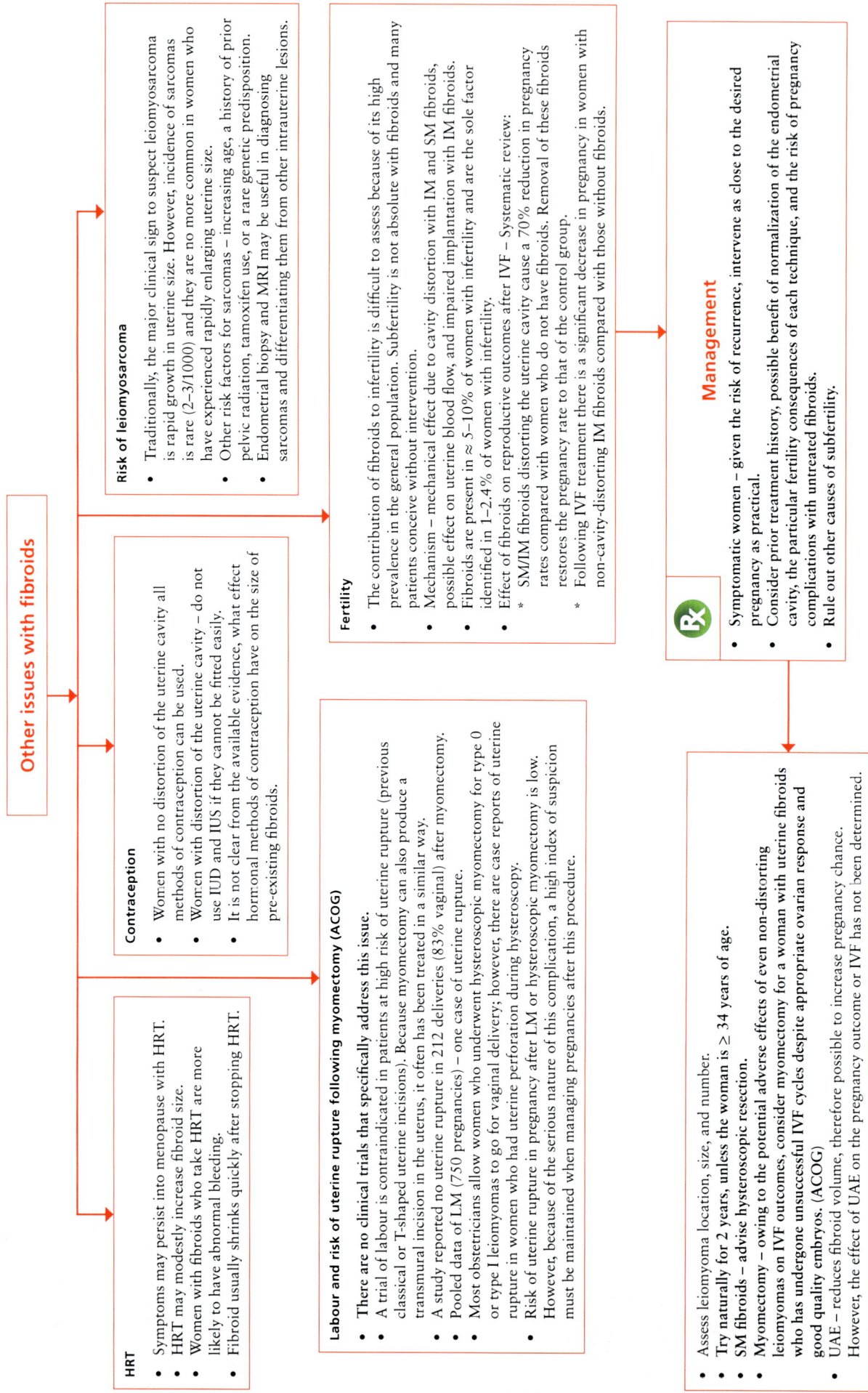

Other issues with fibroids

HRT

- Symptoms may persist into menopause with HRT.
- HRT may modestly increase fibroid size.
- Women with fibroids who take HRT are more likely to have abnormal bleeding.
- Fibroid usually shrinks quickly after stopping HRT.

Contraception

- Women with no distortion of the uterine cavity all methods of contraception can be used.
- Women with distortion of the uterine cavity – do not use IUD and IUS if they cannot be fitted easily.
- It is not clear from the available evidence, what effect hormonal methods of contraception have on the size of pre-existing fibroids.

Risk of leiomyosarcoma

- Traditionally, the major clinical sign to suspect leiomyosarcoma is rapid growth in uterine size. However, incidence of sarcomas is rare (2–3/1000) and they are no more common in women who have experienced rapidly enlarging uterine size.
- Other risk factors for sarcomas – increasing age, a history of prior pelvic radiation, tamoxifen use, or a rare genetic predisposition.
- Endometrial biopsy and MRI may be useful in diagnosing sarcomas and differentiating them from other intrauterine lesions.

Labour and risk of uterine rupture following myomectomy (ACOG)

- There are no clinical trials that specifically address this issue.
- A trial of labour is contraindicated in patients at high risk of uterine rupture (previous classical or T-shaped uterine incisions). Because myomectomy can also produce a transmural incision in the uterus, it often has been treated in a similar way.
- A study reported no uterine rupture in 212 deliveries (83% vaginal) after myomectomy.
- Pooled data of LM (750 pregnancies) – one case of uterine rupture.
- Most obstetricians allow women who underwent hysteroscopic myomectomy for type 0 or type I leiomyomas to go for vaginal delivery; however, there are case reports of uterine rupture in women who had uterine perforation during hysteroscopy.
- Risk of uterine rupture in pregnancy after LM or hysteroscopic myomectomy is low. However, because of the serious nature of this complication, a high index of suspicion must be maintained when managing pregnancies after this procedure.

Fertility

- The contribution of fibroids to infertility is difficult to assess because of its high prevalence in the general population. Subfertility is not absolute with fibroids and many patients conceive without intervention.
- Mechanism – mechanical effect due to cavity distortion with IM and SM fibroids, possible effect on uterine blood flow, and impaired implantation with IM fibroids.
- Fibroids are present in ≈ 5–10% of women with infertility and are the sole factor identified in 1–2.4% of women with infertility.
- Effect of fibroids on reproductive outcomes after IVF – Systematic review:
  * SM/IM fibroids distorting the uterine cavity cause a 70% reduction in pregnancy rates compared with women who do not have fibroids. Removal of these fibroids restores the pregnancy rate to that of the control group.
  * Following IVF treatment there is a significant decrease in pregnancy in women with non-cavity-distorting IM fibroids compared with those without fibroids.

Management

- Symptomatic women – given the risk of recurrence, intervene as close to the desired pregnancy as practical.
- Consider prior treatment history, possible benefit of normalization of the endometrial cavity, the particular fertility consequences of each technique, and the risk of pregnancy complications with untreated fibroids.
- Rule out other causes of subfertility.

- Assess leiomyoma location, size, and number.
- Try naturally for 2 years, unless the woman is ≥ 34 years of age.
- SM fibroids – advise hysteroscopic resection.
- Myomectomy – owing to the potential adverse effects of even non-distorting leiomyomas on IVF outcomes, consider myomectomy for a woman with uterine fibroids who has undergone unsuccessful IVF cycles despite appropriate ovarian response and good quality embryos. (ACOG)
- UAE – reduces fibroid volume, therefore possible to increase pregnancy chance. However, the effect of UAE on the pregnancy outcome or IVF has not been determined.

Evidence round-up – UAE

- Early and mid-term results – it is at least as safe as the surgical alternatives.
- It provides good symptom relief and is particularly affective for HMB.
- The long-term safety and effectiveness of this technique have not been fully evaluated.

Hysterectomy vs UAE

- Equal results for QOL with similar complication rates.
- Hospital stay and recovery are significantly shorter with UAE.
- Around 80–90% have significantly improved symptoms at one year with 40–70% reduction in fibroid volume.
- Up to 10% of women require further treatment (repeat UAE or hysterectomy) within 1 year and 20–25% within 5 years.
- UAE is significantly more cost-effective at the end of one year; however, it may reduce longer term as some patients will require further treatment.
- The faster, shorter recovery period of UAE with uterine conservation needs to be weighed against the need for further treatment in a minority of women.

Myomectomy vs UAE

- Evidence is much less clear.
- Hospital stay and recovery time are significantly shorter with UAE, but it has a high re-intervention rate. Symptom control and complication rates are similar.
- Trend towards higher FSH levels in UAE.
- More pregnancies and significantly fewer miscarriages in myomectomy.
- Obstetric and perinatal outcomes are similar.
- More evidence is needed to establish the role of UAE in patients wishing to maintain fertility.
- Reserve UAE only for patients maintaining fertility, where the option of myomectomy is fully discussed but is felt to be less suitable.

Pregnancy outcome following UAE

- Case series have documented successful pregnancies.
- There is an increased risk of miscarriage (36% vs 10–15%), preterm delivery (16% vs 5–10%), Caesarean section (67% vs 22%), malpresentation (10% vs 5%), and PPH (14% vs 4–6%) compared with the general population. No difference in fetal growth restriction (7% vs 10%) was seen.
- Be cautious when considering UAE for treating symptomatic fibroids in women desiring a future pregnancy.

1. ACOG Practice Bulletin Clinical Management Guidelines for Obstetrician–Gynecologists, Number 96, August 2008.
2. Clinical Knowledge Summaries. http://cks.nice.org.uk/fibroids.
3. Clinical Recommendations on the Use of UAE in the Management of Fibroids – 2nd edition. RCOG/RCR report of a joint working party.
4. Hcmer H, Saridogan E. Pregnancy outcomes after uterine artery embolisation for fibroids. *The Obstetrician and Gynaecologist* 2009; 11:265–270.
5. Kunde D, Khalaf Y. Alternatives to hysterectomy for treatment of uterine fibroids. *The Obstetrician and Gynaecologist* 2004; 6:215–221.
6. Lethaby A, Vollenhoven B, Sowter M. Efficacy of pre-operative gonadotrophin hormone releasing analogues for women with uterine fibroids undergoing hysterectomy or myomectomy: a systematic review. *Brit J Obstet Gynaecol* 2002; 109(10):1097–1108.
7. Kongnyuy EJ, Wiysonge CS. Interventions to reduce haemorrhage during myomectomy for fibroids. *Cochrane Database Syst Rev* 2009; 3:CD005355.
8. Sunkara SK, Khairy M, El-Toukhy T, Khalaf Y, Coomarasamy A. The effect of intramural fibroids without uterine cavity involvement on the outcome of IVF treatment: a systematic review and meta-analysis. *Hum Reprod* 2010; 25(2):418–429.
9. Jin C, Hub Y, Chen X, et al. Laparoscopic versus open myomectomy a meta-analysis of randomized controlled trials. *Eur J Obstet Gynecol Reprod Biol* 2009; 145:14–21.
10. http://en.wikipedia.org/wiki/Uterine_fibroid.

CHAPTER 11 Adenomyosis

Background and definition

- Benign invasion of endometrium into the myometrium, resulting in ectopic, non-neoplastic, endometrial glands and stroma surrounded by the hypertrophic and hyperplastic myometrium.
- Histological diagnosis – widely accepted definition is glandular extension below the endometrial–myometrial interface (EMI) of > 2.5 mm (one low-power field). Adenomyosis sub-basalis – minimally invasive adenomyosis extending < 2 mm beneath the basal endometrium.
- In **diffuse** adenomyosis uteri, the uterus becomes enlarged and globular. Focal lesions can resemble leiomyoma. Adenomyosis has poorly defined margins and cannot be enucleated. The posterior wall is more often affected than the anterior wall.

Prevalence and incidence

- Adenomyosis has been reported to occur in about 30% of the general female population and in up to 5–70% of hysterectomy specimens, depending on the definition.
- Risk factors – multiparity, miscarriage, TOP, endometriosis, HMB, infertility, curettage in pregnancy, endometrial hyperplasia.
- **No difference** – age at menarche, menopausal status, age at first childbirth, COCs, IUCD, tubal sterilization, endometrial carcinoma, caesarean section.

Clinical features

- Asymptomatic in 35%.
- Abnormal uterine bleeding (50%), HMB.
- Secondary dysmenorrhoea (30%).
- Dyspareunia and chronic pelvic pain – less common.
- Frequency and severity of symptoms correlate with the extent and depth of adenomyosis.
- **On examination** – diffusely enlarged, tender uterus.

Investigations

- USS – the normal myometrium has three distinct sonographic layers. The middle layer is the most echogenic and is separated from the thin outer layer by the arcuate venous and arterial plexuses. The inner layer is hypo-echoic relative to the middle and outer layers (the subendometrial halo). Adenomyosis can distort the appearance of these zones.
  TVS criteria:
  * Globular uterine enlargement in the absence of fibroids.
  * Asymmetrical enlargement of the anterior or posterior myometrial wall.
  * Heterogeneous echo texture – lack of homogeneity within the myometrium with architectural disturbance. This finding is the most predictive of adenomyosis.
  * Subendometrial echogenic linear striations – invasion of the endometrial glands into the subendometrial tissue induces a hyperplastic reaction, which appears as echogenic linear striations fanning out from the endometrial layer.
  * Obscure endometrial/myometrial border – invasion of the myometrium by the glands obscures the normally distinct endometrial/myometrial border.
  * Cystic anechoic spaces or lakes in the myometrium of variable size.
  * Thickening of the transition zone (subendometrial hypoechoic halo) of 12 mm or greater has been shown to be associated with adenomyosis.

- HSG – low sensitivity and specificity. Features include multiple, small (< 4 mm) spicules extending from the endometrium into the myometrium, with saccular endings. A local accumulation of contrast material in the myometrium may produce a honeycomb appearance.
- MRI – 3 different zones can be identified within the uterus. The appearance of diffuse or focal widening of the junctional zone is suggestive of adenomyosis.
  * Sensitivity and specificity are comparable to or better than those of TVS. A systematic review reported MRI to be better than TVS – TVS has a sensitivity of 72%, specificity of 81%, whereas MRI has a sensitivity of 77%, specificity of 89%.
  * Cost and limited availability hinders its routine use.
  * MRI is superior to TVS where associated fibroids or additional pathologies are suspected.
- CT – poor diagnostic value owing to similar images portrayed by foci and normal myometrium.
- Hysteroscopic or laparoscopic myometrial biopsy – its role remains limited. Myometrial biopsy of the posterior uterine wall is superior to TVS, but its routine use is not recommended.
- TVS remains the first investigation of choice due to its efficacy, safety, and lower cost.

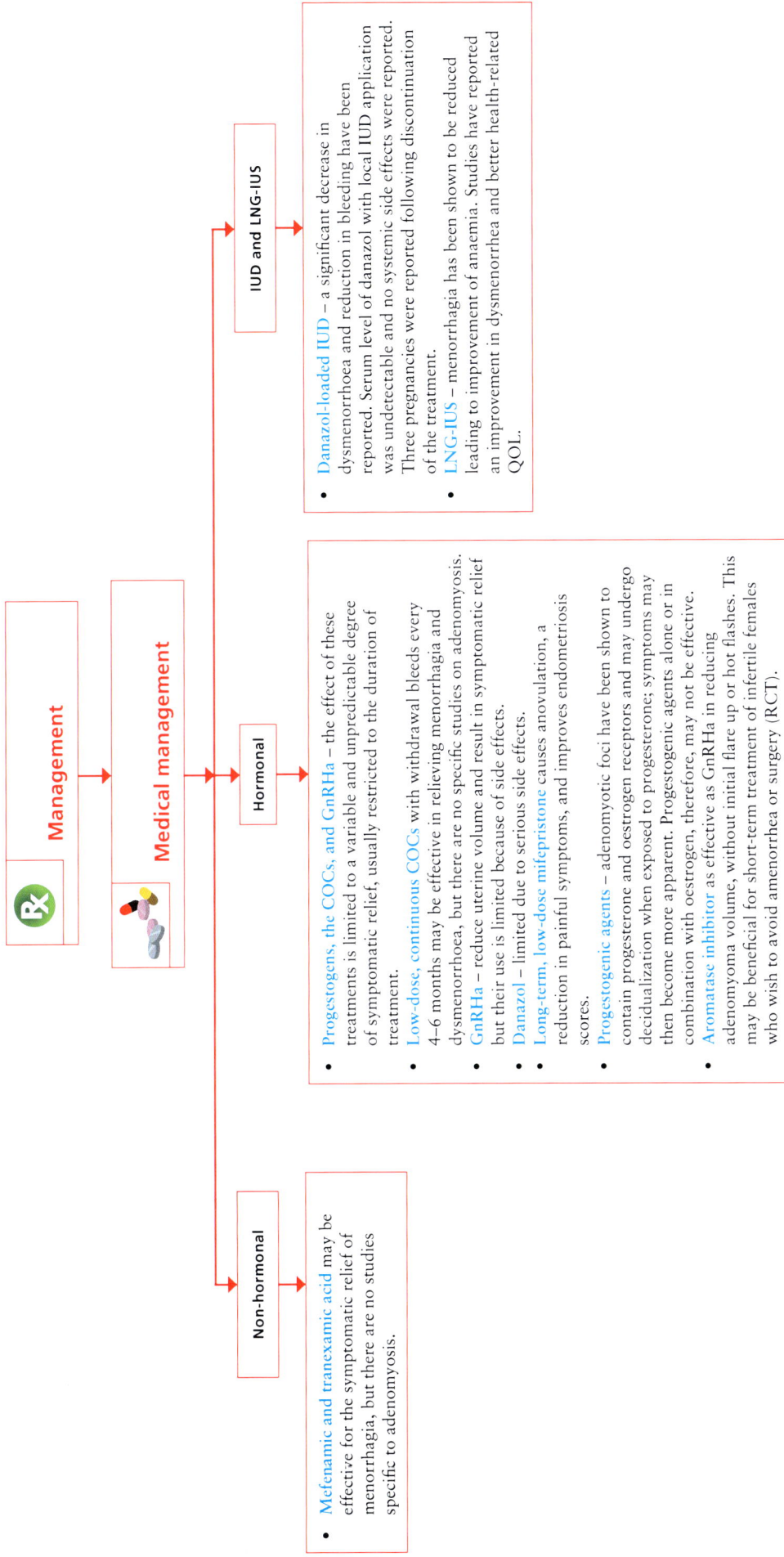

Management

Medical management

Non-hormonal

- **Mefenamic and tranexamic acid** may be effective for the symptomatic relief of menorrhagia, but there are no studies specific to adenomyosis.

Hormonal

- **Progestogens, the COCs, and GnRHa** – the effect of these treatments is limited to a variable and unpredictable degree of symptomatic relief, usually restricted to the duration of treatment.
- **Low-dose, continuous COCs** with withdrawal bleeds every 4–6 months may be effective in relieving menorrhagia and dysmenorrhoea, but there are no specific studies on adenomyosis.
- **GnRHa** – reduce uterine volume and result in symptomatic relief but their use is limited because of side effects.
- **Danazol** – limited due to serious side effects.
- **Long-term, low-dose mifepristone** causes anovulation, a reduction in painful symptoms, and improves endometriosis scores.
- **Progestogenic agents** – adenomyotic foci have been shown to contain progesterone and oestrogen receptors and may undergo decidualization when exposed to progesterone; symptoms may then become more apparent. Progestogenic agents alone or in combination with oestrogen, therefore, may not be effective.
- **Aromatase inhibitor** as effective as GnRHa in reducing adenomyoma volume, without initial flare up or hot flashes. This may be beneficial for short-term treatment of infertile females who wish to avoid amenorrhea or surgery (RCT).

IUD and LNG-IUS

- **Danazol-loaded IUD** – a significant decrease in dysmenorrhoea and reduction in bleeding have been reported. Serum level of danazol with local IUD application was undetectable and no systemic side effects were reported. Three pregnancies were reported following discontinuation of the treatment.
- **LNG-IUS** – menorrhagia has been shown to be reduced leading to improvement of anaemia. Studies have reported an improvement in dysmenorrhea and better health-related QOL.

Surgical management

- **Adenomyomectomy – localized excision of affected myometrium** (cytoreductive surgery) can be performed in localized adenomyosis if the extent of the disease can be accurately defined. The approach is similar to myomectomy and may be useful for women seeking to preserve their fertility.
- There are reports of laparoscopic excision of focal adenomyosis. However, the accurate preoperative localization and meticulous removal of all the lesions are factors associated with the success of the procedure.
- Laparoscopic approach is associated with the concerns of haemostasis and inaccurate assessment of the extent of diffuse disease without palpating the uterus. Open surgery remains the mainstay for extensive disease.
- Excising diffuse disease may result in inadvertent removal of excess myometrial tissue, because of unclear demarcation from surrounding normal myometrium.
- Complete microsurgical resection of the adenomyotic areas, followed by GnRHa, is reported to improve symptoms and fertility. Published series are small, with limited success.
- Consider surgical and obstetric complications of myometrial excision. Excision of a large part of the myometrium may lead to difficulty in wound apposition, decreased expansive capacity of the uterus, and weakening, leading to uterine rupture.

- **Laparoscopic myometrial electrocoagulation** – involves insertion of a monopolar or bipolar needle electrode into the affected myometrium at approximately 1–2 cm intervals, which induces localized coagulation and necrosis.
- Electrocoagulation can be difficult to apply with precision, destruction of all the abnormal tissue may be incomplete and cannot be checked at the time of surgery, and it can reduce the strength of the remaining myometrial tissue.
- There is a risk of emergency hysterectomy for uncontrollable bleeding and a high incidence of adhesion formation.
- Uterine rupture has been reported as early as 12 weeks of gestation, hence it is an undesirable option for women wishing to conceive. This technique may be best suitable for women > 40 years of age who have completed their families but who wish to avoid hysterectomy.

- **UAE** has been shown to reduce the symptoms associated with adenomyosis. The chances of a subsequent successful pregnancy are unclear. A systematic review (15 studies) reported short-term improvement in 83% and long-term satisfaction of 65% with minimal complications.
- **Transcatheter local infusion of MTX combined with UAE** under guidance of digital subtraction angiography – a study reported a decrease in menstrual volume, dysmenorrhoea, reduction of uterine size, with no chemotherapeutic side effects. The efficacy was more evident in diffuse adenomyosis.

- **Laparoscopic uterine artery ligation** has been studied in 20 women with symptomatic uterine adenomyosis. Only 15% of women, however, rated the treatment as satisfactory at 6-month follow-up, suggesting that this approach may not be effective.
- **MRI-guided focused ultrasound ablation** – a case series reported that it is a well-tolerated and effective alternative for selected patients.

- **Hysteroscopic ablation and excision** – the success of the resection depends on the depth of foci. In superficial adenomyosis with penetration < 2 mm, the procedure is more successful. With deep adenomyosis with penetration > 2 mm, it is associated with poor results. It is generally undertaken if the adenomyosis is confined to the superficial 3 mm of the myometrium.
  Ablation or resection of deeper myometrial tissue is associated with risk of bleeding as arteries are situated approximately 5 mm deep to the myometrial surface. Unresected deeper endometrial glands can persist and proliferate to cause recurrence.
- **Endomyometrial ablation** is effective for lesions deeper than the endometrial–myometrial junction whereas the efficacy of hysteroscopic ablation is limited to foci 2–3 mm deep.

- **Hysterectomy remains** the main surgical option for women not wishing to preserve their fertility.

Adenomyosis and infertility

- Adenomyosis is usually diagnosed in the 4th and 5th decades of life in multiparous women and is believed to increase with age. As more women are delaying their pregnancy until later in their 30s or 40s, adenomyosis is encountered more frequently in fertility clinic.
- It is also possible that since its diagnosis by TVS and MRI became possible, it is being encountered more frequently during the diagnostic work-up for infertility.
- There is evidence of a strong association between endometriosis and adenomyosis (25–70%) and that adenomyosis may play a role in infertility in women with endometriosis.
- Possible link between adenomyosis and infertility is also becoming more plausible.

- Possible mechanism of subfertility in women with adenomyosis – gene dysregulation, impaired uterine peristaltic activity, altered endometrial function and receptivity, impaired implantation, altered decidualization, abnormal concentrations of intrauterine free radicals.
- Increase in JZ can be significantly correlated with implantation failure at IVF.
- There are a few reports of higher miscarriage rates in patients with adenomyosis as compared to controls following IVF.
- However, evidence from recipients of sibling oocytes in IVF suggests that adenomyosis has no impact on the rate of embryonic implantation.

Management

- Uterine artery embolization – pregnancy and vaginal delivery has been reported in a small case series.
- High-intensity focused ultrasound (HIFU)) – the safety of transvaginal HIFU is currently being assessed. One case of successful pregnancy has been reported.

- GnRHa – no reports on successful pregnancies following treatment with GnRHa for adenomyosis.
- LNG-IUS – no successful subsequent pregnancies have been reported to date.
- Danazol-loaded IUD – 3 pregnancies have been reported following its use.

- Microsurgical resection of the visible adenomyotic area – (case reports) followed by treatment with GnRHa resulted in the birth of healthy newborns in 4 cases. It is suggested that this cytoreductive surgery results in an increased sensitivity to hormonal treatment due to improved blood supply to the adenomyosis tissue and an improved immune function of the host.
- Risk of surgical and obstetric complications – antepartum bleeding, threatened PTL, and intra-abdominal adhesions.
- Suggested approach – early combined GnRHa treatment after cytoreductive surgery and a delay of 4–6 months before attempting to become pregnant may help to achieve pregnancy.

What not to do

- Routine myometrial biopsy of the uterine wall.
- GnRHa – long-term use.
- Danazol – long-term use.

1. Mahasseb MK, Habiba MA. Adenomyosis – an update. *The Obstetrician and Gynaecologist* 2009;11:41–47.
2. Sunkara1 SK, Khan KS. Adenomyosis and female fertility: a critical review of the evidence. *J Obstet Gynaecol* 2012; 32(2):113–116.
3. Pepas L, Deguara C, Davis C. Update on the surgical management of adenomyosis. *Curr Opin Obstet Gynecol* 2012;24(4):259–264.
4. Elnashar A, Badawy A, Mosbah A. Aromatase inhibitors or gonadotropin-releasing hormone agonists for the management of uterine adenomyosis: a randomized controlled study. *Hum Reprod* 2010;25:i229.
5. Champaneria R, Abedin P, Daniels J, Balogun M, Khan KS. Ultrasound scan and magnetic resonance imaging for the diagnosis of adenomyosis: systematic review comparing test accuracy. *Acta Obstet Gynecol Scand.* 201089(11):1374–1384.
6. Sakhel K, Abuhamad A. Sonography of adenomyosis. *J Ultrasound Med* 2012;31(5):805–808.
7. Campo S, Campo V, Benagiano G. Adenomyosis and infertility. *Reprod BioMed Online* 2012;24:35-46.

CHAPTER 12 Endometriosis

Background and definition

- Definition – presence of endometrial-like tissue outside the uterus, which induces a chronic inflammatory reaction.
- Most commonly affected sites are the pelvic organs and peritoneum (uterosacral ligaments, pouch of Douglas, rectovaginal septum, and ovaries). Extra-pelvic deposits such as the lungs, caesarean section scar, and the bowel are occasionally seen.
- Extent of the disease varies from a few, small lesions on otherwise normal pelvic organs to large ovarian endometriotic cysts (endometriomas), extensive fibrosis in structures such as the uterosacral ligaments, and adhesion formation causing marked distortion of pelvic anatomy.
- All classification systems for endometriosis are subjective and correlate poorly with pain symptoms but may be of value in infertility prognosis and management.

Prevalence and incidence

- Prevalence – 5–10% among the general female population.
- Present in 20–30% of women undergoing investigations for subfertility and in 1–5% of women undergoing sterilization.
- In women with dysmenorrhoea or chronic pelvic pain, the incidence of endometriosis is 40–60%.

- Pathogenesis – poorly understood.
- Theories:
    * Retrograde menstruation.
    * Peritoneal metaplasia.
    * Lymphatic or blood-borne dissemination.

History

- Asymptomatic – incidental finding.
- Symptoms – nonspecific:
    * Secondary dysmenorrhoea (usually before or during menstruation).   * Deep dyspareunia.
    * Chronic pelvic pain.   * Infertility.
    * Cyclical or perimenstrual symptoms, such as bowel or bladder, with or without abnormal bleeding or pain.
    * Dyschezia (pain on defecation).   * Painful caesarean section scar.
- Predictive value of any one symptom or set of symptoms is uncertain, as each of these symptoms can overlap with other causes such as IBS and PID.

Risks or complications

- Dysmenorrhoea.
- Chronic pelvic pain.
- Subfertility.
- Can impact on general physical, mental, and social wellbeing.

Examination

- Can be entirely normal.
- Speculum examination – visible lesions may be seen in the vagina or on the cervix.
- Pelvic examination – there may be:
    * A fixed, retroverted uterus.   * Enlarged ovaries.   * Tender adnexae/uterosacral ligaments.   * Deeply infiltrating nodules may be palpable on the uterosacral ligaments or in the pouch of Douglas.
- Detection of nodules is improved by performing the examination during menstruation.

Differential diagnosis – chronic pelvic pain

- Primary dysmenorrhoea.
- Adenomyosis.   • Uterine fibroids.
- Adhesions.   • PID.
- Congenital anomalies of the reproductive tract.
- Interstitial cystitis or recurrent UTIs.
- IBS or other bowel pathology.
- Cancer (of the cervix, uterus, ovary, rectum, or bladder).
- Musculoskeletal disorders.

Empirical treatment

- Empirical treatment of pain symptoms without a definitive diagnosis – a therapeutic trial of a hormonal drug to reduce menstrual flow is appropriate.
- Counselling, analgesia, progestogens, or the COCs.
- GnRHa may be taken short term.

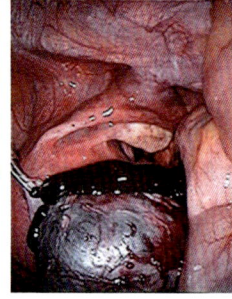

Peritoneal endometriosis

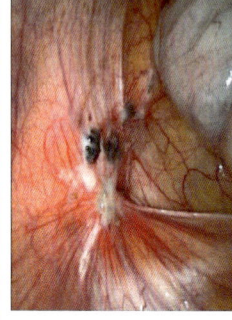

Endometrioma

Investigations

Laparoscopy

- 'Gold standard' – allows visual inspection of the pelvis; palpate lesions to determine their nodularity; document the type, location, and extent of all lesions and adhesions.
- Insufficient evidence to justify scheduling the laparoscopy for a specific time in the menstrual cycle.
- Do not perform during or within 3 months of hormonal treatment, to avoid under-diagnosis.

Others

- Serum CA125 level – may be elevated in endometriosis; has no value as a diagnostic tool.
- Histology:
  - * Positive histology confirms diagnosis; negative histology does not exclude it.
  - * Peritoneal disease – visual inspection is usually adequate but histological confirmation is ideal.
  - * Ovarian endometrioma (> 3 cm in diameter) and in deeply infiltrating disease, obtain histology to identify endometriosis and to exclude rare cases of malignancy.
- TVS – limited value in diagnosing peritoneal endometriosis but is useful in diagnosis of ovarian endometrioma. May have a role in the diagnosis of disease involving bladder or rectum.
- MRI – to assess disease extent, if there is clinical evidence of deeply infiltrating endometriosis, ureteric, bladder, and bowel involvement.

Management

Management of severe/deeply infiltrating disease is complex. Surgery is usually required and multiple organs are sometimes involved. Referral to a centre with the necessary expertise to offer all available treatments in an MDT is recommended.

Suspected endometrioma

Manage as ovarian cyst – see Chapter 36.

Pelvic pain

Subfertility

Medical management

Analgesics

- NSAIDs – inconclusive evidence to show whether NSAIDs are effective in managing pain caused by endometriosis and whether any one NSAID is more effective than another.
  - * Adverse GI side effects including gastric ulceration. Ibuprofen has a lower risk; naproxen and diclofenac are associated with an intermediate risk; mefenamic acid is likely to be associated with a low-to-intermediate risk.
- Paracetamol – no evidence of benefit.
- Codeine – no direct evidence of benefit. Add codeine in women who are unable to take NSAID or who do not get adequate pain relief from paracetamol and NSAID.

Surgical management

See page 57.

Complementary medicine

See page 57.

Hormonal drugs

- Suppression of ovarian function for 6 months reduces pain. Aim is to induce atrophy of ectopic endometrium, and reduce pain by reducing menstrual blood flow or by inducing amenorrhoea.
- Hormonal manipulation does not affect the primary biological mechanisms of the disease process. Therefore, medical treatment does not always provide complete pain relief.
- Symptom recurrence is common.
- Drugs (COCs, danazol, gestrinone, MPA, GnRHa) – equally effective but differ in their adverse effect and cost profile. Duration of therapy is determined by the choice of drug, response to treatment, and adverse effect. The COCs and Depo-Provera can be used long term but the use of danazol and GnRH agonists is restricted to 6 months owing to their side effects.

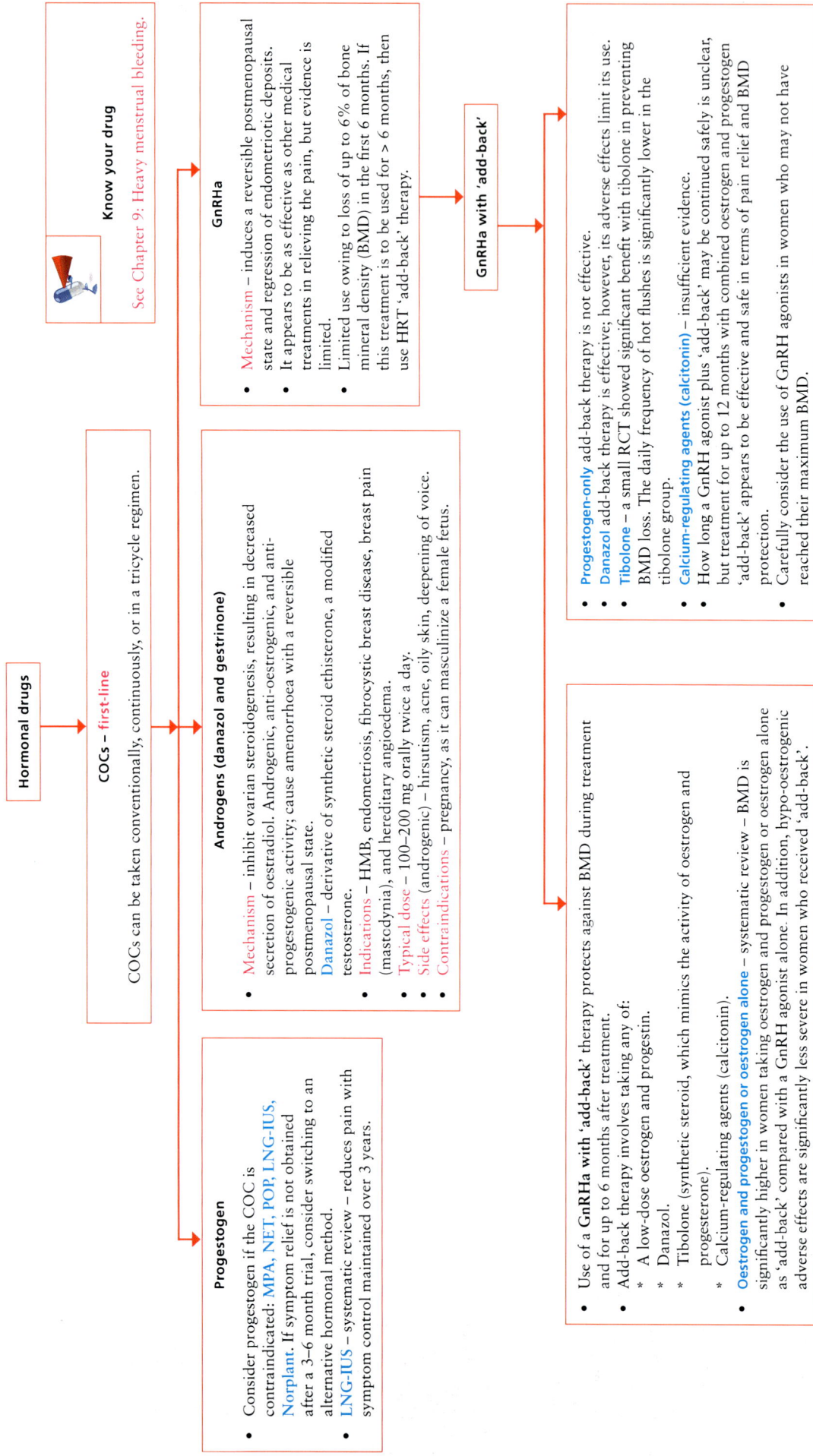

Know your drug

See Chapter 9: Heavy menstrual bleeding.

Hormonal drugs

COCs – first-line

COCs can be taken conventionally, continuously, or in a tricycle regimen.

Progestogen

- Consider progestogen if the COC is contraindicated: MPA, NET, POP, LNG-IUS, Norplant. If symptom relief is not obtained after a 3–6 month trial, consider switching to an alternative hormonal method.
- LNG-IUS – systematic review – reduces pain with symptom control maintained over 3 years.

Androgens (danazol and gestrinone)

- Mechanism – inhibit ovarian steroidogenesis, resulting in decreased secretion of oestradiol. Androgenic, anti-oestrogenic, and anti-progestogenic activity; cause amenorrhoea with a reversible postmenopausal state.
- Danazol – derivative of synthetic steroid ethisterone, a modified testosterone.
- Indications – HMB, endometriosis, fibrocystic breast disease, breast pain (mastodynia), and hereditary angioedema.
- Typical dose – 100–200 mg orally twice a day.
- Side effects (androgenic) – hirsutism, acne, oily skin, deepening of voice.
- Contraindications – pregnancy, as it can masculinize a female fetus.

GnRHa

- Mechanism – induces a reversible postmenopausal state and regression of endometriotic deposits.
- It appears to be as effective as other medical treatments in relieving the pain, but evidence is limited.
- Limited use owing to loss of up to 6% of bone mineral density (BMD) in the first 6 months. If this treatment is to be used for > 6 months, then use HRT 'add-back' therapy.

GnRHa with 'add-back'

- Use of a GnRHa with 'add-back' therapy protects against BMD during treatment and for up to 6 months after treatment.
- Add-back therapy involves taking any of:
  * A low-dose oestrogen and progestin.
  * Danazol.
  * Tibolone (synthetic steroid, which mimics the activity of oestrogen and progesterone).
  * Calcium-regulating agents (calcitonin).
- Oestrogen and progestogen or oestrogen alone – systematic review – BMD is significantly higher in women taking oestrogen and progestogen or oestrogen alone as 'add-back' compared with a GnRH agonist alone. In addition, hypo-oestrogenic adverse effects are significantly less severe in women who received 'add-back'.

- Progestogen-only add-back therapy is not effective.
- Danazol add-back therapy is effective; however, its adverse effects limit its use.
- Tibolone – a small RCT showed significant benefit with tibolone in preventing BMD loss. The daily frequency of hot flushes is significantly lower in the tibolone group.
- Calcium-regulating agents (calcitonin) – insufficient evidence.
- How long a GnRH agonist plus 'add-back' may be continued safely is unclear, but treatment for up to 12 months with combined oestrogen and progestogen 'add-back' appears to be effective and safe in terms of pain relief and BMD protection.
- Carefully consider the use of GnRH agonists in women who may not have reached their maximum BMD.

Surgical treatment for endometriosis-related pain

Conservative (minimally invasive when fertility is required):

- Ideal practice is to diagnose and remove endometriosis surgically.
- Aim – to remove (excise) or destroy (ablate) areas of endometriosis to improve symptoms.

Radical (when continuing fertility is no longer required)

Mild to moderate:

- **Ablation and/or excision** of endometriotic lesions reduce pain compared with diagnostic laparoscopy alone.
- However, some women fail to respond to surgical treatment either because of incomplete excision, postoperative recurrence, or because some of their pain was not due to endometriosis in the first place.

Severe and deeply infiltrating disease:

- **Excisional surgery** involves removing the entire lesions, and results in significant symptomatic improvement as well as general improvement in QOL. Associated with high morbidity.
- Refer to specialized tertiary endometriosis centres with experienced surgeons and MDT care (gynaecologists, radiologists, colorectal surgeons, urologists, anaesthetic pain specialists, and psychologists).

- **Laparoscopic uterine nerve ablation** does not reduce endometriosis-associated pain or dysmenorrhoea associated with endometriosis.
- **Laparoscopic helium plasma coagulation** – used to vaporize endometriotic deposits. Current evidence on the safety and efficacy of this procedure is not adequate to recommend its use outside research.

- **HRT pre- or postoperatively has no evidence of benefit.**
- In a small RCT, the LNG-IUS inserted after laparoscopic surgery significantly reduced the risk of recurrent moderate–severe dysmenorrhoea at 1-year follow-up.

- **TAH + BSO** – hysterectomy and removal of all visible endometriotic tissue, BSO may result in improved pain relief and a reduced chance of future surgery.
- **HRT after BSO** – owing to the overall health benefits and small risk of recurrent disease while taking HRT, advise HRT after BSO in young women.
- Ideal regimen is unclear. There is no good evidence on the type of regimen. These are unopposed oestrogen, combined-continuous regimen, or tibolone. Unopposed oestrogen may reactivate any residual disease. Adding a progestogen is unnecessary but may protect against the unopposed action of oestrogen on any residual disease.
- Adenocarcinoma arising from endometriosis has been reported in women treated with unopposed oestrogen. Limited evidence suggests that combined HRT is associated with a lower risk of malignant change than treatment with unopposed oestrogens.
- **Balance the theoretical benefit of avoiding disease reactivation or malignant transformation against the risk of increase in breast cancer associated with combined oestrogen and progestogen HRT and tibolone.**

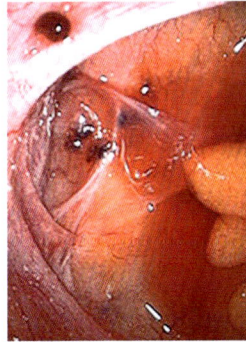

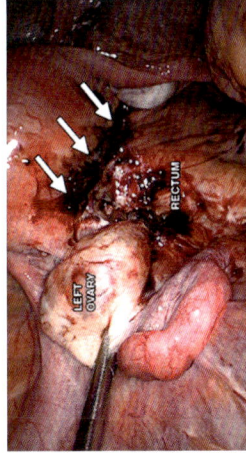

Complementary medicine

- Nutritional and complementary therapies such as homeopathy, reflexology, traditional Chinese medicine, or herbal treatments may improve pain symptoms.
- While there is no evidence from RCTs in endometriosis to support these treatments, they should not be ruled out if the woman feels that they could be beneficial to her overall pain management and/or QOL, or work in conjunction with more traditional therapies.

Endometriosis and infertility

Suggested mechanism for subfertility

- **Mild–moderate** – precise mechanism unclear. Theories:
  * Altered peritoneal milieu may destroy oocytes and spermatozoa and impair fertilization.
  * Increased peritoneal prostaglandin concentrations may interfere with ovulation, tubal peristalsis, sperm motility, or uterine contractility, thereby interfering with implantation.
- **Severe** – adhesions and resulting fibrosis may distort the anatomy of Fallopian tubes and ovaries, thereby impeding the capture of oocytes.
  * Ovarian endometriomas may be extensive and can destroy normal ovarian tissue, causing anovulation.
  * Pelvic pain and dyspareunia may discourage or reduce coital frequency.
- **Effect of endometriosis on IVF** – systematic review – IVF pregnancy rates are lower in women with endometriosis than in those with tubal infertility, predominantly owing to decreased fertilization and implantation rates secondary to abnormalities in oocyte quality and early embryo development. However, ESHRE guidelines reported that endometriosis does not appear to affect pregnancy rates adversely.

Endometriosis and infertility management

Surgical management

- **Minimal–mild disease – laparoscopic ablation plus adhesiolysis** may improve the chance of pregnancy, but the evidence is limited.
- **Moderate–severe disease** – excision/ablation of all visible endometriosis and adhesions, to correct pelvic anatomy. Role of surgery is uncertain. No RCTs are available. There seems to be a negative correlation between the stage of endometriosis and the spontaneous pregnancy rate after surgical removal of endometriosis. Women may improve their chance of conceiving with conservative surgical treatment. (ASRM, 2006)
- **Ovarian endometriomas**   • Drainage.   • Ablation.   • Excision.
  - Risks – recurrence, damaging ovarian reserve secondary to excision of the capsule or to the use of electrosurgery.
  - Do not perform simple drainage as it has a high risk of recurrence.
  - Ablation may carry a higher risk of recurrence and it may result in greater damage to ovarian follicular reserve.
  - Laparoscopic excision is better than drainage and ablation. The risk of recurrence and symptoms are reduced compared to drainage and ablation. Subsequent spontaneous pregnancy rates are also improved.
  - Cochrane review – excision of the endometrioma is preferable to drainage and ablation in regard to recurrence of symptoms, recurrence of endometrioma, and spontaneous pregnancy rates.

ART

Medical management

- Suppression of ovarian function to improve fertility in minimal–mild or severe endometriosis is not effective. More harm than good may result from treatment, because of adverse effects and the lost opportunity to conceive.

Follow-up – relapse

- Systematic review – the absolute benefit on pain relief at short-term follow-up (6 months–1 year) is 30–40%. Relapse is also common after surgical procedures, and up to 50% of women need analgesics or hormonal treatment at 1 year.
- Long-term follow-up – repeat surgery rate up to 50%.
- **Managing relapse** – explain that relapse is common.
  * Exclude other conditions with similar symptoms.
  * Options: NSAIDs and/or medical treatment (such as COCs). Further hormonal treatment under specialist supervision.
  * Consider repeat surgery.

Expectant

Mild–moderate – couples conceive spontaneously with a monthly fecundity rate of 5–10%. **An expectant approach is appropriate in these couples for up to 2 years.**
Severe – probability of spontaneous pregnancy appears to be significantly low with a monthly fecundity rate of approximately 3% or less. **Role of expectant management is therefore limited.**

Evidence round-up – pre- or post-surgical hormonal treatment

- Insufficient evidence to suggest that hormonal suppression in association with surgery will benefit eradication of endometriosis, improve symptoms and pregnancy rates.
- Cochrane review –   • Pre-surgical medical treatment (goserelin) improved fertility compared with surgery alone (1 study),   • Compared with surgery alone, post-surgical medical treatment was no better at 12 months (5 studies).   • There was no significant difference in pain, disease recurrence, or pregnancy rates.

Assisted reproduction

- **Intrauterine insemination (IUI)** with gonadotrophins in minimal to mild endometriosis is not recommended.
- **IVF – indicated:**
  * Especially if tubal function is compromised, there is also male factor infertility, and/or other treatments have failed.
  * Couples with minimal or mild endometriosis and infertility of 2 years' duration or longer.
  * Refer early – women with moderate or severe disease where there is a high chance of impaired tubal-ovarian anatomy.

- **Hormonal treatment before IVF** – limited evidence – Cochrane review (1 RCT) – CPR per woman is significantly higher in women receiving GnRHa for 3–6 months before IVF compared with controls.
- **Surgical treatment of endometriomas before IVF** – no RCTs comparing laparoscopic excision with no treatment before IVF.
- **Ovarian cystectomy** – laparoscopic ovarian cystectomy is recommended if ovarian endometriomas are > 4cm in size, to:
  * Reduce risk of infection.
  * Possibly improve ovarian response.
  * Improve access to follicles.
  * Improve ease of monitoring.
  * Prevent endometriosis progression.
  * However, it is associated with the risks of surgical complications, possibility of reducing ovarian reserve, and risk of loss of the ovary.

What not to do

- Diagnostic laparoscopy during or within 3 months of hormonal treatment.
- Serum CA125 levels as a diagnostic tool.
- Laparoscopic uterine nerve ablation, presacral neurectomy, laparoscopic helium plasma coagulation.
- HRT before or after surgery.
- Expectant management in severe disease.
- Suppression of ovarian function to improve fertility in minimal–mild endometriosis.
- Medical management in more severe disease.
- Endometrioma – simple fenestration with drainage.
- Postoperative hormonal treatment has no beneficial effect on pregnancy rates after surgery.

1. *The Investigation and Management of Endometriosis.* RCOG Green-top Guideline No. 24, October 2006 (minor revisions October 2008).
2. Kenney N, English J. Surgical management of endometriosis. *The Obstetrician and Gynaecologist* 2007;9:147–152.
3. Prasannan-Nair C, Manias T, Mathur R. Management of endometriosis-related subfertility. *The Obstetrician and Gynaecologist* 2011;13:1–6.
4. The Practice Committee of ASRM. Endometriosis and infertility. *Fertil Steril* 2006; 86(Suppl 4).
5. ESHRE guideline for the diagnosis and treatment of endometriosis. *Hum Reprod* 2005; 20(10): 2698–2704.
6. http://en.wikipedia.org/wiki/Endometriosis_of_ovary.
7. http://commons.wikimedia.org/wiki/File:Extragenital_endometriosis.jpg.

CHAPTER 13 Disorders of sexual development (DSD)

Congenital conditions with atypical development of chromosomal, gonadal, or anatomical sex

Background prevalence

- DSD is defined as genital ambiguity at birth or late onset.
- Psychosexual development is influenced by multiple factors such as exposure to androgens, sex chromosome genes, as well as social circumstance and family dynamics.
- Incidence of genital ambiguity is 1/4500 although some degree of male undervirilization or female virilization may be present in as many as 2% of live births.

History

- **Obstetric history:** any evidence of endocrine disturbance during pregnancy. History of maternal virilization may suggest a maternal androgen secreting tumour or aromatase deficiency. Use of any drugs in pregnancy that may cause virilization of a female fetus.
- **Previous neonatal deaths** (which might suggest an undiagnosed adrenal crisis).
- **Family history:**
  * Whether the parents are consanguineous (increased risk of autosomal recessive condition).
  * History of genital ambiguity, abnormal pubertal development, or infertility (X-linked recessive condition such as androgen insensitivity).
- **Gestation of the baby** – in preterm girls, the clitoris and labia minora are relatively prominent; in boys, the testes are usually undescended until about 34 weeks' gestation.

General physical examination

- Any dysmorphic features (syndromes associated with ambiguous genitalia).
- Hypoglycaemia – cortisol deficiency secondary to hypothalamic, pituitary or adrenocortical insufficiency.
- State of hydration and BP – as various forms of CAH can be associated with differing degrees of salt loss or hypertension. Although the cardiovascular collapse with salt loss and hyperkalaemia in CAH does not usually occur until between the 4th and 15th day of life, it should be anticipated until CAH has been excluded.
- Jaundice (both conjugated and unconjugated) may be caused by concomitant thyroid hormone or cortisol deficiency.
- Urine for protein as a screen for any associated renal anomaly.
- Hyperpigmentation, especially of the genital skin and nipples, occurs in the presence of excessive ACTH and pro-opiomelanocortin, and may be apparent in CAH.

Nomenclature

- **International Consensus Conference 2006 nomenclature:**
  * Male pseudohermaphrodite, undervirilization/undermasculinization of XY male – 46,XY DSD.
  * Female pseudohermaphrodite, overvirilization/masculinization of XX female – 46,XX DSD.
  * True hermaphrodite – ovotesticular DSD.
  * XX male or XX sex reversal – 46,XX testicular DSD.
  * XY sex reversal – 46,XY complete gonadal dysgenesis.

Features that suggest DSD

- **Most causes of DSD are recognized in the neonatal period:**
  * Overt genital ambiguity.
  * Apparent female genitalia with an enlarged clitoris, posterior labial fusion, or an inguinal/labial mass.
  * Apparent male genitalia with bilateral undescended testes in a full-term infant, micropenis; isolated perineal hypospadias; mild hypospadias with undescended testis; hypospadias associated with separation of the scrotal sacs.
  * Discordance between genital appearance and a prenatal karyotype.
- **Later presentations in older children and young adults include:**
  * Previously unrecognized genital ambiguity.
  * Inguinal hernia in a female.   * Virilization in a female.
  * Delayed or incomplete puberty.   * Primary amenorrhoea.
  * Breast development in a male.   * Gross and occasionally cyclic haematuria in a male.

Examination of external genitalia

- Whether **gonads** are palpable and the degree of virilization.
- **Gonads** – if both gonads are palpable, they are likely to be testes (or ovotestes), which may be normal or dysgenetic. They may be situated high in the inguinal canal, so careful examination is required.
- **Penis** – assess length of the phallus. A well-developed phallus indicates that significant levels of circulating testosterone were present in utero.
- **Chordee** – this may decrease the apparent length of the phallus, and the penis may be buried in some cases.
- **Urethral meatus** – check for presence of hypospadias and the position of the urethral meatus.
- Note degree of fusion and rugosity of the **labioscrotal folds** and the presence or absence of a separate vaginal opening.

Development and sexual differentiation

The urogenital ridge develops from the mesonephros, which also contains the cells that are the precursors for follicular or Sertoli cells and steroid-producing theca and Leydig cells.

At about 4 weeks after fertilization, primordial germ cells migrate from the yolk sac wall to the urogenital ridge.

Development of the fetal adrenals and gonads occur in parallel; the potential steroidogenic cells of both originate from the mesonephros.

The undifferentiated gonads form on the genital ridges and are capable of developing into either an ovary or a testis.

The theory of the 'default' programme generating an ovary is probably not correct, although the exact role of 'ovarian-determining' genes is unclear at present.

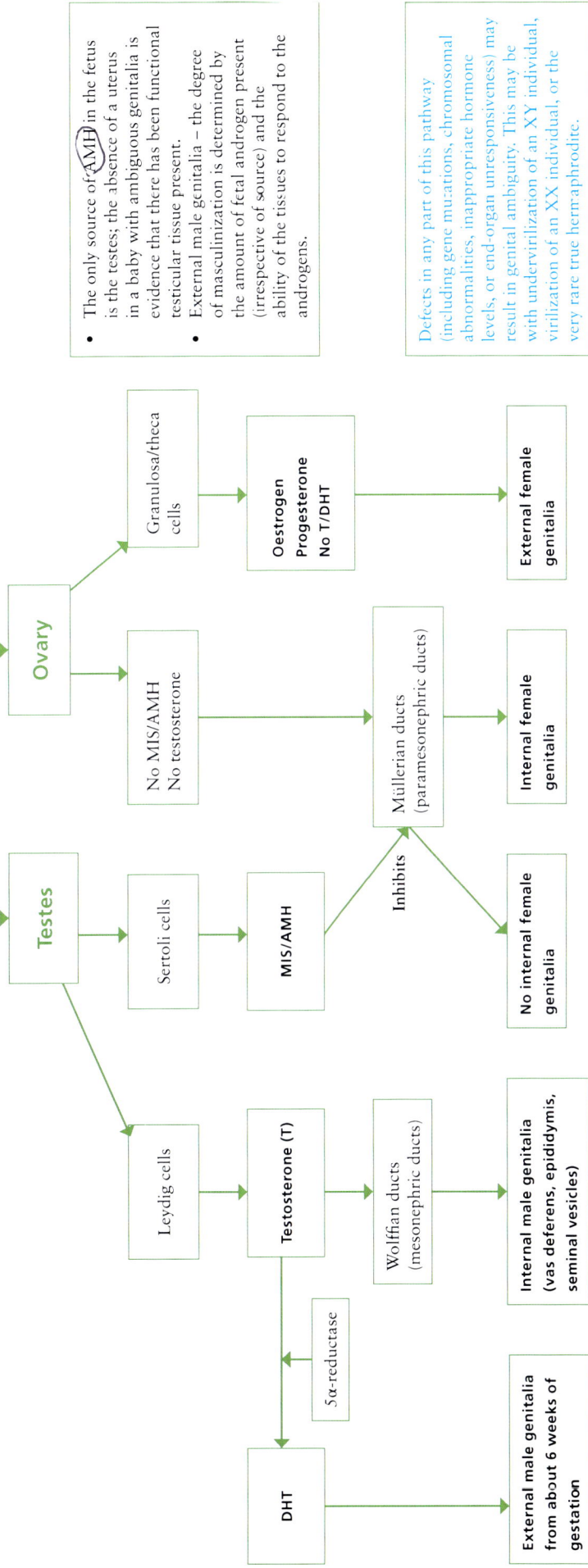

Testicular development is an active process – requires expression of primary testis-determining gene SRY (on Y chromosome).

- The only source of AMH in the fetus is the testes; the absence of a uterus in a baby with ambiguous genitalia is evidence that there has been functional testicular tissue present.
- External male genitalia – the degree of masculinization is determined by the amount of fetal androgen present (irrespective of source) and the ability of the tissues to respond to the androgens.

Defects in any part of this pathway (including gene mutations, chromosomal abnormalities, inappropriate hormone levels, or end-organ unresponsiveness) may result in genital ambiguity. This may be with undervirilization of an XY individual, virilization of an XX individual, or the very rare true hermaphrodite.

Ovary

Granulosa/theca cells

Oestrogen
Progesterone
No T/DHT

External female genitalia

No MIS/AMH
No testosterone

Müllerian ducts (paramesonephric ducts)

Internal female genitalia

Testes

Sertoli cells

MIS/AMH

Inhibits

No internal female genitalia

Leydig cells

Testosterone (T)

Wolffian ducts (mesonephric ducts)

Internal male genitalia (vas deferens, epididymis, seminal vesicles)

5α-reductase

DHT

External male genitalia from about 6 weeks of gestation

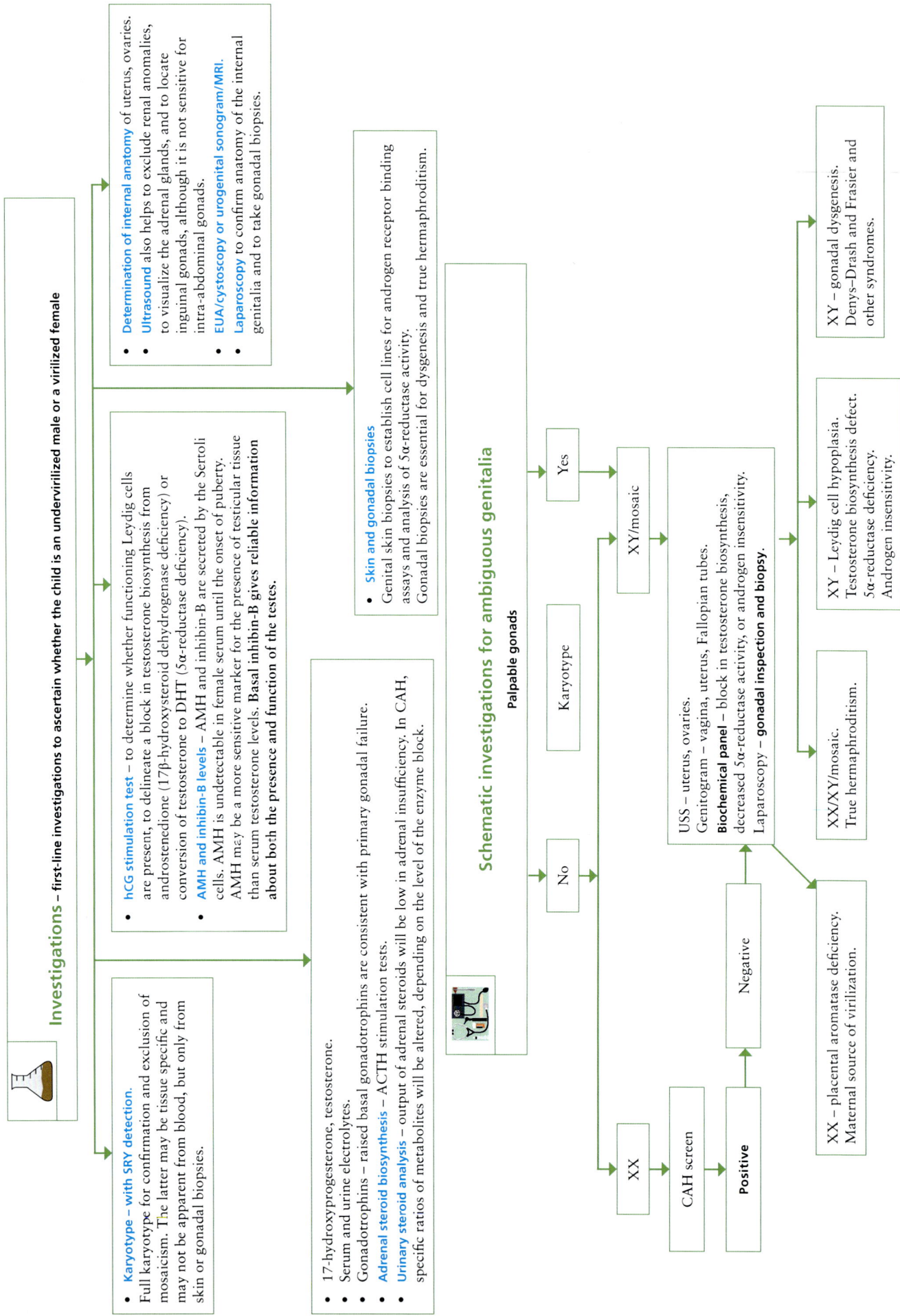

Investigations – first-line investigations to ascertain whether the child is an undervirilized male or a virilized female

- **Karyotype – with SRY detection.**
  Full karyotype for confirmation and exclusion of mosaicism. The latter may be tissue specific and may not be apparent from blood, but only from skin or gonadal biopsies.

- **hCG stimulation test** – to determine whether functioning Leydig cells are present, to delineate a block in testosterone biosynthesis from androstenedione (17β-hydroxysteroid dehydrogenase deficiency) or conversion of testosterone to DHT (5α-reductase deficiency).

- **AMH and inhibin-B levels** – AMH and inhibin-B are secreted by the Sertoli cells. AMH is undetectable in female serum until the onset of puberty. AMH may be a more sensitive marker for the presence of testicular tissue than serum testosterone levels. **Basal inhibin-B gives reliable information about both the presence and function of the testes.**

- 17-hydroxyprogesterone, testosterone.
- Serum and urine electrolytes.
- Gonadotrophins – raised basal gonadotrophins are consistent with primary gonadal failure.
- **Adrenal steroid biosynthesis** – ACTH stimulation tests.
- **Urinary steroid analysis** – output of adrenal steroids will be low in adrenal insufficiency. In CAH, specific ratios of metabolites will be altered, depending on the level of the enzyme block.

- **Determination of internal anatomy** of uterus, ovaries. **Ultrasound** also helps to exclude renal anomalies, to visualize the adrenal glands, and to locate inguinal gonads, although it is not sensitive for intra-abdominal gonads.

- **EUA/cystoscopy or urogenital sonogram/MRI.**
- **Laparoscopy** to confirm anatomy of the internal genitalia and to take gonadal biopsies.

- **Skin and gonadal biopsies**
  Genital skin biopsies to establish cell lines for androgen receptor binding assays and analysis of 5α-reductase activity. Gonadal biopsies are essential for dysgenesis and true hermaphroditism.

Schematic investigations for ambiguous genitalia

Palpable gonads

No → Karyotype

Yes → XY/mosaic

XX

CAH screen

Positive

Negative

XX – placental aromatase deficiency. Maternal source of virilization.

USS – uterus, ovaries. Genitogram – vagina, uterus, Fallopian tubes. **Biochemical panel** – block in testosterone biosynthesis, decreased 5α-reductase activity, or androgen insensitivity. Laparoscopy – **gonadal inspection and biopsy.**

XX/XY/mosaic. True hermaphroditism.

XY – Leydig cell hypoplasia. Testosterone biosynthesis defect. 5α-reductase deficiency. Androgen insensitivity.

XY – gonadal dysgenesis. Denys–Drash and Frasier and other syndromes.

Differential diagnosis according to gonadal histology

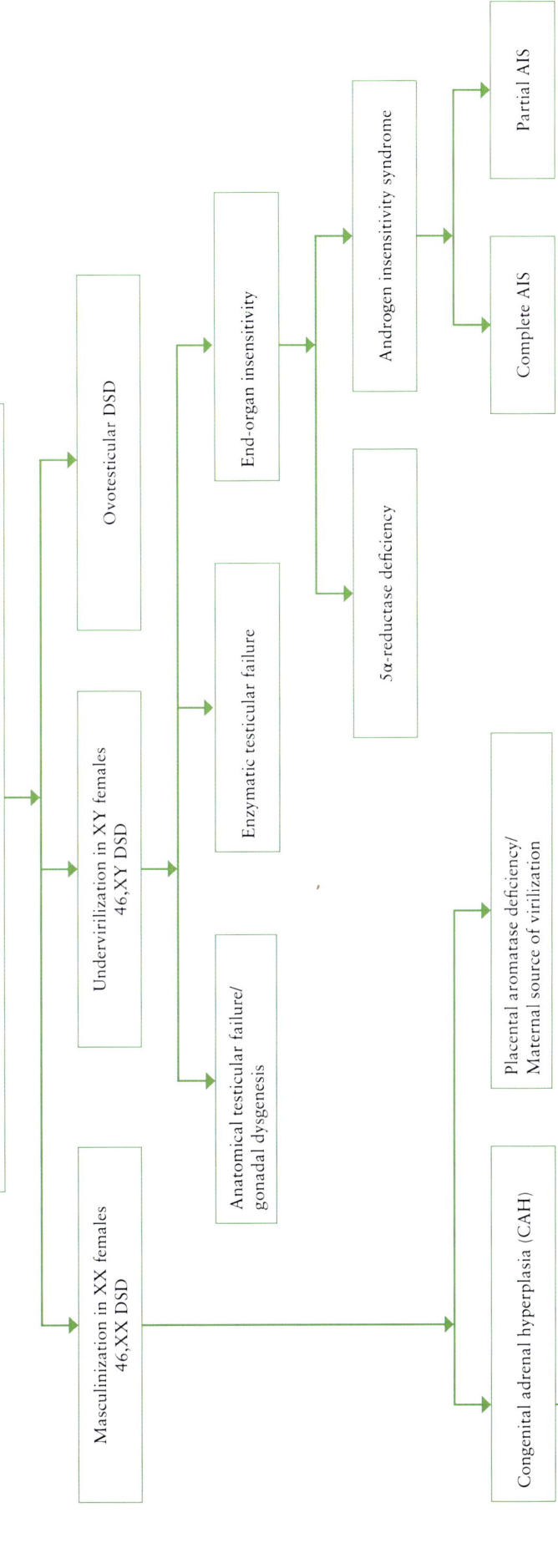

DDx

Differential diagnosis according to gonadal histology

- Masculinization in XX females 46,XX DSD
  - Congenital adrenal hyperplasia (CAH)
    - Classical
    - Late onset
  - Placental aromatase deficiency/Maternal source of virilization

- Undervirilization in XY females 46,XY DSD
  - Anatomical testicular failure/gonadal dysgenesis
  - Enzymatic testicular failure
    - 5α-reductase deficiency
  - End-organ insensitivity
    - Androgen insensitivity syndrome
      - Complete AIS
      - Partial AIS

- Ovotesticular DSD

Differential diagnosis of ambiguous genitalia

(according to gonadal histology – AAP)

- Ovary:
  - CAH.
  - Placental aromatase deficiency.
  - Maternal source of virilization.
- Testis:
  - Leydig cell hypoplasia.
  - Testosterone biosynthesis defect.
  - 5α-reductase deficiency.
  - Androgen insensitivity.
- Ovary and testis:
  - True hermaphroditism.
- Dysgenetic gonads:
  - Gonadal dysgenesis.
  - Denys–Drash and Frasier syndromes.
  - Smith–Lemli–Opitz syndrome.
  - Camptomelic dwarfism.

CHAPTER 13 Disorders of sexual development

Rx Management

General concepts of care

- Tertiary centre (MDT) – paediatric subspecialists in endocrinology, surgery, urology, genetics, neonatology, psychology/ psychiatry, gynaecology, nursing, and medical ethics.
- Psychosocial management to promote positive adaptation.

Risk of gonadal tumour

- Germ cell malignancy only occurs in patients who have Y-chromosomal material.
- Highest risk (up to 60%) is in patients with gonadal dysgenesis and partial AIS with intra-abdominal gonads. Remove intra-abdominal gonads of high-risk patients at diagnosis.
- Lowest risk (< 5%) is found in ovotestis and genetically confirmed CAIS.
- Perform gonadal biopsy at puberty in patients with DSD raised as males with scrotal gonads.

Gender assignment in newborns

- Avoid gender assignment before expert evaluation of newborn. However, it should be made as quickly as thorough diagnostic evaluation permits.
- Factors that influence gender assignment – diagnosis, genital appearance, therapeutic options, need for lifelong replacement therapy, potential for fertility, views of the family, and sometimes circumstances relating to cultural practices.
- Recommendations are to raise infants with
  * 46,XY CAIS and 46,XX CAH as females.
  * 5α-reductase or 17-hydroxysteroid dehydrogenase-3 deficiency as males.

Sex-steroid replacement

- Hypogonadism is common in patients with dysgenetic gonads, defects in sex-steroid biosynthesis, and resistance to androgens.
- Hormonal induction of puberty to induce secondary sexual characteristics, pubertal growth spurt, and optimal bone mineral accumulation.
- Route – IM depot injections, oral, and transdermal.
- PAIS may need supra-physiological doses of testosterone for optimal effect.
- Females with hypogonadism – supplement oestrogen to induce pubertal changes and menses. Add a progestin after breakthrough bleeding develops or within 1–2 years of continuous oestrogen.

Surgical management

- Emphasis is on functional outcome rather than a cosmetic appearance. Rationale for early reconstruction includes beneficial effects of oestrogen on infant tissues, avoiding complications from anatomical anomalies, minimizing family concern and distress, and mitigating the risks of stigmatization and gender-identity confusion of atypical genital appearance.
- However, surgical reconstruction in infancy might need to be refined at the time of puberty.

Masculinizing genital surgery:

- Involves more surgical procedures and difficulties than feminizing genitoplasty.
- Repair involving hypospadias includes chordee correction, urethral reconstruction, and testosterone supplementation.
- If needed, adult-sized testicular prostheses can be inserted after sufficient pubertal scrotal development.

Feminizing genital surgery:

- External genitalia reconstruction and vaginal exteriorization, with early separation of the vagina and urethra.
- Consider clitoral reduction in severe virilization, and perform in conjunction with common urogenital sinus repair.
- Do not advise vaginal dilatation during childhood. Perform vaginoplasty in the teenage years; it has potential for scarring that would require modification before sexual function.

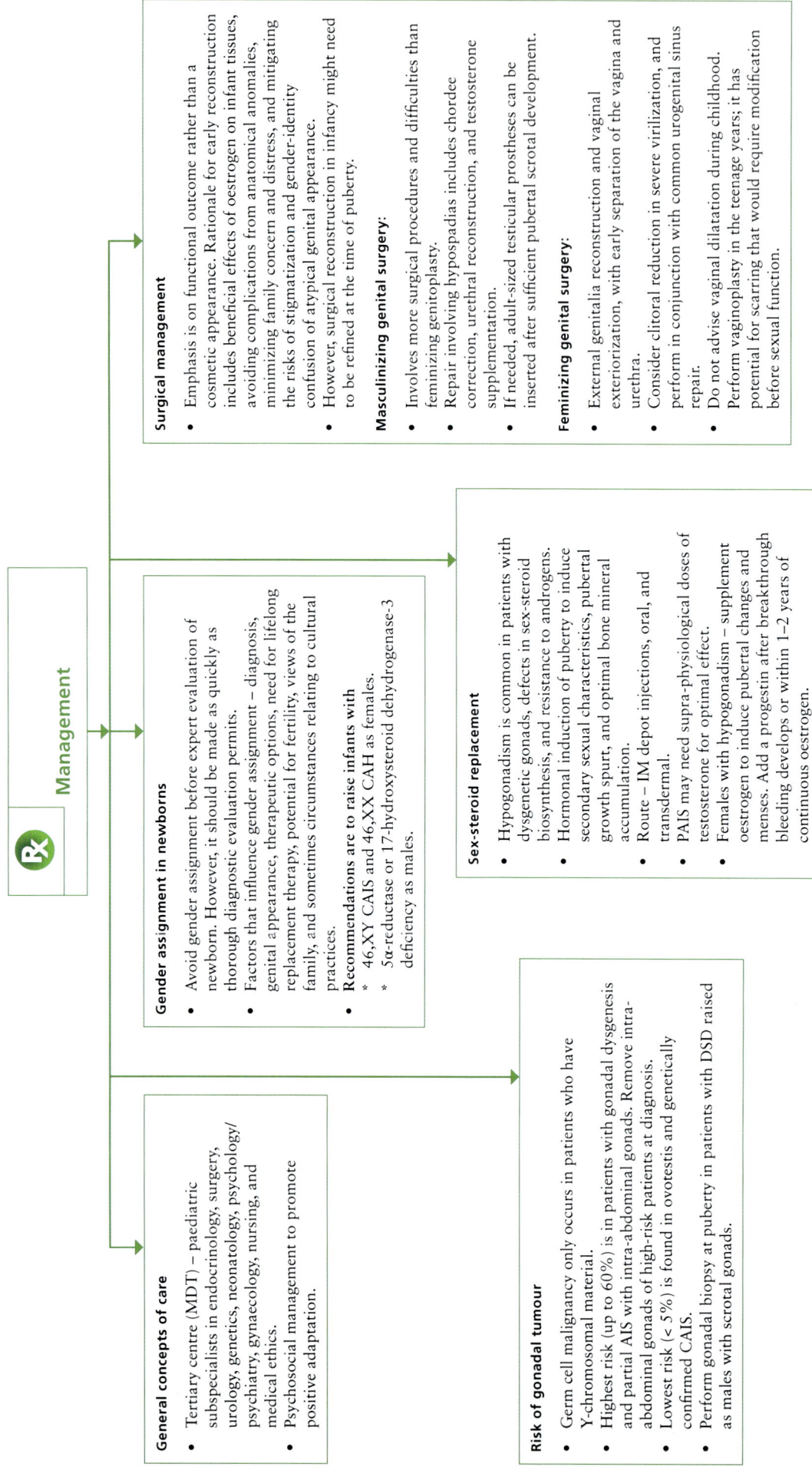

Fertility – females with an adequately formed uterus and males with evidence of functional seminiferous tubules may have fertility potential with assisted-reproduction techniques.
- Fertility-potential considerations include:
  * Expected fertility in virilized females with a well-developed uterus and ovaries.
  * Unlikely fertility in undermasculinized males without assisted-reproduction techniques.
  * Fertility in some patients with ovotesticular DSD.

Congenital adrenal hyperplasia

- Most common cause of female DSD.
- Autosomal recessive.
- Enzyme deficiency related to the biosynthesis of cortisol and aldosterone.
- Severe enzyme deficiency – ambiguous genitalia in the newborn due to virilization.
- Partial enzyme deficiency – presents in adolescence with virilization in the female and (precocious puberty in the male).

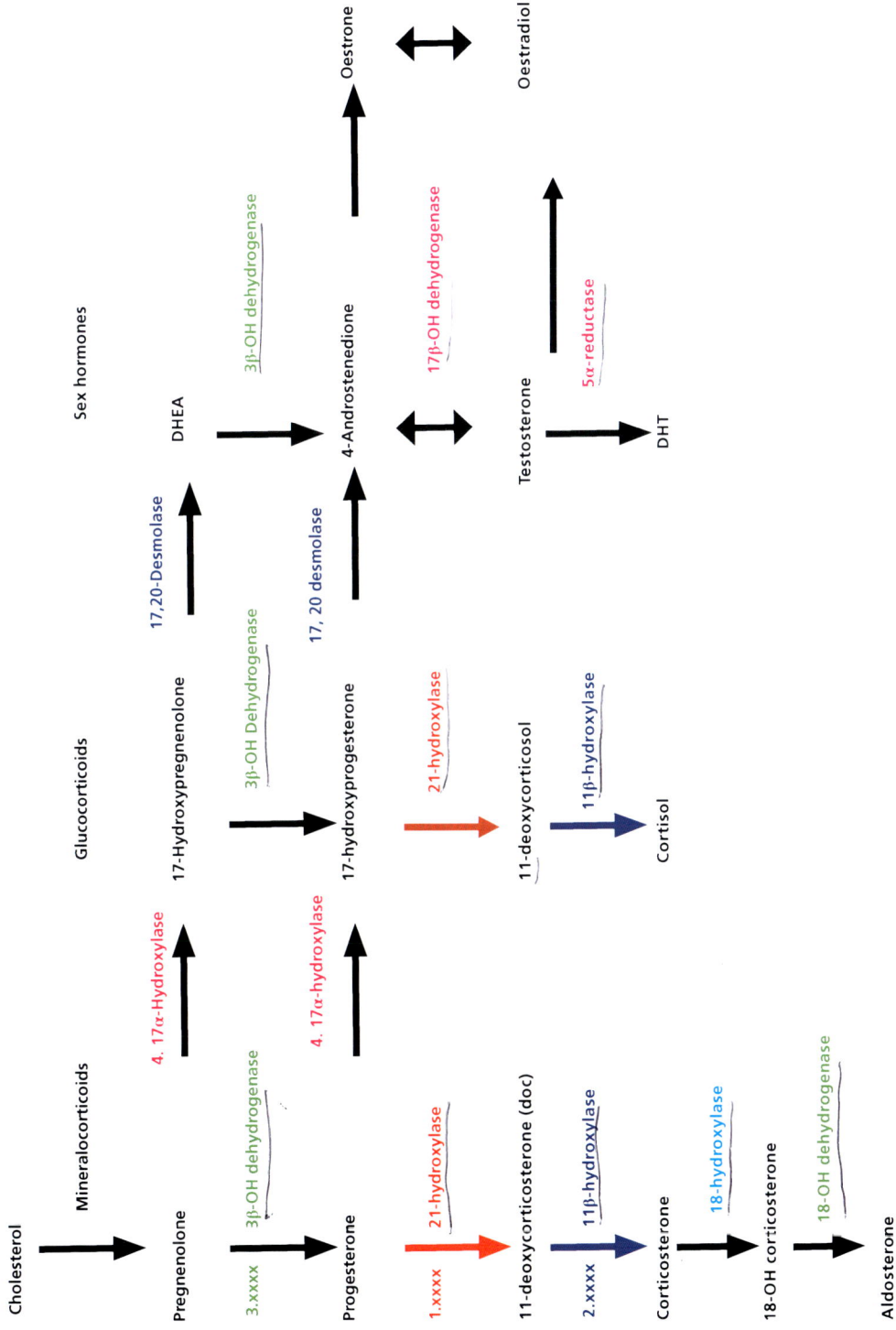

Cholesterol

Mineralocorticoids   Glucocorticoids   Sex hormones

Pregnenolone → (4. 17α-Hydroxylase) → 17-Hydroxypregnenolone → (17,20-Desmolase) → DHEA → (3β-OH dehydrogenase) → Oestrone

Progesterone → (4. 17α-hydroxylase) → 17-hydroxyprogesterone → (17, 20 desmolase) → 4-Androstenedione → (17β-OH dehydrogenase) → Testosterone

Oestrone ↔ Oestradiol

4-Androstenedione ↔ Testosterone → (5α-reductase) → DHT

17-hydroxyprogesterone → (21-hydroxylase) → 11-deoxycorticosol → (11β-hydroxylase) → Cortisol

Pregnenolone → (3β-OH dehydrogenase, 3.xxxx) → Progesterone

Progesterone → (21-hydroxylase, 1.xxxx) → 11-deoxycorticosterone (doc) → (11β-hydroxylase, 2.xxxx) → Corticosterone → (18-hydroxylase) → 18-OH corticosterone → (18-OH dehydrogenase) → Aldosterone

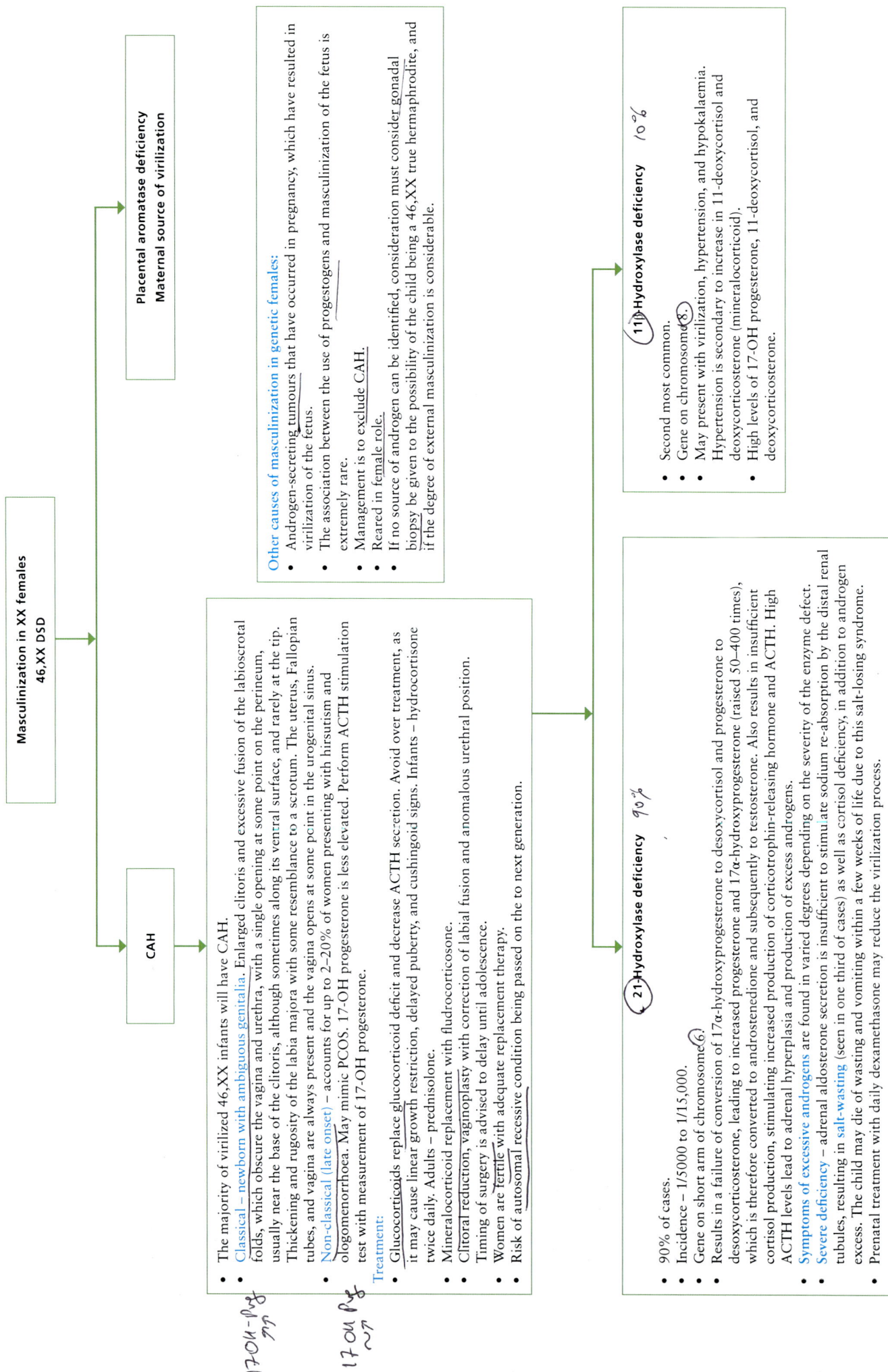

Masculinization in XX females
46,XX DSD

↓

Placental aromatase deficiency
Maternal source of virilization

CAH

- The majority of virilized 46,XX infants will have CAH.
- Classical – newborn with ambiguous genitalia. Enlarged clitoris and excessive fusion of the labioscrotal folds, which obscure the base of the clitoris, although sometimes along its ventral surface, and rarely at the tip. Thickening and rugosity of the labia majora with some resemblance to a scrotum. The uterus, Fallopian tubes, and vagina are always present and the vagina opens at some point in the urogenital sinus.
- Non-classical (late onset) – accounts for up to 2–20% of women presenting with hirsutism and oligomenorrhoea. May mimic PCOS. 17-OH progesterone is less elevated. Perform ACTH stimulation test with measurement of 17-OH progesterone.

Treatment:
- Glucocorticoids replace glucocorticoid deficit and decrease ACTH secretion. Avoid over treatment, as it may cause linear growth restriction, delayed puberty, and cushingoid signs. Infants – hydrocortisone twice daily. Adults – prednisolone.
- Mineralocorticoid replacement with fludrocorticosone.
- Clitoral reduction, vaginoplasty with correction of labial fusion and anomalous urethral position.
- Timing of surgery is advised to delay until adolescence.
- Women are fertile with adequate replacement therapy.
- Risk of autosomal recessive condition being passed on the to next generation.

Other causes of masculinization in genetic females:
- Androgen-secreting tumours that have occurred in pregnancy, which have resulted in virilization of the fetus.
- The association between the use of progestogens and masculinization of the fetus is extremely rare.
- Management is to exclude CAH.
- Reared in female role.
- If no source of androgen can be identified, consideration must consider gonadal biopsy be given to the possibility of the child being a 46,XX true hermaphrodite, and if the degree of external masculinization is considerable.

21-Hydroxylase deficiency 90%

- 90% of cases.
- Incidence – 1/5000 to 1/15,000.
- Gene on short arm of chromosome 6.
- Results in a failure of conversion of 17α-hydroxyprogesterone to desoxycortisol and progesterone to desoxycorticosterone, leading to increased progesterone and 17α-hydroxyprogesterone (raised 50–400 times), which is therefore converted to androstendione and subsequently to testosterone. Also results in insufficient cortisol production, stimulating increased production of corticotrophin-releasing hormone and ACTH. High ACTH levels lead to adrenal hyperplasia and production of excess androgens.
- Symptoms of excessive androgens are found in varied degrees depending on the severity of the enzyme defect.
- Severe deficiency – adrenal aldosterone secretion is insufficient to stimulate sodium re-absorption by the distal renal tubules, resulting in salt-wasting (seen in one third of cases) as well as cortisol deficiency, in addition to androgen excess. The child may die of wasting and vomiting within a few weeks of life due to this salt-losing syndrome.
- Prenatal treatment with daily dexamethasone may reduce the virilization process.

11-Hydroxylase deficiency 10%

- Second most common.
- Gene on chromosome 8.
- May present with virilization, hypertension, and hypokalaemia. Hypertension is secondary to increase in 11-deoxycortisol and deoxycorticosterone (mineralocorticoid).
- High levels of 17-OH progesterone, 11-deoxycortisol, and deoxycorticosterone.

Undervirilization in XY females
46,XY DSD

End-organ insensitivity

Enzymatic testicular failure

- A number of biosynthetic defects can occur at each stage of the testosterone biosynthesis process.
- Clinical features are varied, but as such enzyme defects are incomplete generally, there is external genital ambiguity of varying degree.
- Uterus, Fallopian tubes, and upper vagina are absent as the production of MIS is normal.
- Decision on the sex of rearing depends on the degree of masculinization of the external genitalia but the female role is often chosen.
- hCG stimulation with measurement of various androgens helps to determine the site of the enzyme block.

Gonadal dysgenesis/anatomical testicular failure

- Failure of normal testicular differentiation and development may be the result of a chromosome mosaicism affecting the sex chromosomes but usually the sex chromosomes appear to be normal.
- Most patients have mild masculinization or none at all and, generally, the uterus, Fallopian tubes, and vagina are present.
- Degree of masculinization is often minimal and is limited to a minor clitoral enlargement with little or no fusion of the genital folds. Generally does not need surgery.
- Risk of malignancy in the rudimentary testes is about 30%, therefore gonadal removal during childhood is recommended.
- Around the age of puberty, replace oestrogen–progestogen therapy to induce secondary sexual development and menstruation.

Androgen insensitivity

- Incidence 1/60,000 male births.
- X-linked recessive.
- Karyotype – 46,XY.
- Testosterone levels are normal, but there is insensitivity to secreted androgens owing to complete absence of the gene for the androgen receptor or to mutations in the gene. The condition may be complete in patients who have an absent androgen receptor or, in some cases, where the androgen receptor mutation is not complete, some receptivity may persist and partial androgenization may occur.
- Patients present at or after puberty, but sometimes may be seen earlier in childhood if the defect is incomplete or when a testis is found to occupy a hernial sac.

Complete androgen insensitivity (CAIS):
- Present at or after puberty with primary amenorrhoea despite normal breast development. Absent or scanty pubic and axillary hair, normal vulva but a short blind vagina with no cervix. Antimüllerian factor prevents the development of müllerian structures, therefore no uterus, Fallopian tubes. External genitalia appear female.
- Wolffian structures also fail to develop because of the insensitivity to testosterone.

Partial androgen insensitivity (PAIS): In about 10% of patients the defect is incomplete. The external genitalia may be ambiguous at birth, and virilization may occur before puberty.

Management – depends upon the age at which the patient is seen.
- If seen after puberty when breast development is complete, undertake gonadectomy owing to increased risk of cancer (5%). Provide HRT with oestrogen; need not be cyclical because the uterus is absent.
- If the patient is seen for the first time in childhood, feminization will occur at puberty and nothing needs to be done until that time. If, however, there are heterosexual features, it is very likely that masculinization will occur to some extent at puberty. This will have a profound psychological effect on the patient when she has been brought up in the female role. In these circumstances, advise gonadectomy in childhood and induction of puberty with HRT at the appropriate time.
- Surgery is seldom necessary to elongate the vagina as it is usually functional, but if required, graduated dilatation using Frank's procedure is the treatment of choice.

5α-Reductase deficiency

- Autosomal recessive, history of other affected family members.
- Normal masculinization of the external genitalia requires the conversion of testosterone to dihydrotestosterone by 5α-reductase. The Wolffian structures respond directly to testosterone, therefore internal organs will be male. Uterus, Fallopian tubes, and upper vagina will always be absent because MIS production is normal. There is deficient or absent breast development, yet normal or increased pubic and axillary hair.
- Male infant will have poor masculinization of external genitalia.
- As a rule, the degree of genital masculinization is small or at worst moderate, and most children are initially placed in the female role. At puberty, however, the testes produce increased amounts of testosterone and there is greater virilization.
- Penis size is barely adequate and female gender role is often better.
- Test – hCG stimulation of the gonad – elevated testosterone to DHT ratio.

Phenotypic males with 46,XX karyotype are rarely found. Those who have been appropriately examined have been shown to be H-Y antigen positive and there is little clinical ambiguity in this group, the external genitalia being generally normal, although underdeveloped, and hypospadias may be present.

Isolated deficiency of Müllerian inhibition has also been reported but such cases do not present clinically as examples of doubtful sex, unless some unrelated surgical procedure reveals the surprising presence of Müllerian structures in an otherwise normal or near normal male.

1. Lawson Wilkins Pediatric Endocrine Society and the European Society for Paediatric Endocrinology in collaboration with the participants in the International Consensus Conference on Intersex. Consensus Statement on Management of Intersex Disorders. *Pediatrics* 2006;118(2):e488–e500.

2. American Academy of Pediatrics, Committee on Genetics, Sections on Endocrinology and Urology. Evaluation of the newborn with developmental anomalies of the external genitalia. *Pediatrics* 2000;106(1):138–142.

3. Ogilvy-Stuart AL, Brain CE. Early assessment of ambiguous genitalia. *Arch Dis Child* 2004;89:401–407.

CHAPTER 14 Primary amenorrhoea

Failure to establish menstruation by:

- 16 years of age in girls with normal secondary sexual characteristics (SSC).
- 14 years of age in girls with no secondary sexual characteristics.

History

- Sexual history, exclude pregnancy.
- Cyclical lower abdominal pain – haematocolpos (genital tract malformation).
- Stress, depression, weight loss, disturbance of perception of weight or shape, level of exercise, and chronic systemic illness – hypothalamic dysfunction.
- Headache, visual disturbance, or galactorrhoea – prolactinoma.
- Family history of late menarche – constitutional delay.
- Family history of autoimmune disorders, premature menopause, or genetic anomalies (e.g., androgen insensitivity).
- Medication (such as antipsychotic), previous chemotherapy or radiotherapy, and illicit drug use (opiates and cocaine).

Examination

- Height and weight (BMI).
- Secondary sexual characteristics (Tanner staging).
- Hirsutism, clitoromegaly, virilization, galactorrhoea.
- Signs of thyroid and other endocrine disease.
- External genitalia – haematocolpos.
- Features of Turner's syndrome, androgen insensitivity.
- Pelvic examination – inappropriate in young girls who are not sexually active.

Investigations

- Trans-abdominal USS to assess pelvic anatomy – uterus, ovaries.
- Karyotype.
- Hormonal profile – FSH, LH, prolactin, TSH, testosterone.
- Examination under anaesthesia.
- Bone mineral density.
- CT/MRI of head.

Complications

- Oestrogen deficiency (premature ovarian failure, weight loss, anorexia nervosa, and excessive exercise) – risk of **osteoporosis**. This increased risk persists even if normal menses are resumed.
- Oestrogen deficiency in adolescents – desirable peak bone mass may not be attained.
- Oestrogen deficiency may increase risk of cardiovascular disease.
- Infertility.
- Unpredictable spontaneous ovulation may occur; therefore, contraception is needed.
- Psychological distress – anxiety, altered self-image, and loss of self-esteem.
- Women with a Y-chromosome – increased risk of gonadal tumours. Gonads (residual testes) need removal either at diagnosis or, in women with androgen insensitivity after puberty.

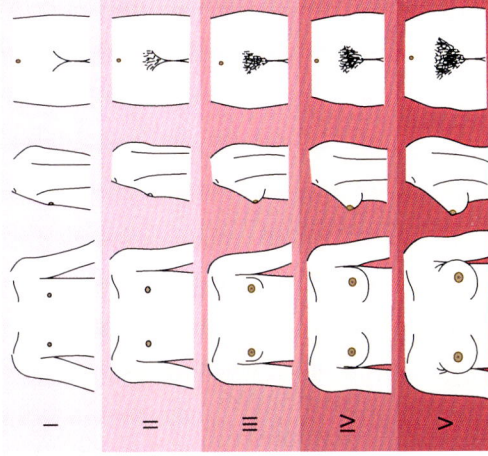

Tanner stages	Breast development	Pubic hair growth
Stage I	Prepubertal.	Prepubertal.
Stage II	Breast buds form.	Few long, downy hairs at the labia majora.
Stage III	Breast buds larger.	Pubic hair growth continues, but mainly central.
Stage IV	Breasts in a 'mound' form.	Pubic hair in the triangular adult shape, but smaller.
Stage V	Breasts fully formed.	Pubic hair adult in shape, quantity, and type, and spread to the inner thighs.

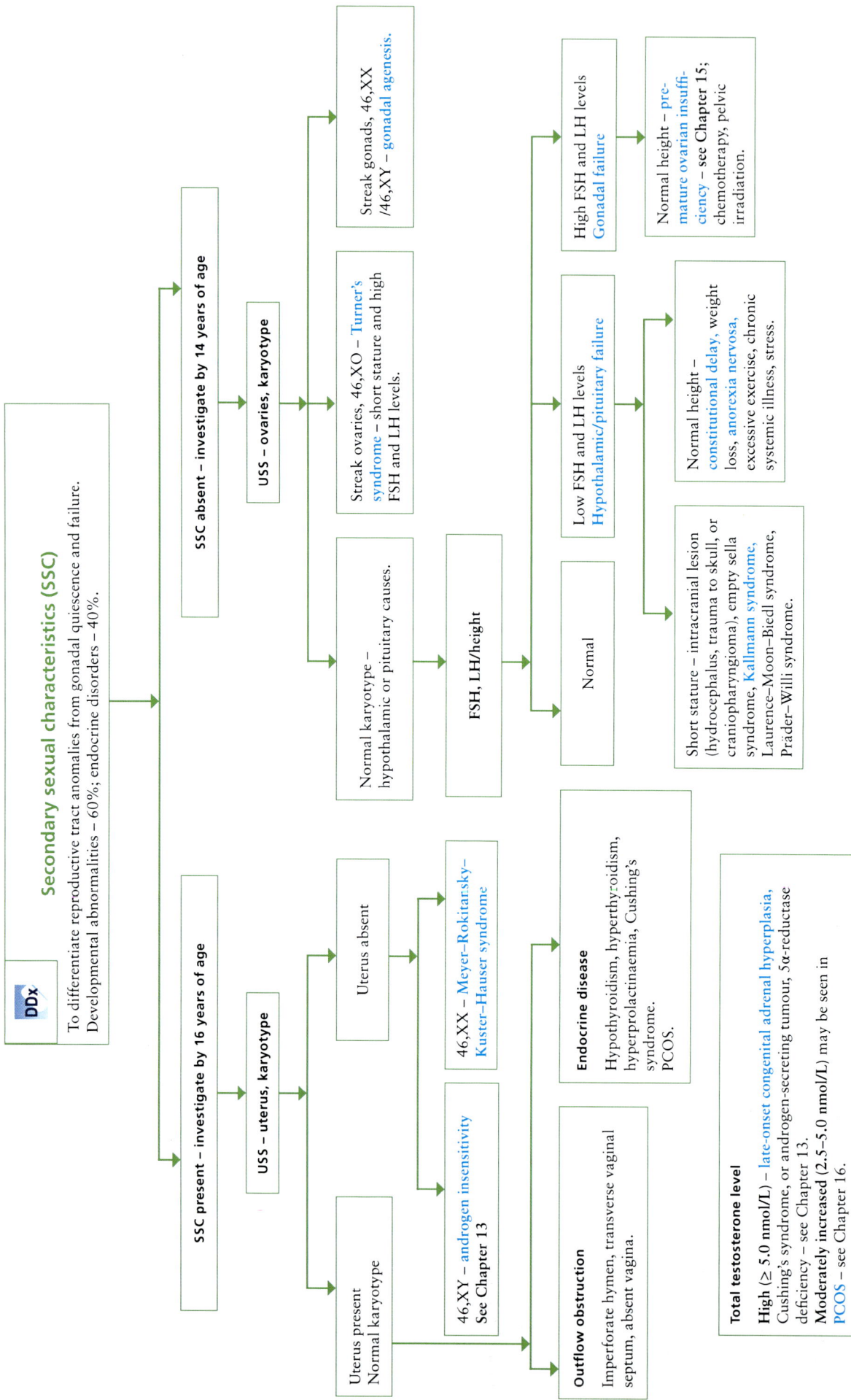

Secondary sexual characteristics (SSC)

DDx

To differentiate reproductive tract anomalies from gonadal quiescence and failure.
Developmental abnormalities – 60%; endocrine disorders – 40%.

SSC present – investigate by 16 years of age

USS – uterus, karyotype

Uterus present
Normal karyotype

46,XY – androgen insensitivity
See Chapter 13

Uterus absent

46,XX – Meyer–Rokitansky–Kuster–Hauser syndrome

Outflow obstruction

Imperforate hymen, transverse vaginal septum, absent vagina.

Endocrine disease

Hypothyroidism, hyperthyroidism, hyperprolactinaemia, Cushing's syndrome.
PCOS.

Total testosterone level

High (≥ 5.0 nmol/L) – late-onset congenital adrenal hyperplasia, Cushing's syndrome, or androgen-secreting tumour, 5α-reductase deficiency – see Chapter 13.
Moderately increased (2.5–5.0 nmol/L) may be seen in PCOS – see Chapter 16.

SSC absent – investigate by 14 years of age

USS – ovaries, karyotype

Streak gonads, 46,XX /46,XY – gonadal agenesis.

Streak ovaries, 46,XO – Turner's syndrome – short stature and high FSH and LH levels.

Normal karyotype – hypothalamic or pituitary causes.

FSH, LH/height

Normal

High FSH and LH levels
Gonadal failure

Normal height – premature ovarian insufficiency – see Chapter 15; chemotherapy, pelvic irradiation.

Low FSH and LH levels
Hypothalamic/pituitary failure

Normal height – constitutional delay, weight loss, anorexia nervosa, excessive exercise, chronic systemic illness, stress.

Short stature – intracranial lesion (hydrocephalus, trauma to skull, or craniopharyngioma), empty sella syndrome, Kallmann syndrome, Laurence–Moon–Biedl syndrome, Präder–Willi syndrome.

Outflow tract obstruction

- Imperforate hymen: * Normal SSC.   * Cyclical lower abdominal pain.
  * Visible haematocolpos with a bulging purple/blue, stretching thin hymen at introitus.
  * USS may show haematometra.
  * Treatment – surgery – simple cruciate incision on the hymen.
- Transverse vaginal septum: * Owing to failure of fusion or canalization between the Müllerian tubercle and sinovaginal bulb.
  * Normal SSC.   * Cyclical lower abdominal pain.
  * Pink bulge at introitus as the septum is thicker than the hymen.
  * Treatment – surgery (risk of annular constriction).

Constitutional delay (physiologically delayed puberty)

- There is no anatomical abnormality, and maturation usually occurs spontaneously by 18 years of age.
- Familial.
- Diagnosis is by exclusion of pathological causes.

Kallman's syndrome

Congenital gonadotrophin deficiency characterized by anosmia and other cranial anomalies.

Mayer–Rokitansky–Kuster–Hauser syndrome

- 46,XX, normal female phenotype.   • Incidence 1/5000 female births.
- Ovarian tissue functions normally, therefore normal SSC.
- Müllerian ducts fail to fuse. Uterine development is rudimentary or absent with uterine remnants. Vaginal agenesis with short and blind ending vagina.
- External genitalia has normal appearance.
- May be associated with renal tract (15–40%) and skeletal anomalies (10–20%).
- Investigations – USS, laparoscopy.
- Treatment: Sexual function – gradual dilatation of vagina (Vecchetti procedure). Surgery to create neovagina – McIndoe vaginoplasty, tissue expansion vaginoplasty, Williams vaginoplasty. Fertility – oocytes retrieval and surrogacy.

Turner's syndrome

- Most common cause of gonadal dysgenesis.
- Pubertal delay.
- 45,XO. Classical features – short stature, webbing of the neck, cubitus valgus, widely spaced nipples, cardiac and renal abnormality, autoimmune hypothyroidism.
- Mosaicism – spontaneous menstruation may occur, but leads to POF.
- Streak gonads.
- Treatment – low-dose oestrogen to promote breast development without affecting linear growth. Cyclical oestrogen and progesterone treatment for maintenance.
- Fertility – egg donation.

Anorexia

- Weight 10–12% less than ideal body weight.
- Growth spurt usually occurs, but SSC are absent.
- Associated features – constipation, hypothermia, cold intolerance, bradycardia, hypotension, lanugo-type hair.
- Low LH, FSH, E2; anaemia; ECG abnormality in 52%, abnormal GTT in 37% of cases.
- Dietary therapy, psychotherapy, antidepressants.
- Oestrogen replacement.

Secondary amenorrhoea

Absence of menstruation for at least 6 consecutive months in women with previously normal and regular menses or for 12 months in women with prior oligomenorrhoea.

History

- History of infertility, contraceptive use.
- Headache, visual disturbances, or galactorrhoea – pituitary tumour.
- Acne and hirsutism – PCOS.
- Weight loss or gain – eating disorders.
- Stress or depression – stress-related hypothalamic amenorrhoea.
- Exercise level – exercise-associated hypothalamic amenorrhoea.
- Symptoms of thyroid and other endocrine disease.
- Menstrual, obstetric, and surgical history such as endometrial curettage – intrauterine adhesions (Asherman's syndrome).
- Hot flushes and vaginal dryness – POI.
- Medical history, including chemotherapy, pelvic radiotherapy – POI.
- Cranial radiotherapy, head injury, or major obstetric haemorrhage – hypopituitarism.
- Medication (such as antipsychotics) and illicit drug use (cocaine and opiates).
- Family history of cessation of menses before 40 years of age – POI.
- Diabetes – associated with PCOS; autoimmune disorders – associated with POI.

Examination

- Measure height and body weight, and calculate BMI.
- Examine for galactorrhoea, if appropriate.
- Signs of excess androgens (hirsutism, acne) or virilization (hirsutism, acne, deep voice, temporal balding, increase in muscle bulk, breast atrophy, and clitoromegaly).
- Acanthosis nigricans (associated with PCOS).
- Signs of thyroid disease.
- Signs of Cushing's syndrome (striae, buffalo hump, significant central obesity, easy bruising, hypertension, and proximal muscle weakness).
- Fundoscopy to assess visual fields if a pituitary tumour is suspected.

Investigations

- FSH, LH, prolactin, TSH.
- Total testosterone and sex hormone-binding globulin.

Evaluate the woman when amenorrhoea has persisted for 3–6 months. This also applies to women with amenorrhoea after stopping the COCs.
Investigate by 6 months after the end of last period. This can be done earlier if it is clinically indicated (e.g. hirsutism) or if the woman is anxious.
Women who are amenorrhoeic after cessation of an injectable progestogen – investigate 9 months after the last injection.
Exclude pregnancy.

FSH, LH, TSH, prolactin, testosterone

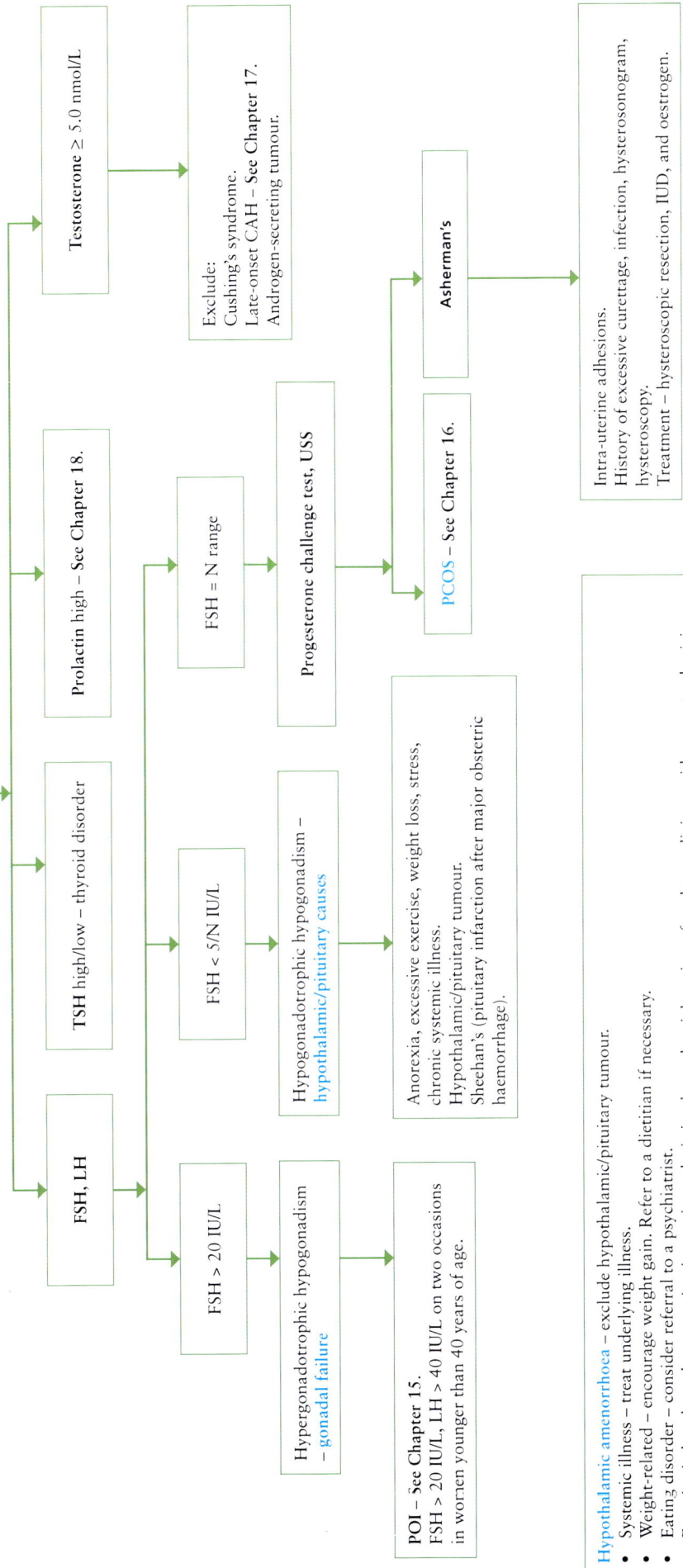

Branches:

FSH, LH

TSH high/low – thyroid disorder

Prolactin high – See Chapter 18.

Testosterone ≥ 5.0 nmol/L
→ Exclude:
Cushing's syndrome.
Late-onset CAH – See Chapter 17.
Androgen-secreting tumour.

From **FSH, LH**:

FSH > 20 IU/L
→ Hypergonadotrophic hypogonadism – gonadal failure
→ POI – See Chapter 15.
FSH > 20 IU/L, LH > 40 IU/L on two occasions in women younger than 40 years of age.

FSH < 5/N IU/L
→ Hypogonadotrophic hypogonadism – hypothalamic/pituitary causes
→ Anorexia, excessive exercise, weight loss, stress, chronic systemic illness.
Hypothalamic/pituitary tumour.
Sheehan's (pituitary infarction after major obstetric haemorrhage).

FSH = N range
→ Progesterone challenge test, USS
→ PCOS – See Chapter 16.

Asherman's
→ Intra-uterine adhesions.
History of excessive curettage, infection, hysterosonogram, hysteroscopy.
Treatment – hysteroscopic resection, IUD, and oestrogen.

Hypothalamic amenorrhoea – exclude hypothalamic/pituitary tumour.

- Systemic illness – treat underlying illness.
- Weight-related – encourage weight gain. Refer to a dietitian if necessary.
- Eating disorder – consider referral to a psychiatrist.
- Exercise-induced – reduce exercise, increasing calorie intake and weight gain; referral to or liaison with a sports physician.
- Stress-related – consider measures to manage stress and improve coping strategies, such as cognitive behavioural therapy.
- Inform the woman that they are at increased risk of osteoporosis and cardiovascular disease because of low oestrogen levels.

1. The Practice Committee of ASRM. Current evaluation of amenorrhoea. *Fertil Steril* 2006;86:S148–155.
2. Illustration by Michal Komorniczak (Wikipedia). http://en.wikipedia.org/wiki/Tanner_scale#mediaviewer/ File:Tanner_scale-female.svg.

What not to do

- Pelvic examination in young girls who are not sexually active.

CHAPTER 14 Primary amenorrhoea

CHAPTER 15 Premature ovarian insufficiency (POI)

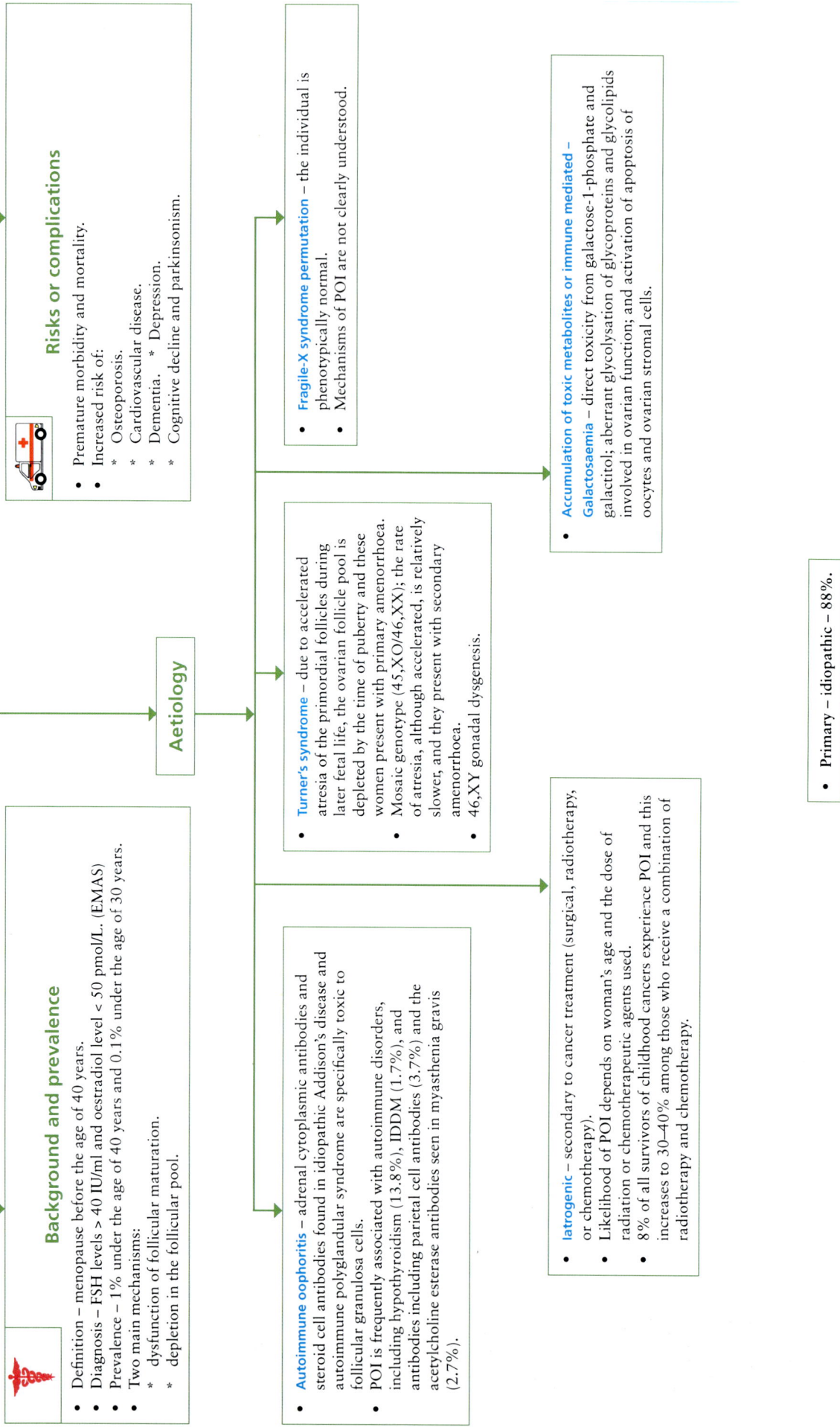

Background and prevalence

- Definition – menopause before the age of 40 years.
- Diagnosis – FSH levels > 40 IU/ml and oestradiol level < 50 pmol/L. (EMAS)
- Prevalence – 1% under the age of 40 years and 0.1% under the age of 30 years.
- Two main mechanisms:
  * dysfunction of follicular maturation.
  * depletion in the follicular pool.

Risks or complications

- Premature morbidity and mortality.
- Increased risk of:
  * Osteoporosis.
  * Cardiovascular disease.
  * Dementia.   * Depression.
  * Cognitive decline and parkinsonism.

Aetiology

- **Autoimmune oophoritis** – adrenal cytoplasmic antibodies and steroid cell antibodies found in idiopathic Addison's disease and autoimmune polyglandular syndrome are specifically toxic to follicular granulosa cells.
- POI is frequently associated with autoimmune disorders, including hypothyroidism (13.8%), IDDM (1.7%), and antibodies including parietal cell antibodies (3.7%) and the acetylcholine esterase antibodies seen in myasthenia gravis (2.7%).

- **Turner's syndrome** – due to accelerated atresia of the primordial follicles during later fetal life, the ovarian follicle pool is depleted by the time of puberty and these women present with primary amenorrhoea. Mosaic genotype (45,XO/46,XX); the rate of atresia, although accelerated, is relatively slower, and they present with secondary amenorrhoea.
- 46,XY gonadal dysgenesis.

- **Iatrogenic** – secondary to cancer treatment (surgical, radiotherapy, or chemotherapy).
- Likelihood of POI depends on woman's age and the dose of radiation or chemotherapeutic agents used.
- 8% of all survivors of childhood cancers experience POI and this increases to 30–40% among those who receive a combination of radiotherapy and chemotherapy.

- **Fragile-X syndrome permutation** – the individual is phenotypically normal. Mechanisms of POI are not clearly understood.

- **Accumulation of toxic metabolites or immune mediated – Galactosaemia** – direct toxicity from galactose-1-phosphate and galactitol; aberrant glycolysation of glycoproteins and glycolipids involved in ovarian function; and activation of apoptosis of oocytes and ovarian stromal cells.

- Primary – idiopathic – 88%.

History

- Amenorrhoea or oligomenorrhoea – most common presentation is secondary amenorrhoea with normal pubertal development. In 20% of cases, there is primary amenorrhoea with pubertal development delay.
- Symptoms of oestrogen deficiency – vasomotor symptoms of hot flushes, night sweats, and loss of libido.
- Past history of chemotherapy, radiotherapy, or pelvic surgery.
- History of autoimmune disorders, including hypothyroidism or adrenal insufficiency.
- Family history of POI (14–31% of cases) and a familial disorder can be identified, e.g., Perrault syndrome (XX gonadal dysgenesis with sensorineural deafness), FSH receptor mutations, and fragile-X permutations.

Examination

- Height, weight, and BMI.
- Any dysmorphic features suggesting a chromosomal or genetic cause.
- Skin for hirsutism, acne, striae, acanthosis nigrans, and vitiligo.

Investigations

To confirm diagnosis

- Serum FSH, LH, and oestradiol. Repeat after 3–4 weeks to confirm diagnosis.
- Endocrine screen for serum prolactin and thyroxine levels.
- If there are signs of hyperandrogenism measure serum DHEA and testosterone.
- USS to assess endometrial thickness, ovarian volume, and antral follicle count.
- A progestogen withdrawal test has less clinical significance because approximately 50% of women with secondary amenorrhoea and 20% with primary amenorrhoea will have withdrawal bleeding. This can give women a sense of reassurance but may be misleading.

Differential diagnosis

DDx

- Diagnose POI by excluding other common causes of primary and secondary amenorrhoea.
- Rule out pregnancy.

Second-line investigations – once the diagnosis of POI is confirmed

- Karyotyping and FMR-1 pre-mutation analysis.
- Screen for autoimmune diseases (anti-adrenal, anti-21-hydroxylase, anti-thyroid peroxidase, and anti-thyroglobulin antibodies).
- Ovarian antibody screen.
- Antimullerian hormone (AMH) to assess ovarian reserve.
- Ovarian biopsy – clinical significance is uncertain, as pregnancy has been reported even when a specimen has shown an absence of follicles.
- Dual-emission X-ray absorptiometry (DEXA) scan for baseline assessment, due to risk of osteopenia.

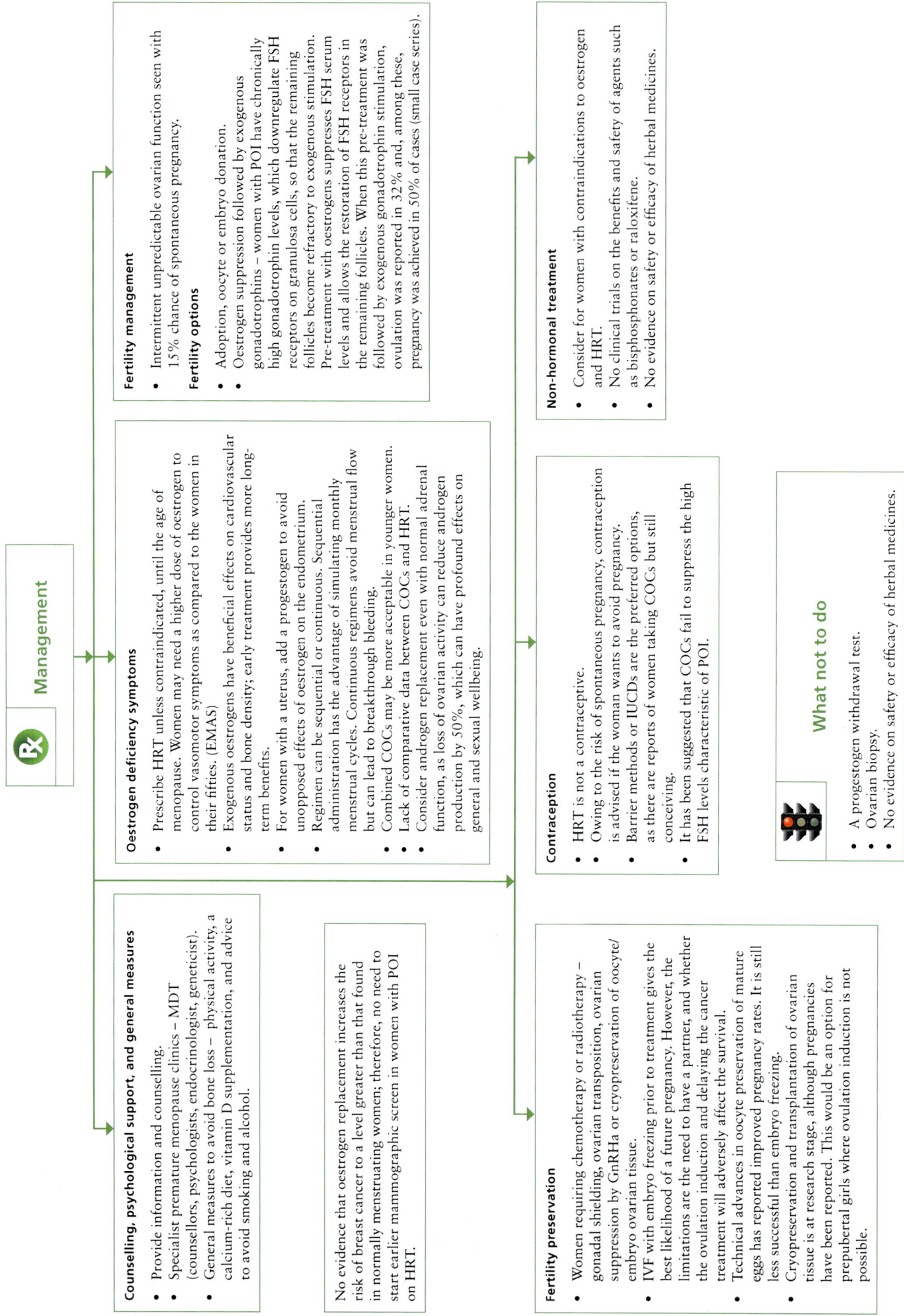

℞ Management

Counselling, psychological support, and general measures

- Provide information and counselling.
- Specialist premature menopause clinics – MDT (counsellors, psychologists, endocrinologist, geneticist).
- General measures to avoid bone loss – physical activity, a calcium-rich diet, vitamin D supplementation, and advice to avoid smoking and alcohol.

No evidence that oestrogen replacement increases the risk of breast cancer to a level greater than that found in normally menstruating women; therefore, no need to start earlier mammographic screen in women with POI on HRT.

Oestrogen deficiency symptoms

- Prescribe HRT unless contraindicated, until the age of menopause. Women may need a higher dose of oestrogen to control vasomotor symptoms as compared to the women in their fifties. (EMAS)
- Exogenous oestrogens have beneficial effects on cardiovascular status and bone density; early treatment provides more long-term benefits.
- For women with a uterus, add a progestogen to avoid unopposed effects of oestrogen on the endometrium. Regimen can be sequential or continuous. Sequential administration has the advantage of simulating monthly menstrual cycles. Continuous regimens avoid menstrual flow but can lead to breakthrough bleeding.
- Combined COCs may be more acceptable in younger women. Lack of comparative data between COCs and HRT.
- Consider androgen replacement even with normal adrenal function, as loss of ovarian activity can reduce androgen production by 50%, which can have profound effects on general and sexual wellbeing.

Fertility preservation

- Women requiring chemotherapy or radiotherapy – gonadal shielding, ovarian transposition, ovarian suppression by GnRHa or cryopreservation of oocyte/ embryo ovarian tissue.
- IVF with embryo freezing prior to treatment gives the best likelihood of a future pregnancy. However, the limitations are the need to have a partner, and whether the ovulation induction and delaying the cancer treatment will adversely affect the survival.
- Technical advances in oocyte preservation of mature eggs has reported improved pregnancy rates. It is still less successful than embryo freezing.
- Cryopreservation and transplantation of ovarian tissue is at research stage, although pregnancies have been reported. This would be an option for prepubertal girls where ovulation induction is not possible.

Fertility management

- Intermittent unpredictable ovarian function seen with 15% chance of spontaneous pregnancy.

Fertility options

- Adoption, oocyte or embryo donation.
- Oestrogen suppression followed by exogenous gonadotrophins – women with POI have chronically high gonadotrophin levels, which downregulate FSH receptors on granulosa cells, so that the remaining follicles become refractory to exogenous stimulation. Pre-treatment with oestrogens suppresses FSH serum levels and allows the restoration of FSH receptors in the remaining follicles. When this pre-treatment was followed by exogenous gonadotrophin stimulation, ovulation was reported in 32% and, among these, pregnancy was achieved in 50% of cases (small case series).

Contraception

- HRT is not a contraceptive.
- Owing to the risk of spontaneous pregnancy, contraception is advised if the woman wants to avoid pregnancy.
- Barrier methods or IUCDs are the preferred options, as there are reports of women taking COCs but still conceiving.
- It has been suggested that COCs fail to suppress the high FSH levels characteristic of POI.

Non-hormonal treatment

- Consider for women with contraindications to oestrogen and HRT.
- No clinical trials on the benefits and safety of agents such as bisphosphonates or raloxifene.
- No evidence on safety or efficacy of herbal medicines.

What not to do

- A progestogen withdrawal test.
- Ovarian biopsy.
- No evidence on safety or efficacy of herbal medicines.

Fragile-X syndrome (FXS)

Background and incidence

- FXS is the most common cause of 'inherited learning difficulty' and the most common known genetic cause of autism.
- X-linked dominant condition.
- Prevalence – full mutation seen in approximately 1/4000 men and 1/8000 women.
- Women carriers – about 1/154 if no family history of 'inherited learning difficulty', developmental problems, or autism; and 1/128 if there is a positive family history.
- Caused by mutations of the FMR-1 (fragile-X mental retardation-1) gene on the X-chromosome. The FMR-1 gene can be present in different allelic sizes. These different sizes correlate with the phenotype and risk of transmission.

- Intermediate fragile-X alleles have a small risk of expansion, estimated to be 6.6%.
- However, no intermediate allele has been reported to expand to a full mutation (FM).
- Carriers of intermediate alleles are not at risk of having an affected child; therefore, do not offer prenatal diagnosis for FXS.

- Permutation (PM) – the FMR-1 gene is active.
- Some PM carriers, primarily males but also females, are at risk of developing late-onset tremor/ataxia syndrome or psychological symptoms.
- Females who are PM carriers may develop POI.
- When a PM allele is transmitted from a carrier mother to her offspring, there is usually an increase in the CGG-repeat size of the mutant allele. Thus, pre-mutation women are at risk of having children with FM.

- Full mutation (FM) – the gene is silenced, and is responsible for the 'inherited learning difficulty'.
- Because males have only one X-chromosome, a male with an FM will always have FXS, but the manifestations vary significantly, even within members of a single family.
- In females who carry an FM, clinical manifestations are even more variable than in males, because they have two X-chromosomes, one of which is inactive. The proportion of the cells with the active X-chromosome carrying the fragile-X mutation determines the clinical manifestations, which cannot be predicted by routine testing.

Fragile-X tremor ataxia syndrome (FXTAS)

- Neurodegenerative disorder occurs in male PM carriers aged > 50 years.
- Prevalence is unclear; 30% of all male carriers might develop FXTAS although many will not present until the 8th decade of life. As the PM is thought to occur in 1/813 men, it could affect a significant percentage of the population.
- Men with the PM do not have the intellectual impairment.
- Progressive cerebellar ataxia and intention tremor, loss of sensation in the lower extremities, and autonomic dysfunction in the form of impotence, faecal and urinary incontinence. Dementia risk increases with increased allele length.
- Female PM carriers have a much lower risk of FXTAS. Women affected by FXTAS, may have additional co-morbidities, such as thyroid disease, hypertension, peripheral neuropathy, and fibromyalgia.

Premature ovarian insufficiency

- Up to 26% of women who are carriers of the PM develop POI, compared with the general population risk of 1%.
- A woman who has POI has a 2–4% risk of being a carrier of the fragile-X PM; this risk rises to 8–15% if there is also a family history of POI.
- There is a non-linear relationship between the number of trinucleotide repeats and the risk of POI. The highest risk occurs with repeats of 59–99. The risk plateaus or even decreases with repeat sizes of > 100.
- Women with the FM do not have an increased risk of POI.
- PM carriers report irregular menses and shorter cycles more frequently.
- There is no validated test for assessing the risk of altered ovarian function in asymptomatic women who carry the PM.

Full mutation – fragile-X syndrome

- Both men and women can be affected. Invariably all males, and some carrier females, present with significant 'learning difficulty' and behavioural problems.
- Women with the syndrome are more mildly affected, possibly as a result of X-chromosome inactivation. They often have a normal or borderline IQ but they are at higher risk of depression, mood lability, and social anxiety compared with the general population.
- Most affected men do not reproduce but it is not known whether this is due to the severity of cognitive difficulty or as a direct effect of the syndrome, which is known to cause macro-orchidism.

- Men – symptoms range from mild learning difficulties to severe intellectual disability and autistic behaviour.
  * Developmental delay – intellectual disability, speech delay.
  * Behavioural features – attention-deficit disorders, autistic features.
  * Medical conditions – epilepsy (20%), mitral valve prolapse, recurrent ear infections, eye problems, e.g., strabismus.
  * Physical characteristics – long face, large prominent ears, high broad forehead, large testicles after puberty.
- Almost all affected men have a degree of learning difficulty.

FXS and screening

- A woman with the FM can reproduce and transmit the mutation to her offspring.
- Identification of an FM or PM would allow counselling about reproductive options.
- Screening for PM in males would indicate a significant risk of being affected by a late-onset neurodegenerative disease.
- Screening for PM in women – FXTAS is less common and less debilitating in women than in men. Identification of a PM indicates a higher risk of POI; therefore, women may try to complete their family early while still young or by using techniques such as oocyte storage.
- Various strategies for screening – there is no evidence as to the efficacy of the different strategies.

Recommendations (SOGC)

- Thorough counselling and informed consent.
- Fragile-X testing (FXT) is indicated for a woman:
  * With a family history of FXS, FXTAS, or POI (in > 1 family member) if the family history indicates that she is at risk of inheriting the mutated gene.
  * Who has a personal history of autism or mental retardation/developmental delay of an unknown aetiology, or who has at least one male relative with these conditions within a three-generation pedigree.
  * Who has reproductive or fertility problems associated with an elevated level of FSH before the age of 40 years.
- Offer prenatal fetal testing via CVS or amniocentesis to women who are confirmed to be carriers of a PM or FM of the FMR-1 gene.
- American College of Medical Genetics – screen women who present with elevated FSH levels, a family history of POI, or have relatives with an undiagnosed learning difficulty.

Reproductive options

Prenatal diagnosis

- Fetal sex testing – cell-free fetal DNA in maternal blood at 9 weeks' gestation.
- CVS or amniocentesis.
- Diagnosis raises difficult ethical questions about TOP.
- PM-carrier fetus:
  * Does a 30% risk of FXTAS in middle age in a male fetus constitute grounds for TOP?
  * Does the risk of POI or FTXAS in a female offspring constitute appropriate grounds for consideration of TOP?
- FM-carrier female fetus – only 50% of females with FM will have a learning disability. It is a difficult decision whether or not to terminate such potentially healthy fetuses?

Pre-implantation genetic diagnosis

- Can be used to allow the selection of embryos without the mutation; however, the molecular techniques applied do not allow distinction between PM and FM.
- Women with PM often have elevated FSH levels and may not respond well to gonadotrophin stimulation, limiting the number of embryos available for selection.

1. EMAS Position Statement. Managing women with premature ovarian failure. *Maturitas* 2010;67(1):91–93.
2. Clinical Knowledge Summaries. http://www.cks.nhs.uk/menopause.
3. Arora P, Polson DW. Diagnosis and management of premature ovarian failure. *The Obstetrician and Gynaecologist* 2011;13:67–72.
4. Genetics Committee of SOGC; Prenatal Diagnosis Committee of CCMG. Fragile X testing in obstetrics and gynaecology in Canada. *J Obstet Gynaecol Can.* 2008;30(9):837–846.
5. Bambang K, Metcalfe K, Newman W, McFarlane T. Fragile X syndrome: an overview. *The Obstetrician and Gynaecologist* 2011;13:92–97.

Prevalence and incidence

- A complex disorder, with clinical manifestation of oligomenorrhoea, hirsutism, and acne, often complicated by chronic anovulatory infertility and hyperandrogenism.
- Prevalence – 6–7%.
- PCOS presents at a younger age, has more severe symptoms, and a higher prevalence in women of South Asian origin.

History

- Symptoms vary widely, with symptoms of hyperandrogenism and severe menstrual disturbances at one end of the spectrum and mild symptoms at the other.
- Symptoms:
  - * Infrequent or no ovulation. * Infertility.
  - * Hirsutism or acne. * Alopecia.
- Family history of PCOS.

Diagnosis

- Rotterdam Criteria – two of the three following criteria is diagnostic:
- Polycystic ovaries (≥ 12 peripheral follicles) or increased ovarian volume (> 10 cm³).
- Oligo- or anovulation.
- Clinical and/or biochemical signs of hyperandrogenism.
- A raised LH/FSH ratio is no longer a diagnostic criterion for PCOS owing to its inconsistency.

Examination

- Women may have indirect evidence of insulin resistance as acanthosis nigricans – skin is dry and rough, with grey–brown pigmentation, palpably thickened and covered by a papillomatous elevation, giving it a velvety texture. The condition commonly affects the axillae, perineum, or extensor surfaces of the elbows and knuckles.
- Obesity – especially central obesity.
- Hirsutism, acne, or alopecia.

Risks and issues

- **Risks** – obesity and higher prevalence of:
  - * Impaired glucose tolerance, type 2 diabetes.
  - * Sleep apnoea.
  - * Adverse cardiovascular risk profile with cardiometabolic syndrome (HT, dyslipidaemia, visceral obesity, insulin resistance, and hyperinsulinaemia).
- **Health issues:**
  - * Irregular menstrual cycles – oligomenorrhea, amenorrhea.
  - * Hirsutism. * Acne.
  - * Subfertility – anovulation.
  - * Long-term health issues.

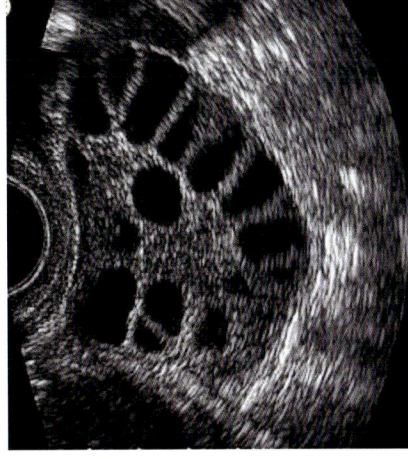

The Androgen Excess and PCOS Society Task Force

PCOS should be defined by two criteria:
- Presence of hyperandrogenism (biochemical or clinical).
- Ovarian dysfunction (oligo- or anovulation or polycystic ovaries).

Pathophysiology

Cause of PCOS is unknown.
Multifactorial – genetic and environmental factors.

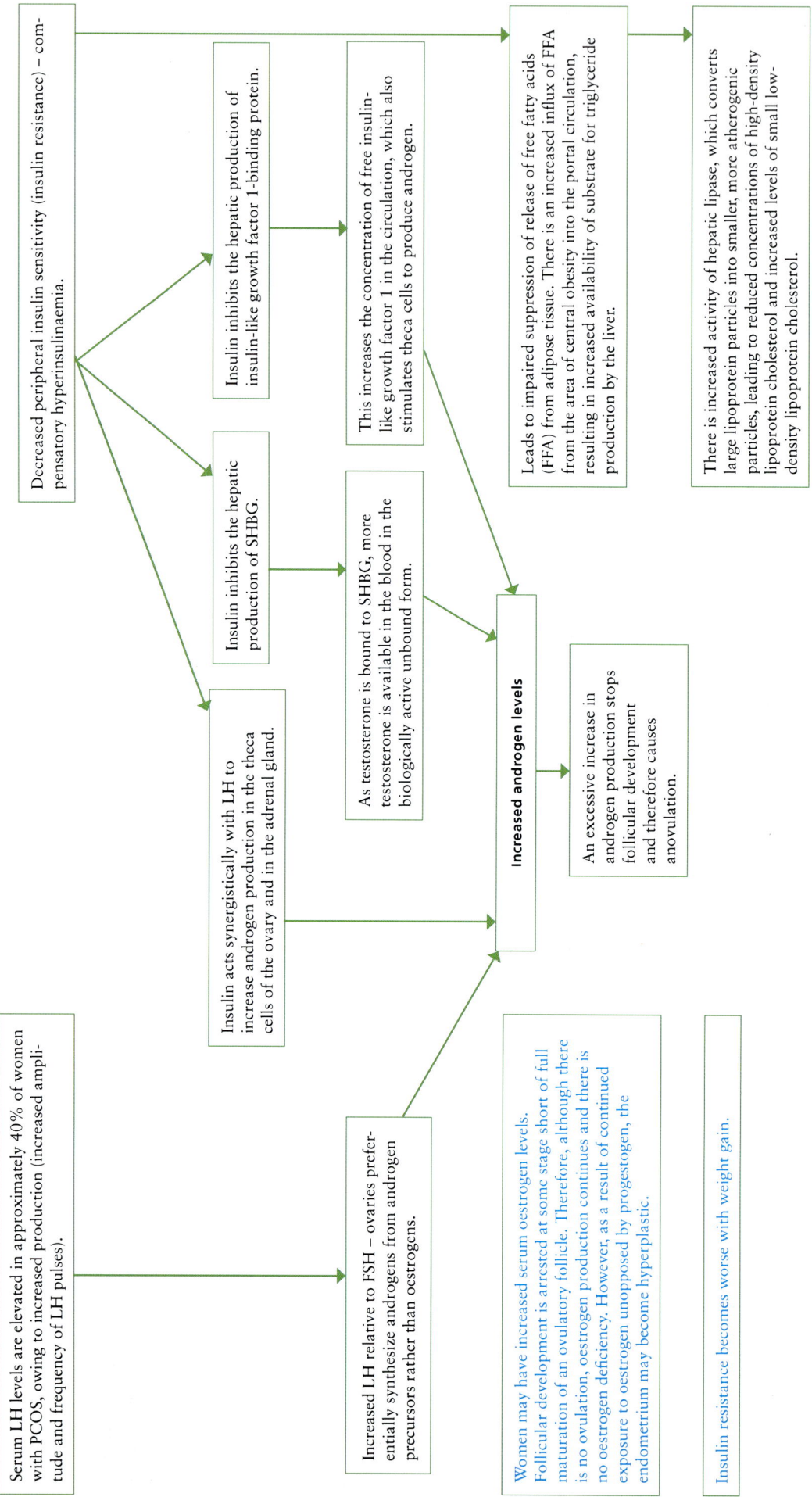

Decreased peripheral insulin sensitivity (insulin resistance) – compensatory hyperinsulinaemia.

Insulin inhibits the hepatic production of insulin-like growth factor 1-binding protein.

This increases the concentration of free insulin-like growth factor 1 in the circulation, which also stimulates theca cells to produce androgen.

Leads to impaired suppression of release of free fatty acids (FFA) from adipose tissue. There is an increased influx of FFA from the area of central obesity into the portal circulation, resulting in increased availability of substrate for triglyceride production by the liver.

There is increased activity of hepatic lipase, which converts large lipoprotein particles into smaller, more atherogenic particles, leading to reduced concentrations of high-density lipoprotein cholesterol and increased levels of small low-density lipoprotein cholesterol.

Insulin inhibits the hepatic production of SHBG.

As testosterone is bound to SHBG, more testosterone is available in the blood in the biologically active unbound form.

Insulin acts synergistically with LH to increase androgen production in the theca cells of the ovary and in the adrenal gland.

Increased androgen levels

An excessive increase in androgen production stops follicular development and therefore causes anovulation.

Serum LH levels are elevated in approximately 40% of women with PCOS, owing to increased production (increased amplitude and frequency of LH pulses).

Increased LH relative to FSH – ovaries preferentially synthesize androgens from androgen precursors rather than oestrogens.

Women may have increased serum oestrogen levels. Follicular development is arrested at some stage short of full maturation of an ovulatory follicle. Therefore, although there is no ovulation, oestrogen production continues and there is no oestrogen deficiency. However, as a result of continued exposure to oestrogen unopposed by progestogen, the endometrium may become hyperplastic.

Insulin resistance becomes worse with weight gain.

Investigations

- Total testosterone – normal to moderately elevated.
- SHBG – normal to low, provides a surrogate measurement of the degree of hyperinsulinaemia.
- Free androgen index (total testosterone/SHBG × 100) – normal or elevated, provides an assessment of physiologically active testosterone. The most sensitive method of assessing hyperandrogenaemia.
- LH, FSH – not needed for the diagnosis of PCOS but essential to rule out other causes of oligomenorrhoea and amenorrhoea. LH/FSH ratios are not useful in diagnosing PCOS because of their inconsistency. LH level may be moderately elevated.
- Prolactin – may be mildly elevated.
- TSH – to rule out thyroid dysfunction.
- USS – to look for the classic picture of polycystic ovaries (PCO – 12 or more follicles in at least one ovary, measuring 2–9 mm in diameter) or increased ovarian volume (> 10 mL). Finding of PCO alone does not establish the diagnosis. Do not measure oestradiol as levels can be normal or low in both PCOS and hypothalamic amenorrhoea.

Differential diagnosis
Signs of hyperandrogenaemia

DDx

Oligomenorrhoea, amenorrhea/hyperandrogenaemia
FSH, LH, TFT, prolactin, testosterone

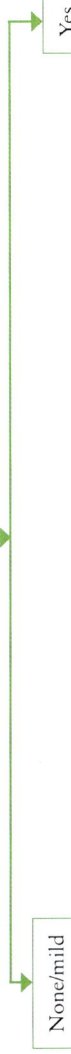

None/mild

Yes

- Total testosterone > 5 nmol/L.
- Check 17-hydroxyprogesterone.

Androgen-secreting tumours, virilizing adrenal or ovarian tumours
- Extremely elevated plasma androgen levels.
- Clitoromegaly, extreme hirsutism, or male pattern alopecia.
- Oligo/amenorrhoea.

Cushing's syndrome
- Elevated 24-hour urinary free cortisol level.
- Hypertension, striae, easy bruising.
- Oligo/amenorrhoea.

- Raised prolactin.
- Hyperprolactinaemia.
- Oligo/amenorrhoea.
- See Chapter 18.

Late-onset congenital adrenal hyperplasia
- Deficiency of 21-hydroxylase.
- Elevated 17-hydroxyprogesterone level in the morning or on stimulation.
- Oligo/amenorrhoea – not often.
- See Chapter 14.

- Raised TSH.
- Hypothyroidism.
- Oligo/amenorrhoea.

- Raised FSH, LH – POI.
- Oligo/amenorrhoea.
- See Chapter 15.

Acromegaly
- Increased plasma insulin-like growth factor level.
- Enlargement of the extremities, coarse features, prognathism.
- Oligo/amenorrhoea – often.

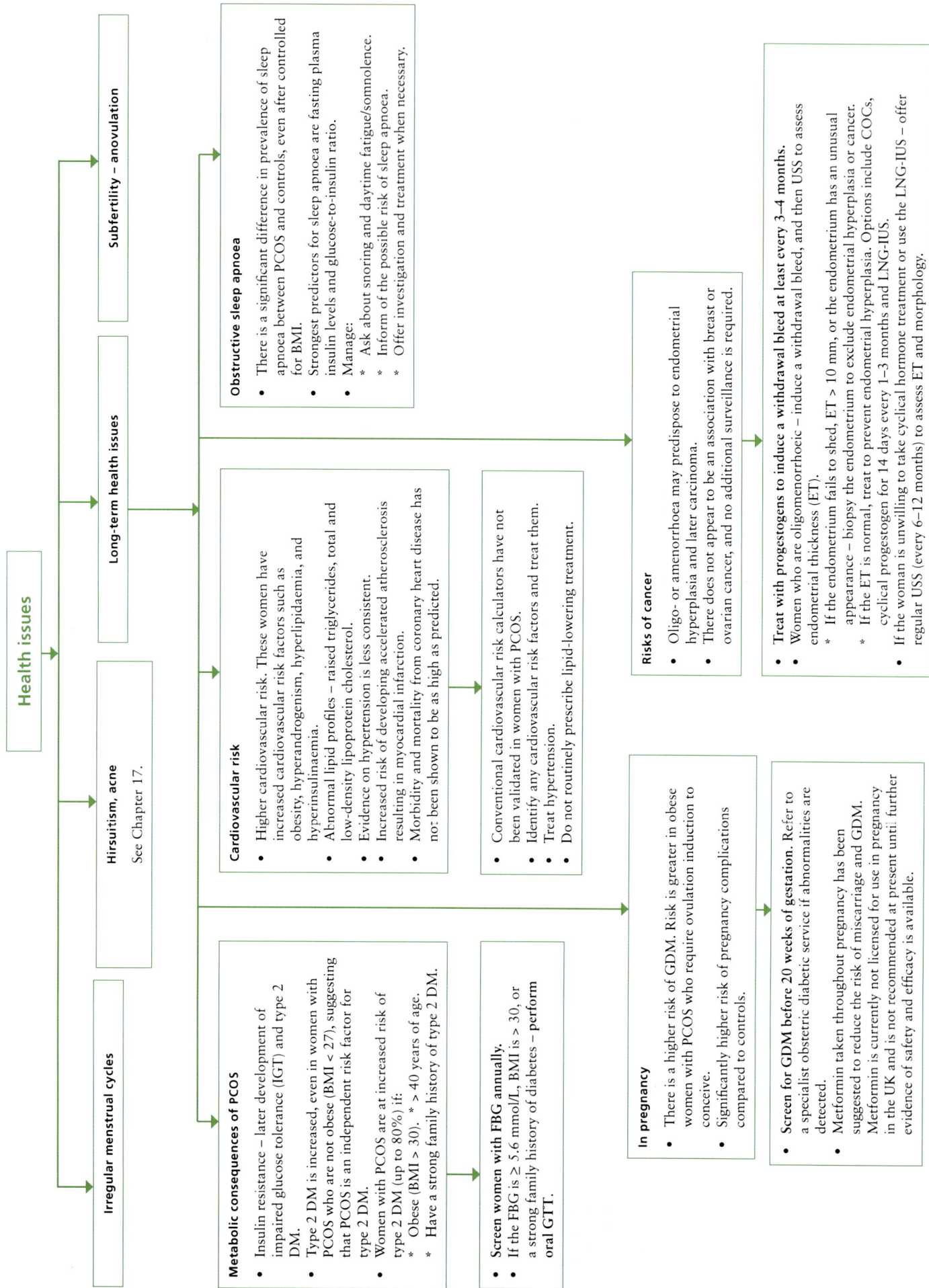

Health issues

Irregular menstrual cycles

Hirsuitism, acne
See Chapter 17.

Long-term health issues

Subfertility – anovulation

Obstructive sleep apnoea

- There is a significant difference in prevalence of sleep apnoea between PCOS and controls, even after controlled for BMI.
- Strongest predictors for sleep apnoea are fasting plasma insulin levels and glucose-to-insulin ratio.
- Manage:
  * Ask about snoring and daytime fatigue/somnolence.
  * Inform of the possible risk of sleep apnoea.
  * Offer investigation and treatment when necessary.

Cardiovascular risk

- Higher cardiovascular risk. These women have increased cardiovascular risk factors such as obesity, hyperandrogenism, hyperlipidaemia, and hyperinsulinaemia.
- Abnormal lipid profiles – raised triglycerides, total and low-density lipoprotein cholesterol.
- Evidence on hypertension is less consistent.
- Increased risk of developing accelerated atherosclerosis resulting in myocardial infarction.
- Morbidity and mortality from coronary heart disease has not been shown to be as high as predicted.

- Conventional cardiovascular risk calculators have not been validated in women with PCOS.
- Identify any cardiovascular risk factors and treat them.
- Treat hypertension.
- Do not routinely prescribe lipid-lowering treatment.

Risks of cancer

- Oligo- or amenorrhoeic may predispose to endometrial hyperplasia and later carcinoma.
- There does not appear to be an association with breast or ovarian cancer, and no additional surveillance is required.

- **Treat with progestogens to induce a withdrawal bleed at least every 3–4 months.**
- Women who are oligomenorrhoeic – induce a withdrawal bleed, and then USS to assess endometrial thickness (ET).
  * If the endometrium fails to shed, ET > 10 mm, or the endometrium has an unusual appearance – biopsy the endometrium to exclude endometrial hyperplasia or cancer.
  * If the ET is normal, treat to prevent endometrial hyperplasia. Options include COCs, cyclical progestogen for 14 days every 1–3 months and LNG-IUS.
- If the woman is unwilling to take cyclical hormone treatment or use the LNG-IUS – offer regular USS (every 6–12 months) to assess ET and morphology.

Metabolic consequences of PCOS

- Insulin resistance – later development of impaired glucose tolerance (IGT) and type 2 DM.
- Type 2 DM is increased, even in women with PCOS who are not obese (BMI < 27), suggesting that PCOS is an independent risk factor for type 2 DM.
- Women with PCOS are at increased risk of type 2 DM (up to 80%) if:
  * Obese (BMI > 30). * > 40 years of age.
  * Have a strong family history of type 2 DM.

- **Screen women with FBG annually.**
- If the FBG is ≥ 5.6 mmol/L, BMI is > 30, or a strong family history of diabetes – **perform oral GTT.**

In pregnancy

- There is a higher risk of GDM. Risk is greater in obese women with PCOS who require ovulation induction to conceive.
- Significantly higher risk of pregnancy complications compared to controls.

- **Screen for GDM before 20 weeks of gestation.** Refer to a specialist obstetric diabetic service if abnormalities are detected.
- Metformin taken throughout pregnancy has been suggested to reduce the risk of miscarriage and GDM. Metformin is currently not licensed for use in pregnancy in the UK and is not recommended at present until further evidence of safety and efficacy is available.

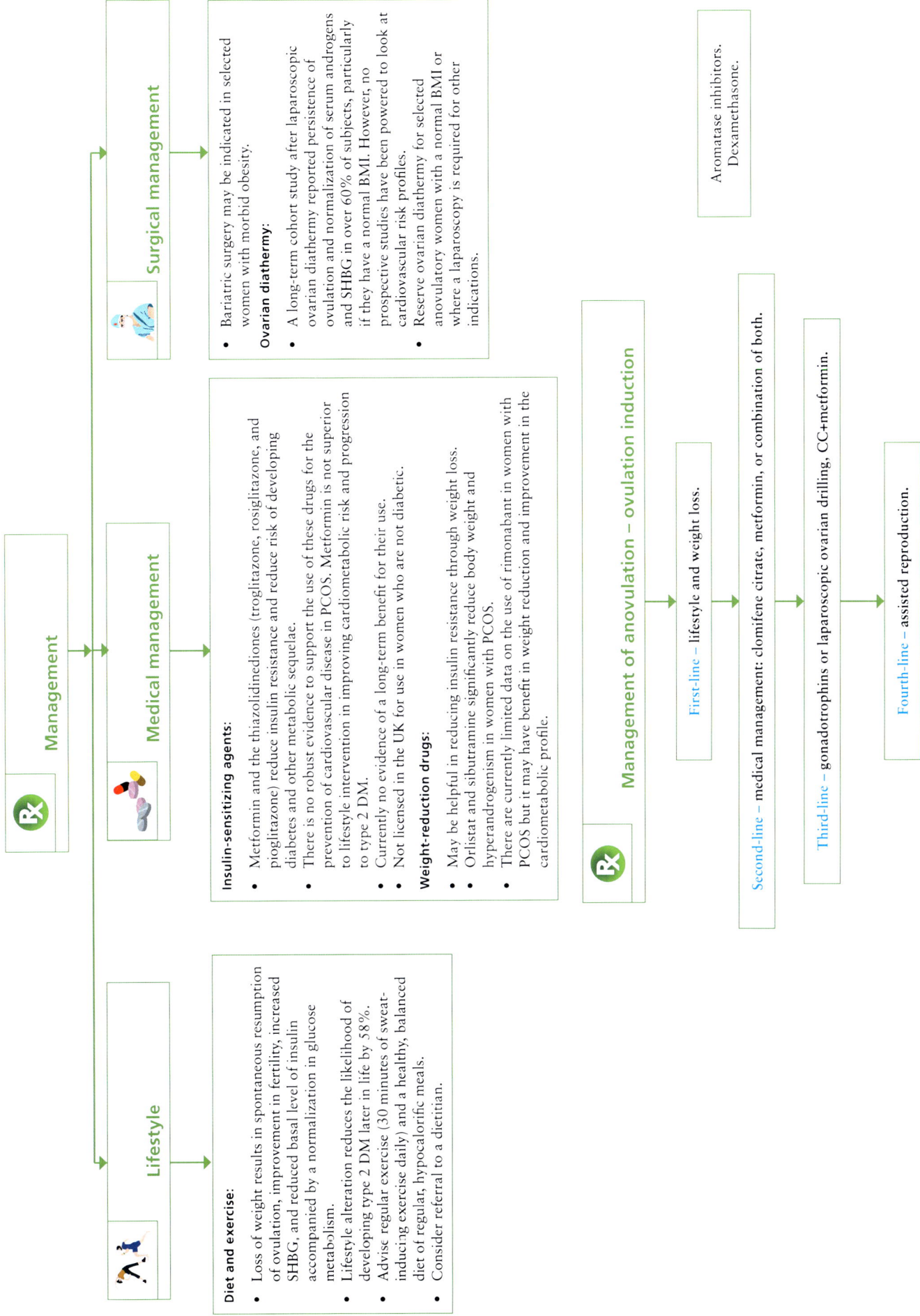

Management

Lifestyle

Diet and exercise:

- Loss of weight results in spontaneous resumption of ovulation, improvement in fertility, increased SHBG, and reduced basal level of insulin accompanied by a normalization in glucose metabolism.
- Lifestyle alteration reduces the likelihood of developing type 2 DM later in life by 58%.
- Advise regular exercise (30 minutes of sweat-inducing exercise daily) and a healthy, balanced diet of regular, hypocalorific meals.
- Consider referral to a dietitian.

Medical management

Insulin-sensitizing agents:

- Metformin and the thiazolidinediones (troglitazone, rosiglitazone, and pioglitazone) reduce insulin resistance and reduce risk of developing diabetes and other metabolic sequelae.
- There is no robust evidence to support the use of these drugs for the prevention of cardiovascular disease in PCOS. Metformin is not superior to lifestyle intervention in improving cardiometabolic risk and progression to type 2 DM.
- Currently no evidence of a long-term benefit for their use.
- Not licensed in the UK for use in women who are not diabetic.

Weight-reduction drugs:

- May be helpful in reducing insulin resistance through weight loss.
- Orlistat and sibutramine significantly reduce body weight and hyperandrogenism in women with PCOS.
- There are currently limited data on the use of rimonabant in women with PCOS but it may have benefit in weight reduction and improvement in the cardiometabolic profile.

Surgical management

- Bariatric surgery may be indicated in selected women with morbid obesity.

Ovarian diathermy:

- A long-term cohort study after laparoscopic ovarian diathermy reported persistence of ovulation and normalization of serum androgens and SHBG in over 60% of subjects, particularly if they have a normal BMI. However, no prospective studies have been powered to look at cardiovascular risk profiles.
- Reserve ovarian diathermy for selected anovulatory women with a normal BMI or where a laparoscopy is required for other indications.

Management of anovulation – ovulation induction

First-line – lifestyle and weight loss.

Second-line – medical management: clomifene citrate, metformin, or combination of both.

Third-line – gonadotrophins or laparoscopic ovarian drilling, CC+metformin.

Fourth-line – assisted reproduction.

Aromatase inhibitors.
Dexamethasone.

Management of anovulation – lifestyle and weight loss – first-line

- Obese women with PCOS are more likely than thin women with PCOS to suffer from anovulation and less likely to respond to pharmacological OI methods.
- Women with a BMI of ≥ 30 – advise to lose weight as it may restore ovulation, improve their response to ovulation induction agents, and have a positive impact on pregnancy outcomes. Weight loss of even 5–10% of body weight often restores ovulatory cycles.

Medical management – second-line – clomiphene citrate

- 60–85% ovulate but only about half conceive.
- Monitor cycle in at least the first cycle and when the treatment dose needs to be increased to minimize the risk of multiple pregnancy.
- Approximately 50% of conceptions will occur on 50 mg; with another 20–25% and 10% on 100 mg and 150 mg, respectively.
- Most pregnancies occur within first six ovulatory cycles; although a constant monthly pregnancy rate is noted, do not continue treatment for longer than 6 months.
- Lack of conception despite evidence of ovulation may be due to anti-oestrogenic effects of CC on the endometrium, which may manifest as a thin endometrium on TVS.
- Risk of over-response and OHSS.
- CC has been proven effective in OI for women with PCOS and is the first-line medical therapy.
- Consider alternatives for OI if:
  * Endometrium is persistently thin on CC therapy.
  * Pregnancy does not occur within six ovulatory cycles.

Know your drug

- Mechanism – selective oestrogen receptor modulator, stimulates endogenous FSH secretion by interrupting oestrogen feedback to the hypothalamus and pituitary.
- Dose – 50 mg per day for 5 days, starting from day 2 to 5 of menses. If this produces multiple follicular development, dose can be lowered to 25mg. If ovulation is not achieved, dose can be increased in increments of 50 mg up to 150 mg.
- Side effects – vasomotor hot flashes, visual symptoms (visual blurring or persistent after-images) in 1–2%, which are likely due to anti-oestrogenic effect on the visual cortex. Risk of OHSS, multiple pregnancy (twin – 7–9% and triplet – 0.3%).
- Although more studies are required, it is best to limit a patient's lifetime exposure to CC to 12 treatment cycles, as additional cycles may place the patient at increased risk of borderline ovarian tumours.

Metformin

- Metformin alone increased the odds of ovulation compared with placebo but does not result in a significantly higher CBR.
- Metformin combined with CC may increase ovulation rates and pregnancy rates.
- Offer metformin combined with CC to CC-resistant women, who have a BMI of > 25, because this increases ovulation and pregnancy rates. (NICE)

Know your drug

- Mechanism – insulin-sensitizing agent, acts by inhibiting hepatic glucose production and increasing peripheral glucose uptake.
- Dose – start with 250–500 mg daily and increase as tolerated to the optimal daily dose of 500–750 mg three times daily.
- Side effects – nausea, bloating, cramps, and diarrhoea.
- Not currently licensed for the treatment of ovulatory disorders in the UK.

Aromatase inhibitors (letrozole and anastrozole)

- Ovulation and pregnancy rates are promising, they appear to have less of an anti-oestrogenic effect on the endometrium, and most studies show equivalence with CC.
- Mechanism – block the conversion of testosterone and androstenedione to oestradiol and oestrone, respectively, and inhibit the oestrogen-negative feedback on the hypothalamic–pituitary axis. This leads to increased gonadotrophin secretion, which results in ovarian follicular growth.
- Advantages – shorter half-life than CC, potentially higher implantation rates and lower multiple pregnancy rates.
- 2.4% incidence of congenital malformations and chromosomal abnormalities in the letrozole group compared to 4.8% in the CC group.
- However, until aromatase inhibitors have been approved for OI by the Government, use with caution, and counsel patients carefully.(SOGC, ACOG)

Dexamethasone and growth hormone

- Dexamethasone as adjuvant therapy to CC has been shown to increase pregnancy rates in CC resistant PCOS. (ACOG)
- Use of adjuvant growth hormone treatment with GnRHa and/or hMG during OI in women with PCOS who do not respond to CC is not recommended because it does not improve pregnancy rates. (NICE)

Gonadotrophins

- Human menopausal gonadotrophin (hMG), urinary FSH, and recombinant FSH are equally effective in achieving pregnancy.
- Pregnancy rates are 20–25% per cycle.
- Very expensive and require monitoring to minimize the risks of excessive follicular growth.
- High risk of OHSS, multiple pregnancy, and treatment cancellation.
- Use low-dose regimen when using gonadotrophins in PCOS women because of significantly lower risk of OHSS. (ACOG)

Laparoscopic ovarian drilling/diathermy (LOD)

- Surgical ovarian wedge resection was thought to induce ovulation by decreasing the ovarian theca and thus reducing androgen production. Because of the operative morbidity of the procedure and the risk of postoperative adhesions, ovarian wedge resection by laparotomy has been abandoned.
- LOD – uses either cautery or laser to create approximately four superficial perforations per ovary. Less destructive to the ovary with lower risk of adhesion formation.
- Cochrane review – there is no difference in the rates of miscarriage or LBR between patients who undergo LOD and patients treated with gonadotropins. There are significantly fewer multiple pregnancies in the LOD than in the gonadotrophin treatment groups (1% vs 16%).
- Fertility benefit with LOD may be temporary and adjuvant therapy with CC or gonadotrophins may be necessary.
- Risks – surgical risks and concerns about adhesion formation. The long-term effects on ovarian function are unclear.
- **Consider LOD in women with clomiphene-resistant PCOS, particularly when there are other indications for laparoscopy.**

GnRHa

- Effectiveness of pulsatile GnRH in women with CC-resistant PCOS is uncertain; therefore, do not use outside a research context.
- Women with PCOS who are being treated with gonadotrophins – do not offer GnRHa concomitantly because it does not improve pregnancy rates, and it is associated with an increased risk of OHSS.

IVF – fourth-line Management

- IVF/ICSI – for women who fail to conceive with gonadotropin treatment or in the presence of other indications for ART.
- Pregnancy rates – 40–50% per cycle with IVF.
- Side effects – multiple pregnancy and a higher risk of OHSS.

Guideline comparator

Androgen Excess Society:

- All women with PCOS should have an oral GTT.
- All women with IGT should be screened annually.
- Oral GTT more frequently than once every 2 years in women at particular risk of type 2 DM.

What not to do

- LH, FSH, and oestradiol measurement for the diagnosis of PCOS.
- Fasting insulin and HOMA-IR.
- Routine lipid-lowering treatment.
- Metformin is currently not licensed for use in pregnancy in the UK.
- Osteoporosis prophylaxis is unnecessary as PCOS women are not oestrogen deficient.

1. *Long-Term Consequences of Polycystic Ovary Syndrome*. RCOG Green-top Guideline No. 33, December 2007.
2. Clinical Knowledge Summaries. http://www.cks.nhs.uk/polycystic_ovary_syndrome.
3. *Polycystic Ovarian Syndrome*. ACOG Practice Bulletin, Clinical Management Guidelines for Obstetricians and Gynaecologists, Number 108, 2009.
4. *Ovulation Induction in Polycystic Ovary Syndrome*. SOGC Clinical Practice Guideline No. 242, May 2010.
5. *Fertility: Assessment and Treatment for People with Fertility Problems*. NICE Clinical Guideline 11, February 2004.

CHAPTER 16 Polycystic ovarian syndrome

CHAPTER 17 Hirsutism

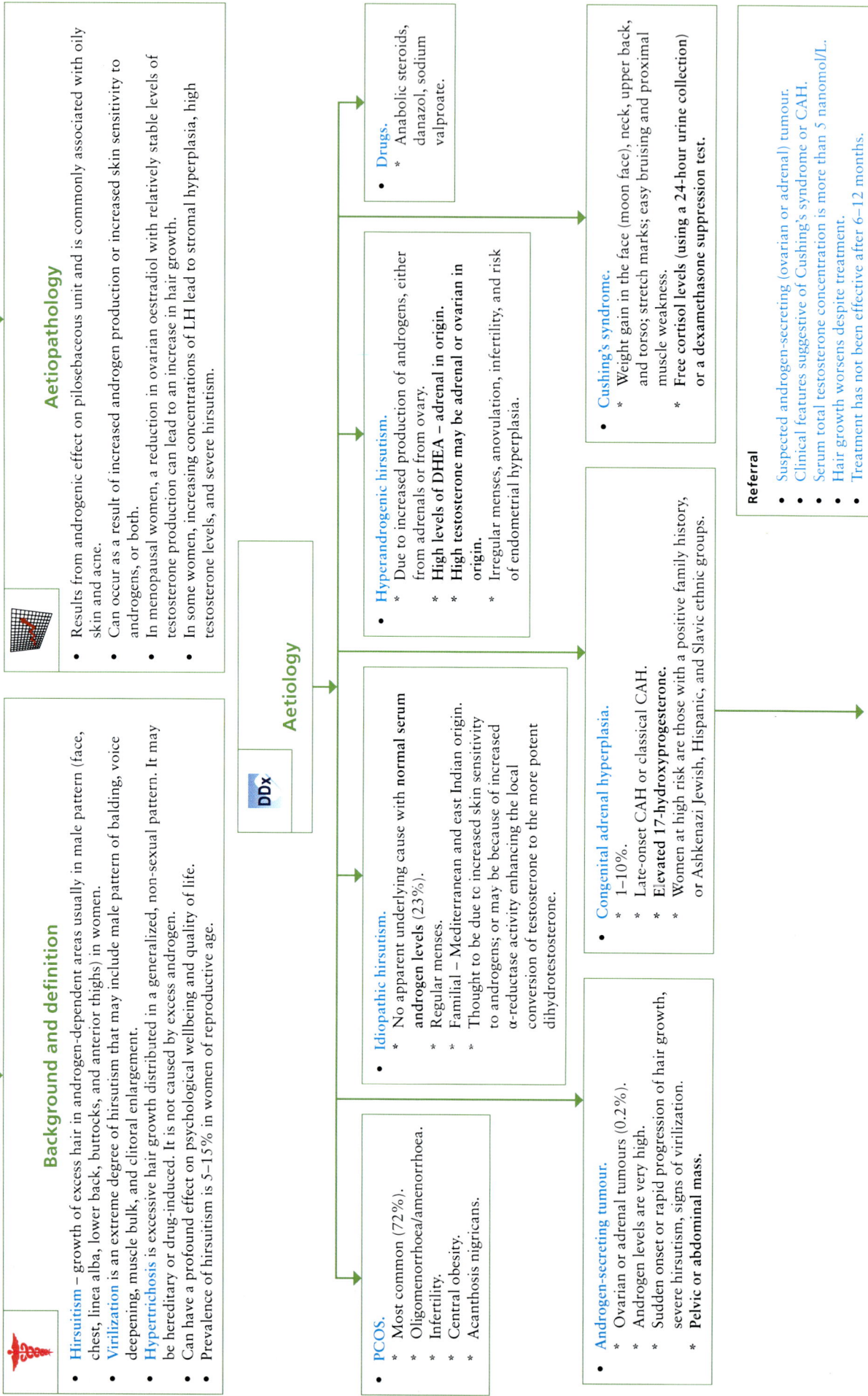

Background and definition

- Hirsutism – growth of excess hair in androgen-dependent areas usually in male pattern (face, chest, linea alba, lower back, buttocks, and anterior thighs) in women.
- Virilization is an extreme degree of hirsutism that may include male pattern of balding, voice deepening, muscle bulk, and clitoral enlargement.
- Hypertrichosis is excessive hair growth distributed in a generalized, non-sexual pattern. It may be hereditary or drug-induced. It is not caused by excess androgen.
- Can have a profound effect on psychological wellbeing and quality of life.
- Prevalence of hirsutism is 5–15% in women of reproductive age.

Aetiopathology

- Results from androgenic effect on pilosebaceous unit and is commonly associated with oily skin and acne.
- Can occur as a result of increased androgen production or increased skin sensitivity to androgens, or both.
- In menopausal women, a reduction in ovarian oestradiol with relatively stable levels of testosterone production can lead to an increase in hair growth.
- In some women, increasing concentrations of LH lead to stromal hyperplasia, high testosterone levels, and severe hirsutism.

Aetiology

DDx

- **PCOS.**
  * Most common (72%).
  * Oligomenorrhoea/amenorrhoea.
  * Infertility.
  * Central obesity.
  * Acanthosis nigricans.

- **Idiopathic hirsutism.**
  * No apparent underlying cause with **normal serum androgen levels** (23%).
  * Regular menses.
  * Familial – Mediterranean and east Indian origin.
  * Thought to be due to increased skin sensitivity to androgens; or may be because of increased α-reductase activity enhancing the local conversion of testosterone to the more potent dihydrotestosterone.

- **Androgen-secreting tumour.**
  * Ovarian or adrenal tumours (0.2%).
  * Androgen levels are very high.
  * Sudden onset or rapid progression of hair growth, severe hirsutism, signs of virilization.
  * **Pelvic or abdominal mass.**

- **Congenital adrenal hyperplasia.**
  * 1–10%.
  * Late-onset CAH or classical CAH.
  * **Elevated 17-hydroxyprogesterone.**
  * Women at high risk are those with a positive family history, or Ashkenazi Jewish, Hispanic, and Slavic ethnic groups.

- **Hyperandrogenic hirsutism.**
  * Due to increased production of androgens, either from adrenals or from ovary.
  * **High levels of DHEA – adrenal in origin.**
  * **High testosterone may be adrenal or ovarian in origin.**
  * Irregular menses, anovulation, infertility, and risk of endometrial hyperplasia.

- **Drugs.**
  * Anabolic steroids, danazol, sodium valproate.

- **Cushing's syndrome.**
  * Weight gain in the face (moon face), neck, upper back, and torso; stretch marks; easy bruising and proximal muscle weakness.
  * **Free cortisol levels (using a 24-hour urine collection) or a dexamethasone suppression test.**

Referral

- Suspected androgen-secreting (ovarian or adrenal) tumour.
- Clinical features suggestive of Cushing's syndrome or CAH.
- Serum total testosterone concentration is more than 5 nanomol/L.
- Hair growth worsens despite treatment.
- Treatment has not been effective after 6–12 months.

Assessment of severity

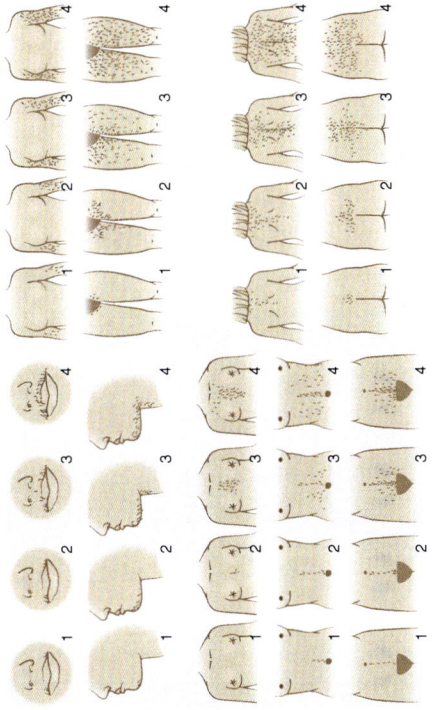

Ferriman–Gallwey scoring system – designed to assess the severity of hirsutism (See Figure).

- Each of the nine body areas most sensitive to androgen production is assigned a score from 0 (no hair) to 4 (heavy hair growth). The nine areas are: upper lip, chin, chest, upper back, lower back, upper abdomen, lower abdomen, upper arms, and thighs.
- The separate scores are added to provide a total score (0–36). A score of >15 is considered to indicate moderate to severe hirsutism.
- It is a validated tool. Although it is valuable as a clinical research tool, it has a number of limitations, and is impractical for routine use in clinical practice.
- Assess woman's own perception of her condition and the extent it impacts on her quality of life, as this may guide treatment.

Investigations

Mild hirsutism

- With no other signs of PCOS or other underlying condition. Investigations are not usually necessary because the likelihood of identifying a medical disorder that would change management or outcome is low. (ESCP)

Moderate to severe hirsutism

- Plasma testosterone.
- Pelvic USS to detect an ovarian neoplasm or PCO.
- DHEAS, 17-hydroxyprogesterone to rule out adrenal hyperandrogenism.
- Assess for Cushing's syndrome, thyroid dysfunction, or acromegaly, if other features of these conditions are present.

Management

- The choice between these options depends on:
  * Patient preferences.
  * Extent to which the area of hirsutism that affects wellbeing is amenable to direct hair removal.
  * Access to and affordability of these alternatives.
- Give a trial of at least 6 months before making changes in dose, changing medication, or adding medication. Because of the life span of hair, at least 6 months of medical therapy is required to notice any effect.

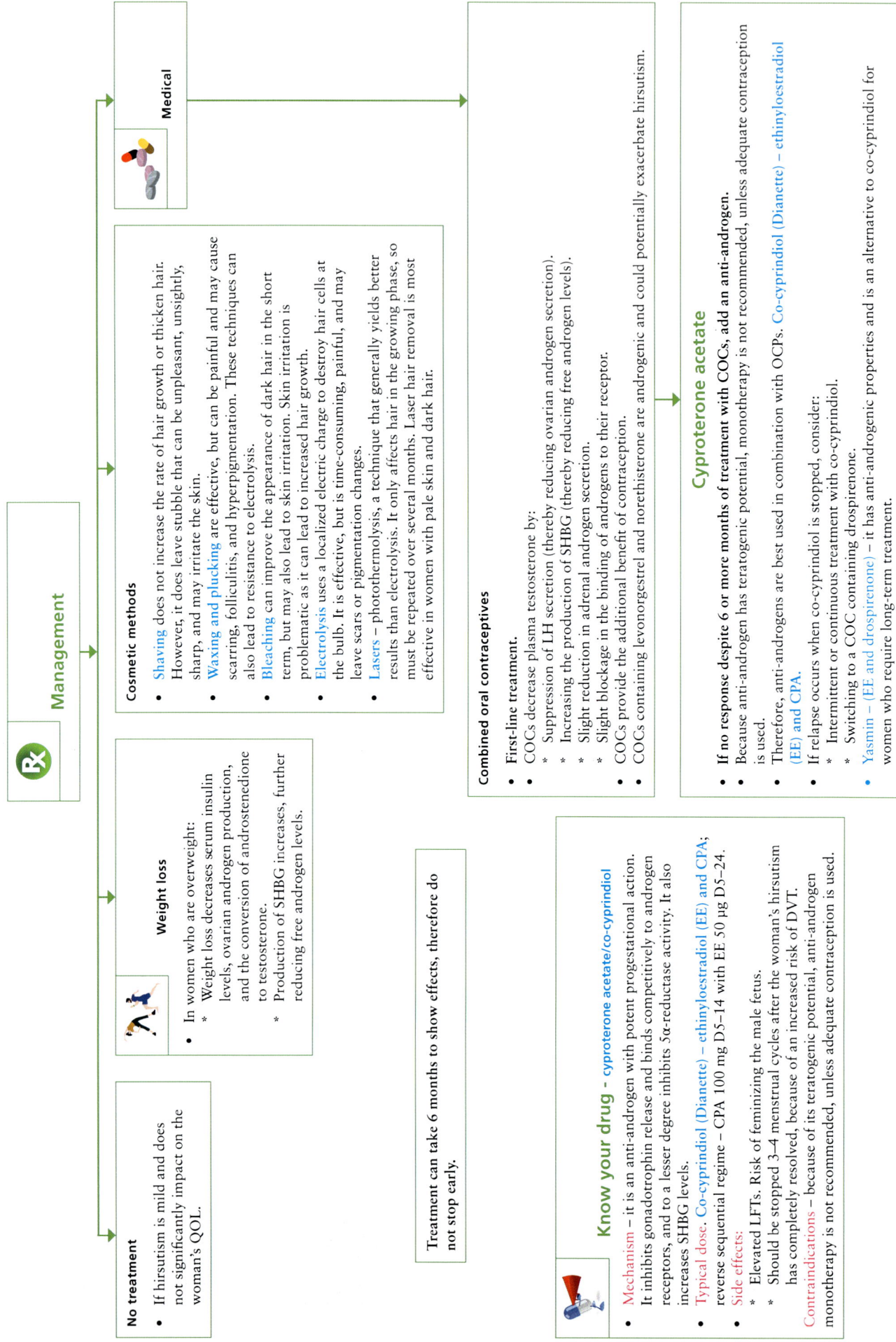

Management

No treatment

- If hirsutism is mild and does not significantly impact on the woman's QOL.

Weight loss

- In women who are overweight:
  * Weight loss decreases serum insulin levels, ovarian androgen production, and the conversion of androstenedione to testosterone.
  * Production of SHBG increases, further reducing free androgen levels.

Treatment can take 6 months to show effects, therefore do not stop early.

Cosmetic methods

- Shaving does not increase the rate of hair growth or thicken hair. However, it does leave stubble that can be unpleasant, unsightly, sharp, and may irritate the skin.
- Waxing and plucking are effective, but can be painful and may cause scarring, folliculitis, and hyperpigmentation. These techniques can also lead to resistance to electrolysis.
- Bleaching can improve the appearance of dark hair in the short term, but may also lead to skin irritation. Skin irritation is problematic as it can lead to increased hair growth.
- Electrolysis uses a localized electric charge to destroy hair cells at the bulb. It is effective, but is time-consuming, painful, and may leave scars or pigmentation changes.
- Lasers – photothermolysis, a technique that generally yields better results than electrolysis. It only affects hair in the growing phase, so must be repeated over several months. Laser hair removal is most effective in women with pale skin and dark hair.

Medical

Combined oral contraceptives

- First-line treatment.
- COCs decrease plasma testosterone by:
  * Suppression of LH secretion (thereby reducing ovarian androgen secretion).
  * Increasing the production of SHBG (thereby reducing free androgen levels).
  * Slight reduction in adrenal androgen secretion.
  * Slight blockage in the binding of androgens to their receptor.
- COCs provide the additional benefit of contraception.
- COCs containing levonorgestrel and norethisterone are androgenic and could potentially exacerbate hirsutism.

Cyproterone acetate

- If no response despite 6 or more months of treatment with COCs, add an anti-androgen.
- Because anti-androgen has teratogenic potential, monotherapy is not recommended, unless adequate contraception is used.
- Therefore, anti-androgens are best used in combination with OCPs. Co-cyprindiol (Dianette) – ethinylestradiol (EE) and CPA.
- If relapse occurs when co-cyprindiol is stopped, consider:
  * Intermittent or continuous treatment with co-cyprindiol.
  * Switching to a COC containing drospirenone.
- Yasmin – (EE and drospirenone) – it has anti-androgenic properties and is an alternative to co-cyprindiol for women who require long-term treatment.

Know your drug - cyproterone acetate/co-cyprindiol

- Mechanism – it is an anti-androgen with potent progestational action. It inhibits gonadotrophin release and binds competitively to androgen receptors, and to a lesser degree inhibits 5α-reductase activity. It also increases SHBG levels.
- Typical dose. Co-cyprindiol (Dianette) – ethinyloestradiol (EE) and CPA; reverse sequential regime – CPA 100 mg D5–14 with EE 50 µg D5–24.
- Side effects:
  * Elevated LFTs. Risk of feminizing the male fetus.
  * Should be stopped 3–4 menstrual cycles after the woman's hirsutism has completely resolved, because of an increased risk of DVT.
- Contraindications – because of its teratogenic potential, anti-androgen monotherapy is not recommended, unless adequate contraception is used.

Medical management – others

Insulin-sensitizing drugs

- Metformin and the glitazones.
- Systematic review (16 RCTs) – limited efficacy.
- Not recommended.

Androgen receptor blockers

- Individual anti-androgens (spironolactone, finasteride, and flutamide) are each more effective than placebo, and there did not appear to be differences among the three anti-androgens.

Gonadotrophin-releasing hormone analogues

- Induce medical oophorectomy.
- GnRH agonists can be used for women with refractory hirsutism due to ovarian hyperandrogenism.
- Owing to the hypo-oestrogenic side effects, COCs or oestrogen/progesterone add-back therapy is necessary.

Facial topical eflornithine

- Benefit should be noticed in 6–8 weeks. Discontinue eflornithine if no benefit is seen within 4 months. If improvement is seen, continue treatment to maintain the benefits. Once the cream is discontinued, hair growth returns to pre-treatment levels within about 8 weeks.
- Eflornithine is contraindicated during pregnancy and breastfeeding.
- Evidence from small RCTs suggests that eflornithine may improve the appearance of facial hair in the short term (up to 6 months), but its efficacy in the longer term remains unclear.

Know your drug – spironolactone

- Mechanism – an aldosterone antagonist; competes for the androgen receptors in skin fibroblasts and produces limited suppression of gonadal and adrenal androgen biosynthesis, as well as inhibition of 5α-reductase activity.
- Typical dose – 100–200 mg daily. It can be used alone or in combination with COCs.
- Side effects – menstrual irregularity, transient diuresis, hyperkalaemia, postural hypotension, fatigue, headache, gastric upset, and breast tenderness. Feminization of male fetus if pregnant while on medication.
- Contraindications – pregnancy.

Know your drug – flutamide

- Mechanism – nonsteroidal anti-androgen. Equally effective as spironolactone and finasteride.
- Typical dose – 250–500 mg daily. Used alone or in combination with COGs.
- Side effects – hepatotoxicity is rare, but liver failure and death have been reported. Therefore, mandates LFT monitoring.

Know your drug – finasteride

- Mechanism – blocks 5α-reductase enzyme responsible for conversion of testosterone to dihydrotestosterone.
  * 30–60% effect in reducing hirsutism scores.
- Side effects – very low side-effect profile.
  * Teratogenic potential.

What not to do

- COCs containing levonorgestrel and norethisterone are androgenic and could potentially exacerbate hirsutism.
- Insulin-sensitizing drugs.

Evidence round-up

- Limited evidence from Cochrane review – some laser and photoepilation treatments may lead to short-term hair reduction. There is less evidence of long-term benefit.
- Evidence from one RCT – COCs containing drospirenone are at least as effective as those containing CPA.
- Insulin-sensitizing drugs – systematic review (16 RCTs) has shown limited efficacy, therefore not recommended.

1. Evaluation and treatment of hirsutism in premenopausal women: an Endocrine Society Clinical Practice Guideline. *J Clin Endocrinol Metab* 2008;93:1105–1120.
2. Clinical Knowledge Summaries: Guidelines on Hirsutism. http://www.cks.nhs.uk/hirsutism.
3. *Hirsutism – Evaluation and Treatment.* SOGC Clinical Practice Guidelines, No.110, 2002.
4. ASRM Practice Committee Report. The evaluation and treatment of androgen excess. *Fertil Steril* 2006;86(4):S241–247.
5. http://www.hakanbuzoglu.com/killar-ve-killarin-yapisi/.

CHAPTER 17 Hirsutism

CHAPTER 18 Hyperprolactinaemia

Pathogenesis

Prolactinomas

- Pituitary adenomas that secrete prolactin (PRL).
- Invariably benign. Over 90% are small, intrasellar tumours that rarely increase in size.
- Microadenomas (< 10 mm in diameter); macroadenomas (> 10 mm in diameter).
- Occasionally, can be aggressive or locally invasive and cause compression of vital structures. Malignant prolactinomas that are resistant to treatment and disseminate inside and outside the CNS are very rare.
- Prolactinomas secrete PRL, which is enhanced by oestrogen and inhibited by dopamine (synthesized by the hypothalamus and transported to the pituitary by portal vessels). PRL stimulates milk production and also has secondary effects on gonadal function.
- PRL-secreting adenomas may also produce TSH or ACTH – uncommon.
- Prolactinomas may be a component of multiple endocrine neoplasia syndrome type I (MEN I) – very rare.
- Age – 2–80 years. More common in women, with a peak incidence during the child-bearing years.
- Microadenomas are present in about 10% of the normal population.

Other causes of hyperprolactinaemia

- **Drugs or situations that inhibit:**
  - * Hypothalamic production of dopamine.
  - * Its transport to the pituitary due to the compression of the pituitary stalk.
  - * Its effectiveness at dopaminergic receptors.
- Craniopharyngioma and other sellar or parasellar masses, granulomatous infiltration of the hypothalamus, head trauma, and large pituitary adenomas.
- Large nonfunctional tumour in the hypothalamus or pituitary.
- Mixed growth hormone and PRL secreting tumours – acromegaly in association with hyperprolactinaemia.
- Chronic renal or hepatic failure – due to decreased clearance of PRL.
- PCOS is commonly associated with elevated PRL levels.
- Primary hypothyroidism – some cases have mild hyperprolactinaemia. This is a result of increased synthesis of, or sensitivity to, hypothalamic TRH, which is able to stimulate pituitary lactotroph cells; but the true cause is unknown.
- During pregnancy there is a progressive increase in prolactin levels (as high as 10 times normal) because of pituitary lactotroph hyperplasia induced by the high oestrogen levels secreted by the placenta.
- PRL levels can also rise modestly after exercise, meals, stress, chest wall/breast stimulation, or sexual intercourse.
- Idiopathic hyperprolactinaemia.
- Drugs that reduce dopamine secretion or action – metoclopramide, phenothiazines, butyrophenones, risperidone, serotonin reuptake inhibitors (rare), sulpiride, domperidone, and verapamil.

History

- Premenopausal women present with oligo-/amenorrhoea (90%), galactorrhoea (80%), and anovulatory infertility.
- Women with amenorrhoea present with symptoms of oestrogen deficiency.
- Women with PCOS will have symptoms of PCOS.
- Postmenopausal women – usually pressure effects owing to large adenoma.
- Children – uncommon, greater proportion of macroadenomas compared to adults. Delayed puberty in both sexes and primary amenorrhoea and galactorrhoea in girls. Because of the increased prevalence of macroadenomas, prolactinomas in children are more frequently accompanied by neurological symptoms.
- Evidence on the effect of hyperprolactinaemia as a risk factor for recurrent miscarriage is insufficient and is not a part of the routine investigations. (RCOG)

Risks or complications

- Hyperprolactinaemia – interrupts the pulsatile secretion of GnRH, inhibits the release of LH and FSH, and directly impairs gonadal steroidogenesis, leading to primary or secondary amenorrhoea.
- Chronic hyperprolactinaemia-induced hypogonadism – reduces spinal bone mineral density (BMD). After prolactin normalization, BMD increases but does not always return to normal.
- Pressure symptoms – very large tumours result in compression of other pituitary cells or of the hypothalamic–pituitary stalk, leading to hypopituitarism.
- Neurological manifestations are common with macroadenomas or giant adenomas, because they are space-occupying lesions with possible compression of the optic chiasma. Neurological symptoms include headaches, and visual impairment ranging from quadrantanopia to classical bitemporal hemianopia or scotomas.
- Visual field defects are seen in up to 5% of cases.
- Blindness owing to an expanding prolactinoma may occur in pituitary apoplexy.

DDx Differential diagnosis

rule out secondary causes:

- Pregnancy.
- Drugs.

Investigations

Prolactinoma – requires both radiographic evidence of pituitary adenoma and laboratory evidence of sustained hyperprolactinaemia, and exclusion of other causes of hyperprolactinaemia.

Measurement of prolactin level

- PRL values are not absolute; prolactinomas can present with variable elevation in PRL, and there may be dissociation between tumour mass and hormonal secretion.
- Normal levels in women and men are < 500 mIU/L and 400 mIU/L, respectively (1 µg/L = 21.2 mIU/L).
- Microadenoma – most patients have moderately elevated PRL levels of > 3000 mIU/L.
- Macroadenoma – levels of > 5000 mIU/L.
- Large nonfunctional tumours – PRL levels of < 3000 mIU/L.
- PRL values between the upper limits of normal to 2000 mIU/L – may be due to psychoactive drugs, oestrogen, or idiopathic causes, but can also be caused by microprolactinomas.
- A single measurement is usually adequate for diagnosis. When initial PRL values are not diagnostic, repeat the test. To avoid the effect of pulsatile secretion, get 2–3 samples separated by at least 15–20 min.
- **Repeat if PRL level is > 1000 mIU/L, and if still elevated investigate further with MRI.**

Diagnostic pitfalls: macroprolactin and the 'hook effect'

- Macroprolactin is a complex of PRL, an IgG antibody. Serum PRL concentrations are elevated secondary to a reduced rate of clearance of this complex. Macroprolactin has reduced bioactivity and is present in significant amounts in up to 20%, resulting in pseudo-hyperprolactinaemia and potential misdiagnosis.
- Rule out the presence of macroprolactin in patients with moderately elevated PRL levels (500–3000 mIU/L) and less typical symptoms.
- The 'hook effect' may be observed when the serum PRL concentration is extremely high, as in some cases of giant prolactinomas. The high amount of circulating PRL causes antibody saturation in the immunoradiometric assay, leading to artefactually low results. Exclude the hook effect in all new patients with large pituitary macroadenomas who have normal or mildly elevated PRL levels.

Pituitary imaging

- Gadolinium-enhanced MRI – extent of tumour, suprasellar extension, and compression of optic chiasma or invasion of the cavernous sinus.
- CT with intravenous contrast enhancement is less effective than MRI in diagnosing small adenomas and in defining the extension of large tumours, but may be used if MRI is unavailable or contraindicated.
- Normal MRI does not necessarily exclude a microadenoma.

Formal visual-field examination – for patients with macroadenomas that abut the optic chiasm.

Diagnosis

- Hyperprolactinaemia in the presence of an MRI-detected pituitary adenoma is consistent with but not unequivocally diagnostic of a prolactinoma, because any pituitary mass that compresses the pituitary stalk may cause hyperprolactinaemia.
- Unequivocal diagnosis requires pathological analysis, but prolactinomas are rarely surgically removed.
- Empirical confirmation of the diagnosis can be obtained by medical treatment with dopamine agonists with serial assessment of serum PRL levels and adenoma size.
- Following a course of therapy:
  * Normalization of PRL plus a substantial reduction (≥ 75%) of the initial adenoma size confirms the diagnosis of a prolactinoma.
  * Normalization of PRL with no change or only a small reduction in tumour volume may suggest a pituitary adenoma other than a prolactinoma.
  * No change in serum PRL and no reduction in tumour volume indicate a resistant prolactinoma.
- Large tumour on the scan with only moderately elevated PRL levels (2000–3000) suggests a nonfunctioning tumour.

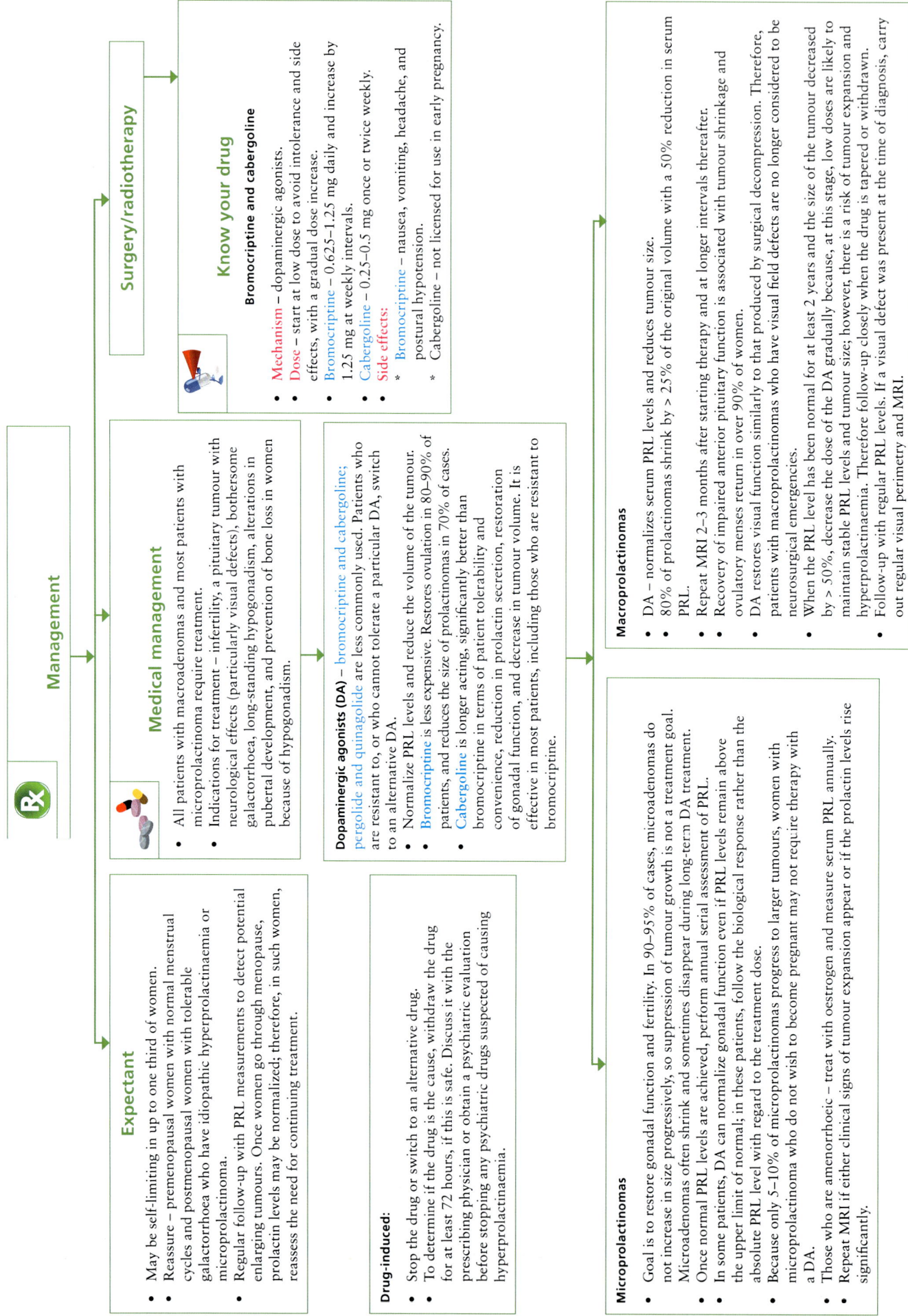

Management

Surgery/radiotherapy

Know your drug

Bromocriptine and cabergoline

* **Mechanism** – dopaminergic agonists.
* **Dose** – start at low dose to avoid intolerance and side effects, with a gradual dose increase.
* Bromocriptine – 0.625–1.25 mg daily and increase by 1.25 mg at weekly intervals.
* Cabergoline – 0.25–0.5 mg once or twice weekly.
* **Side effects:**
  * Bromocriptine – nausea, vomiting, headache, and postural hypotension.
  * Cabergoline – not licensed for use in early pregnancy.

Medical management

* All patients with macroadenomas and most patients with microprolactinoma require treatment.
* Indications for treatment – infertility, a pituitary tumour with neurological effects (particularly visual defects), bothersome galactorrhoea, long-standing hypogonadism, alterations in pubertal development, and prevention of bone loss in women because of hypogonadism.

Dopaminergic agonists (DA) – bromocriptine and cabergoline; pergolide and quinagolide are less commonly used. Patients who are resistant to, or who cannot tolerate a particular DA, switch to an alternative DA.

* Normalize PRL levels and reduce the volume of the tumour.
* Bromocriptine is less expensive. Restores ovulation in 80–90% of patients, and reduces the size of prolactinomas in 70% of cases.
* Cabergoline is longer acting, significantly better than bromocriptine in terms of patient tolerability and convenience, reduction in prolactin secretion, restoration of gonadal function, and decrease in tumour volume. It is effective in most patients, including those who are resistant to bromocriptine.

Expectant

* May be self-limiting in up to one third of women.
* Reassure – premenopausal women with normal menstrual cycles and postmenopausal women with tolerable galactorrhoea who have idiopathic hyperprolactinaemia or microprolactinoma.
* Regular follow-up with PRL measurements to detect potential enlarging tumours. Once women go through menopause, prolactin levels may be normalized; therefore, in such women, reassess the need for continuing treatment.

Drug-induced:

* Stop the drug or switch to an alternative drug.
* To determine if the drug is the cause, withdraw the drug for at least 72 hours, if this is safe. Discuss it with the prescribing physician or obtain a psychiatric evaluation before stopping any psychiatric drugs suspected of causing hyperprolactinaemia.

Microprolactinomas

* Goal is to restore gonadal function and fertility. In 90–95% of cases, microadenomas do not increase in size progressively, so suppression of tumour growth is not a treatment goal. Microadenomas often shrink and sometimes disappear during long-term DA treatment.
* Once normal PRL levels are achieved, perform annual serial assessment of PRL.
* In some patients, DA can normalize gonadal function even if PRL levels remain above the upper limit of normal; in these patients, follow the biological response rather than the absolute PRL level with regard to the treatment dose.
* Because only 5–10% of microprolactinomas progress to larger tumours, women with microprolactinoma who do not wish to become pregnant may not require therapy with a DA.
* Those who are amenorrhoeic – treat with oestrogen and measure serum PRL annually.
* Repeat MRI if either clinical signs of tumour expansion appear or if the prolactin levels rise significantly.

Macroprolactinomas

* DA – normalizes serum PRL levels and reduces tumour size.
* 80% of prolactinomas shrink by > 25% of the original volume with a 50% reduction in serum PRL.
* Repeat MRI 2–3 months after starting therapy and at longer intervals thereafter.
* Recovery of impaired anterior pituitary function is associated with tumour shrinkage and ovulatory menses return in over 90% of women.
* DA restores visual function similarly to that produced by surgical decompression. Therefore, patients with macroprolactinomas who have visual field defects are no longer considered to be neurosurgical emergencies.
* When the PRL level has been normal for at least 2 years and the size of the tumour decreased by > 50%, decrease the dose of the DA gradually because, at this stage, low doses are likely to maintain stable PRL levels and tumour size; however, there is a risk of tumour expansion and hyperprolactinaemia. Therefore follow-up closely when the drug is tapered or withdrawn.
* Follow-up with regular PRL levels. If a visual defect was present at the time of diagnosis, carry out regular visual perimetry and MRI.

Resistant prolactinoma – no adequate response to a dopamine agonist

Treatment options

- Achieve the maximally tolerated dose.
- Change to a different dopamine agonist.
- Surgery or radiotherapy.

Surgical management

- Indications:
  * Up to 10% of patients who do not respond to DA.
  * If visual field deficits do not improve.
  * Apoplexy with neurological signs in macroadenomas.
  * Cystic macroprolactinomas (which generally do not shrink in response to DA) causing neurological symptoms.
  * Intolerance to DA.
  * Patient preference.
  * Nonfunctional tumours.
  * If there is suprasellar extension of the tumour that has not regressed with medical treatment and a pregnancy is desired.
- Trans-sphenoidal adenectomy – does not reliably lead to a long-term cure, and recurrence of hyperprolactinaemia is frequent.
  * Microadenomas – the success rate is about 75%.
  * Macroprolactinomas – success rate is much lower. Recurrence in about 20%.

Radiotherapy

- External radiation – significant side effects, including hypopituitarism, damage to the optic nerve, neurological dysfunction, and increased risks of stroke and secondary brain tumours. Therefore, reserved for:
  * Those who do not respond to DA.
  * Those who are not cured by surgery.
  * Very rare cases of malignant prolactinoma.

- Malignant prolactinomas – present as:
  * Resistant prolactinomas.
  * Dissociation between serum PRL levels and tumour mass.
  * Recurrence after surgery.
  * Extension to non-contiguous areas of the CNS.
  * Metastasis to areas outside the CNS.
  Surgery and radiotherapy are only palliative, and chemotherapy seems to provide little or no benefit. These cancers are uniformly fatal.

Follow-up

- Minimal length of DA therapy is one year. There are no signs to predict whether drug discontinuation will be successful, but DA can be withdrawn safely in patients with long-term normalization of prolactin levels.
- If a patient has normal PRL levels after therapy with DA for at least three years and the tumour volume is markedly reduced, initiate a trial of tapering and discontinuation of these drugs. Carefully follow such patients to detect recurrence of hyperprolactinaemia and tumour enlargement so that treatment can be resumed promptly.

Hyperprolactinaemia and fertility

- No treatment is necessary if regular menstrual cycles. Treat only if anovulatory cycles and fertility is desired.
- Anovulatory women – DA restore ovulation in approximately 90% of cases, and result in a pregnancy in 80–85%.
- Treat to correct amenorrhoea and its sequelae, rather than just for normalization of serum levels of PRL.
- Association between hyperprolactinaemia and infertility in the presence of ovulation and regular menstrual cycles is controversial. The incidence of raised prolactin in infertile but ovulatory women ranges from 4–12%.
- NICE – there is no evidence to support an association between prolactin and conception rates in ovulatory women; measure PRL levels in anovulatory women or those with symptoms of galactorrhoea or a pituitary tumour.
- When a patient with a macroprolactinoma wishes to become pregnant – plan pregnancy once serum PRL is normalized and the tumour volume significantly reduced to avoid or reduce the risk of compression of the optic chiasm during pregnancy.
- Surgery before pregnancy in women with macroprolactinomas to reduce the likelihood of major tumour expansion is a less preferable option, as medical therapy during pregnancy is probably less harmful than surgery.
- Trans-sphenoidal surgery is an option in an infertile patient with a prolactinoma who cannot tolerate/is resistant to dopaminergic drugs.

Hyperprolactinaemia and pregnancy

- Serum PRL in pregnancy does not reliably reflect an increase in the size of prolactinomas.
- Microprolactinomas – the risk of clinically relevant tumour expansion is < 2% during pregnancy. Therefore, stop DA as soon as pregnancy is confirmed. Advise patient to report for urgent assessment in the event of a severe headache or visual disturbance. Serial PRL monitoring is not necessary.
- Macroadenomas – symptomatic tumour expansion occurs in 20–30% of women. Options include stopping the DA when pregnancy is confirmed, with close surveillance, or continuing the DA through the pregnancy.
- If visual field defects or progressive headaches develop, perform an MRI without gadolinium and restart a DA if the tumour has grown significantly. Monitor visual fields every 2–3 months.
- If the enlarged tumour does not respond to DA therapy, alternatives include delivery if the pregnancy is far enough advanced or trans-sphenoidal surgery.

Safety of dopamine agonists in pregnancy and lactation

- Bromocriptine – incidence of miscarriage or congenital malformations is no higher than that in the general population.
- Cabergoline – similar reports; however, data are limited.
- Pergolide and quinagolide – limited experience; do not use these two drugs in this setting.
- Bromocriptine and cabergoline – best to limit the exposure of the embryo to such drugs as much as possible. Teratogenicity most often occurs during the first trimester and the first trimester is associated with the period of lowest growth of a macroadenoma in pregnant women who have stopped therapy. **Therefore, stop bromocriptine or cabergoline once a pregnancy test is positive.**
- Lactation – do not prescribe DA in women wishing to breastfeed because the resulting decrease in serum PRL levels will **impair lactation.** There are no data to suggest that breastfeeding leads to an increase in tumour size.

1. Guidelines of the Pituitary Society for the diagnosis and management of prolactinomas. *Clin Endocrinol* 2006;65:265–273.

Definition and prevalence

- Defined as puberty occurring in those younger than 2 standard deviations before the average age.
- Normal age of pubertal onset is 8–13 years in girls. The traditional threshold for PP is 8 years.
- Recent cross-sectional data (USA) – pubertal milestones are reached earlier by black girls and to a lesser extent by Mexican–American and white girls; therefore, suggested PP when it occurs before the ages of 6 years in black girls and 7 years in all other girls.
- Current UK/European guidelines remain as 8 years.

- Prevalence – girls: 0.2%, boys: < 0.05%.
- Factors affecting onset of puberty – earlier in girls with:
  * Black race.
  * Early maternal menarche.
  * Low birth weight.
  * Excessive weight gain or obesity in infancy and childhood.
  * Improved socioeconomic status and nutrition, after international adoption (the risk is 10–20 times higher).
  * Exposure to oestrogenic endocrine-disrupting chemicals.
  * Child abuse, particularly sexual abuse.

Risks or complications

- Early menarche – difficult to predict the age at which menarche will occur after the onset of puberty.
- Short adult stature owing to early epiphyseal fusion leads to loss of about 12 cm compared to normal adult height. Height loss is inversely correlated with the age at the onset of puberty.
- Adverse psychosocial outcomes – disruptive behaviour, difficulties in interpersonal relationships, and an earlier onset of sexual behaviour.

Classification

Progressive central precocious puberty

- Characterized by a sustained activation of the gonadotropic axis.
- Progression of pubertal stages from one stage to the next in 3–6 months.
- Growth velocity is accelerated (> about 6 cm/year).
- Bone age – usually advanced by at least 1 year.
- Predicted adult height – below target height range or declining.
- Uterine volume > 2.0 ml or length > 34 mm, pear-shaped uterus, endometrial thickening.
- Usually measurable oestradiol level with advancing pubertal development.
- LH peak after GnRH or GnRHa in the pubertal range.

Non-progressive precocious puberty

- Gonadotropic axis is not activated.
- Stabilization or regression of pubertal signs.
- Growth velocity – usually normal for age.
- Bone age – usually within 1 year of chronological age.
- Predicted adult height – within target height range.
- Uterine volume of ≤ 2.0 ml or length of ≤ 34 mm; prepubertal tubular-shaped uterus.
- Oestradiol not detectable or close to the detection limit.
- LH peak after GnRH or GnRH agonist in the prepubertal range.

In at least 50% of cases of PP, pubertal manifestations will regress or stop progressing and no treatment is necessary. The mechanism underlying these cases of non-progressive PP is unknown. When these features are inconsistent, wait a few months and reassess in order to avoid unnecessary treatment.

Precocious puberty

Central or gonadotrophin-dependent
- Premature activation of the hypothalamopituitary–gonadal axis – serum gonadotrophins are elevated with same pattern of endocrine change as in normal puberty (consonant).
- Breast with or without pubic hair development.
- Increased growth velocity, possible acne, oily skin and hair, and emotional changes.
- Variable serum oestradiol.
- Peak LH level after GnRHa stimulation – in pubertal range.
- Advanced bone age. • Developed uterus on USS.

Peripheral or gonadotrophin-independent precocious puberty (GIPP)
- Premature activation of the ovaries or adrenal glands independent of gonadotrophin secretion. • Secretion of sex steroids is autonomous with loss of normal feedback regulation. Sex steroid concentrations are elevated with low gonadotrophins.
- Pubertal development does not follow the pattern of normal puberty (disconsonant).
- Varied pubertal symptoms depending on nature of sex steroid produced.
- High/markedly elevated serum oestradiol in girls.
- Low peak serum LH after GnRHa stimulation.
- Advanced bone age. • Developed uterus on USS.
- May have advanced pubic and axillary hair growth prior to breast development, or menstruation with minimal breast development.

Benign variants of precocious pubertal development
- Usually isolated secondary sexual characteristic.
- No/slightly increased growth velocity.
- Bone age within normal range.
- Low serum levels of sex steroids.
- Peak LH levels after GnRHa stimulation in prepubertal range.
- Normal pelvic USS.

Early exposure to sex steroids
- Prolonged sex steroid exposure in GIPP has a direct maturational effect on the hypothalamus and can accelerate the onset of centrally mediated puberty, leading to GDPP.

Idiopathic
- 90% of girls.
- Diagnosis of exclusion. May have:
  * Positive family history.
  * History of adoption.
- Can be part of a developmental syndrome (Williams–Beuren syndrome).
- MRI – no hypothalamic abnormality.

CNS lesions
- Hypothalamic tumour (glioma involving the hypothalamus or optic chiasm, germ-cell tumour, etc.).
  * Possible headache, cognitive changes, symptoms or signs of anterior or posterior pituitary deficiency (decreased growth velocity, polyuria, or polydipsia), fatigue, visual-field defects. * Mass on MRI. * Evidence of intracranial hypertension.
- Hypothalamic hamartoma – focal, or tonic–clonic seizures. * Mass on floor of third ventricle on MRI.
- Injury – cranial irradiation, head injury, infection such as meningitis or encephalitis, perinatal insult.
  * Relevant history, possible symptoms and signs of anterior or posterior pituitary deficiency.
  * Moderate radiation doses used for the treatment of brain tumours in children are associated with PP, whereas higher doses are associated with gonadotrophin deficiency and a delay in puberty.
- Cerebral malformations involving the hypothalamus – suprasellar arachnoid cyst, hydrocephalus, etc.

- Autonomous gonadal activation – McCune–Albright syndrome – classic triad: PP, café au lait spots, and fibrous dysplasias of bone. Rapid progression of breast development and early vaginal bleeding. Autonomous hyperfunctioning most commonly involves the ovary, but other endocrine involvement includes the thyroid (thyrotoxicosis), adrenals (Cushing's syndrome), pituitary (gigantism/acromegaly or hyperprolactinaemia), and parathyroid glands (hyperparathyroidism). • Large ovarian cysts on USS.
- Exposure to exogenous agents:
  * Sex steroids – COCs or testosterone gels.
  * Oestrogenic endocrine-disrupting chemicals – oestrogenic agents in cosmetics and food products can lead to premature thelarche.
- Severe primary hypothyroidism – signs of hypothyroidism, no increase in growth velocity, low levels of free thyroxine, no advancement in bone age.

- Ovarian tumours:
  * Granulosa-cell tumour – rapid progression of breast development and possible abdominal pain.
  * Androgen-producing tumour – Leydig cell tumours, and gonadoblastoma. Progressive virilization.
- Abdominal examination – mass on USS or CT scan; may be palpable. Adrenal disorders – increased androgen production leading to virilization.
  * CAH.
  * Adrenal tumour – mass on USS or CT scan; elevated DHEA or adrenal steroid precursors.
  * Cushing's syndrome.

- Isolated precocious thelarche:
  * Unilateral or bilateral breast development is frequent before the age of 2 years. No further evaluation needed in most cases.
- Isolated precocious pubarche:
  * Pubic hair development, sometimes associated with adult body odour, axillary hair, or mild acne.
  * Normal cortisol precursors in serum
  * Normal levels of 17-hydroxyprogesterone after corticotropin stimulation.
- Isolated precocious menarche:
  * Isolated vaginal bleeding without breast or pubic-hair development.
  * Evaluate clinically for a vaginal lesion (sexual abuse, foreign body, tumour).
  * Normal bone age and prepubertal uterus on USS.

History

- Age at onset of puberty and of menarche; SSCs and their pattern of progression. Take detailed history to determine if the pattern of endocrine change is the same as in normal puberty.
- Any history of recent rapid growth.
- Family history – parents' age and height at onset of puberty; age of menarche in mother.
- Symptoms suggesting possible CNS dysfunction – headache, increased head circumference, visual impairment, or seizures.
- Social history – any history of adoption, child abuse, or sexual abuse.
- Drug history – to rule out an exogenous drug.

Examination

- Height – increased growth velocity; may precede the onset of pubertal manifestations.
- Stage of pubertal development (Tanner staging – See Chapter 14):
  * Breast development.
  * Pubic hair results from the effects of androgens, which may be produced by ovaries in central PP. Pubic hair in the absence of breast development is suggestive of adrenal disorders, premature pubarche, or exposure to androgens.
- Hyper-pigmented skin lesions in neurofibromatosis or McCune–Albright syndrome.
- Presence of dysmorphic features in multisystem syndromes.
- Visual fields and fundoscopy; focal motor deficits in intracranial tumours, injury.

Evaluate if

- Precocious breast development at stage 3 or higher.
- Precocious breast development at stage 2 with additional criteria such as increased growth velocity.
- Symptoms or signs suggestive of CNS dysfunction or of peripheral PP.

Investigations

- Oestradiol (E2):
  * Elevated levels suggest oestrogen production or exposure.
  * Markedly elevated levels (> 100 pg/ml) suggest ovarian cyst/tumour.
  * Highly variable and has a low sensitivity in discriminating early pubertal and prepubertal levels.
  * Levels can be normal in progressive central PP.
- FSH – not useful, as varies little throughout pubertal development.
- Serum testosterone – elevated levels suggest adrenal disorder.
- DHEAS – produced by adrenals; marker of androgen-producing adrenal tumours or of adrenal enzymatic defect.
- 17-hydroxy progesterone – marker of adrenal enzymatic defects (CAH); occasionally elevated with adrenal tumours.
- Urinary steroid profile and ACTH stimulation test.
- Last four are indicated if there are signs of hyperandrogenism.

- Basal LH – poorly discriminates prepubertal and early pubertal levels. Values > 0.3–0.4 IU/L suggest central PP (high specificity and low sensitivity). However, if levels of LH are not clearly elevated, it needs to be confirmed with a stimulation test.
- GnRH or GnRHa stimulation – the gold standard.
- Peak LH above the pubertal cutoff (5–8 IU/L) with elevated sex steroids suggests progressive central PP; suppressed peak LH level with elevated sex steroid levels indicates peripheral PP.
- Peak LH:FSH ratio typically increases during puberty; high ratio was used as a criterion for progressive central PP; not in common use now as more sensitive LH assays are available.

- Bone age with an X-ray of non-dominant hand/wrist. It is generally greater than their chronological age.
- Pelvic USS – ovarian cysts/tumours; the multicystic ovary is a classic feature of early puberty.
- Uterine changes due to oestrogen exposure such as uterine size and shape (pear shape); endometrial echo.
- Uterine volume > 2.0 ml – 89% sensitivity and specificity.
- Brain MRI – in all cases of progressive central PP, determine whether a hypothalamic lesion is present.
- CT scan or MRI of the adrenal glands.
- TFTs to rule out primary hypothyroidism.
- Genetic testing, e.g., neurofibromatosis type 1.

Investigations

Bone age, oestradiol, and random LH levels

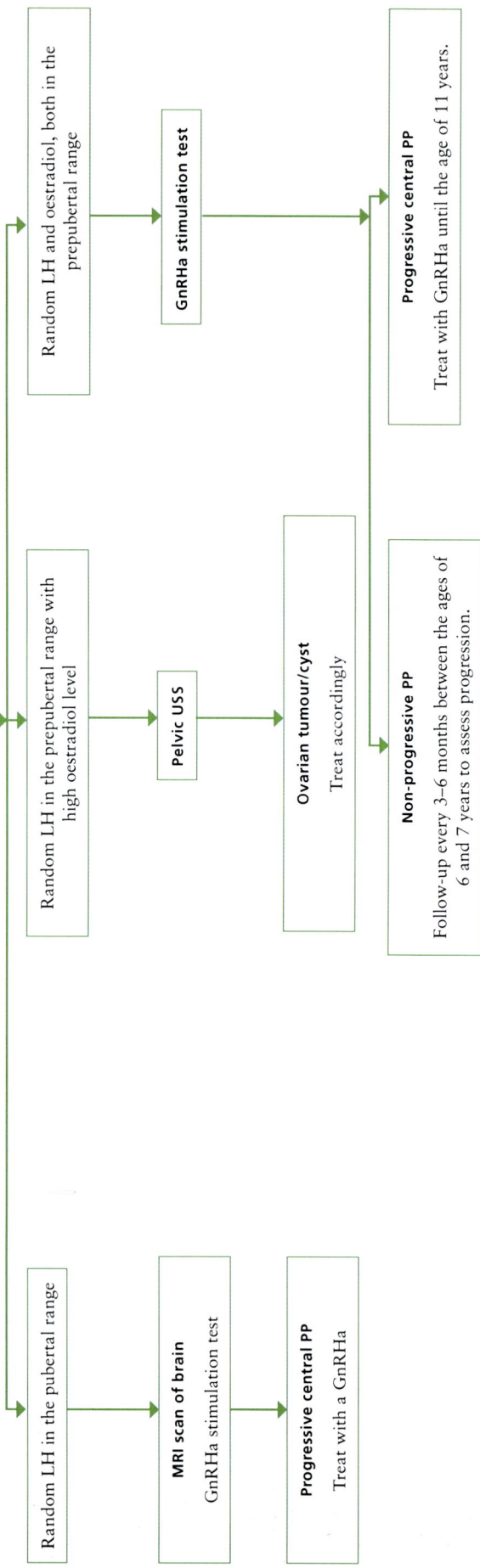

Random LH in the pubertal range

→ **MRI scan of brain**
GnRHa stimulation test

→ **Progressive central PP**
Treat with a GnRHa

Random LH in the prepubertal range with high oestradiol level

→ **Pelvic USS**

→ **Ovarian tumour/cyst**
Treat accordingly

→ **Non-progressive PP**
Follow-up every 3–6 months between the ages of 6 and 7 years to assess progression.

Random LH and oestradiol, both in the prepubertal range

→ **GnRHa stimulation test**

→ **Progressive central PP**
Treat with GnRHa until the age of 11 years.

Management

- Aim – to prevent progression of SSC and onset of menarche; maximize the growth potential and psychosocial wellbeing.
- Monitor for progression of pubertal development and growth velocity for 6 months before a decision to treat is made.
- Treat the underlying cause, if any. Refer to paediatric endocrinologist for evaluation and treatment.

Central precocious puberty – GnRHa

- Reasons for GnRHa therapy – potential for compromise in adult height, inability to adapt oneself to menarche, and psychosocial difficulties.
- Provides continuous stimulation of the pituitary gonadotrophs, leading to desensitization and decrease in the release of LH and FSH; results in the regression or stabilization of pubertal symptoms, as it is only the pulsatile exposure that triggers pubertal progression.
- Most important clinical criterion for GnRHa treatment is:
  * Documented progression of pubertal development, because many patients with CPP have a slowly progressive or non-progressive form and achieve normal adult height without GnRHa.
  * Accelerated growth velocity and skeletal maturation. However, some patients with slowly progressive CPP and advanced bone age reach normal adult height without intervention.
- Document progressive pubertal development and growth acceleration over a 3–6-month period before GnRHa therapy. This may not be necessary if the child is at or past Tanner stage III (breast), particularly with advanced skeletal maturation.
- Height gain varies. Girls with onset of progressive CPP before 6 years of age benefit most in terms of height from GnRHa treatment. Individualize the decision to initiate therapy in girls with onset after the age of 6 years.

Central lesion (mass or malformation)

- Refer for management of any brain neoplasms.
- Managing the causal lesion generally has no effect on the course of pubertal development.
- Remove hypothalamic hamartomas surgically.
- Cyproterone – it is a peripherally acting anti-androgen that suppresses both gonadotrophin and gonadal function. Can be used in combination with GnRHa or alone.
- Growth hormone – treatment with GnRH agonists can lead to a reduction in the growth rate owing to a reduction in GH and insulin-like growth factor 1 levels. Addition of GH may lead to a better growth velocity, although data are limited.

Peripheral precocious puberty

- Manage underlying cause.
- Use agents to inhibit steroidogenesis, so as to reduce oestrogen formation, which is a prime driver of bone maturation acceleration.
- Surgery for tumours of ovary or adrenals.
- CAH – hydrocortisone with/without fludrocortisone.
- Withdraw if any exogenous sex steroids.
- McCune–Albright syndrome – drugs to prevent the synthesis or action of gonadal steroids. Options:
  * Ketoconazole – an inhibitor of steroid synthesis and suppresses both gonadal and adrenal steroid production. It decreases testosterone levels and achieves good growth.
  * Aromatase inhibitors inhibit the production of oestrogens, and selective oestrogen-receptor modulators interfere with the action of oestrogens and are effective in some cases.
  * Aromatase inhibitors – inhibit functions of testosterone that are dependent upon its conversion to oestrogen. If aromatase inhibitors are used, anti-androgen agents may be needed to reduce testosterone effects on pubic hair and genital development (spironolactone and bicalutamide).

1. Carel J-C, Leger J. Precocious puberty. Clinical practice. *N Engl J Med* 2008;358:2366–2377.
2. Carel J-C, Eugster EA, Rogol A, Ghizzoni L, Palmert MR. Consensus statement on the use of gonadotropin-releasing hormone analogs in children. *Pediatrics* 2009;123:e752.

CHAPTER 20 Infertility – female

Background and prevalence

- Failure to conceive after regular unprotected sexual intercourse for 1 year in the absence of known reproductive pathology. One in 7 couples has difficulty conceiving.
- Primary – couples who have never conceived. Secondary – couples who have previously conceived.
- About 80% of couples conceive within 1 year of regular unprotected sexual intercourse (UPSI). Of those who do not conceive in the first year, about half will do so in the second year (cumulative pregnancy rate > 90%).
- Female fertility and male fertility decline with age.
- With regular UPSI, 94% of fertile women aged 35 years, and 90% of those aged 39 years, will conceive after 2 years of trying.
- Sexual intercourse every 2 to 3 days optimizes the chance of pregnancy. Timed intercourse has no added benefit and can result in stress.

Initial assessment and referral

- Investigate couples who have not conceived after 1 year of regular UPSI.
- Investigate earlier if there is a history of predisposing factors such as in:
  * Women – aged ≥ 36 years, amenorrhoea, oligomenorrhoea, history of PID or STI, abdominal or pelvic surgery, known or suspected tubal disorder or endometriosis.
  * Men – history of – undescended testes, urogenital surgery, STIs.
- Refer early to specialist centre, if there is a known reason for infertility (such as prior treatment for cancer).
- Evaluate both partners at the same time.
- Discuss the options for attempting conception with people who are unable to or would find it very difficult to have vaginal intercourse.

General advice and lifestyle

- **Smoking:**
  * Women – smoking reduces fertility. Offer women referral to a smoking cessation programme. Passive smoking is likely to affect their chance of conceiving.
  * Men – there is an association between smoking and reduced semen quality.
- **Alcohol:**
  * Women – should drink no more than 1 or 2 units of alcohol once or twice per week and avoid episodes of binge drinking to reduce the risk of harming a fetus.   * Men – 3 to 4 units per day is unlikely to affect the semen quality; excessive alcohol intake is detrimental to semen quality.
- **Body weight – women with:**
  * BMI > 30 are likely to take longer to conceive.
  * BMI > 30 and not ovulating – losing weight will increase the chance of conception.
  * BMI < 19 and who have irregular menstruation or amenorrhea – increasing body weight improves the chance of conception.
  * Group programme of exercise and diet leads to more pregnancies than weight loss advice alone.
  * Men with BMI > 29 are likely to have reduced fertility.
- **Tight underwear** – there is an association between elevated scrotal temperature and reduced semen quality, but it is not clear whether wearing loose-fitting underwear improves fertility.
- **Occupation** – some occupations involve exposure to hazards that can reduce fertility, therefore enquire about occupation.
- **Folic acid** – dietary supplementation with folic acid (0.4 mg/day) before conception and up to 12 weeks' gestation reduces the risk of having a baby with NTDs. For women who had an infant with an NTD, and who are diabetic, or who are receiving antiepileptic medication, 5 mg/day is recommended.
- **Rubella** – offer rubella susceptibility screening and vaccination for women who are susceptible to rubella and advise not to become pregnant for at least 1 month following vaccination.

Psychological effects of fertility problems

- Stress can affect the couple's relationship, and is likely to reduce libido and frequency of intercourse, which can contribute to fertility problems.
- Fertility problems, investigations, and treatment can cause psychological stress. Offer counselling before, during, and after investigation and treatment, irrespective of the outcome of these procedures.

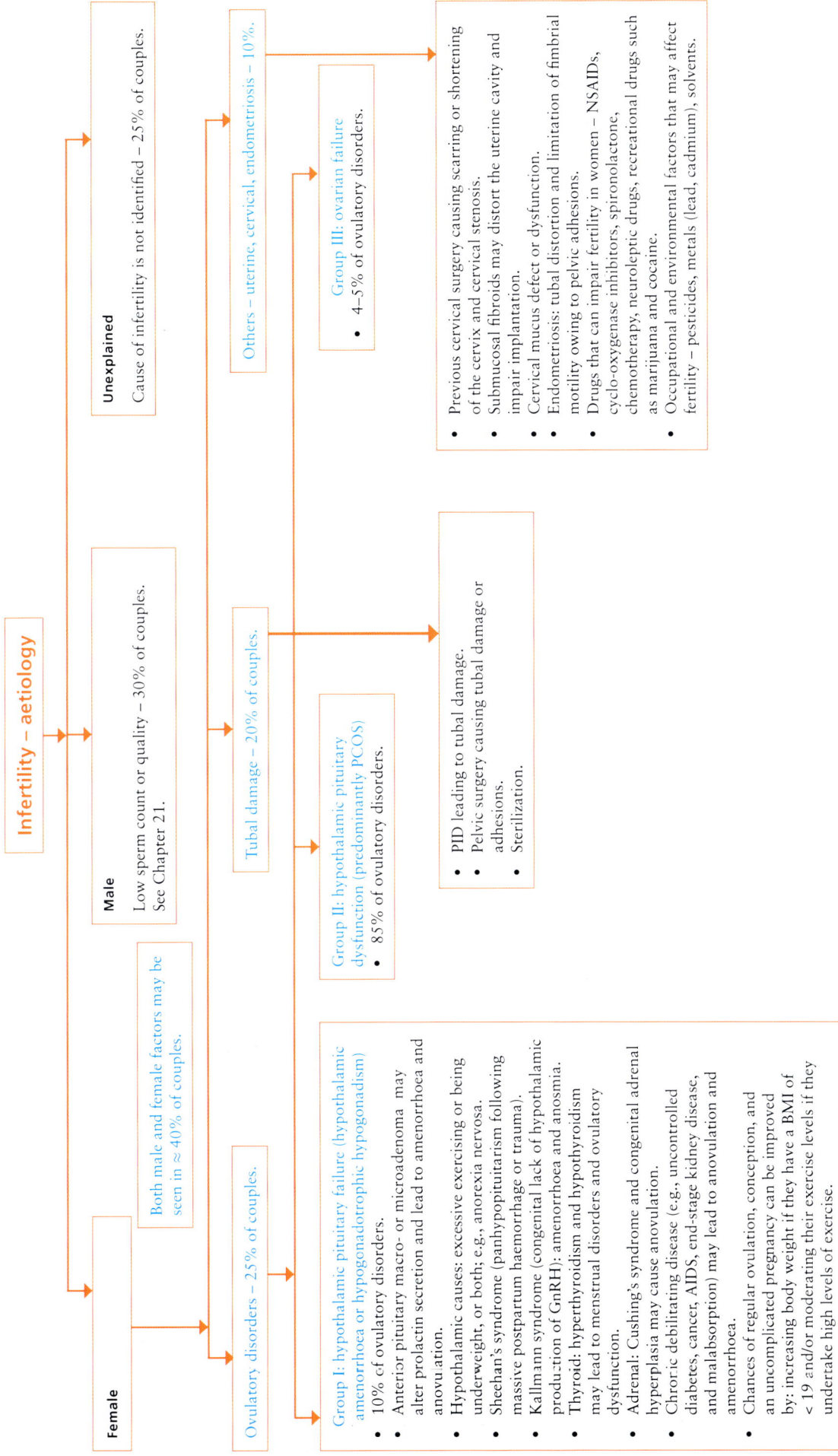

Infertility – aetiology

Female

Both male and female factors may be seen in ≈ 40% of couples.

Male

Low sperm count or quality – 30% of couples. See Chapter 21.

Unexplained

Cause of infertility is not identified – 25% of couples.

Ovulatory disorders – 25% of couples.

Group I: hypothalamic pituitary failure (hypothalamic amenorrhoea or hypogonadotrophic hypogonadism)
- 10% of ovulatory disorders.

- Anterior pituitary macro- or microadenoma may alter prolactin secretion and lead to amenorrhoea and anovulation.
- Hypothalamic causes: excessive exercising or being underweight, or both; e.g., anorexia nervosa.
- Sheehan's syndrome (panhypopituitarism following massive postpartum haemorrhage or trauma).
- Kallmann syndrome (congenital lack of hypothalamic production of GnRH): amenorrhoea and anosmia.
- Thyroid: hyperthyroidism and hypothyroidism may lead to menstrual disorders and ovulatory dysfunction.
- Adrenal: Cushing's syndrome and congenital adrenal hyperplasia may cause anovulation.
- Chronic debilitating disease (e.g., uncontrolled diabetes, cancer, AIDS, end-stage kidney disease, and malabsorption) may lead to anovulation and amenorrhoea.
- Chances of regular ovulation, conception, and an uncomplicated pregnancy can be improved by: increasing body weight if they have a BMI of < 19 and/or moderating their exercise levels if they undertake high levels of exercise.

Tubal damage – 20% of couples.

Group II: hypothalamic pituitary dysfunction (predominantly PCOS)
- 85% of ovulatory disorders.

- PID leading to tubal damage.
- Pelvic surgery causing tubal damage or adhesions.
- Sterilization.

Others – uterine, cervical, endometriosis – 10%.

Group III: ovarian failure
- 4–5% of ovulatory disorders.

- Previous cervical surgery causing scarring or shortening of the cervix and cervical stenosis.
- Submucosal fibroids may distort the uterine cavity and impair implantation.
- Cervical mucus defect or dysfunction.
- Endometriosis: tubal distortion and limitation of fimbrial motility owing to pelvic adhesions.
- Drugs that can impair fertility in women – NSAIDs, cyclo-oxygenase inhibitors, spironolactone, chemotherapy, neuroleptic drugs, recreational drugs such as marijuana and cocaine.
- Occupational and environmental factors that may affect fertility – pesticides, metals (lead, cadmium), solvents.

Female infertility

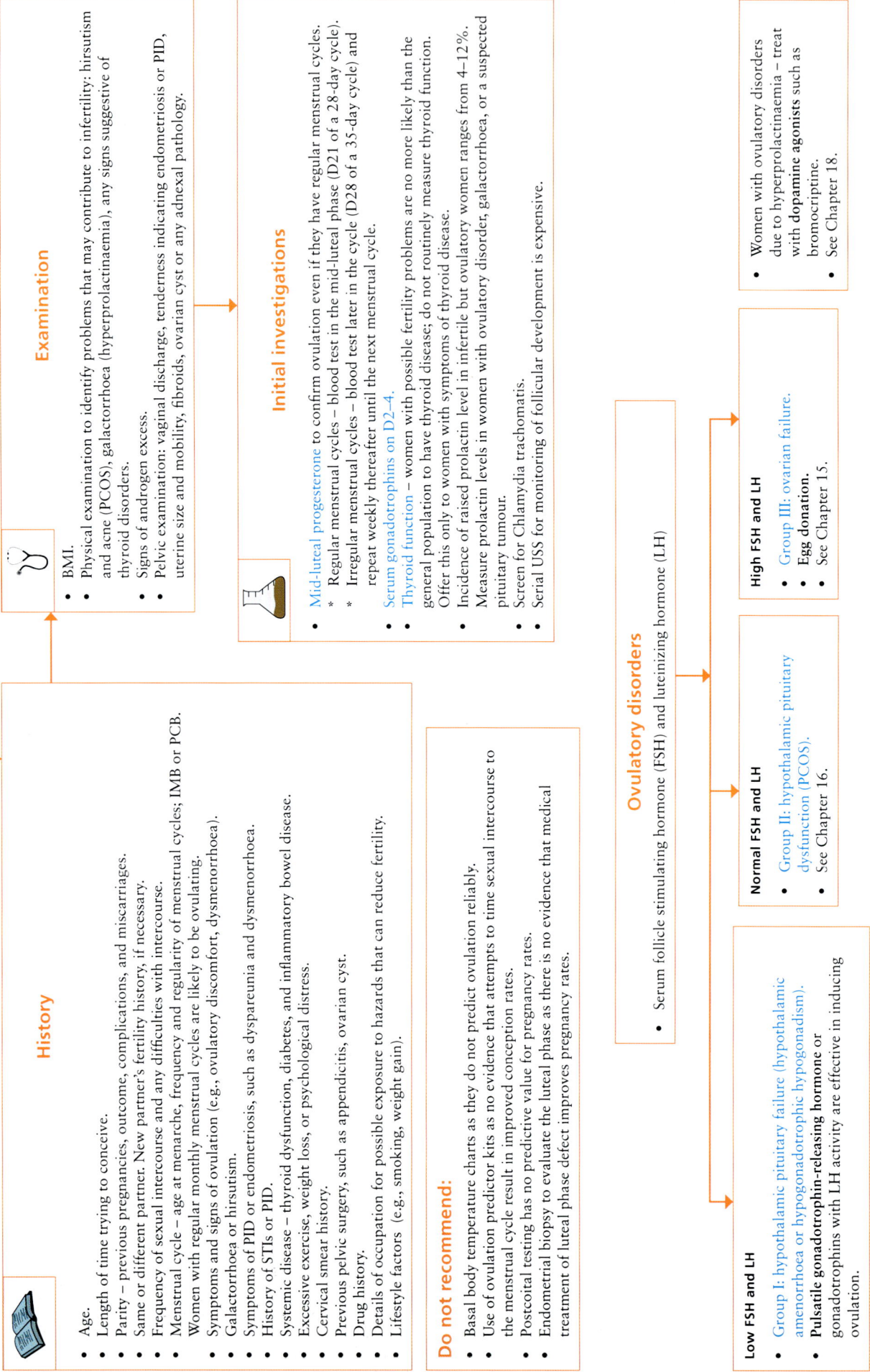

History

- Age.
- Length of time trying to conceive.
- Parity – previous pregnancies, outcome, complications, and miscarriages.
- Same or different partner. New partner's fertility history, if necessary.
- Frequency of sexual intercourse and any difficulties with intercourse.
- Menstrual cycle – age at menarche, frequency and regularity of menstrual cycles; IMB or PCB.
  Women with regular monthly menstrual cycles are likely to be ovulating.
- Symptoms and signs of ovulation (e.g., ovulatory discomfort, dysmenorrhoea).
- Galactorrhoea or hirsutism.
- Symptoms of PID or endometriosis, such as dyspareunia and dysmenorrhoea.
- History of STIs or PID.
- Systemic disease – thyroid dysfunction, diabetes, and inflammatory bowel disease.
- Excessive exercise, weight loss, or psychological distress.
- Cervical smear history.
- Previous pelvic surgery, such as appendicitis, ovarian cyst.
- Drug history.
- Details of occupation for possible exposure to hazards that can reduce fertility.
- Lifestyle factors (e.g., smoking, weight gain).

Do not recommend:

- Basal body temperature charts as they do not predict ovulation reliably.
- Use of ovulation predictor kits as no evidence that attempts to time sexual intercourse to
  the menstrual cycle result in improved conception rates.
- Postcoital testing has no predictive value for pregnancy rates.
- Endometrial biopsy to evaluate the luteal phase as there is no evidence that medical
  treatment of luteal phase defect improves pregnancy rates.

Examination

- BMI.
- Physical examination to identify problems that may contribute to infertility: hirsutism
  and acne (PCOS), galactorrhoea (hyperprolactinaemia), any signs suggestive of
  thyroid disorders.
- Signs of androgen excess.
- Pelvic examination: vaginal discharge, tenderness indicating endometriosis or PID,
  uterine size and mobility, fibroids, ovarian cyst or any adnexal pathology.

Initial investigations

- Mid-luteal progesterone to confirm ovulation even if they have regular menstrual cycles.
  * Regular menstrual cycles – blood test in the mid-luteal phase (D21 of a 28-day cycle).
  * Irregular menstrual cycles – blood test later in the cycle (D28 of a 35-day cycle) and
    repeat weekly thereafter until the next menstrual cycle.
- Serum gonadotrophins on D2–4.
- Thyroid function – women with possible fertility problems are no more likely than the
  general population to have thyroid disease; do not routinely measure thyroid function.
  Offer this only to women with symptoms of thyroid disease.
- Incidence of raised prolactin level in infertile but ovulatory women ranges from 4–12%.
  Measure prolactin levels in women with ovulatory disorder, galactorrhoea, or a suspected
  pituitary tumour.
- Screen for Chlamydia trachomatis.
- Serial USS for monitoring of follicular development is expensive.

Ovulatory disorders

- Serum follicle stimulating hormone (FSH) and luteinizing hormone (LH)

Low FSH and LH
- Group I: hypothalamic pituitary failure (hypothalamic
  amenorrhoea or hypogonadotrophic hypogonadism).
- **Pulsatile gonadotrophin-releasing hormone** or
  gonadotrophins with LH activity are effective in inducing
  ovulation.

Normal FSH and LH
- Group II: hypothalamic pituitary
  dysfunction (PCOS).
- See Chapter 16.

High FSH and LH
- Group III: ovarian failure.
- **Egg donation.**
- See Chapter 15.

- Women with ovulatory disorders
  due to hyperprolactinaemia – treat
  with **dopamine agonists** such as
  bromocriptine.
- See Chapter 18.

Tubal disorders

Investigations

- SA and assessment of ovulation should be known before a test for tubal patency.
- **Hysterosalpingography (HSG)** - for women at low risk of co-morbidities (PID, previous ectopic pregnancy, or endometriosis) to screen for tubal occlusion. It is a reliable test for ruling out tubal occlusion, and is less invasive and makes more efficient use of resources than laparoscopy.
- **Laparoscopy and dye** – for women at risk of co-morbidities so that tubal and other pelvic pathology can be assessed at the same time.
- **Hysterosalpingo-contrast ultrasonography (HYCOSY)** – consider screening for tubal occlusion with HYCOSY because it is an effective alternative to HSG for women who are at low risk of co-morbidities.
- **Screen for Chlamydia trachomatis:**
  * Screen women before any uterine instrumentation. See Chapter 44.
  * Consider prophylactic antibiotics if screening has not been carried out.

Management

- **Tubal catheterization or cannulation** – for women with proximal tubal obstruction, selective salpingography plus tubal catheterization or hysteroscopic tubal cannulation may be treatment options because these treatments improve the chance of pregnancy.
- **Tubal microsurgery and laparoscopic tubal surgery** – for women with mild tubal disease, tubal surgery may be more effective than no treatment.
- **Surgery for hydrosalpinges before in vitro fertilization treatment:**
  * LBR with IVF in women with hydrosalpinges is about one half compared to women without hydrosalpinges. Offer laparoscopic salpingectomy or proximal tubal occlusion to women with hydrosalpinges before IVF because this improves the chance of a live birth.
  * For every six women with hydrosalpinges, one more pregnancy will be achieved if salpingectomy or tubal occlusion is performed before IVF. (ASRM)
  * Insufficient data on the effectiveness of alternative treatments such as neosalpingostomy, transvaginal aspiration of hydrosalpingeal fluid, hysteroscopic tubal occlusion, or antibiotic therapy. (ASRM)

Investigations

- **Assessing uterine abnormalities – HSG, USS, hysteroscopy:**
  * Examination of uterine cavity – tailor to the needs of the individual patient. (ASRM)
  * Do not offer hysteroscopy routinely as part of the initial investigation unless clinically indicated because the effectiveness of surgical treatment of uterine abnormalities on improving CPR is not established.
- **Peritoneal factors (adhesions, endometriosis):**
  * **USS, laparoscopy** – laparoscopy if there is evidence or suspicion of endometriosis, pelvic/ adnexal adhesions, or tubal disease. (ASRM)
  * **Post-coital testing of cervical mucus** – do not offer routine post-coital testing of cervical mucus because it has no predictive value on CPR.
- Tests of ovarian reserve currently have limited sensitivity and specificity in predicting fertility. However, inform women who have high levels of gonadotrophins that they are likely to have reduced fertility.
- Evaluate ovarian reserve in selected patients to obtain prognostic information that may have a significant influence on treatment. (ASRM)

Management

- **Uterine surgery:**
  * Hysteroscopic adhesiolysis – for women with amenorrhoea with intrauterine adhesions. This may restore menstruation and improve the chance of pregnancy.
- **Endometriosis** – See Chapter 12.
  * **Medical management (ovarian suppression)** – medical treatment of minimal and mild endometriosis does not enhance fertility in subfertile women.
  * **Surgical ablation** – women with minimal or mild endometriosis who undergo laparoscopic surgical ablation or resection of endometriosis and adhesiolysis, it improves the chance of pregnancy.
  * Ovarian endometriomas – laparoscopic cystectomy improves chance of pregnancy.
  * Moderate or severe endometriosis – surgical treatment improves chance of pregnancy.
  * Postoperative medical treatment does not improve pregnancy rates in women with moderate to severe endometriosis.

Unexplained infertility

- Do not offer oral ovarian stimulation agents (such as clomifene citrate, anastrozole, or letrozole) as a standalone treatment as this does not increase the chances of a pregnancy.
- Offer IVF treatment if women do not conceive after 2 years of regular UPSI.

Intrauterine insemination

- **Do not offer IUI** for:
  * Mild male factor infertility.
  * Unexplained infertility.
  * Minimal to mild endometriosis.
  * Advise them to try to conceive for a total of 2 years, then consider IVF.

IVF – NICE

Factors affecting the outcome of IVF

- **Female age** – chance of a live birth following IVF declines with female age. Use a woman's age as an initial predictor of her overall chance of success through natural conception or with IVF.
- Can **predict the ovarian response** to gonadotrophin stimulation in IVF with:
  * Total antral follicle count of ≤ 4 for a low response and > 16 for a high response.
  * AMH ≤ 5.4 pmol/L for a low response and ≥ 25.0 pmol/L for a high response.
  * FSH > 8.9 IU/L for a low response and < 4 IU/L for a high response.
- Do not use ovarian volume, ovarian blood flow, inhibin B, or oestradiol (E2) to predict any outcome of fertility treatment.
- **Number of embryos to be transferred and multiple pregnancy** – the chance of multiple pregnancy depends on the number of embryos transferred per cycle of treatment. To balance the chance of a live birth and the risk of multiple pregnancy and its consequences, do not transfer more than two embryos during any one cycle.
- **Number of previous treatment cycles** – chance of a live birth falls as the number of unsuccessful cycles increases.
- **Pregnancy/obstetric history** – IVF is more effective in women who have previously been pregnant and/or had a live birth.
- **Alcohol, smoking, and caffeine consumption:**
  * Consumption of > 1 unit of alcohol per day reduces the effectiveness of ART.
  * Male and female smoking can adversely affect the success rates of ART.
  * Caffeine consumption has adverse effects on the success rates of ART.
- **Body weight** – female BMI outside 19–30 is likely to reduce the success of ART.

Ovulation induction

- Using **pre-treatment** (with either the OCPs or a progestogen) as part of IVF does not affect the chances of having a live birth. Consider pre-treatment to schedule IVF in women who are not undergoing long down-regulation protocols.
- **Down-regulation** – regimens to avoid premature LH surges in gonadotrophin-stimulated IVF cycles. Use either GnRH agonist down-regulation (long protocol) or GnRH antagonists.
- Use GnRH agonists in women who have a low risk of OHSS.
- **Controlled ovarian stimulation** – urinary and recombinant gonadotrophins are equally effective. Individualize the starting dose of FSH based on age, BMI, presence of PCO, and ovarian reserve. Do not use a dosage of FSH > 450 IU/day.
- Natural cycle IVF has lower pregnancy rates than stimulated IVF (CC or gonadotrophins). For women who have regular ovulatory cycles, the likelihood of a live birth after replacement of frozen–thawed embryos is similar in natural or stimulated cycles.
- Use of adjuvant growth hormone or dehydroepiandrosterone (DHEA) with gonadotrophins does not improve pregnancy rates.
- Monitor the cycle with USS (with or without oestradiol levels) for efficacy and safety.
- **Triggering ovulation** – use hCG (urinary or recombinant) to trigger ovulation.
- Women at high risk of OHSS – do not use hCG for oocyte maturation or luteal support.

Referral, medical assessment, and screening for IVF in the UK

- **Screen** for HIV, hepatitis B and hepatitis C viruses; manage and counsel people found to test positive.
- **Referral** – women who have not conceived after 2 years of regular UPSI or 12 cycles of artificial insemination (where 6 or more are by IUI):
  * Women aged < 40 years – offer 3 full cycles of IVF/ICSI. If woman reaches the age of 40 years during treatment, complete the current full cycle but do not offer further full cycles.
  * Women aged 40 to 42 years – offer 1 full cycle of IVF/ICSI, provided they have never previously had IVF treatment, there is no evidence of low ovarian reserve, risks and implications of IVF and pregnancy at this age have been discussed.

- **Oocyte retrieval:**
  * Women undergoing transvaginal retrieval of oocytes – offer conscious sedation because it is a safe and acceptable analgesia.
  * Do not use follicle flushing in women who have developed at least three follicles because it does not increase the numbers of oocytes retrieved or pregnancy rates, and it increases the duration of oocyte retrieval and associated pain.
- **Assisted hatching** does not improve pregnancy rates.
- **Embryo transfer** – ultrasound-guided ET improves pregnancy rates.
  * ET on D2 or D3 and D5 or D6 appear to be equally effective.
  * Replacement of embryos into a uterine cavity with an endometrium of < 5 mm thickness is unlikely to result in a pregnancy.
  * Bed rest of more than 20 minutes' duration following ET does not improve the outcome.
- **Number of fresh or frozen embryos to transfer in IVF:**
  * For women aged < 37 years: 1st IVF cycle, use single embryo transfer (SET); 2nd IVF cycle, use SET if 1 or more top-quality embryos are available. Consider using 2 embryos if no top-quality embryos are available; 3rd IVF cycle, transfer no more than 2 embryos.
  * For women aged 37–39 years: 1st and 2nd IVF cycles, use SET if there are one or more top-quality embryos. Consider double embryo transfer if there are no top-quality embryos; 3rd IVF cycle, transfer no more than 2 embryos.
  * For women aged 40–42 years, consider double embryo transfer.
  * No more than 2 embryos should be transferred during any one cycle of IVF. Where a top-quality blastocyst is available, use SET.
  * Women using donor eggs – embryo transfer strategy based on the age of the donor.
  * Cryopreserve to store any remaining good-quality embryos after embryo transfer.
  * If ≥ 2 embryos are frozen then transfer them before the next stimulated cycle because this will minimize ovulation induction and egg collection, both of which carry risks for the woman and use more resources.
  * Women with regular ovulatory cycles – chances of live birth after replacement of frozen–thawed embryos is similar for natural cycles and hormone-supplemented cycles.
- **Luteal support** – use progesterone for luteal support.
  * Do not routinely use hCG for luteal support because of the increased risk of OHSS.
  * No evidence to support continuing any form of treatment for luteal phase support beyond 8 weeks' gestation.

Long-term safety of ARTs for women and children

- OI and ovarian stimulation:
  - * No direct association is seen between these treatments and invasive cancer.
  - * No association is seen in the short- to medium-term between these treatments and adverse outcomes (including cancer) in children born.
  - * Information on long-term health outcomes in women and children is still awaited.
- IVF – while the absolute risks of long-term adverse outcomes of IVF treatment with or without ICSI are low, a small increased risk of borderline ovarian tumours cannot be excluded. The absolute risks of long-term adverse outcomes in children born as result of IVF are low.
- Limit drugs used for OI or ovarian stimulation agents and controlled ovarian stimulation in IVF treatment to the lowest effective dose and duration of use.

Virology issues

HIV positive

- If male is HIV positive – risk of HIV transmission to the female partner is negligible through UPSI if all the below criteria are met:
  - * Male is compliant with HAART.
  - * Male has had a plasma viral load of < 50 copies/ml for more than 6 months.
  - * There are no other infections present.
  - * UPSI is limited to the time of ovulation.
- If all the above criteria are met, sperm washing may not reduce the risk of infection further and may reduce the likelihood of pregnancy.
- If couples who meet the above criteria still perceive an unacceptable risk of HIV transmission, consider sperm washing.
- There is insufficient evidence to recommend that HIV negative women use pre-exposure prophylaxis, when all the above criteria are met.
- If male is HIV positive and either he is not compliant with HAART or his plasma viral load is ≥ 50 copies/ml, offer sperm washing.
- Sperm washing reduces, but does not eliminate, the risk of HIV transmission.

Hepatitis B positive

- Offer and vaccinate partners with hepatitis B before starting fertility treatment.
- Do not offer sperm washing as part of fertility treatment.

Hepatitis C – where the man has hepatitis C:

- The risk of transmission through UPSI is low.
- MDT care – the couple, a fertility specialist, and a hepatitis specialist. Men can consider treatment options to eradicate the hepatitis C with their appropriate specialist before conception is considered.

Intrauterine insemination

- Consider unstimulated IUI in those:
  - * Who are unable to, or find it very difficult to, have vaginal intercourse because of a clinically diagnosed physical disability or psychosexual problem.
  - * Who are using partner or donor sperm.
  - * People with a specific condition (e.g., after sperm washing where the man is HIV positive).
  - * People in same-sex relationships.
- Success rate: > 50% of women aged under 40 years will conceive within 6 cycles of IUI. Of those who do not conceive within 6 cycles of IUI, about half will do so with a further 6 cycles (cumulative pregnancy rate over 75%).
- Fresh sperm is associated with higher conception rates than frozen–thawed sperm. However, IUI even using frozen–thawed sperm is associated with higher conception rates than intracervical insemination.
- Advise insemination to time around ovulation.
- If the woman does not conceive after 6 cycles, assess clinically and investigate. If partner sperm is being used, partner also needs assessment and investigations.
- If not conceived after 6 cycles of donor or partner insemination, despite evidence of normal ovulation, tubal patency, and semen analysis, offer a further 6 cycles of unstimulated IUI before IVF is considered.

Intracytoplasmic sperm injection

- Indications:
  - * Severe deficits in semen quality.
  - * Obstructive azoospermia.
  - * Non-obstructive azoospermia.
  - * Previous IVF cycle – failed or very poor fertilization.
- Consider genetic issues including appropriate genetic counselling and testing.
- ICSI vs IVF – ICSI improves fertilization rates compared to IVF alone, but once fertilization is achieved, the pregnancy rate is no better than with IVF.

Gamete intra-Fallopian transfer and zygote intra-Fallopian transfer:

- There is insufficient evidence for the use of GIFT or ZIFT in preference to IVF in couples with unexplained fertility problems or male factor fertility problems.

Oocyte donation

- Indications:
  - * Premature ovarian insufficiency.
  - * Gonadal dysgenesis including Turner's syndrome.
  - * Bilateral oophorectomy.
  - * Ovarian failure following chemotherapy or radiotherapy.
  - * Certain cases of IVF treatment failure.
  - * High risk of transmitting a genetic disorder to the offspring.
- Screen oocyte donors for infectious and genetic diseases.
- Offer counselling for oocyte recipients and donors regarding the physical and psychological implications of treatment for themselves and their genetic children, including any potential children resulting from donated oocytes.

What not to do

- Basal body temperature charts to predict ovulation.
- Use of ovulation predictor kits.
- Post-coital testing of cervical mucus.
- Endometrial biopsy to evaluate the luteal phase.
- Routine measurement of TFT and prolactin levels.
- Hysteroscopy on its own as part of the initial investigation.
- Medical treatment of minimal and mild endometriosis.
- Postoperative medical treatment in women with moderate to severe endometriosis.
- Use of GnRH antagonists.
- Natural cycle IVF.
- Use of adjuvant growth hormone with gonadotrophins.
- Monitoring oestrogen levels during OI.
- Assisted hatching.
- Embryo replacement into a uterine cavity with an endometrium of < 5 mm thickness.
- Routine use of hCG for luteal support.

1. *Fertility: Assessment and Treatment for People with Fertility Problems.* NICE Clinical Guideline 11, February 2004.
2. The Practice Committee of ASRM. Optimum evaluation of the infertile female. *Fertil Steril* 2006;86(5):S264–267. Please also refer to updated guidelines from Feb 2013.
3. The Practice Committee of ASRM. Effectiveness and treatment for unexplained infertility. *Fertil Steril* 2006;86(5):S111–114.
4. The Practice Committee of ASR. Salpingectomy for hydrosalpinx prior to IVF. *Fertil Steril* 2008;90(5):S66–68.

CHAPTER 21 Infertility – male

Male factor is responsible in about 30% of infertile couples and contributory in another 30–40%.

Investigate if pregnancy fails to occur within one year of regular unprotected intercourse.

Evaluate before one year if male infertility risk factors are present.

Initial screening evaluation

Semen analysis

WHO 2010 normal semen parameters

Parameter	Lower reference limit
Semen volume (ml)	1.5 (1.4–1.7)
Total sperm number (10⁶/ejaculate)	39 (33–46)
Sperm concentration (10⁶/per ml)	15 (12–16)
Total motility (progressive + non-progressive, %)	
Progressive motility (%)	40 (38–42)
Vitality (live spermatozoa, %)	32 (31–34)
Sperm morphology (normal, %)	58 (55–63)
	4 (3.0–4.0)

- If the first semen analysis (SA) is abnormal, repeat it in 3 months after the initial analysis to allow time for the cycle of spermatozoa formation to be completed (not mandatory and can be done earlier if it generates anxiety).
- A single-sample analysis will falsely identify about 10% of men as abnormal, but repeating the test reduces this to 2%.
- If azoospermia or severe oligozoospermia is detected, repeat the test as soon as possible (within 2–4 weeks).

Normal SA → Unexplained subfertility/female factor

Abnormal SA

History

- Duration of infertility and prior fertility.
- Sexual history – coital frequency and timing.
- Childhood illnesses and developmental history such as viral orchitis or cryptorchidism.
- Infections such as epididymitis or urethritis, including STIs.
- Genital trauma or prior pelvic or inguinal surgery.
- Gonadal toxin exposure such as prior radiation therapy/chemotherapy, recent fever, or heat exposure.
- Family history of birth defects, mental disability, reproductive failure, or cystic fibrosis.
- Medical and surgical history.
- Drug history, over-the-counter and recreational drugs.
- Agents such as heat, X-rays, metals, and pesticides – evidence suggestive of a harmful effect. Therefore, enquire about occupation; e.g., radiotherapists, engine drivers, diggers, agricultural workers, chemists, laboratory workers, painters.

Full evaluation – examination and investigations

- If the sperm concentration is ≤ 5 × 10⁶/ml, impaired sexual function or other clinical findings suggestive of any specific concern from history.
- Azoospermia – complete absence of sperm from the ejaculate (1%) of all men and in approximately 15% of infertile men).

Examination

- Secondary sexual characteristics – body habitus, hair distribution, and gynaecomastia.
- Examination of the penis; location of the urethral meatus; testis size (normal volume > 19 ml), mass, and consistency; presence of a varicocele; presence and consistency of vasa and epididymides.

General advice

- Alcohol consumption of 3–4 units per day is unlikely to affect fertility. Excessive alcohol intake is detrimental to semen quality.
- There is an association between smoking and reduced semen quality (although the impact of this on male fertility is uncertain), and stopping smoking will improve general health.
- BMI of > 29 – likely to have reduced fertility.
- There is an association between elevated scrotal temperature and reduced semen quality, but it is uncertain whether wearing loose-fitting underwear improves fertility.

Investigations

- **Serum FSH and testosterone levels.** If the testosterone level is low, repeat total and free testosterone, LH, and prolactin levels.
- Scrotal USS – if, on palpation, scrotum is difficult or inadequate to assess, or a testicular mass is suspected.

Low FSH and testosterone

Pre-testicular – secondary testicular failure

- Hypogonadotropic hypogonadism.
- Bilateral testicular atrophy, low semen volume, low LH levels.
- Congenital abnormalities such as Kallmann syndrome.
- Acquired – functioning and nonfunctioning pituitary tumours.
- **Perform serum prolactin levels and pituitary CT or MRI.**

High FSH and normal/low testosterone

Testicular – primary testicular failure

- Bilateral testicular atrophy, low semen volume.
- Chromosomal abnormalities found in 7% of male infertility. Sex chromosome aneuploidy is most common (Klinefelter syndrome in 2/3 cases). Karyotype all patients with non-obstructive azoospermia and severe oligospermia (sperm count: < 5 × 10⁶/ml).
- **Y-chromosome microdeletions** – may be found in 10–15% of men with azoospermia or severe oligozoospermia. Prognostic significance – with deletions in AZFa or AZFb regions, sperm are normally not found, whereas up to 80% with AZFc deletions may have retrievable sperm. (AUA)
- Counsel regarding inheritance of the compromised fertility potential in male offspring.

Normal FSH and testosterone

Post-testicular – 40%

Erectile/ejaculatory

- Anejaculation.
- Retrograde ejaculation – perform a post-ejaculatory urinalysis.
- Erectile dysfunction.

Obstruction

Epididymal/vasal obstruction

- Vasa and testes are normal, semen volume normal.
- * Bilateral epididymal obstruction – identified only by surgical exploration.
- * Vasal obstruction – vasectomy (most common), severe genitourinary infections, iatrogenic.
- Vasography – to diagnose whether the obstruction is in vas deferens or ejaculatory ducts. It should not be done unless reconstructive surgery is undertaken at the same surgical procedure.

Ejaculatory duct obstruction

- Semen volume low (< 1.0 ml).
- Seminal pH low and fructose low, as the seminal vesicle secretions are alkaline and contain fructose.
- TRUS – minimally invasive and avoids the risk of vasal injury associated with vasography. With or without seminal vesicle aspiration and seminal vesiculography – determine the anatomical site of the obstruction.
- Vasography.

Obstructive

Vasal agenesis

Congenital bilateral absence of the vas deferens

- 70% of men with CBAVD and no clinical evidence of cystic fibrosis have an abnormality of CFTR gene. (Almost all males with clinical cystic fibrosis have CBAVD).
- Seminal vesicle hypoplasia or agenesis – owing to embryological association between the vasa and seminal vesicles.
- Low semen volume – since majority of semen is derived from seminal vesicles.
- Both partners – genetic counselling and test for CFTR gene. Failure to identify a CFTR abnormality in a man with CBAVD does not rule out the presence of a mutation, as many mutations may not be detected by routine testing methods; therefore, test the spouse for CFTR gene abnormalities because she may be a carrier.
- In patients who have CBAVD and CFTR mutations, the prevalence of renal anomalies is extremely rare. Therefore, imaging of the kidneys with USS or CT scan is only indicated in men with CBAVD with no mutations in CFTR.

Unilateral vasal agenesis

- Transrectal USS (TRUS) – to evaluate the ampullary portion of the contralateral vas deferens and the seminal vesicles, because unilateral vasal agenesis can be associated with contralateral atresia of the vas deferens or seminal vesicle, leading to obstruction azoospermia.
- There is a strong association between unilateral vasal agenesis and ipsilateral renal anomalies; therefore, organize USS or CT scan of the kidneys.

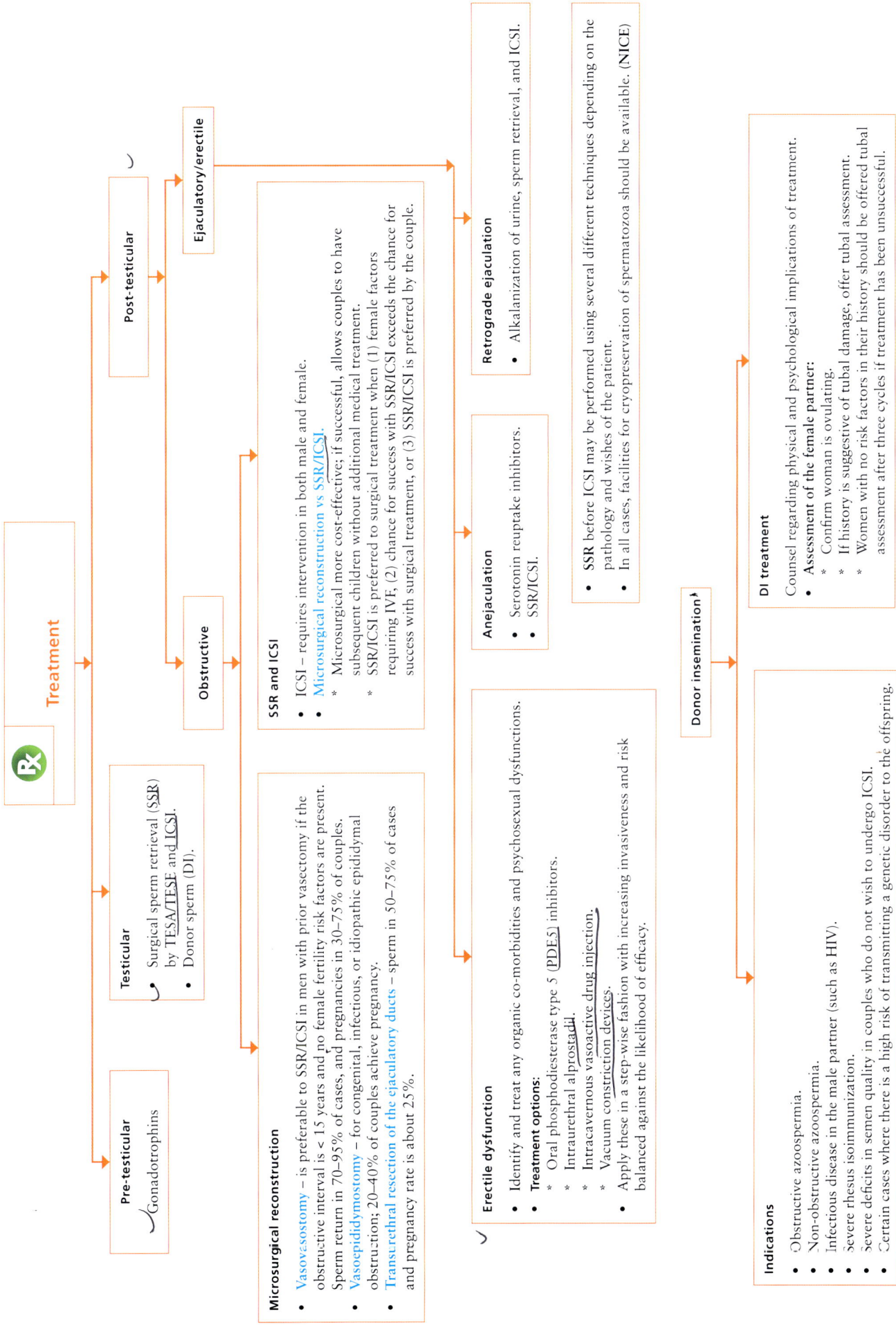

Treatment

Pre-testicular
- Gonadotrophins

Testicular
- Surgical sperm retrieval (SSR) by TESA/TESE and ICSI.
- Donor sperm (DI).

Post-testicular

Obstructive

Ejaculatory/erectile

Microsurgical reconstruction
- **Vasovasostomy** – is preferable to SSR/ICSI in men with prior vasectomy if the obstructive interval is < 15 years and no female fertility risk factors are present. Sperm return in 70–95% of cases, and pregnancies in 30–75% of couples.
- **Vasoepididymostomy** – for congenital, infectious, or idiopathic epididymal obstruction; 20–40% of couples achieve pregnancy.
- **Transurethral resection of the ejaculatory ducts** – sperm in 50–75% of cases and pregnancy rate is about 25%.

SSR and ICSI
- ICSI – requires intervention in both male and female.
- **Microsurgical reconstruction vs SSR/ICSI.**
  * Microsurgical more cost-effective; if successful, allows couples to have subsequent children without additional medical treatment.
  * SSR/ICSI is preferred to surgical treatment when (1) female factors requiring IVF, (2) chance for success with SSR/ICSI exceeds the chance for success with surgical treatment, or (3) SSR/ICSI is preferred by the couple.

Erectile dysfunction
- Identify and treat any organic co-morbidities and psychosexual dysfunctions.
- **Treatment options:**
  * Oral phosphodiesterase type 5 (PDE5) inhibitors.
  * Intraurethral alprostadil.
  * Intracavernous vasoactive drug injection.
  * Vacuum constriction devices.
- Apply these in a step-wise fashion with increasing invasiveness and risk balanced against the likelihood of efficacy.

Retrograde ejaculation
- Alkalanization of urine, sperm retrieval, and ICSI.

Anejaculation
- Serotonin reuptake inhibitors.
- SSR/ICSI.

- **SSR** before ICSI may be performed using several different techniques depending on the pathology and wishes of the patient.
- In all cases, facilities for cryopreservation of spermatozoa should be available. (NICE)

Donor insemination

Indications
- Obstructive azoospermia.
- Non-obstructive azoospermia.
- Infectious disease in the male partner (such as HIV).
- Severe rhesus isoimmunization.
- Severe deficits in semen quality in couples who do not wish to undergo ICSI.
- Certain cases where there is a high risk of transmitting a genetic disorder to the offspring.

DI treatment
Counsel regarding physical and psychological implications of treatment.
- **Assessment of the female partner:**
  * Confirm woman is ovulating.
  * If history is suggestive of tubal damage, offer tubal assessment.
  * Women with no risk factors in their history should be offered tubal assessment after three cycles if treatment has been unsuccessful.

- **IUI vs intracervical insemination** – couples using donor sperm should be offered IUI in preference to intracervical insemination because it improves pregnancy rates.
- **Unstimulated vs stimulated DI** – women who are ovulating regularly should be offered a minimum of six cycles of DI without ovarian stimulation to reduce the risk of multiple pregnancy and its consequences.
- **Timing of DI** – timing of insemination using either urinary LH or basal body temperature changes is equally effective in donor cycles. However, using urinary LH detection reduces the number of clinic visits per cycle.
- **Maximum number of cycles** – couples should be offered other treatment options after six unsuccessful cycles of DI.

Guideline comparator

AUA:

- If the first semen analysis is abnormal, repeat test in 1 month after the initial analysis.
- Examination and investigations if the sperm concentration is $< 10 \times 10^6$/ml.
- **Tests for anti-sperm antibodies (ASA):**
  - * Pregnancy rates may be reduced by ASA in the semen. Risk factors for ASA include ductal obstruction, prior genital infection, testicular trauma, and prior vasovasostomy or vasoepididymostomy.
  - * Consider ASA test when there is isolated asthenospermia with normal sperm concentration, sperm agglutination, or an abnormal post-coital test.
  - * Some recommend ASA test for couples with unexplained infertility.
  - * ASA test is not needed if sperm are to be used for ICSI.
- **Sperm viability tests** – determine whether non-motile sperm are viable by identifying which sperm have intact cell membranes. Non-motile but viable sperm, as determined by the HOS test, may be used successfully for ICSI.
- Quantitation of leucocytes in semen – true pyospermia leukocytes: 1×10^6/ml) should be evaluated for a genital tract infection or inflammation. (AUA)

NICE:

- Do not routinely test for Y-chromosome microdeletions before ICSI.

What not to do

- Screening for antisperm antibodies.
- Routine use of post-coital testing of cervical mucus.
- Routine use of sperm DNA integrity testing. (AUA).
- Routine test of reactive oxygen species (ROS).
- Complementary therapies.
- Use of anti-oestrogens, gonadotrophins, androgens, bromocriptine, or kinin-enhancing drugs in men with idiopathic semen abnormalities.
- Use of antibiotics for men with leucocytes in their semen unless there is an identified infection.
- Surgery for men for varicocele.

1. *WHO Laboratory Manual for the Examination and Processing of Human Semen, Fifth edition*, 2010.
2. *Fertility: Assessment and Treatment for People with Fertility Problems*. NICE Clinical Guideline 11, February 2004. Please also refer to updated guidelines from Feb 2013.
3. *The Evaluation of the Azoospermic Male*. AUA Best Practice Statement; Revised, 2010.
4. British Fertility Society Guidelines for Practice. Impact of Chlamydia trachomatis in the reproductive setting. *Hum Fertil (Camb)* 2010;13(3):115–125.
5. AUA Guidelines on the Pharmacological Management of Premature Ejaculation. *J Urol* 2004:172(1):290–294.
6. *Guideline on the Management of Erectile Dysfunction*. AUA Diagnosis and Treatment Recommendations, 2005.
7. ASRM. Evaluation of azoospermic man. *Fertil Steril* 2008;90:S74–77.
8. ASRM. Genetic considerations related to ICSI. *Fertil Steril* 2008;90:S182–184.
9. ASRM. ICSI. *Fertil Steril* 2008;90:S187.
10. *The Management of Obstructive Azoospermia*. AUA Best Practice Statement; Revised, 2010.
11. *The Optimal Evaluation of the Infertile Male*. AUA Best Practice Statement; Revised, 2010.
12. ASRM. Report on varicocele and subfertility. *Fertil Steril* 2008;90:S247–249.
13. ASRM. Sperm retrieval for obstructive azoospermia. *Fertil Steril* 2008;90:S213–218.
14. ASRM. The clinical utility of the sperm DNA integrity testing. *Fertil Steril* 2008;90:S178–180.
15. ASRM. The management of infertility due to obstructive azoospermia. *Fertil Steril* 2008;90:S121–124.
16. Report on varicocele and infertility. AUA Best Practice Policy, Reviewed, 2011.
17. ASRM. Vasectomy reversal. *Fertil Steril* 2008;90:S78–82.

Background and incidence

- A systemic disease resulting from vasoactive products released by hyperstimulated ovaries.
- Increased capillary permeability leads to leakage of fluid from the vascular compartment, with third-space fluid accumulation and intravascular dehydration.
- It can occur after any form of supra-physiological ovarian stimulation, including clomifene citrate (CC), gonadotrophin ovulation induction, and IVF.
- Incidence – variable incidence reported owing to the variety of classification schemes used.
  * Mild OHSS – up to 33% of IVF cycles.
  * Moderate or severe OHSS 3–8%.

Risk factors – women at higher risk of OHSS

- Women with polycystic ovaries.
- Women < 30 years of age.
- Use of GnRH agonists.
- Exposure to LH/hCG.
- Development of multiple follicles.
- Previous episodes of OHSS.
- Cycles where pregnancy occurs, particularly multiple pregnancies.

History

- Ovarian stimulation.
- Abdominal distension, abdominal pain.
- Nausea and vomiting.
- Breathlessness.

Examination

- Body weight and abdominal girth.
- Abdominal examination – degree of distension, palpable ovaries, presence or absence of ascites, any tenderness.
- Heart rate, blood pressure, chest examination.
- Hydration – intake and output.

Risks or complications

- Morbidity – thrombosis, renal and liver dysfunction, acute respiratory distress syndrome, prolonged hospitalization.
- Mortality – very rare.
- Although reduced renal perfusion secondary to hypovolaemia or tense ascites may lead to oliguria in about one third of women with severe OHSS, acute renal failure is rare.

Differential diagnosis

- Complication of an ovarian cyst (torsion, haemorrhage). Suspect torsion in the presence of worsening, particularly of unilateral pain and nausea. Colour Doppler assessment of ovarian blood flow may help in diagnosis.
- Pelvic infection.
- Intra-abdominal haemorrhage.
- Ectopic pregnancy.
- Appendicitis.

HFEA (UK) standards

- Provide all women undergoing ovarian stimulation clear advice about the symptoms and risks of OHSS.
- Assisted Conception centers should have agreed protocols for referral of women with suspected OHSS to hospital care, and written protocols for initial OHSS management.

Investigations

- Full blood count: haemoglobin, haematocrit, white cell count to assess haemoconcentration.
- CRP, urea and electrolytes, LFTs.
- Serum β-hCG.
- Baseline clotting studies.
- Pelvic ultrasound for ascites and ovarian size.
- Chest X-ray and ultrasonography if respiratory symptoms.

'Early' and 'late' OHSS – may be useful in determining the prognosis.

- Early – OHSS presenting within 9 days after the ovulatory dose of hCG; is likely to reflect excessive ovarian response and the precipitating effect of exogenous hCG administered for final follicular maturation.
- Late – OHSS presenting after this period reflects endogenous hCG stimulation from an early pregnancy. Late OHSS is more likely to be severe and to last longer than early OHSS.

Grading – to aid management

The severity could worsen over time as the condition evolves.

Mild

- Abdominal bloating.
- Mild abdominal pain.
- Ovarian size usually < 8 cm.

Moderate

- Moderate abdominal pain.
- Nausea ± vomiting.
- Ultrasound evidence of ascites.
- Ovarian size usually 8–12 cm.

Severe

- Clinical ascites (occasionally hydrothorax). • Oliguria.
- Haemoconcentration; haematocrit > 45%.
- Hypoproteinaemia.
- Ovarian size usually >12 cm.

Critical

- Tense ascites or large hydrothorax.
- Haematocrit > 55%.
- White cell count > 25,000/ml.
- Oligo-/anuria.
- Thromboembolism.
- Acute respiratory distress syndrome.

Management

Essentially supportive care until the condition resolves spontaneously.

Outpatient

- Mild OHSS and majority of moderate OHSS.
- Analgesia – paracetamol or codeine.
- Encourage to drink to thirst, rather than to excess. It is the most physiological approach to replace volume avoiding the risk of hypervolaemia and worsening ascites that may occur with vigorous intravenous therapy.
- Continue progesterone luteal support.
- Review every 2–3 days.
- Urgent review if increasing severity of pain, increasing abdominal distension, shortness of breath, and a subjective impression of reduced urine output as signs of worsening OHSS.

Inpatient

- Severe OHSS.
- Moderate OHSS if unable to achieve control of pain and/or nausea with oral treatment.
- Where there are difficulties in ensuring adequate ongoing monitoring.
- Assess at least daily.

Intensive care

- Critical OHSS.
- Specific complications – ARDS, renal failure, and thromboembolism.
- Severe OHSS where initial crystalloid and colloid therapy fails to correct dehydration and haemoconcentration.
- Needs more frequent than daily assessment.

Inpatient care

- Experienced clinicians.
- MDT care – anaesthetic, medical colleagues, specialists with expertise in intensive care.

Assessment

- History – pain, breathlessness.
- Examination – degree of distension of abdomen, palpable ovaries, presence of ascites and paralytic ileus.
- Abdominal girth and weight – admission and daily until resolution.
- Cardiovascular – heart rate, blood pressure.
- Hydration – monitor intake and output chart at least on daily basis, with more frequent assessment if the woman is dehydrated or receiving intravenous fluids. Urine output of <1000 ml/day or a persistent positive fluid balance is a cause for concern.

Investigations

- FBC – haemoconcentration is a measure of the severity of OHSS and may be measured by raised haemoglobin and haematocrit.
- White cell count – an increase may indicate an ongoing systemic stress response.
- Urea and electrolytes – hyponatraemia, may be dilutional as a result of antidiuretic hormone hypersecretion.
- LFTs may be abnormal in 25–40% of severe OHSS cases and usually normalize with resolution of the disease.
- Baseline clotting studies.
- Pelvic ultrasound for ascites and ovarian size.
- Chest X-ray if respiratory symptoms and signs are suggestive of hydrothorax, pulmonary infection, or pulmonary embolism.
- Chest ultrasonography can assist diagnosis of hydrothorax.
- ECG and echocardiogram if suspected pericardial effusion or pulmonary embolism.

Inpatient management

Symptomatic relief

- Antiemetics if necessary. Nausea is usually related to the accumulation of ascites, so measures to reduce abdominal distension should provide relief.
- Analgesia – paracetamol, opiates.
- Do not use NSAIDs because they may compromise renal function in patients with OHSS.

Fluid management

- Drink to thirst, rather than to excess.
- Where oral intake cannot be maintained, IV crystalloids, such as normal saline 2–3 L in 24 hours, guided by a strict fluid balance chart.
- Colloids – women with persistent haemoconcentration and/or UOP < 0.5 ml/kg/hour may benefit from colloids; e.g., human albumin, 6% hydroxyethyl starch (HES), dextran, mannitol, and Haemaccel.
- HES – reported to be associated with a higher mean daily UOP, fewer paracenteses, and shorter hospital stay than human albumin.
- Avoid diuretics as they deplete intravascular volume. They may have a role with careful haemodynamic monitoring in cases where oliguria persists despite adequate intravascular volume expansion and a normal intra-abdominal pressure.

Prevention of thrombosis

- Incidence of thrombosis is 0.7–10% with an apparent preponderance of upper body sites and frequent involvement of the arterial system. Unusual neurological symptoms should raise the possibility of a thrombotic episode in an uncommon location.
- Thromboprophylaxis to all women admitted to hospital.
  * Full-length venous support stockings and prophylactic heparin.
  * Intermittent pneumatic compression device if patient is confined to bed.
- In women who do not conceive, discontinue thromboprophylaxis with resolution of OHSS. In women who conceive, the risk of thrombosis persists into the first trimester of pregnancy; therefore, consider the risks and benefits of heparin prophylaxis until the end of the first trimester, or even longer, depending on the presence of risk factors and course of the OHSS.
- Therapeutic anticoagulation if thromboembolism is suspected, and manage accordingly.

Surgical management

- Paracentesis – indications:
  * Women distressed with significant discomfort or respiratory compromise due to severe abdominal distension.
  * Oliguria persisting despite adequate volume replacement. Relief of intra-abdominal pressure may promote renal perfusion and improve UOP.
  * Under USS guidance to avoid inadvertent puncture of vascular ovaries distended by large luteal cysts.
  * Avoid repeated paracenteses.
  * To avoid cardiovascular collapse from massive fluid shifts, control the rate of ascitic fluid drainage, administer IV colloids, and monitor BP and pulse.
- Symptomatic hydrothorax – drainage of ascites may suffice to resolve hydrothorax; however, if it persists, may be drained directly.
- Adnexal torsion or coincident problems requiring surgery:
  * Experienced surgeon following careful assessment.
  * Untwisting of the twisted adnexa followed by observation of improved colour at laparoscopy or laparotomy is associated with a favourable prognosis for ovarian function.

What not to do

- NSAIDs for analgesia.
- Strenuous exercise and sexual intercourse.
- hCG for luteal support.
- Diuretics.
- Routine screening for thrombophilia in all women undergoing assisted conception.

1. *The Management of Ovarian Hyperstimulation Syndrome.* RCOG Green-top Guideline No. 5; September 2006.
2. SOGC. The diagnosis and management of ovarian hyperstimulation syndrome. *J Obstet Gynaecol (Can)* 2011;33(11):1156–1162.
3. The Practice Committee of ASRM. Ovarian hyperstimulation syndrome. *FertilSteril* 2008;90:S188–193.

CHAPTER 23 Fertility sparing treatments in gynaecological cancers

Annually in the UK, over 1000 women with cervical cancer, 120 with endometrial cancer, and over 500 with ovarian cancer present before the age of 45 years.

Cervical cancer

Up to 43% of all cervical cancers diagnosed are in women under the age of 45 years.

Stage IA1 – cone biopsy

- Stage IA1 squamous cell carcinoma – risk of < 1% of lymph node involvement compared with 5% in women with tumour invading to a depth > 3 mm. Manage with knife/laser cone biopsy or LLETZ, provided the excisional margins are free of dysplasia or invasive disease and there is no lymphovascular space invasion. Further cone biopsy may be performed if the surgical margins are involved.
- Stage IA1 adenocarcinoma – knife cone biopsy with the depth of the cone being at least 25 mm and clear margins of 5 mm or more.
- LLETZ – diathermy can make pathological assessment difficult because of the heat artefact. To obtain a 2.5 cm depth of cervical tissue, two loop specimens may be necessary, whereas with a knife or laser cone one specimen can be obtained. Staging can be more accurately assessed with one intact specimen.
- Knife cone biopsy – increased risk of PTD, LBW and CS. Meta-analysis – PTD rate is related to the proportion of the cervix removed; delivery before 37 weeks of gestation is 11% vs 7% in controls.

Stage IA2 – cone biopsy and laparoscopic pelvic node dissection

- Stage IA2 squamous cell carcinoma and adenocarcinoma of the cervix – large cone biopsy and laparoscopic pelvic node dissection. Tumour < 1 cm in diameter have a 0.6% chance of parametrial involvement and lymph node spread is up to 5%. Therefore, a pelvic node dissection is required as part of the treatment. However, the lesion on the cervix is very small and local treatment need not be radical.

Stage IB1

Radical vaginal trachelectomy (RVT)

- **Laparoscopic lymph node dissection and radical removal of the upper vagina, cervix, and paracervical tissue vaginally,** leaving the body and fundus of the uterus to allow conception. A permanent cerclage suture is placed around the isthmic portion of the uterus to decrease the incidence of mid and late pregnancy loss. Any subsequent pregnancies are delivered by CS.
- Tumour diameter should be < 2 cm, grade 1–2, with no lymphovascular space invasion.
- 10–12% of patients require adjunctive treatment for positive margins, positive lymph nodes, or poor prognostic features. No significant difference in recurrence rates after RVT compared with radical hysterectomy (5.8% vs 4.4%) with a 5-year survival of 97% in both groups.
- A significantly higher recurrence rate with tumours > 2 cm in diameter; therefore, restrict the use of RVT to those with smaller tumours.
- Intraoperative and postoperative complication rates similar to radical hysterectomy. Approximately 15% of RVT patients develop cervical stenosis, which can lead to dysmenorrhoea or infection.
- 41–7% conception rate is reported. The rate of miscarriage in first trimester is similar to the background population at 16–20%, but there is 8–10% risk of second trimester miscarriage. Only 70–75% of pregnancies deliver at term (> 37 weeks of gestation), but the risk of significant prematurity is only 12%.

Radical abdominal trachelectomy (RAT)

- Similar to radical hysterectomy. Dissect the parametrium and remove the paracervical tissue as a radical hysterectomy; by laparotomy or laparoscopically.
- Whereas RVT should be restricted to tumours ≤ 2 cm in diameter, this technique may be useful in tumours > 2 cm that would otherwise need a radical hysterectomy.
- Data from 94 women – 3 recurrences, 2 deaths, and 5/20 women successfully conceived.
- Simple hysterectomy with pelvic lymph node dissection may be an option for Stage IB1 tumours, with possibility of ovarian preservation.

Cervical cancer (contd.)

Stage IB2 and above – ovarian transposition and oocyte retrieval

- Advanced cervical cancers (pelvic nodal metastasis or parametrial invasion) are treated with pelvic radiation and chemotherapy. Radiation destroys ovarian function.
- Ovarian transposition – repositioning the ovaries outside the field of radiation, relocating them into the paracolic gutters at the level of the lower ribs with preserved blood supply to preserve ovarian function. It can be performed at laparotomy during the time of surgical treatment, or laparoscopically prior to chemoradiation. It does not protect against the risks associated with chemotherapy.
- It may prevent early menopause and ovaries may be used later for oocyte retrieval, IVF, and surrogate pregnancy. However, there is still a high risk of ovarian failure. There have been reports of ovarian cyst formation in the transposed ovary as well as vascular injuries.
- There have been reports of pregnancy.
- IVF – oocyte or embryo freezing. Disadvantage of delaying the treatment in order for hormonal stimulation. Transposition of the ovaries can be performed after egg retrieval, but may be complicated due to the increased size of the ovaries caused by the hormonal stimulation required.

Endometrial cancer

6% of endometrial cancers are diagnosed in women under the age of 50 years.

Stage IA endometrial cancer – progesterone treatment

- Case reports of stage IA grade 1 being treated with MPA, megestrol acetate, tamoxifen, and gonadotrophin-releasing hormone analogue.
- **Concerns:**
  - * Accurate staging – hysteroscopy, dilatation and curettage, and MRI (MRI has a 90% accuracy) may lead to underestimation of the staging. Disease that is curable with hysterectomy may progress to advanced incurable disease.
  - * 10–29% of young women with endometrial cancer will have coexisting ovarian cancer.
- LNG-IUS – very limited evidence. There are reports of disease progression while the LNG-IUS was in place and, therefore, it is not recommended on its own.
- No consensus on the appropriate duration of treatment. Endometrium may need to be sampled at 3-monthly intervals and the time to response varies between 3 and 12 months.
- There is no consensus on long-term treatment. It is likely that a hysterectomy after childbearing will decrease the risk of long-term disease.

- Response rate is 75% and there is no evidence that those who do not respond have a poorer prognosis than if they had proceeded to hysterectomy initially.
- Recurrence rate is 23% can be re-treated 3 or 4 times in order to give a window of opportunity to conceive.
- There is a high risk of recurrence and survival chances may be compromised.
- Fertility rates tend to be lower and most series have offered assisted conception immediately following complete response.
- A total of 89 live births have been recorded in the 278 women in these studies.
- There is currently no evidence to suggest a difference in the pregnancy outcomes once conception has been achieved.

Ovarian cancer

Approximately 10% of ovarian cancers are in women of reproductive age. The most common ovarian tumours in young women are germ cell tumours.

Stage I germ cell tumours confined to one ovary – unilateral salpingo-oophorectomy (USO)

- Survival rate – 98% for dysgerminoma, 90% for endodermal sinus, 100% for mixed types, and 100% for immature teratoma. Survival rates are not significantly different from those of women who were not treated conservatively.
- 88% of women were able to conceive and 69% had a full-term delivery.
- Metastatic germ cell ovarian tumours – unilateral oophorectomy or guided biopsy should be taken to confirm the diagnosis and neoadjuvant chemotherapy should be given. Germ cell tumours are very chemosensitive and an excellent response is expected. If the diagnosis is made by biopsy and the ovary still appears abnormal on scanning at the end of chemotherapy, then a unilateral oophorectomy should be performed.

Borderline epithelial ovarian tumours – USO

- Epithelial ovarian tumours account for 85% of ovarian cancers. Approximately 10% are borderline tumours and about 25% of these are in women of childbearing age.
- Most are confined to the ovaries and can be managed conservatively with preservation of the uterus and contralateral ovary.
- The survival rates are 95–97% at 5 years, recurrences tend to occur late and this can give a false sense of reassurance.
- If the tumour is bilateral, bilateral ovarian cystectomy may be performed.
- Successful pregnancy outcomes have been documented.
- Recurrence rates are generally higher; however, survival rates are similar to those in women who have undergone hysterectomy and BSO.

Stage I epithelial ovarian cancer – USO

- USO to women who wish to retain their fertility. However, these women will need full surgical staging, as metastasis occurs in 15–20% of women with apparent stage I ovarian cancer.
- Endometrial biopsy is needed as 10–29% of women have a coexisting endometrial cancer.
- Full staging may be performed laparoscopically. The incidence of laparoscopic tumour rupture is similar to laparotomy and port site metastasis is low. If the diameter of the ovarian cyst exceeds a 15 mm endobag, then perform a laparotomy.
- No additional benefit with taking a biopsy from a normal contralateral ovary. However, if the uterus and the contralateral ovary are to be preserved, there is presumably a risk that microscopic metastatic disease will not be recognized, leading to an increased risk of recurrence. In 2.5% the contralateral ovary has microscopic disease.
- A review (507 women) – 10% chance of recurrence and 5.5% chance of death from disease, which is comparable to historical controls. A total of 186 full-term deliveries were recorded. Recurrent disease confined to the preserved ovary in 4–6%.
- European Society of Gynecologic Oncology – Stage IA grade 1 and possibly grade 2 tumours of mucinous, endometrioid, or serous types are suitable for fertility sparing surgery. Grade 1 stage IC could also be considered.

Fertility preservation

- Where fertility sparing surgery is not appropriate, undertake embryo cryopreservation.
- There are no guarantees that this method will result in a successful pregnancy.
- Surrogacy will be required if the uterus is removed.
- Provision of sex hormone replacement should be in line with other long-term replacement therapies.

Sperm banking

- Consider for all males prior to treatment that carries a risk of long-term gonadal damage.
- Testicular sperm extraction is sometimes possible even when azoospermia is present.

Oocyte/embryo cryopreservation

- Technically challenging and requires ovarian stimulation, with a potential delay in cancer treatment.
- It may be contraindicated if the tumour is thought to be hormone sensitive although there are no scientific data.

Ovarian tissue cryopreservation

- Can be performed without significant delay, but success rates from its use remain unclear.

Oocyte cryopreservation

- Oocyte vitrification may offer increased success rates in comparison with slow freezing, but is limited by the number of oocytes that can be obtained.
- This technique carries only a 3–5% chance of resulting in a successful pregnancy per frozen egg.

Embryo cryopreservation

- Embryo storage prior to treatment is possible for the minority of patients with a partner and sufficient time for IVF.
- Limited data on its success rates in achieving pregnancy.

People with cancer who wish to preserve fertility

- There is no fixed lower age limit for cryopreservation for fertility preservation in people diagnosed with cancer.
- Consider – diagnosis, treatment plan, expected outcome of subsequen: fertility treatment, prognosis of the cancer treatment, viability of stored/post-thawed material.
- Sperm cryopreservation for men and adolescent boys who are preparing for chemotherapy that is likely to make them infertile. Use freezing in liquid nitrogen vapour as the preferred cryopreservation technique for sperm.
- Oocyte or embryo cryopreservation for women of reproductive age who are preparing for chemotherapy that is likely to make them infertile if: they are well enough to undergo ovarian stimulation and egg collection and this will not worsen their condition, and enough time is available before the start of their cancer treatment. Use vitrification instead of controlled-rate freezing if the necessary equipment and expertise is available.
- Store cryopreserved material for an initial period of 10 years. Do not continue to store cryopreserved sperm beyond 10 years for a man whose normal fertility has been restored by the time he is discharged from oncology follow-up.

1. *Fertility Sparing Treatments in Gynaecological Cancers.* RCOG Scientific Impact Paper No. 35, February 2013.
2. Ellis P, Mould T. Fertility-saving treatment in gynaecological oncology. *The Obstetrician and Gynaecologist* 2009;11:239–244.
3. *The Effects of Cancer Treatment on Reproductive Functions. Guidance on Management.* RCOG Report of a Working Party, November 2007.

CHAPTER 24 Urinary incontinence (UI)

Background and definition

- Urodynamic SUI – demonstration of involuntary leakage of urine during increased abdominal pressure but in the absence of detrusor contraction during filling cystometry.
- UUI – involuntary urine leakage accompanied by or immediately preceded by urgency.
- Overactive bladder (OAB) syndrome – urgency, with or without UUI, usually with frequency and nocturia. OAB wet is where UUI is present, and OAB dry is where incontinence is absent.
- Mixed urinary incontinence (MUI) – involuntary leakage associated with urgency and also with exertion, effort, sneezing, or coughing.
- Chronic urinary retention (overflow incontinence) occurs when the bladder cannot empty completely and becomes over-distended.
- Detrusor over-activity is a urodynamic observation characterized by involuntary detrusor contractions during the filling phase, which may be spontaneous or provoked.

Risk factors

- Age.
- Obstetric factors – risk of SUI is increased in women who developed SUI for the first time during their first pregnancy or during the first 6 weeks postpartum. There is an association of vaginal delivery, increased parity, and heavier birth weight with SUI.
- Menopause, hysterectomy.
- Obesity. • Smoking.
- Lower urinary tract symptoms.
- Functional impairment, cognitive impairment.
- Family history. • Diet and genetics. • Neurological disease.

Risks or complications

- Psychological problems: depression, feelings of shame, loss of self confidence, poor self-rated health, low self esteem, impairment in QOL.
- Social isolation.
- Sexual problems: loss of urine during sexual intercourse may cause embarrassment and relationship problems.
- Loss of sleep: nocturia is associated with sleep disruption.
- Constipation: owing to limiting fluid intake.
- Falls and fractures: particularly in older people.

Prevalence and incidence

- Definition: any involuntary urinary leakage (International Continence Society (ICS)).
- Prevalence underreported.
- Stress UI (SUI) is reported in 50%, only urge UI (UUI) in 11% and mixed UI in 36%.
- UK – UI is reported in 20% of people aged ≥ 40 years, increases to 36% at age ≥ 80.

History

- Urinary symptoms – determine storage and voiding patterns.
  * Storage symptoms: frequency, nocturia, urgency, UUI, SUI, constant leakage (fistula).
  * Voiding symptoms: hesitancy, straining to void, poor or intermittent urinary stream.
  * Post-micturition symptoms: sensation of incomplete emptying, post-micturition dribbling.
  * Symptoms such as haematuria, persisting bladder or urethral pain may indicate a more serious diagnosis.
- Bowel symptoms:
  * Constipation and straining can contribute to loss of bladder control by weakening pelvic floor muscles and may predispose to UI and adversely affect the outcome of continence surgery.
  * Faecal incontinence may suggest the presence of cognitive impairment, neurological and/ or anatomical damage.
- Obstetric and gynaecological history:
  * Number and type of deliveries and their outcome, woman's desire for further childbearing.
  * Menstrual history, menopausal status, symptoms of prolapse, sexual function.
- Medical history – conditions that may exacerbate or coexist with UI or OAB – neurological system (e.g., multiple sclerosis, spinal cord injury), metabolic system (e.g., diabetes), cardiorespiratory system, renal system.
- Surgical history – previous surgery for UI or for prolapse may complicate diagnosis and treatment. Any surgery that might have interfered with normal nerve supply to the bladder or urethra, e.g., low spinal surgery, radical hysterectomy.
- Drug history – drugs may be associated with UI. Drugs that affect:
  * CNS, e.g., sedatives, hypnotics, anxiolytics, and smooth muscle relaxants.
  * Autonomic nervous system, e.g., drugs with antimuscarinic action, sympathomimetics, and sympatholytics.
  * Fluid balance, e.g., diuretics and alcohol.
  * Previous medication for UI symptoms.
- Occupational, social, personal history – assess social and functional impact of UI, expectations, and motivation.
- Lifestyle factors such as smoking and BMI.

Comparison of urinary history with urodynamic assessment (UDA)

- If there is no history of mixed UI (i.e., pure SUI or pure UUI), the probability of finding SUI plus detrusor overactivity on cystometry is small (10%), therefore UDA offers little additional diagnostic value.
- If no pure UUI, the probability of finding DO on cystometry is small (10%), therefore UDA offers little added diagnostic value.
- Pure SUI – 15–51% of women who do not report pure SUI may be found to have SUI on cystometry.
- Low level of agreement between a history of urinary symptoms and UDA.
- However, women who do not report mixed or UUI are unlikely to have findings of mixed UI or DO on UDA.
- In the absence of evidence that UDA improves the outcome of women treated conservatively, and without robust evidence that UDA provides additional valuable information to the history alone in the initial assessment of women with UI, UDA is not required before initiating conservative treatment.

Referral indications

Urgent
- Microscopic haematuria in women aged ≥ 50 years. • Visible haematuria.
- Recurrent or persisting UTI associated with haematuria in women aged ≥ 40 years.
- Suspected malignant mass arising from the urinary tract.

Routine
- Symptomatic prolapse that is visible at or below the vaginal introitus.
- Palpable bladder after voiding. • Persisting bladder or urethral pain.
- Clinically benign pelvic masses. • Associated faecal incontinence.
- Suspected neurological disease. • Symptoms of voiding difficulty.
- Suspected urogenital fistulae.
- Previous continence surgery, pelvic cancer surgery, pelvic radiotherapy.

Urine dipstick test

- Urine dipstick for blood, glucose, protein, leucocytes, and nitrites.
- Urine dipstick test for leucocytes and nitrites has low sensitivity and high specificity for the diagnosis of UTI. A negative test excludes a UTI with a high degree of certainty. However, only one third of positive tests are associated with bacteriologically proven UTI.
- False negatives can arise when infection occurs with organisms that do not convert nitrates to nitrites. Hence, in symptomatic patients with a negative test, consider prescribing antibiotics before results of urine culture are available.
- In patients with symptoms of UTI and a positive urine test for leucocytes and nitrites, infection is highly likely and prescribe antibiotics immediately.
- MSU for culture and antibiotic sensitivities before prescribing in all.
- Women with symptoms of UTI with urine test:
  - * Positive for both leucocytes and nitrites – prescribe antibiotics pending culture.
  - * Negative for leucocytes or nitrites – consider antibiotics pending culture results.
- Women who do not have symptoms of UTI with urine test
  - * Positive for both leucocytes and nitrites – do not offer antibiotics without the results of MSU culture.
  - * Negative for leucocytes or nitrites – unlikely UTI, do not send a urine culture.

Examination and assessment

- Assess cognitive impairment.
- Abdominal examination – enlarged bladder (chronic urinary retention) or pelvic mass.
- Speculum/vaginal examination – identify and assess prolapse, atrophic changes, infection and excoriation, uterine and ovarian enlargement, urine leak on straining. Ask women to cough and bear down, which may demonstrate SUI or presence of cystocele or rectocele.
- Rectal examination – evaluate posterior vaginal wall prolapse.
- Neurophysiology – where history suggests neurological disease, examination of lower limbs together with sacral sensation and sacral reflexes.
- Pelvic floor muscle assessment: * Digital palpation.   * EMG.   * Perineometry.
- There is a lack of evidence as to whether digital assessment of pelvic floor muscle contraction affects the outcome of pelvic floor muscle training (PFMT). However, the determination of whether a woman can contract pelvic floor muscles will direct treatment decisions. Assess pelvic floor muscle contraction digitally before the use of supervised PFMT for the treatment of UI.
- Assess residual urine in women suspected of voiding dysfunction. Large post-void residual urine may indicate the presence of underlying bladder outlet obstruction, neurological disease, or detrusor failure.
- Methods used to measure post-void residual urine – abdominal palpation, USS, and catheterization.
  The sensitivity and specificity of USS in comparison with catheterization are within clinically acceptable limits. USS is less invasive with fewer side effects. Measure post-void residual volume by bladder scan or catheterization in women with symptoms suggestive of voiding dysfunction or recurrent UTI. Use a bladder scan in preference to catheterization on the grounds of acceptability and less adverse events.

Initial assessment and referral

- At the initial clinical assessment, categorize woman's UI as SUI, mixed UI, or UUI/OAB.
- Commence initial treatment on this basis.
- In mixed UI, treat the predominant symptom.
- Identify relevant predisposing and precipitating factors and other diagnoses that may require referral for additional investigation and treatment.

Assessment

- Bladder diaries – a reliable method of quantifying urinary frequency and incontinence.
  - These are used to document each cycle of filling and voiding over a number of days and can provide information about urinary frequency, urgency, diurnal and nocturnal cycles, functional bladder capacity, fluid intake, urine output, leakage episodes, pad changes, and give an indication of the severity of wetness. They may also be used for monitoring the effects of treatment.
  - Optimum duration of bladder diaries is unclear. They should be used in the initial assessment with a minimum of 3 days of the diary covering variations in their usual activities.
- Symptom scoring and QOL assessment – to quantify the impact of urinary symptoms and to provide a measure that can be used to assess outcomes of treatment.
- Pad tests – to detect and quantify urine loss. Where there is no evidence of diagnostic value or clinical utility, the pad tests may be useful for evaluating therapies for incontinence. They are not recommended in the routine assessment of women with UI.
- Cystoscopy – the direct visualization of the bladder and urethral lumen. It identifies areas of inflammation, tumour, stones, and diverticula, all of which will require referral.
  - Evidence does not support the role of cystoscopy in the assessment of women with UI. It may be of value in women with pain or recurrent UTI following previous pelvic surgery, or where a fistula is suspected; its place in recurrent SUI without these additional features is less clear.
  - Cystoscopy is not recommended in the initial assessment of women with UI alone.

Investigations and assessment of severity

Urodynamic assessment (UDA) – a number of varied physiological tests of bladder and urethral function, which aim to demonstrate an underlying abnormality of storage or voiding.

Cystometry

Measurement of intra-vesical pressure – by single recording channel (simple cystometry) or by multichannel cystometry (measurement of both bladder and intra-abdominal pressures by means of catheters inserted into the bladder and the rectum or vagina). The aim is to replicate the woman's symptoms by filling the bladder and observing pressure changes or leakage caused by provocation tests. Multichannel cystometry may reveal the underlying pathophysiological explanation of incontinence. Single-channel cystometry is less reliable.

- A clinical stress test may be as accurate as multichannel cystometry in the diagnosis of USI.
- There is no evidence that pre-treatment multichannel cystometry will improve the outcomes of treatments for UI. Although some urodynamic parameters have been found to correlate with adverse outcomes of surgery, no test has been shown to reliably predict beneficial or adverse outcomes of surgery.
- **Uroflowmetry** entails a free-flow void into a recording device, which provides the information about the volume of urine passed and the rate of urine flow.
- **Videourodynamics** – synchronous radiographic screening of the bladder with multichannel cystometry. It has the benefit of simultaneous structural and functional assessment; however, it is not clear whether this adds any relevant diagnostic accuracy, compared with multichannel cystometry.
- **Ambulatory urodynamics** involves multichannel cystometry carried out with physiological bladder filling rates and using portable recording devices. It demonstrates functional abnormalities more often than multichannel cystometry, but the significance of this is unclear.
- Use of multichannel cystometry, ambulatory urodynamics, or videourodynamics is not recommended before starting conservative treatment.
- For women with a clearly defined clinical diagnosis of pure SUI the use of multichannel cystometry is not routinely recommended.
- Multichannel cystometry is recommended in women before surgery if:
  * There is clinical suspicion of detrusor overactivity. DOA
  * There has been previous surgery for USI or anterior compartment prolapse. ?/0 جرى
  * There are symptoms suggestive of voiding dysfunction. Voids
  * Ambulatory urodynamics or videourodynamics may also be considered in these circumstances.

Tests of urethral function

- **Urethral pressure profilometry and leak point pressure measurement.** These are used to derive values that reflect the ability of the urethra to resist urine flow, expressed as maximum urethral closure pressure (MUCP); or as abdominal, cough, or Valsalva leak point pressures (ALPP, CLPP, VLPP).
- Q-tip, POP-Q, Bonney, Marshall, and fluid-bridge tests have been developed to evaluate the mobility or competence of the urethrovesical junction.
- **Q-tip test** – placing a sterile Q-tip in the urethra and the woman is asked to bear down. If the Q-tip moves more than 30°, the test is considered positive.
- **Bonney and Marshall tests** – pressing either the index and middle finger of the examiner's hand (Bonney test) or the jaws of a forceps (Marshall test) against the anterior vaginal wall, without pressing on the urethra. The stress provocation test is repeated and if no leakage occurs, the Bonney or Marshall test is said to be positive.
- **Fluid-bridge test is** designed to test bladder neck competence by testing for the presence of fluid within the urethra, by demonstrating continuity between two channels of a pressure-recording catheter (one in the bladder and the other in the urethra).
- Q-tip, Bonney, Marshall and fluid-bridge tests demonstrate no evidence to support their role in the clinical assessment of UI, therefore these tests are not recommended in the assessment of women with UI.

Imaging

- USS, X-ray, CT, MRI – for confirmation of alternative pelvic pathology which is an indication for referral.
- Imaging may be used to characterize the extent and anatomical contents of a prolapse, especially in the standing position, with MRI.
- USS – diagnosis of post-void residual urine, bladder wall thickness, bladder neck positioning, specific urethral measurements, and the posterior urethrovesical angle.
- Bladder wall thickness of > 5 mm has sensitivity of 84%, specificity 89%, and PPV 94% for diagnosing DO.
- Correlation of anatomical shape or movement with SUI is not clear.
- There is a lack of evidence regarding the use of MRI or CT in the assessment of women with UI.
- Imaging is not recommended for the routine assessment of women with UI.
- USS is not recommended other than for the assessment of residual urine volume.

Management

Lifestyle – general measures

- There is a lack of data on the effects of modifying lifestyle factors such as bowel habit and dietary factors in women with UI or OAB.
- Constipation and increased straining in early adult life may be associated with an increased tendency to prolapse and UI, but no evidence on the effect of modifying bowel habit on continence is identified.
- Increased caffeine intake may be associated with OAB and UI. There is some evidence that caffeine reduction leads to less urgency and frequency when used in addition to bladder training. **Give a trial of caffeine reduction for the treatment of OAB.**
- There is evidence of an association between obesity and UI or OAB. Weight reduction of at least 5% is associated with relief of UI symptoms. **Advise women with UI or OAB who have a BMI > 30 to lose weight.**
- Smoking is associated with an increased risk of UI and OAB although there is no evidence relating to smoking cessation in the management of these symptoms.

Non-therapeutic interventions

- Acupuncture, hypnosis, herbal medicines – poor-quality evidence shows that acupuncture may reduce nocturia and both SUI and UUI in the short term.
- Hypnotherapy – limited evidence of some benefit over the short term for UUI.
- Lack of evidence on herbal medicines for UI or OAB.
- Do not recommend complementary therapies for the treatment of UI or OAB.
- Catheters – intermittent catheterization is associated with reduced risk of UTI compared with indwelling catheterization.
- Bladder catheterization (intermittent or indwelling urethral or suprapubic) – consider for women in whom persistent urinary retention is causing incontinence, symptomatic infections, or renal dysfunction.
- Products to prevent leakage – intravaginal devices: continence guard, bladder neck support prosthesis, meatal devices, a urethral plug. Intravaginal and intraurethral devices are not recommended. Do not advise women to consider such devices other than for occasional use when necessary to prevent leakage, for example during physical exercise.
- Pessaries – the limited evidence does not support the use of ring pessaries for the treatment of UI in women whether or not there is prolapse present.

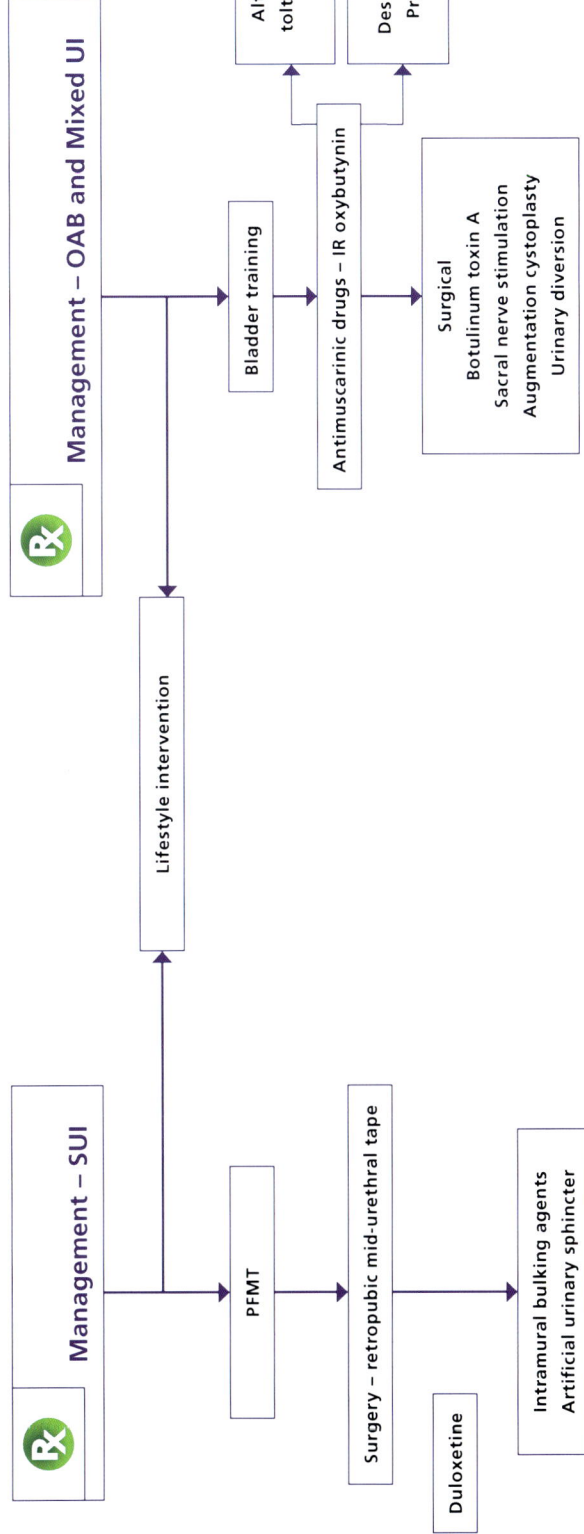

Management – OAB and Mixed UI

Lifestyle intervention → Bladder training → Antimuscarinic drugs – IR oxybutynin

→ Alternatives – darifenacin, solifenacin, tolterodine, trospium, or ER/transdermal oxybutynin

→ Desmopressin – for troublesome nocturia
Propiverine to treat frequency in OAB

→ Surgical
Botulinum toxin A
Sacral nerve stimulation
Augmentation cystoplasty
Urinary diversion

Management – SUI

Lifestyle intervention → PFMT → Surgery – retropubic mid-urethral tape → Intramural bulking agents
Artificial urinary sphincter

Duloxetine

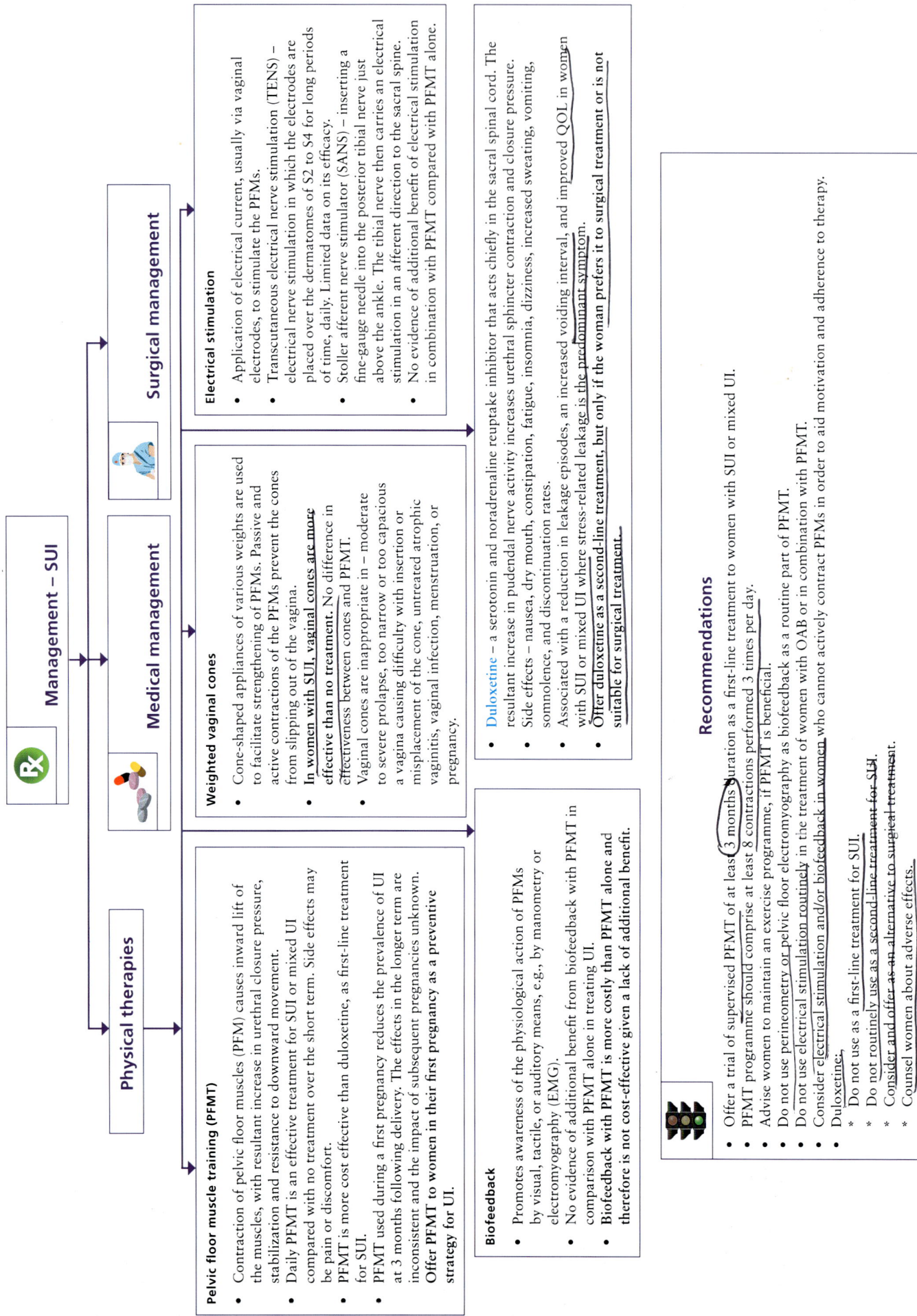

Management – SUI

Physical therapies

Medical management

Surgical management

Pelvic floor muscle training (PFMT)

- Contraction of pelvic floor muscles (PFM) causes inward lift of the muscles, with resultant increase in urethral closure pressure, stabilization and resistance to downward movement.
- Daily PFMT is an effective treatment for SUI or mixed UI compared with no treatment over the short term. Side effects may be pain or discomfort.
- PFMT is more cost effective than duloxetine, as first-line treatment for SUI.
- PFMT used during a first pregnancy reduces the prevalence of UI at 3 months following delivery. The effects in the longer term are inconsistent and the impact of subsequent pregnancies unknown. **Offer PFMT to women in their first pregnancy as a preventive strategy for UI.**

Biofeedback

- Promotes awareness of the physiological action of PFMs by visual, tactile, or auditory means, e.g., by manometry or electromyography (EMG).
- No evidence of additional benefit from biofeedback with PFMT in comparison with PFMT alone in treating UI.
- **Biofeedback with PFMT is more costly than PFMT alone and therefore is not cost-effective given a lack of additional benefit.**

Weighted vaginal cones

- Cone-shaped appliances of various weights are used to facilitate strengthening of PFMs. Passive and active contractions of the PFMs prevent the cones from slipping out of the vagina.
- **In women with SUI, vaginal cones are more effective than no treatment.** No difference in effectiveness between cones and PFMT.
- Vaginal cones are inappropriate in – moderate to severe prolapse, too narrow or too capacious a vagina causing difficulty with insertion or misplacement of the cone, untreated atrophic vaginitis, vaginal infection, menstruation, or pregnancy.

- **Duloxetine** – a serotonin and noradrenaline reuptake inhibitor that acts chiefly in the sacral spinal cord. The resultant increase in pudendal nerve activity increases urethral sphincter contraction and closure pressure.
- Side effects – nausea, dry mouth, constipation, fatigue, insomnia, dizziness, increased sweating, vomiting, somnolence, and discontinuation rates.
- Associated with a reduction in leakage episodes, an increased voiding interval, and improved QOL in women with SUI or mixed UI where stress-related leakage is the predominant symptom.
- **Offer duloxetine as a second-line treatment, but only if the woman prefers it to surgical treatment or is not suitable for surgical treatment.**

Electrical stimulation

- Application of electrical current, usually via vaginal electrodes, to stimulate the PFMs.
- Transcutaneous electrical nerve stimulation (TENS) – electrical nerve stimulation in which the electrodes are placed over the dermatomes of S2 to S4 for long periods of time, daily. Limited data on its efficacy.
- Stoller afferent nerve stimulator (SANS) – inserting a fine-gauge needle into the posterior tibial nerve just above the ankle. The tibial nerve then carries an electrical stimulation in an afferent direction to the sacral spine.
- No evidence of additional benefit of electrical stimulation in combination with PFMT compared with PFMT alone.

Recommendations

- Offer a trial of supervised PFMT of at least 3 months duration as a first-line treatment to women with SUI or mixed UI.
- PFMT programme should comprise at least 8 contractions performed 3 times per day.
- Advise women to maintain an exercise programme, if PFMT is beneficial.
- Do not use perineometry or pelvic floor electromyography as biofeedback as a routine part of PFMT.
- Do not use electrical stimulation routinely in the treatment of women with OAB or in combination with PFMT.
- Consider electrical stimulation and/or biofeedback in women who cannot actively contract PFMs in order to aid motivation and adherence to therapy.
- Duloxetine:
  * Do not use as a first-line treatment for SUI.
  * Do not routinely use as a second-line treatment for SUI.
  * Consider and offer as an alternative to surgical treatment.
  * Counsel women about adverse effects.

Surgical management

To support or stabilize bladder neck or urethra
Objective is to prevent the downward displacement of the urethra

- **Retropubic suspension procedures** secure the paraurethral or vaginal tissues to a fixed structure by sutures. Burch colposuspension, Marshall–Marchetti–Krantz (MMK) and vagino-obturator shelf procedure.
- **Colposuspension** – open or laparoscopic.
- Open colposuspension is an effective treatment and has longevity. There is no difference in effectiveness between laparoscopic and open colposuspension. However, laparoscopic colposuspension consumes more resources and skills take longer to acquire.
- Complications are common – voiding difficulty, urgency syndrome, development of vaginal vault and posterior wall prolapse.
- No evidence that the MMK procedure offers any advantage over open colposuspension. MMK procedure is no longer in routine clinical practice owing to the serious additional complication of osteitis pubis.
- **Minimally invasive procedures** that suspend the paraurethral tissues by means of a suspensory suture, usually inserted under endoscopic control and secured to the rectus sheath to provide support. These include the Raz, Pereyra, Stamey, and Gittes procedures.

To augment urethral closure

- **Sling operations** aim to stabilize the urethra by placing a strip of material around the underside of the urethra and securing the ends to a fixed structure above, with 'no tension' under the urethra.
- These could be classified according to:
  * The tissues to which they are fixed (pubic arch or rectus sheath).
  * The route by which they are inserted: open abdominal, combined abdominovaginal; minimally invasive.
  * Retropubic space (from bottom upwards or from top downwards).
  * Obturator foramen (from outside inwards/from inside outwards).
  * The materials used.
- Most RCT data regarding synthetic slings for the treatment of SUI relate to a macroporous (type 1) polypropylene mesh inserted through the retropubic space using a bottom-up approach (TVT). This has comparable efficacy to colposuspension, less use of hospital resources, more cost-effective, and shorter recovery time. Limited data on outcomes beyond 3 years.
- Higher prevalence of prolapse in open colposuspension would increase the relative cost effectiveness of TVT.
- Slings inserted through the obturator foramen appear to be effective in the short term.
- Intraoperative complications are rare except for bladder perforation, which, although common, has no long-term sequelae provided it is recognized and repaired at the time of surgery.
- Long-term complications – voiding difficulties and development of urgency and UUI.

To augment urethral closure

- **Operations to augment sphincter closure:**
  * Injection of urethral bulking agents and implants that aim to occlude the urethra.
  * Intramural urethral bulking procedures.
  * Extraurethral retropubic adjustable compression devices.
- **Artificial urinary sphincter** – a complex device that comprises an occlusive cuff inserted around the urethra, which, while inflated, will exert a constant closure pressure. Pressure is maintained by means of an inflated pressure-regulating balloon. A small pump located in the labium is manually operated by the woman whenever she wishes to pass urine.
- Data supporting the use of an artificial urinary sphincter are limited. Subjective cure rates are high although complications requiring removal or revision are common.
- **Bulking agents** may be less effective than open surgery, but are associated with fewer postoperative complications. Any benefit observed declines with time, and complications, although common, are transient; include acute retention, dysuria, haematuria, frequency, and UTI. De novo DO with urge UI is the only long-term complication.

Others

- Anterior colporrhaphy and abdominal paravaginal repair are aimed primarily at treating prolapse but may have a secondary effect in preventing associated SUI.
- Most suspension procedures are effective in the short term but the longer-term outcomes for anterior colporrhaphy, abdominal paravaginal repair, and needle suspension are poor when used for SUI alone.

Surgical management

Recommendations

- Retropubic mid-urethral tape procedures using a 'bottom-up' approach with macroporous (type 1) polypropylene meshes.
- Open colposuspension and autologous rectus fascial sling are alternatives.
- Synthetic slings using a retropubic 'top-down' or a transobturator foramen approach provided women are made aware of the lack of long-term outcome data.
- Intramural bulking agents (glutaraldehyde cross-linked collagen, silicone, carbon-coated zirconium beads, or hyaluronic acid/dextran co-polymer). Inform women that repeat injections may be required to achieve efficacy; efficacy diminishes with time; efficacy is inferior to that of retropubic suspension or sling.
- In view of the associated morbidity, consider the use of an artificial urinary sphincter only if previous surgery has failed. Life-long follow-up is recommended.

What not to do

- Synthetic slings using materials other than polypropylene that are not of a macroporous (type 1) construction.
- Laparoscopic colposuspension as a routine procedure.
- Anterior colporrhaphy, needle suspensions, paravaginal defect repair, and the Marshall–Marchetti–Krantz procedure.
- Autologous fat and polytetrafluoroethylene as intramural bulking agents.

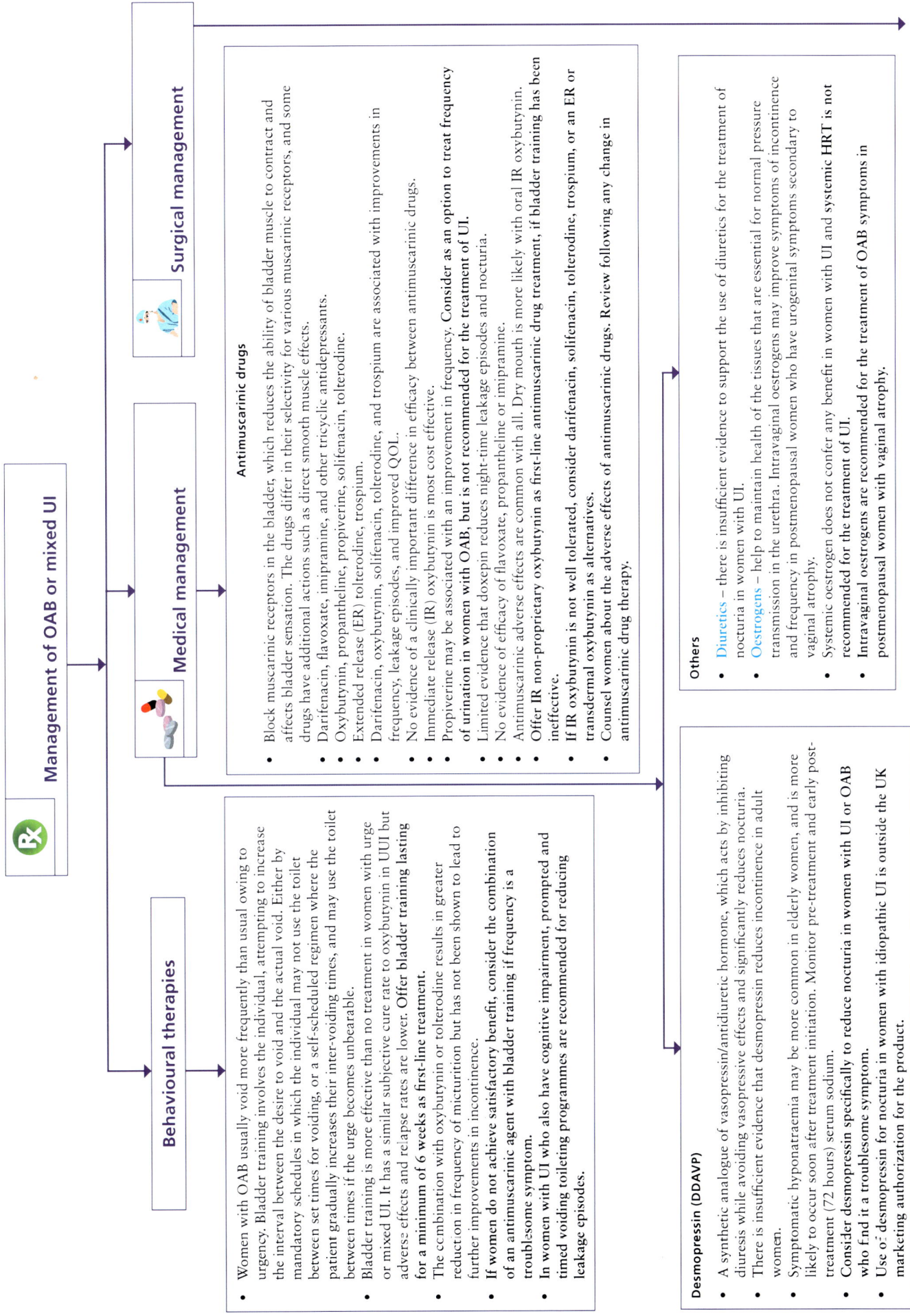

Management of OAB or mixed UI

Behavioural therapies

- Women with OAB usually void more frequently than usual owing to urgency. Bladder training involves the individual, attempting to increase the interval between the desire to void and the actual void. Either by mandatory schedules in which the individual may not use the toilet between set times for voiding, or a self-scheduled regimen where the patient gradually increases their inter-voiding times, and may use the toilet between times if the urge becomes unbearable.
- Bladder training is more effective than no treatment in women with urge or mixed UI. It has a similar subjective cure rate to oxybutynin in UUI but adverse effects and relapse rates are lower. **Offer bladder training lasting for a minimum of 6 weeks as first-line treatment.**
- The combination with oxybutynin or tolerodine results in greater reduction in frequency of micturition but has not been shown to lead to further improvements in incontinence.
- **If women do not achieve satisfactory benefit, consider the combination of an antimuscarinic agent with bladder training if frequency is a troublesome symptom.**
- In women with UI who also have cognitive impairment, prompted and timed voiding toileting programmes are recommended for reducing leakage episodes.

Medical management

Antimuscarinic drugs

- Block muscarinic receptors in the bladder, which reduces the ability of bladder muscle to contract and affects bladder sensation. The drugs differ in their selectivity for various muscarinic receptors, and some drugs have additional actions such as direct smooth muscle effects.
- Darifenacin, flavoxate, imipramine, and other tricyclic antidepressants.
- Oxybutynin, propantheline, propiverine, solifenacin, tolterodine.
- Extended release (ER) tolterodine, trospium.
- Darifenacin, oxybutynin, solifenacin, tolterodine, and trospium are associated with improvements in frequency, leakage episodes, and improved QOL.
- No evidence of a clinically important difference in efficacy between antimuscarinic drugs.
- Immediate release (IR) oxybutynin is most cost effective.
- Propiverine may be associated with an improvement in frequency. **Consider as an option to treat frequency of urination in women with OAB, but is not recommended for the treatment of UI.**
- Limited evidence that doxepin reduces night-time leakage episodes and nocturia.
- No evidence of efficacy of flavoxate, propantheline or imipramine.
- Antimuscarinic adverse effects are common with all. Dry mouth is more likely with oral IR oxybutynin.
- Offer IR non-proprietary oxybutynin as first-line antimuscarinic drug treatment, if bladder training has been ineffective.
- If IR oxybutynin is not well tolerated, consider darifenacin, solifenacin, tolterodine, trospium, or an ER or transdermal oxybutynin as alternatives.
- Counsel women about the adverse effects of antimuscarinic drugs. Review following any change in antimuscarinic drug therapy.

Desmopressin (DDAVP)

- A synthetic analogue of vasopressin/antidiuretic hormone, which acts by inhibiting diuresis while avoiding vasopressive effects and significantly reduces nocturia.
- There is insufficient evidence that desmopressin reduces incontinence in adult women.
- Symptomatic hyponatraemia may be more common in elderly women, and is more likely to occur soon after treatment initiation. Monitor pre-treatment and early post-treatment (72 hours) serum sodium.
- Consider desmopressin specifically to reduce nocturia in women with UI or OAB who find it a troublesome symptom.
- Use of desmopressin for nocturia in women with idiopathic UI is outside the UK marketing authorization for the product.

Surgical management

Others

- Diuretics – there is insufficient evidence to support the use of diuretics for the treatment of nocturia in women with UI.
- Oestrogens – help to maintain health of the tissues that are essential for normal pressure transmission in the urethra. Intravaginal oestrogens may improve symptoms of incontinence and frequency in postmenopausal women who have urogenital symptoms secondary to vaginal atrophy.
- Systemic oestrogen does not confer any benefit in women with UI and systemic HRT is not recommended for the treatment of UI.
- Intravaginal oestrogens are recommended for the treatment of OAB symptoms in postmenopausal women with vaginal atrophy.

Surgical management

Aims to increase the capacity of the bladder, alter or modulate its nerve supply and contractility, or bypass the lower urinary tract completely. The contractility of the detrusor is reduced, leading to difficulty in voiding, a very common adverse effect.

Sacral nerve stimulation (SNS) neuromodulation

- Appropriate electrical stimulation of the sacral reflex pathway will inhibit the reflex behaviour of the bladder.
- Permanently implantable sacral root stimulators provide chronic stimulation directly to the S3 nerve roots.
- Up to two thirds of patients achieve continence or substantial improvement after SNS, and the beneficial effects appear to persist for up to 3–5 years after implantation.
- Around one third of patients may require re-operation, owing to pain at the implant site, infection, or the need for adjustment and modification of the lead system.
- Permanent removal of the electrodes may be required in 1/10 patients.
- Offer sacral nerve stimulation for the treatment of UI owing to DO in women who have not responded to conservative treatments. Offer sacral nerve stimulation on the basis of their response to preliminary percutaneous nerve evaluation. Life-long follow-up is recommended.

Detrusor myectomy

- Aims to improve the functional bladder capacity by excising bladder muscle from the fundus of the bladder while leaving the mucosa intact, thus creating a permanent wide-necked diverticulum. The defect is usually covered with a segment of mobilized omentum.
- While urodynamic parameters may improve in some patients, the clinical outcomes are unclear; hence its role in the treatment of DO is not yet established.

Augmentation cystoplasty

- Aims to increase functional bladder capacity by bivalving the bladder wall and incorporating a segment of bowel into the resultant defect.
- Limited data. Improvement in at least half of patients with idiopathic DO.
- Complications – bowel disturbance, metabolic acidosis, mucus production and/or retention in the bladder, UTI, and urinary retention are common and many patients will need to self-catheterize.
- Malignant transformation in the bowel segment or urothelium has been reported. Life-long follow-up is recommended.
- Augmentation cystoplasty for the management of idiopathic detrusor overactivity should be restricted to women who have not responded to conservative treatments and who are willing and able to self-catheterize.

Urinary diversion

- Urine drainage is re-routed away from the urethra by means of transposing the ureters to an isolated segment of ileum, which is used to create a permanent cutaneous stoma (ileal conduit).
- Limited data; vesical infection, stoma-related problems, and the need for surgical revisions occur very commonly.
- Consider urinary diversion for a woman with OAB only when conservative treatments have failed, and if sacral nerve stimulation and augmentation cystoplasty are not appropriate or are unacceptable.
- Life-long follow-up is recommended.

Botulinum toxin

- A potent neurotoxin derived from the bacterium Clostridium botulinum. Two strains – types A and B. Botulinum toxin blocks the release of acetylcholine and it will temporarily paralyse any muscle into which it is injected. However, the precise mechanism of action when injected into the detrusor muscle is unknown.
- Can be injected directly into the bladder wall using a flexible cystoscope.
- Botulinum toxin A – limited data show improvement in about half of patients, with duration of benefit between 3 and 12 months.
- Botulinum toxin B appears to be effective only in the short term (up to 6 weeks).
- Botulinum toxin A should be used in the treatment of idiopathic DO only in women who have not responded to conservative treatments and who are willing and able to self-catheterize.
- Use of botulinum toxin A for this indication is outside the UK marketing authorization for the product.
- Botulinum toxin B is not recommended for the treatment of women with idiopathic OAB.

What not to do

- UDA before conservative treatment.
- Use of multichannel cystometry, ambulatory urodynamics or videourodynamics, before starting conservative treatment.
- For women with a clearly defined clinical diagnosis of pure SUI, the use of multichannel cystometry.
- Routine ultrasound, except to assess residual urine volume.
- Routine use of pad tests or MRI, CT, and X-ray.
- Cystoscopy in the initial assessment of women with UI alone.
- Q-tip, Bonney, Marshall, and fluid-bridge tests in the assessment of women with UI.
- Complementary therapies for the treatment of UI or OAB.

- Combining oxybutynin treatment with posterior tibial nerve stimulation.
- Posterior tibial nerve stimulation for UI/OAB.
- Electrical stimulation in combination with PFMT.
- Sham electrical stimulation in the treatment of UUI.
- Absorbent products, hand-held urinals, and toileting aids for UI.
- Intravaginal and intraurethral devices for the routine management of UI in women.

1. *Urinary Incontinence. The Management of Urinary Incontinence in Women.* NICE, 2006.
2. *Management of Urinary Incontinence in Primary Care. A National Clinical Guideline.* Scottish Intercollegiate Guidelines Network, 2004.
3. *IUGA Guidelines for Research and Clinical Practice.* Evaluation and outcome measures in the treatment of female urinary stress incontinence. *Int Urogynecol J* 2008;19:5–33.
4. Recommendations arising from the 42nd Study Group: Incontinence in Women. RCOG *Press* 2002; 433–441.

CHAPTER 25 Uterovaginal prolapse

Background and prevalence

- Life-time risk for undergoing surgery for prolapse or urinary incontinence is 11%.
- Most common indication for hysterectomy in women aged ≥ 50 years.
- Descent of one or more pelvic structures:
  * Uterine cervix or vagina apex – **apical/uterine prolapse.**
  * Anterior vagina usually with the bladder – **cystocele.**
  * Posterior vagina usually with the rectum – **rectocele.**
  * Peritoneum of the cul-de-sac usually with the small intestine – **enterocele.**
  * Vaginal apex after hysterectomy– **vaginal vault prolapse.**

Risk factors

- Age – prolapse is more common in older women.
- Parity – particularly with history of long or difficult labour, multiple births, or delivery of a large baby. It is rare in women who have not had children.
- Menopause – owing to low levels of oestrogen resulting in weakening of tissue.
- High BMI – being overweight or obese creates extra pressure in the pelvic area.
- Previous pelvic surgery, such as hysterectomy or bladder repair.
- Factors associated with increased intra-abdominal pressure – heavy lifting and manual work, long-term coughing (smoking), long-term constipation.
- Genetic predisposition.
- Conditions that cause weakening of the tissues and connective tissue disorder – joint hypermobility syndrome, Marfan syndrome, Ehlers–Danlos syndrome, etc.

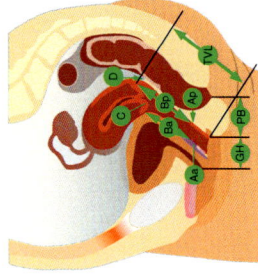

Aa – anterior wall	Ba – anterior wall	C – cervix or cuff
GH – genital hiatus	PB – perineal body	TVL – total vaginal length
Ap – posterior wall	Bp – posterior wall	D – posterior fornix

POP-Q scoring system

Baden–Walker system for evaluation of prolapse

- Grade 0 – normal position.
- Grade 1 – descent halfway to the hymen.
- Grade 2 – descent to the hymen.
- Grade 3 – descent halfway past the hymen.
- Grade 4 – maximum possible descent/procidentia.

History

- Asymptomatic – incidental finding in some women. Up to half of all women who have had children are affected by some degree of prolapse; however, most are clinically not affected.
- A sensation of something coming down or out of the vagina – progressive protrusion of the bulge as the day goes on, or after long periods of physical exertion (lifting/standing).
- An uncomfortable feeling of fullness or heaviness.
- Difficulty having sex and difficulty walking.
- Backache or dragging sensation.
- Stress incontinence – severe prolapse may mask the symptoms of incontinence.
- Difficulty voiding or incomplete emptying of bladder/rectum. Might require manual pressure for complete voiding.
- It can have a significant impact on a woman's QOL.

The only symptom specific to prolapse is the awareness of a vaginal bulge or protrusion. For all other pelvic symptoms, resolution with prolapse treatment cannot be assumed. (ACOG)

Assessment

- Severity of the symptoms and affect on QOL.
- Nature and extent of the prolapse needs to be assessed – the maximum degree of descent may be observed on examination with the patient supine in heel stirrups, performing a Valsalva maneuver. (ACOG)
- All pelvic floor defect assessment should be based on standard tools such as POP-Q.
- Assess occult urinary stress incontinence after reducing the prolapse with a pessary – **prolapse reduction stress test.** Currently there is no consensus on how to best reduce prolapse for SUI testing.
- Assess efficiency of bladder emptying – by assessing post-void residual urine volume.
- Baden–Walker system or POP-Q system – POP-Q system may be more detailed than necessary for clinical practice and may be better suited for clinical research purposes.

Management

Depends on: the stage of the prolapse, severity of symptoms, age, general health of the patient, and desire for future childbearing.

Non-surgical management

Expectant

- If asymptomatic or mildly symptomatic prolapse.

Symptom-directed therapy

- Weight loss if overweight.
- Avoid standing for long periods of time.
- Defaecatory problems – behavioural training, dietary modification (high-fibre diet), and laxatives to prevent constipation and straining.

Hormone replacement therapy (HRT)

- There is no evidence to support the use of oestrogen replacement to prevent or treat prolapse.

Pessaries

- Indicated in pregnant women, physically frail women, those unfit for surgery, or when surgery is declined.
- Change every 6–8 months to prevent ulceration of the vaginal vault. If left for a long period, there is a risk of calcium deposition, erosion, and fistula formation.
- Various shapes and sizes. Supportive (ring) or space-occupying (donut pessary).
- Shelf pessaries preclude sexual intercourse and are therefore suitable for women who are not sexually active.
- Ring pessaries tend to fail in women with deficient perineum, who may require shelf pessaries instead.
- Side effects – vaginal discharge, irritation, bleeding.
- Pessarie scan be fitted in most women with prolapse, regardless of prolapse stage or site. (ACOG)

Pelvic floor muscle training

PFMT may improve pelvic function and is recommended as an adjunct therapy for women with prolapse and associated symptoms.

Evidence round-up

Cochrane review (2013) – pessaries (mechanical devices) for pelvic organ prolapse in women found only one RCT comparing ring and Gellhorn pessaries. Both pessaries are effective in 60% of women, with no differences between the two types of pessary.

Cochrane review (2011) – PFMT improves in prolapse stage by 17% compared to no PFMT. There is some evidence indicating a positive effect of PFMT for prolapse symptoms and severity; 6 months of supervised PFMT has anatomical and symptom improvement.

Cochrane reviews (2010) – oestrogen – use of local oestrogen in conjunction with PFMT before surgery may reduce the incidence of postoperative cystitis within 4 weeks after surgery.

Surgical management

Anterior vaginal prolapse/cystocele

- Anterior colporrhaphy with or without mesh/graft material.
- Paravaginal repair – vaginally or retropubically (open/laparoscopic).
  Studies comparing the above approaches are lacking.
- Retrospective case series – recurrence rate of 15–37%.
- Cochrane review (2010):
  * Standard anterior repair is associated with more recurrent cystoceles than with a polyglactin mesh or porcine dermis mesh inlay, polypropylene mesh overlay, or armed transobturator mesh; but data on morbidity and other clinical outcomes are lacking.
  * No differences in subjective outcomes, QOL data, de novo dyspareunia, stress incontinence, re-operation rates for prolapse, or incontinence.
  * Blood loss with transobturator meshes was significantly higher than for native tissue anterior repair.
  * Mesh erosions – 10% of anterior repairs with polypropylene mesh.

Posterior vaginal prolapse/rectocele

- Posterior colporrhaphy with or without mesh/graft material.
- Site-specific repair – a specific defect in the vaginal muscularis or adventitia is repaired.
- Levator myorraphy (plication of the medial portion of levator ani) – insufficient evidence to judge the value of levatormyorraphy during vaginal repair. Its use has been largely abandoned because of dyspareunia except when postoperative sexual activity is not anticipated. (ACOG)
- Sacral colpoperineopexy – performed in conjuction with sacral colpopexy, where a mesh is placed along the posterior vagina, all the way to perineal body (open/laparoscopic). Main complication is dyspareunia.
- Transanal approach with plication of redundant rectal mucosa and anterior rectal muscle.
  Transvaginal repair was more effective for subjective symptom relief and recurrence of prolapse.
- Cochrane review (2010) – vaginal approach was associated with a lower rate of recurrent rectocele, or enterocele, or both, than the transanal approach, although there was a higher blood loss and postoperative narcotic use. No data on efficacy of polypropylene mesh in the posterior vaginal compartment.

Apical prolapse

Abdominal/laparoscopic sacrocolpopexy (ASC)
Vaginal sacrospinous fixation/colpopexy (SSF)
Vaginal uterosacral ligament suspension
Iliococcygeus fixation
Sling procedures/hysteropexy
Colpocleisis

- See Chapter 26.
- Hysterectomy – the traditional surgical approach. However, hysterectomy alone or hysterectomy with anterior or posterior colporrhaphy does not address the underlying problem of deficient apical support. When hysterectomy is performed for prolapse, apical support should be restored.
- Cochrane review (2010) – surgical management of pelvic organ prolapse – ASC is better than vaginal SSF in terms of a lower rate of recurrent vault prolapse (RR 0.23) and less dyspareunia (RR 0.39). However, there is no difference in re-operation rates for prolapse. The vaginal SSF is quicker and cheaper to perform and associated with quicker recovery.
- Whether the results are superior with uterosacral vs SSF is unknown as these procedures have not been compared in RCTs.

What can be done

Young women with childbearing potential or women who prefer to avoid hysterectomy

Vaginal suspension procedures:
- Utero-scaral or SSF; ASC.

Hysteropexy/sling procedures:
- Sacral hysteropexy (abdominal/laparoscopic attachment of lower uterus to sacral promontory with synthetic mesh); sacrospinous hysteropexy. Prolapse recurrence – 7–30%.
- Hysteropexy should not be performed by using the ventral abdominal wall for support because of the high risk of recurrent prolapse, mainly enterocele.

Round ligament suspension:
- It is not effective in treating uterine prolapse.

Future pregnancy:
- Limited data on pregnancy outcome.
- Ideally, childbearing should be completed before considering surgery for prolapse to avoid the theoretical risk of recurrence after subsequent pregnancy and delivery.
- For women who become pregnant after prolapse repair, decision regarding mode of delivery should be made on case-to-case basis.

What can be done

To anticipate or prevent occurrence of urinary stress incontinence after surgery for uterovaginal prolapse

- Many women with severe degree of prolapse (particularly with cystocele) will not have symptoms of USI because:
  - * Sphincter mechanism is intact.
  - * Prolapse kinks the urethra, masking the USI.

Therefore, some of these urinary continent women will become incontinent following surgery (occult USI).

- Investigation – prolapse reduction stress test – women with positive test more frequently have USI following prolapse repair compared with negative test.
- Postoperative USI is significantly reduced with the addition of anti-continence procedure along with the prolapse surgery in women with positive prolapse reduction stress test. The TVT mid-urethral sling rather than sub-urethral fascial plication offers better prevention from postoperative USI. However, this prophylaxis against postoperative USI is not perfectly effective as some women continue to have urinary incontinence, both stress and urge incontinence, after the surgery.
- Cochrane review (2012) – continence surgery at the time of prolapse surgery in continent women does not significantly reduce the rate of postoperative SUI.

Use of mesh in prolapse repair surgery

NICE
- Surgical repair of vaginal wall prolapse using mesh may be more efficacious than traditional surgical repair without mesh. Both efficacy and safety vary with different types of mesh, and the data on efficacy in the long term are limited. There is a risk of complications that can cause significant morbidity.
- Insertion of mesh uterine suspension sling (including sacrohysteropexy), infracoccygeal sacropexy using mesh – current evidence on the safety and efficacy is inadequate.
- Therefore, the above procedures should only be used with special arrangements for clinical governance, consent, and audit or research.

ACOG
- Based on currently available limited data, although many patients undergoing mesh augmented vaginal repairs heal well without problems, there seems to be a small but significant group of patients who experience permanent life altering sequelae including pain and dyspareunia.
- Range of mesh-related complications available from RCTs – mesh erosions 5–19%; buttock, groin, pelvic pain 0–10%; de novo dyspareunia 8–28%; re-operation (excluding operation of USI) 3–22%.
- Pelvic organ prolapse: mesh repair should be reserved for high-risk individuals in whom the benefit of mesh replacement may justify the risk, such as individuals with recurrent prolapse (particularly of anterior compartment) or with medical co-morbidities that preclude more invasive lengthier open and endoscopic procedures.

Consent – vaginal surgery for prolapse, with or without vaginal hysterectomy

Discuss

- Describe the nature of the patient's complaint and the significance of the prolapse, extent of the planned surgery, locations of incisions and possible effects on fertility.
- Intended benefits – to improve or resolve the symptoms of prolapse.
- Procedure is likely to involve – pelvic floor repair ± vaginal hysterectomy and attempt at restoring normal pelvic anatomy.
- Discuss the benefits and risks of any available alternative treatments, including no treatment and other therapies, such as physiotherapy and pessaries.

Risks

Very common	1/1 to 1/10.
Common	1/10 to 1/100.
Uncommon	1/100 to 1/1000.
Rare	1/1000 to 1/10,000.
Very rare	< 1/10,000.

Extra procedures

- Any extra procedures:
  * Blood transfusion: 2/100 undergoing vaginal hysterectomy.
  * Repair to bladder and bowel.
  * Laparotomy and conversion to abdominal approach.

- **Serious risks: 4/100:**
  * Damage to bladder/urinary tract – 2/1000.
  * Damage to bowel – 5/1000.
  * Bleeding requiring transfusion or return to theatre – 2/100.
  * New or continuing bladder dysfunction (variable).
  * Pelvic abscess – 3/1000.
  * Failure to achieve desired results; recurrence of prolapse (common).
  * Although DVT (common) and PE (uncommon) may contribute to mortality, the overall risk of death within 6 weeks is 37/100,000.

- **Frequent risks:**
  * Urinary infection, retention, and/or frequency.
  * Vaginal bleeding.
  * Postoperative pain and difficulty and/or pain with intercourse.
  * Wound infection.
  * Both surgical and anaesthetic risks are increased with obesity; patients who have significant pathology, who have had previous surgery, or who have pre-existing medical conditions.

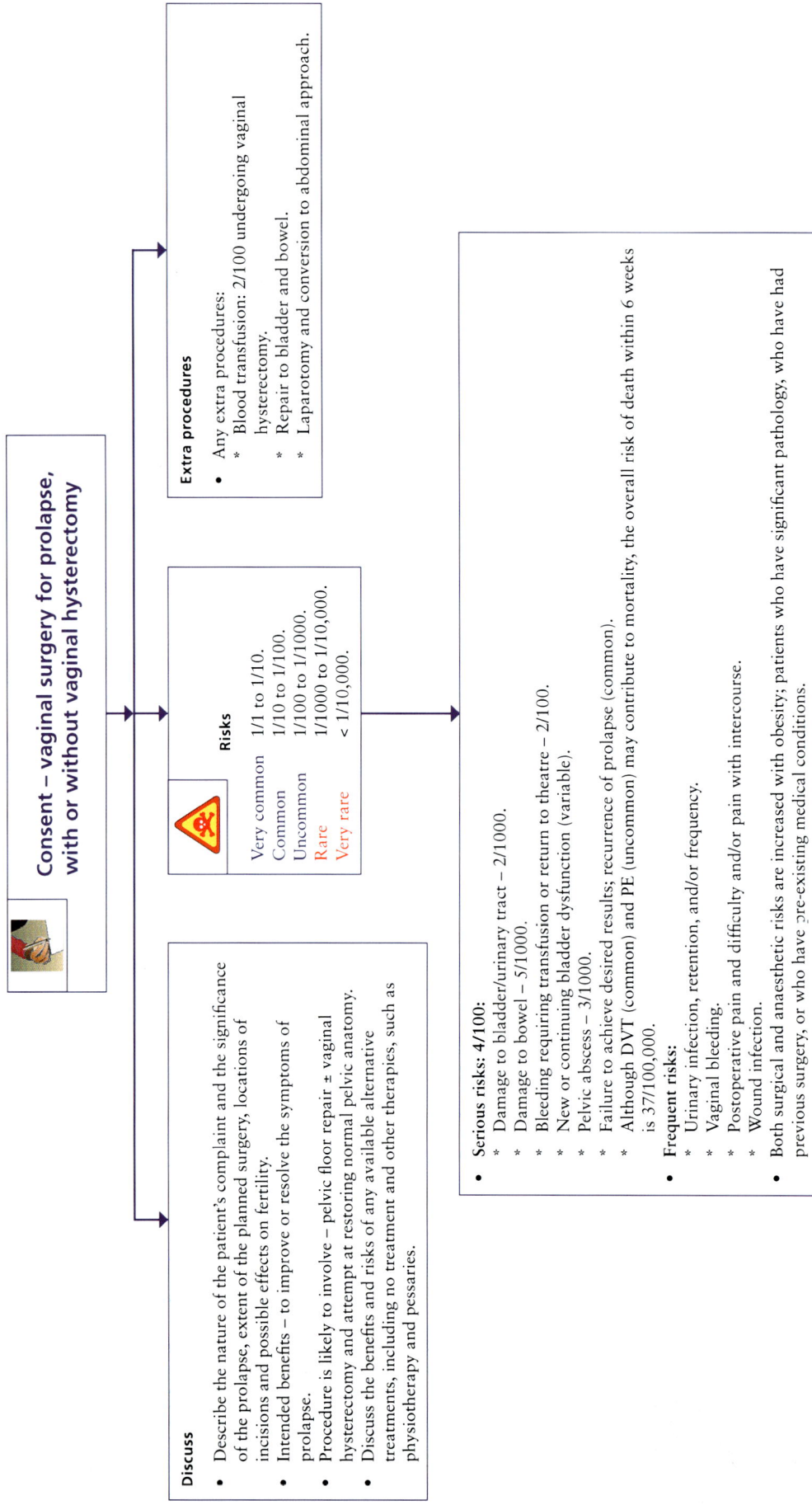

1. *Pelvic Organ Prolapse.* ACOG Practice Bulletin, Clinical Management Guidelines for Obstetricians and Gynaecologists, Number 79, 2007.
2. Bugge C, Adams EJ, Gopinath D, Reid F. Pessaries (mechanical devices) for pelvic organ prolapse in women. *Cochrane Database Syst Rev* 2013;2:CD004010.
3. Ismail SI, Bain C, Hagen S. Oestrogens for treatment or prevention of pelvic organ prolapse in postmenopausal women. *Cochrane Database Syst Rev* 2010;9:CD007063.
4. Hagen S, Stark D. Conservative prevention and management of pelvic organ prolapse in women. *Cochrane Database Syst Rev* 2011;12:CD003882.
5. Maher C, Feiner B, Baessler K, Glazener CMA. Surgical management of pelvic organ prolapse in women. *Cochrane Database Syst Rev* 2010;4:CD004014.
6. *Insertion of Mesh Uterine Suspension Sling (including Sacrohysteropexy) for Uterine Prolapse Repair.* NICE Interventional Procedure Guidance, 2009.
7. *Sacrocolpopexy with Hysterectomy Using Mesh for Uterine Prolapse Repair.* NICE Interventional Procedure Guidance, 2009.
8. *Vaginal Placement of Synthetic Mesh for Pelvic Organ Prolapse.* ACOG Committee Opinion, Number 513, 2011.
9. "<a href="http://commons.wikimedia.org/wiki/File:Pelvic_Organ_Prolapse_Quantification_System.

Background and prevalence

- Definition – descent of the vaginal cuff scar below a point that is 2 cm less than the total vaginal length above the plane of the hymen.
- Incidence – follows 12% of hysterectomies performed for prolapse and 2% of those performed for other indications.

Assessment

- Symptoms – pressure and discomfort; effect on urinary, bowel and sexual function.
- Can affect QOL.
- Assess all pelvic floor defects on standard tools such as POP-Q.
- Assess occult stress incontinence of urine after reducing the prolapse with a pessary.

Prevention at the time of hysterectomy

- McCall culdoplasty at the time of vaginal hysterectomy to prevent enterocele formation. It involves approximating the uterosacral ligaments using continuous sutures, to obliterate the peritoneum of the posterior cul-de-sac as high as possible. It is more effective than vaginal Moschowitz or simple closure of the peritoneum in preventing enterocele.
- Attaching the uterosacral and cardinal ligaments to the vaginal cuff and high circumferential obliteration of the pouch of Douglas at the time of hysterectomy to prevent vault prolapse and enterocele formation.
- Prophylactic sacrospinous fixation (SSF) at the time of vaginal hysterectomy is recommended when the vault (point C on the POP-Q system) descends to the introitus during closure.

Management

Non-surgical management

- Pessaries – require change every 6–8 months to prevent ulceration of the vaginal vault. If left for a long period, there is a risk of calcium deposition, erosion, and fistula formation. Therefore, they are reserved for physically frail women, those considered unfit for surgery, or when surgery is declined.
- Shelf pessaries preclude sexual intercourse and, therefore, are more suitable for women who are not sexually active.
- Ring pessaries tend to fail in women with deficient perineum, who may require shelf pessaries instead.
- Pelvic-floor exercises – no evidence to suggest that pelvic-floor exercises are helpful in vault prolapse.

Surgical management

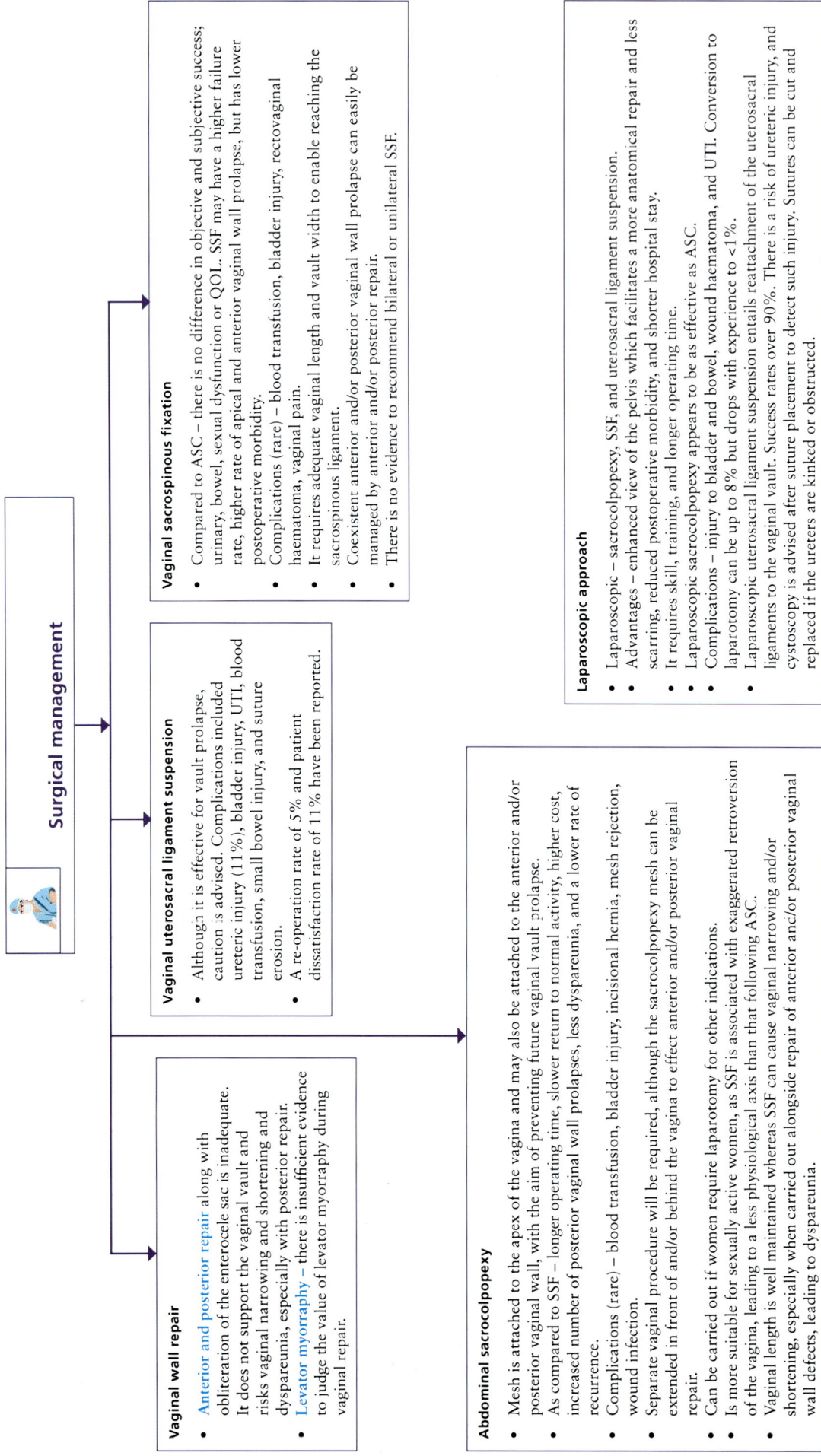

Surgical management

Vaginal wall repair

- **Anterior and posterior repair** along with obliteration of the enterocele sac is inadequate. It does not support the vaginal vault and risks vaginal narrowing and shortening and dyspareunia, especially with posterior repair.
- **Levator myorraphy** – there is insufficient evidence to judge the value of levator myorraphy during vaginal repair.

Vaginal uterosacral ligament suspension

- Although it is effective for vault prolapse, caution is advised. Complications included ureteric injury (11%), bladder injury, UTI, blood transfusion, small bowel injury, and suture erosion.
- A re-operation rate of 5% and patient dissatisfaction rate of 11% have been reported.

Vaginal sacrospinous fixation

- Compared to ASC – there is no difference in objective and subjective success; urinary, bowel, sexual dysfunction or QOL. SSF may have a higher failure rate, higher rate of apical and anterior vaginal wall prolapse, but has lower postoperative morbidity.
- Complications (rare) – blood transfusion, bladder injury, rectovaginal haematoma, vaginal pain.
- It requires adequate vaginal length and vault width to enable reaching the sacrospinous ligament.
- Coexistent anterior and/or posterior vaginal wall prolapse can easily be managed by anterior and/or posterior repair.
- There is no evidence to recommend bilateral or unilateral SSF.

Abdominal sacrocolpopexy

- Mesh is attached to the apex of the vagina and may also be attached to the anterior and/or posterior vaginal wall, with the aim of preventing future vaginal vault prolapse.
- As compared to SSF – longer operating time, slower return to normal activity, higher cost, increased number of posterior vaginal wall prolapses, less dyspareunia, and a lower rate of recurrence.
- Complications (rare) – blood transfusion, bladder injury, incisional hernia, mesh rejection, wound infection.
- Separate vaginal procedure will be required, although the sacrocolpopexy mesh can be extended in front of and/or behind the vagina to effect anterior and/or posterior vaginal repair.
- Can be carried out if women require laparotomy for other indications.
- Is more suitable for sexually active women, as SSF is associated with exaggerated retroversion of the vagina, leading to a less physiological axis than that following ASC.
- Vaginal length is well maintained whereas SSF can cause vaginal narrowing and/or shortening, especially when carried out alongside repair of anterior and/or posterior vaginal wall defects, leading to dyspareunia.

Laparoscopic approach

- Laparoscopic – sacrocolpopexy, SSF, and uterosacral ligament suspension.
- Advantages – enhanced view of the pelvis which facilitates a more anatomical repair and less scarring, reduced postoperative morbidity, and shorter hospital stay.
- It requires skill, training, and longer operating time.
- Laparoscopic sacrocolpopexy appears to be as effective as ASC.
- Complications – injury to bladder and bowel, wound haematoma, and UTI. Conversion to laparotomy can be up to 8% but drops with experience to <1%.
- Laparoscopic uterosacral ligament suspension entails reattachment of the uterosacral ligaments to the vaginal vault. Success rates over 90%. There is a risk of ureteric injury, and cystoscopy is advised after suture placement to detect such injury. Sutures can be cut and replaced if the ureters are kinked or obstructed.

Surgical management (contd.)

Iliococcygeus fixation

- Involves bilateral fixation of the vaginal vault to the iliococcygeus fascia.
- Reduces the exaggerated retroversion of the vagina, and thus the subsequent increase in anterior vaginal wall prolapse, and avoids the risk of injury to pudendal and sacral nerves and vessels associated with SSF.
- No significant difference in postoperative complications or subsequent development of anterior vaginal wall prolapse compared to vaginal SSF; therefore, is not routinely recommended.

Total mesh reconstruction

- A number of techniques, where a sheet of synthetic mesh material is fixed at a number of points to act as a new pelvic floor ('total mesh').
- Insufficient evidence to judge the safety and effectiveness.
- Complications – mesh erosion and infection.
- Data on long-term effectiveness are limited.

Infracoccygeal sacropexy with mesh

- An incision is made in the posterior wall of the vagina and a small puncture incision is made in each buttock. A tape (mesh) is introduced through one buttock and, using a tunnelling device, the tape is passed around the rectum. The tape is then passed up the side of the vagina, across the top, and down the other side, and out through the incision in the other buttock. The tape is sutured to the top of the vagina to act as a tension-free sling that aims to suspend the vault.
- Limited evidence – uncertainty about the procedure's safety, including mesh erosion and the risk of recurrence.
- Failure rate 9–10%. Symptomatic relief is reported in 85%.
- Complications – mesh erosion, infection, rectal perforation.

Sling procedures

- Uterine suspension sling using mesh involves attaching the uterus (or cervix) either to the sacrum (sacrohysteropexy) or to the ileopectineal ligaments.
- The mesh can be attached to the uterus either in the midline of the posterior cervix or bilaterally, where the uterosacral ligaments join the uterus; or to the front of the cervix and to the ileopectineal ligaments.
- Can also be used for women with cervical prolapse after supracervical hysterectomy.
- Significantly longer operating times and more blood loss compared to SSF.
- Complications – mesh erosion, infection, rectal perforation, bleeding, incisional hernia, small bowel obstruction.

Vault suspension to the anterior abdominal wall

- Simple measure; however, data are limited.
- Techniques include suspending the vaginal vault to anterior rectus sheath, to pectineal (Cooper's) ligament; plus the use of a rectus sheath fascial sling, using a transverse or a midline incision or an abdominovaginal approach.
- Minimal operative complications.
- Failure rate of 10%.
- Main concern – unphysiological axis of the vagina.

Colpocleisis

- Safe and effective procedure.
- It entails closure of the vagina, which is suitable for frail women who do not want to retain sexual function.
- Short operating time and low incidence of complications.
- Success rates of 97% and above.
- Can also be performed under local anaesthesia.

1. *The Management of Post-Hysterectomy Vaginal Vault Prolapse.* RCOG Green-top Guideline No. 46, October 2007.
2. *Infracoccygeal Sacropexy Using Mesh for Vaginal Vault Prolapse Repair.* NICE Interventional Procedure Guidance, January 2009.
3. *Insertion of Mesh Uterine Suspension Sling (including Sacrohysteropexy) for Uterine Prolapse Repair.* NICE Interventional Procedure Guidance, January 2009.
4. *Sacrocolpopexy with Hysterectomy Using Mesh for Uterine Prolapse Repair.* NICE Interventional Procedure Guidance, January 2009.

CHAPTER 27 Menopause and hormone replacement therapy

Background and prevalence

- Menopause – when menstruation ceases permanently owing to the loss of ovarian follicular activity. It is diagnosed with certainty after 12 months of spontaneous amenorrhoea.
- The average age of menopause is 52 years.
- Peri-menopause is the period before the menopause when the endocrinological, biological, and clinical features of approaching menopause commence because of decreasing oestrogen levels.
- Premature ovarian insufficiency (POI) is menopause that occurs at an age less than two standard deviations below the mean established for the reference population. In practice, in developed countries, 45 years of age is the cut-off point.
- About 80% of women in the UK experience menopausal symptoms and 45% find the symptoms distressing.
- Hot flushes occur in 70–80% of peri-menopausal women. They are most common in the first year after the final menstrual period.
- Vaginal symptoms occur in about 30% of women during the early post-menopausal period and in up to 47% of women during the later post-menopausal period.
- Only 10% seek medical advice.
- Racial, cultural, religious, sociological, and nutritional factors modify the quality and incidence of menopausal symptoms.

Risks or complications

- Can affect QOL. Without treatment menopausal symptoms are usually self-limiting (2–5 years), although some women experience symptoms for many years. Hot flushes are usually present for less than 5 years; however, some women may continue to flush beyond the age of 60 years.
- Vaginal symptoms, including dryness, discomfort, itching, and dyspareunia, generally persist or worsen with ageing.
- **Risk of chronic disease:**
  * Risk of osteoporosis, urogenital atrophy, cardiovascular disease, and stroke all increase after the menopause.
  * It is unclear whether dementia is associated directly with decreased oestrogen levels.

History – symptoms

- Menstrual cycle length may shorten to 2–3 weeks or lengthen to many months. The amount of menstrual blood loss may change.
- Most common symptoms are hot flushes, night sweats, vaginal dryness, and sleep disturbance.
- Hot flushes and night sweats – hot flushes arise as a sudden feeling of heat in the upper body (face, neck, and chest) and spread upwards and downwards. Diffuse or patchy flushing of the skin is followed by sweating and tachycardia/palpitations. Hot flushes generally last only a few minutes.
- Sleep disturbance is often due to night sweats but may also be associated with mood disorders or primary sleep disorders. Chronically disturbed sleep can lead to irritability and to difficulties with short-term memory and concentration.
- Urinary and vaginal symptoms, such as vaginal discomfort and dryness, dyspareunia, and recurrent lower urinary tract infection, are common in the menopause.

Assessment at primary care

- Assess the stage of menopause – whether peri-menopausal, post-menopausal, or a POI.
- Assess the symptoms – hot flushes, night sweats, vaginal dryness; primary depression or primary insomnia.
- Determine severity of the symptoms and the extent to which they are affecting the woman's QOL.
- Discuss woman's expectations.
- Assess the risk of cardiovascular disease and of osteoporosis.
- Rule out any contraindications (history of breast cancer, VTE).
- Discuss the risks and benefits of HRT.
- Record BMI and BP.
- Breast examination is not routinely necessary; however, discuss the national mammography screening programme and personal breast awareness before starting HRT.
- Pelvic examination is not routinely required unless clinically indicated.
- Investigations are not routinely indicated.
- Women who are not suitable for HRT or do not want to use HRT discuss alternatives to HRT.
- Encourage all women to participate in the national cervical screening programme.
- Discuss the perceived benefits and possible risks for their individual situations, including consideration of alternative therapies.
- Discuss the risk of VTE and the signs and symptoms of VTE. Advise to access medical help rapidly if they suspect that they have developed a thrombosis.

Contraindications to starting HRT

- Hormone-dependent cancer (endometrial cancer, current or past breast cancer).
- Active or recent arterial thromboembolic disease (angina or myocardial infarction).
- VTE, PE. • Severe active liver disease.
- Undiagnosed breast mass. • Uninvestigated abnormal vaginal bleeding.

Investigations

Do not offer routine investigations before starting HRT unless:

- Change in menstrual pattern, IMB, PCB, or PMB: consider an endometrial assessment.
- Personal or family history of VTE: consider a thrombophilia screen.
- High risk of breast cancer: mammography or MRI as appropriate for the woman's age.
- Woman has arterial disease or other risk markers for arterial disease: a lipid profile may be useful.

- Do not routinely measure FSH levels for diagnosing the menopause. The diagnosis is clinical.
- Measurement of LH, oestradiol, progesterone, or testosterone is of no value.
- Measurement of FSH is of limited value as:
  * FSH levels fluctuate during the peri-menopause.
  * Normal results do not exclude the menopause.
  * An increased concentration is suggestive of ovarian failure but does not indicate an inability to conceive.
- Measurement of FSH may be useful in (≥ 2 occasions at least 1–2 months apart):
  * Women < 45 years of age with suspected POI.
  * Women who have had a hysterectomy with ovarian conservation before 40 years of age.
  * Women using hormonal contraception. As the COC suppresses gonadotrophins, a low level may be impossible to interpret. Measure FSH when the woman is not taking oestrogen-based contraception either by stopping the COC or by changing to a progesterone only preparation. Allow 6 weeks between terminating therapy and measuring FSH.

Routes and regimens

- Oestrogen – transdermal (gels or patches) and subcutaneous (implants) routes avoid the first-pass effect through the liver and are not associated with an increased risk of VTE.
- Progestogen – vaginal route, e.g., levonorgestrel IUS and progesterone gel and pessaries, provide adequate endometrial protection with reduced systemic side effects. Progesterone is available in an oral micronized form, vaginal pessaries, and gel.
- Continuous combined regimens avoid the need for regular withdrawal bleeds but may be associated with continuous low-grade progestogenic side effects. Ultra low-dose oestradiol/progestogen continuous combined regimens appear to maintain the benefits of higher-dose regimens while allowing minimal use of progestogen to reduce side effects.
- Low-dose vaginal oestrogenic creams, rings, tablets, and pessaries should be considered for all women with symptoms of urogenital atrophy. Local oestrogenic preparations may be more effective than systemic therapy and can be used in conjunction with oral/transdermal HRT. Indefinite usage is usually required as symptoms often return when treatment is discontinued. Progestogenic opposition is not required as systemic absorption is minimal with oestradiol and oestriol preparations.
- Drospirenone, a spironolactone analogue, has anti-androgenic and anti-mineralocorticoid properties. It has been incorporated with low-dose oestrogen in a continuous combined formulation.
- With both cyclical and continuous regimens, there may be some erratic bleeding to begin with, but 90% of these women will eventually be completely bleed free.

Progestonic side effects

Non-hysterectomized women require 12–14 days of progestogen to avoid endometrial hyperplasia and minimize the risk of endometrial cancer with unopposed oestrogen.

- One of the main factors for reduced compliance with HRT is that of progestogen intolerance.
- Progestogens – symptoms of fluid retention are produced by the sodium-retaining effect of the renin–aldosterone system, triggered by stimulation of the aldosterone receptors.
- Androgenic side effects such as acne and hirsutism are a problem of the testosterone-derived progestogens owing to stimulation of the androgen receptors.
- Mood swings and PMS-like side effects result from adverse stimulation of the central nervous system progesterone receptors.
- Dose can be halved and duration of progestogen can be reduced to 7–10 days to minimize progestogenic side effects. This may result in bleeding problems and hyperplasia, so keep a low threshold for ultrasound scanning and endometrial sampling if clinically indicated.
- Progesterone and dydrogesterone generally have fewer side effects.
- Progestogenic side effects may be reduced by transvaginal pessaries or gels and LNG-IUS. LNG-IUS provides adequate endometrial protection in women receiving oestrogen therapy. Systemic side effects are reduced, although not completely eliminated. The impact on breast cancer risk remains unclear with preliminary data showing no significant difference when compared to systemic progestogens.

Benefits of HRT – immediate effects of HRT

Vasomotor symptoms – oestrogen remains the most effective treatment. Decide the optimum dose and duration according to the severity of symptoms and response to therapy.
Mood – short-term use of HRT may improve mood and depressive symptoms during the menopausal transition and in the early menopause. Women with severe depression and those who do not respond to HRT will require psychiatric assessment.
Sexual function – HRT, systemic or topical, may improve sexual function in women with dyspareunia secondary to vaginal atrophy, through its proliferative effect on the vulval and vaginal epithelium and by improving vaginal lubrication. Systemic testosterones result in significant improvement in sexual function, including sexual desire, and orgasm.

Urogenital symptoms – oestrogen has a proliferative effect on the bladder and urethral epithelium and may help relieve symptoms of urinary frequency, urgency, and possibly reduce the risk of recurrent UTIs in women with urogenital atrophy. Low-dose vaginal oestrogen preparations can be used long-term in symptomatic women as required, and all topical oestrogen preparations are effective. There is no requirement to combine this with systemic progestogen treatment for endometrial protection, as low-dose vaginal oestrogen preparations do not result in significant systemic absorption. However, there is little evidence to prove the safety of vaginal preparations beyond one year of use; therefore, clinicians should aim to use the lowest effective dose for symptom control.

Musculoskeletal effects – oestrogen deficiency after the menopause has a negative effect on connective tissue metabolism in the bone matrix, skin, intervertebral discs, and elsewhere in the body. Oestrogen therapy has a protective effect against connective tissue loss and may possibly reverse this process in menopausal women receiving HRT.
Colorectal cancer – reduced risk of colorectal cancer with the use of oral combined HRT.
WHI – colorectal cancer risk was reduced in women taking combined conjugated equine oestrogens (CEE) and MPA, but there was no effect of CEE-only therapy.
There are no data on the effect of transdermal HRT and risk of colorectal cancer.

Long-term effects of HRT

Osteoporosis

- HRT is effective in preserving bone density and preventing osteoporosis in both spine and hip, as well as reducing the risk of osteoporosis-related fractures. • HRT is the first-line therapeutic intervention for the prevention and treatment of osteoporosis in women with POI and menopausal women < 60 years, particularly those with menopausal symptoms.
- Initiating HRT after the age of 60 years for the sole purpose of the prevention of osteoporotic fractures is not recommended.
- The bone-protective effect of oestrogen is dose related. The bone-preserving effect of HRT on bone mineral density declines after discontinuation of treatment.
- Use of HRT for a few years around the menopause may provide a long-term protective effect many years after stopping HRT.

Cardiovascular

- Early cohort studies suggested that HRT is associated with a significant reduction in the incidence of heart disease, whether oestrogen alone or combined with progestogen.
- WHI – women using CEE 0.625 mg alone or with MPA 2.5mg had a small increase in incidence of coronary heart disease in the first 12 months.
- 'Early harm' can occur when therapy is commenced in women > 60 years of age with relative overdoses of oral oestrogen. When prescribing HRT for the first time in women over the age of 60 years, use the lowest effective dose.
- RCT data from the Danish Osteoporosis Trial have shown that hormone therapy reduces the incidence of coronary heart disease by around 50% if commenced within 10 years of the menopause – this is referred to as the 'window of opportunity' for primary prevention.

Cognition

- Observational data show an improvement in cognitive function with HRT started in early menopause and a possible reduction in the long-term risk of Alzheimer's disease and all causes of dementia. Further evidence is needed to confirm this.
- Other studies, including the WHI, showed no significant improvement in memory or cognitive function with HRT in older post-menopausal women, with a reported increase in the risk of dementia in women aged 65–79 years.
- Do not initiate HRT for the sole purpose of improving cognitive function or reducing the risk of dementia in post-menopausal women.

Risks of HRT

(handwritten note in margin: lifetime cases 14/1000)

Breast cancer

- WHI – oestrogen and progesterone has a small increase in risk of breast cancer after 5 years of use of approximately one extra case per 1000 women per annum.
- WHI – oestrogen alone has a small but statistically significant decrease in risk.
- The Million Women Study (MWS) raised concerns over the long-term safety of HRT from the perspective of breast cancer.
- The data from these trials are too limited to establish a causal association between HRT and breast cancer.
- Combined HRT has been associated with the highest risk.
- Risk is lower with oestrogen-only HRT than with combined HRT.
- Risk increases with duration of use and returns to baseline within 5 years of stopping treatment.

Endometrial cancer

- Unopposed oestrogen therapy increases the incidence of endometrial cancer; largely avoided by the use of combined sequential oestrogen/progestogen therapy.
- Long-term use of sequential combined HRT for > 5 years may be associated with a small increase in risk of endometrial cancer. Continuous combined regimens are associated with a significantly lower risk of endometrial cancer than an untreated population.

Ovarian cancer – conflicting data.

- Several case–control studies reported a significant increase in risk associated with the use of oestrogen replacement therapy and either a smaller or no increased risk with combined oestrogen and progestogen therapy.
- WHI reported no increased risk.
- Recent data from the Danish National Cancer Registry showed a small but significant increase in the incidence of ovarian cancer following 8 years' use of unopposed oestrogen and oestrogen/progestogen therapy.
- Long-term use of oestrogen-only or combined HRT may be associated with a small increased risk of ovarian cancer. This risk returns to baseline a few years after stopping treatment.

Venous thromboembolism

- Oral HRT increases the risk of VTE 2–4 fold, with the highest risk in the first year of use. The absolute risk, particularly in the absence of other risk factors, remains low. VTE incidence rate is 4.2/1030 patient–years in women who are never exposed to HRT, compared to 5.8/1000 patient–years in women of a similar age exposed to combination HRT with conjugated oestrogen.
- VTE risk is further increased if there is a personal or family history of VTE or other risk factors.
- Oestrogen-type – risk of VTE may be less with esterified oestrogens compared with CEE; there is still a significant VTE risk with both types of oestrogen.
- Combination HRT – there may be a greater risk of VTE with combination therapy. However, HRT with oestrogen alone is also associated with a significant VTE risk.
- Progestogen type – micronized progesterone and pregnane derivatives may carry a lower thrombotic risk compared with norpregnane derivatives and MPA.
- Oestrogen dose – the effect of oestrogen may be dose related. With no significant VTE risk associated with doses of oral oestrogen of around 0.3 mg; a higher VTE risk with oestrogen doses of ≈ 1.25 mg or more (ORs 2.4–6.9) compared with 0.625 mg (ORs 1.7–4.3).
- Transdermal preparations are associated with a substantially lower risk of VTE than oral preparations. A systematic review revealed a nonsignificant OR of VTE in association with transdermal oestrogen of 1.2 (95% CI 0.9–1.7).
- Duration of therapy – risk of VTE is highest in the first year of HRT use, with no evidence of continuing risk on stopping HRT.
- Past use of HRT – there is no significant pooled VTE risk with those who had used oral oestrogen HRT in the past.

Stroke

- Conflicting data.
- WHI – increased incidence of stroke in women using oestrogen and progestogen therapy or oestrogen alone; a smaller increase in incidence of stroke in women who commenced HRT between the ages of 50 and 59 years.
- HERS study – no increased risk of stroke with HRT.
- HRT is not recommended for the primary or secondary prevention of stroke.
- Oestrogen-only and combined HRT increased the risk of stroke (mostly ischaemic).
- Although the increase in relative risk seems to be similar irrespective of age, baseline risk of stroke increases with age and therefore older women have a greater absolute risk.
- Be cautious when prescribing HRT in women > 60 years, particularly when they have a risk factor for stroke or VTE. In these groups, transdermal route may be advantageous. The effects of HRT may be dose related; prescribe the lowest effective dose in women with significant risk factors.

VTE – history and assessment of risk factors (RCOG)

Family history of VTE – heritable thrombophilia

- Combination of HRT and one prothrombotic mutation gives a combined OR of 8.0 for VTE compared with women without exposure to either risk factor. Asymptomatic carriers of FVL mutation – incidence of VTE related to HRT is 3%/year.
- Do not offer universal screening for thrombophilic defects before prescribing HRT. Screening of 795 women would be required to prevent one episode of VTE in 5 years. Screening selected women is the most cost-effective method.
- A history of VTE in a first-degree relative is a relative contraindication to HRT. Discuss alternatives to HRT or consider transdermal preparations. Given the polygenic nature of VTE, the risk of VTE may still be increased in those members of the family who do not carry that thrombophilia. Consequently, a negative thrombophilia result does not necessarily exclude an increased risk.
- If a heritable thrombophilia is detected in an affected family member testing for thrombophilia does not provide a definitive estimate of risk in most cases; therefore, do not offer routinely. However, where a high-risk heritable thrombophilia is identified in a symptomatic family member (e.g., deficiency of anti-thrombin, protein C, or protein S) testing for thrombophilia may assist in the counselling of overall thrombotic risk.
- In women without a personal history of VTE but with a high-risk thrombophilic trait (deficiency of anti-thrombin, protein C or protein S, or combination of defects) that has been identified through screening because of a symptomatic family member, avoid oral HRT and seek specialist advice. With other thrombophilic defects, there is insufficient evidence at present to indicate that HRT should be completely avoided. In the presence of multiple-risk factors for VTE, avoid HRT.

Other risk factors

- Avoid HRT in women with multiple pre-existing risk factors for VTE. Additional risk factors:
  * Increasing age.   * Obesity (BMI > 30).   * Post-thrombotic syndrome.
  * Varicose veins with phlebitis.   * Immobility for > 3 days.
  * Surgical procedures (anaesthesia and surgical time > 60 minutes).
  * Other disorders, e.g., malignancy, myeloproliferative disorders, cardiac disease, paralysis of lower limbs, systemic infection, inflammatory bowel disease, nephritic syndrome, sickle cell disease.
- Age – compared with women aged 50–59 years, those aged 60–69 years had a doubling of risk, and those aged 70–79 years had an almost 4-fold increase in risk.
- Obesity – increased risk of VTE associated with increasing weight. OR of 2.7 associated with BMI 25 to < 30 and an OR of 4.0 with BMI > 30 kg/m². The use of transdermal HRT does not increase the risk associated with weight.

Personal/previous history of VTE

- A personal history of thrombosis is a contraindication to oral HRT.
- Oral combined HRT has a 4–5-fold higher risk of recurrent VTE.
- If QOL is so severely affected that the benefits of HRT outweigh the risks:
  * Use a transdermal preparation.
  * Discuss the risk of recurrence.
  * Consider prophylactic anticoagulant therapy while the woman is taking HRT. However, it has risk of major haemorrhage at around 1% per year of treatment and 25% of these bleeds are fatal.
  * Seek specialist advice.
- Testing for thrombophilia in selected women (e.g., those with previous severe unprovoked or recurrent VTE indicating a severe defect such as deficiency of anti-thrombin, protein C, or protein S) may be helpful in assessing the overall thrombotic risk in women with a personal history of VTE; however, the result will not alter the advice that oral HRT should be avoided.
- Do not routinely offer testing for thrombophilia in unselected women who have experienced a first episode of VTE, as there is insufficient evidence that testing reduces the risk of recurrence, or that the results should influence the duration of anticoagulant therapy.

- Assess risk of VTE prior to commencing HRT. Routine thrombophilia testing is not required, but consider if there is a family history of thrombosis.
- In 'high-risk' individuals who require HRT, use transdermal preparations, and if a progestogen is required, suitable options are micronized progesterone or dydrogesterone.
- Review and provide thromboprophylaxis if a woman on HRT is hospitalized.

6/1000 Teplak Rx (E)
(E+Pg Rx) | x2 jj104/Sy.
14/1000
(E1hg cont)
20/1000

Management

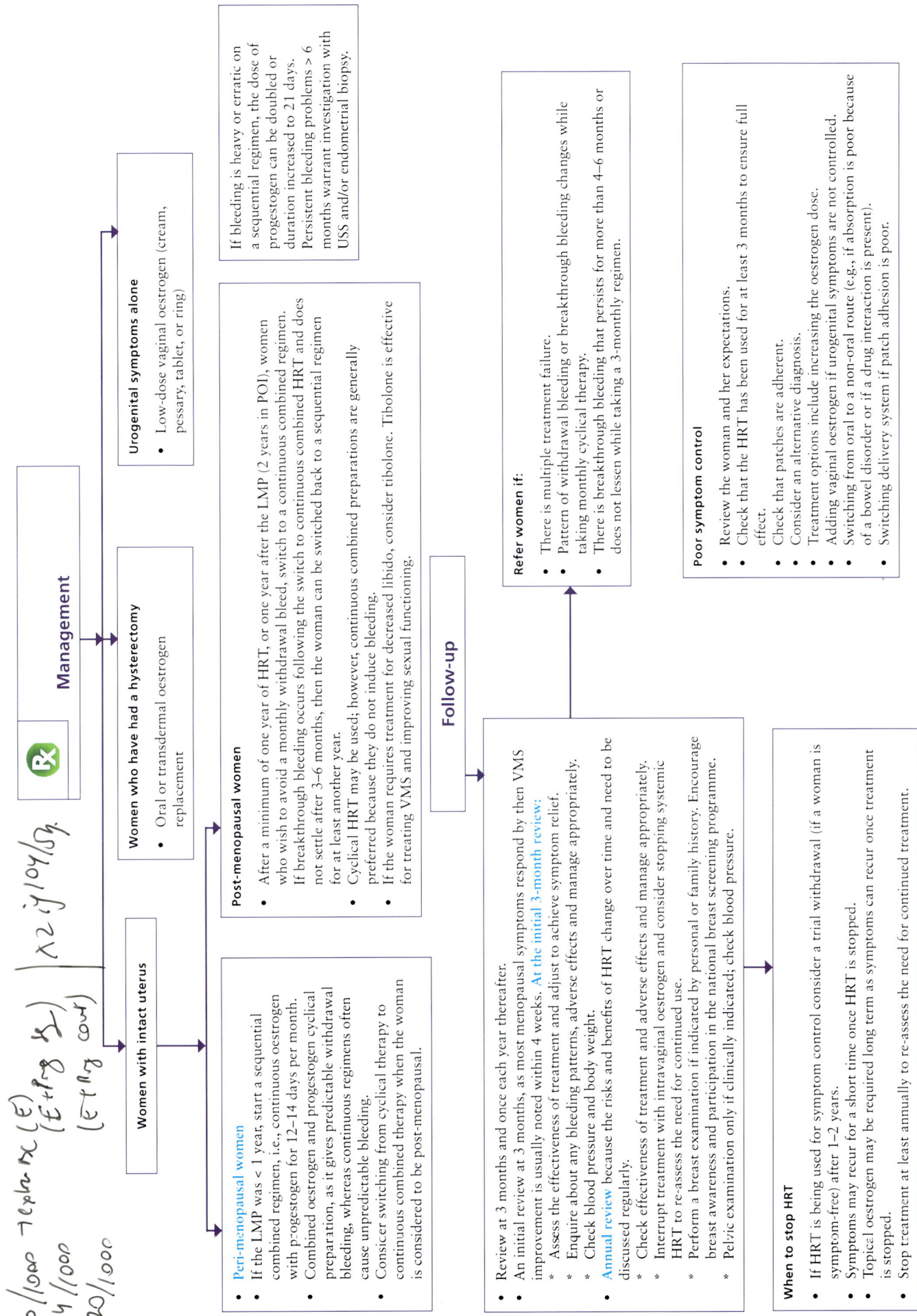

Women with intact uterus

Peri-menopausal women

- If the LMP was < 1 year, start a sequential combined regimen, i.e., continuous oestrogen with progestogen for 12–14 days per month.
- Combined oestrogen and progestogen cyclical preparation, as it gives predictable withdrawal bleeding, whereas continuous regimens often cause unpredictable bleeding.
- Consider switching from cyclical therapy to continuous combined therapy when the woman is considered to be post-menopausal.

Women who have had a hysterectomy

- Oral or transdermal oestrogen replacement

Post-menopausal women

- After a minimum of one year of HRT, or one year after the LMP (2 years in POI), women who wish to avoid a monthly withdrawal bleed, switch to a continuous combined regimen. If breakthrough bleeding occurs following the switch to continuous combined HRT and does not settle after 3–6 months, then the woman can be switched back to a sequential regimen for at least another year.
- Cyclical HRT may be used; however, continuous combined preparations are generally preferred because they do not induce bleeding.
- If the woman requires treatment for decreased libido, consider tibolone. Tibolone is effective for treating VMS and improving sexual functioning.

Urogenital symptoms alone

- Low-dose vaginal oestrogen (cream, pessary, tablet, or ring)

If bleeding is heavy or erratic on a sequential regimen, the dose of progestogen can be doubled or duration increased to 21 days. Persistent bleeding problems > 6 months warrant investigation with USS and/or endometrial biopsy.

Follow-up

- Review at 3 months and once each year thereafter.
- An initial review at 3 months, as most menopausal symptoms respond by then VMS improvement is usually noted within 4 weeks. **At the initial 3-month review:**
  * Assess the effectiveness of treatment and adjust to achieve symptom relief.
  * Enquire about any bleeding patterns, adverse effects and manage appropriately.
  * Check blood pressure and body weight.
- **Annual review** because the risks and benefits of HRT change over time and need to be discussed regularly.
  * Check effectiveness of treatment and adverse effects and manage appropriately.
  * Interrupt treatment with intravaginal oestrogen and consider stopping systemic HRT to re-assess the need for continued use.
  * Perform a breast examination if indicated by personal or family history. Encourage breast awareness and participation in the national breast screening programme.
  * Pelvic examination only if clinically indicated; check blood pressure.

Refer women if:

- There is multiple treatment failure.
- Pattern of withdrawal bleeding or breakthrough bleeding changes while taking monthly cyclical therapy.
- There is breakthrough bleeding that persists for more than 4–6 months or does not lessen while taking a 3-monthly regimen.

Poor symptom control

- Review the woman and her expectations.
- Check that the HRT has been used for at least 3 months to ensure full effect.
- Check that patches are adherent.
- Consider an alternative diagnosis.
- Treatment options include increasing the oestrogen dose.
- Adding vaginal oestrogen if urogenital symptoms are not controlled.
- Switching from oral to a non-oral route (e.g., if absorption is poor because of a bowel disorder or if a drug interaction is present).
- Switching delivery system if patch adhesion is poor.

When to stop HRT

- If HRT is being used for symptom control consider a trial withdrawal (if a woman is symptom-free) after 1–2 years.
- Symptoms may recur for a short time once HRT is stopped.
- Topical oestrogen may be required long term as symptoms can recur once treatment is stopped.
- Stop treatment at least annually to re-assess the need for continued treatment.

Alternatives to HRT for the management of symptoms of the menopause (RCOG)

Lifestyle measures

- Aerobic exercise – limited evidence. Can improve psychological health, QOL, and can result in significant improvements in vasomotor symptoms and other menopause-related symptoms (e.g., mood and insomnia). Low-intensity exercise such as yoga may be beneficial. The best activity appears to be regular sustained aerobic exercise such as swimming or running.
- Hot flushes and night sweats – take regular exercise, wear lighter clothing, sleep in a cooler room, and reduce stress. Avoid possible triggers, such as spicy foods, caffeine, smoking, and alcohol. Smoking cigarettes and having a BMI > 30 kg/m^2 increases the likelihood of flushing.
- Sleep disturbances – avoiding exercise late in the day and maintaining a regular bedtime.
- Mood and anxiety disturbances – adequate sleep, regular physical activity, and relaxation exercises.
- Cognitive symptoms – exercise and good sleep hygiene may improve subjective cognitive symptoms.

Non-pharmacological agents for vaginal dryness

- Lubricants and vaginal moisturizers (Replens and Sylk) – limited evidence.
- Lubricants – a combination of protectants and thickening agents in a water-soluble base used to relieve vaginal dryness during intercourse.
- Moisturizers may contain a bioadhesive polycarbophil-based polymer that attaches to mucin and epithelial cells on the vaginal wall and retains water. May provide longer-term relief of vaginal dryness.

Pharmacological alternatives

Selective serotonin and noradrenaline reuptake inhibitors

- SSRIs (fluoxetine and paroxetine) – study on citalopram and fluoxetine showed no benefit.
- SNRIs – most convincing data are for venlafaxine (37.5 mg BD).
- High incidence of nausea, reduced libido and sexual response.
- Analogue of venlafaxine (desvenlafaxine succinate) – symptom relief can be maintained while adverse effects are reduced.
- Further research is required.

Progestogens

- Megestrol acetate has benefit for VMS over placebo.
- WHI – safety of progestogens is questionable, as the increase in risk of breast cancer with HRT is due to the combination of oestrogen and progestogen (rather than oestrogen alone). Therefore, it is inappropriate to treat women who are at increased risk of breast cancer with progestogens, particularly women with progesterone-receptor-positive tumours.
- Doses of progestogens that achieve VMS control can increase the risk of VTE.

Clonidine

- Centrally active α2 agonist.
- The trial data are contradictory.
- Oral/ transdermal – by avoiding first-pass metabolism, will increase efficacy.
- A systematic review – marginally significant benefit over placebo; however, the effects of clonidine are not as great as those of oestrogen, and adverse effects may restrict its use.

Diet and supplements

- Vitamins such as E and C, and minerals such as selenium are present in various supplements. The evidence that they are of any benefit is limited.
- Vitamin E – a statistically significant reduction in hot flush frequency is reported with vitamin E 800 IU/day compared with placebo; however, this reduction was only small and might not be clinically significant.

- β-blockers – trials have been disappointing.
- Gabapentin – showed efficacy for hot flush reduction compared with placebo, but oestrogen is more effective. Adverse effect profile (drowsiness, dizziness, fatigue) may restrict use.
- Dehydroepiandrosterone – a pilot study showed a modest reduction in hot flushes.

Stellate ganglion blockade

- Local anaesthetic injection into the stellate ganglion. Recently emerged as a new technique against hot flushes and sweating refractory to other treatments or where HRT is contraindicated.
- Preliminary studies report encouraging efficacy with minimal complications.

Homeopathy

- Mechanisms that underlie the biological response to ultra-molecular dilutions are unclear.
- Data from case histories, observational studies, and a small number of randomized trials are encouraging, but more research is needed.

Alternatives to HRT (contd.)

Complementary therapies

Botanicals – evidence is limited and conflicting. Herbal medicines have pharmacological actions and thus can cause unwanted effects and have potentially dangerous interactions with other medicines.

Other complementary interventions – further research is needed. Acupressure, acupuncture, Alexander technique, Ayurveda, osteopathy, hypnotherapy, reflexology, magnetism, and Reiki.

- Phyto-oestrogens – soy and red clover.
  * Plant substances that have similar effects to oestrogens.
- Isoflavones – found in soybeans, chickpeas, red clover, and in other legumes (beans and peas).
- Lignans – oilseeds such as flaxseed are rich in lignans; also found in cereal bran, whole cereals, vegetables, legumes, and fruit.
  * Evidence is conflicting.
  * Systematic review – no evidence that they help to relieve symptoms.
- Isoflavone supplementation may produce a slight to modest reduction in the number of daily flushes in menopausal women.
  * Unwanted effects are not increased.
  * Owing to the oestrogenic actions, concerns about safety in hormone-sensitive tissues such as breast and uterus.

- Black cohosh (Actaea racemosa).
  * There is no consensus as to the mechanism by which it relieves hot flushes. Whether it has any oestrogenic actions is debated; raises concerns about its use in women with hormone-sensitive conditions.
  * Evidence is conflicting.
  * Little is known about the long-term safety. Possible liver toxicity has been reported.
- Evening primrose oil – rich in γ-linolenic and linolenic acid.
  * No evidence for its efficacy.
- Ginseng – has not been found to be superior to placebo for VMS, PMB, and mastalgia.

- Chinese herbs
  * Dong quai (Angelica sinensis) – not superior to placebo, but may be effective when combined with other herbs. Interactions with warfarin and photosensitization are reported.
  * Trial on Danggui Buxue Tang – benefit over placebo was found only for mild hot flushes.
  * St John's wort – shown to be efficacious in mild to moderate depression because of its SSRI-type effect, but its efficacy for VMS remains to be proved. It interacts with many other medications. It may cause breakthrough bleeding and contraceptive failure when used concomitantly with oral contraceptives.
  * Agnus castus (chasteberry) – limited data.

- Reflexology
  * Aims to relieve stress or treat health conditions through the application of pressure to specific points or areas of the feet, hands, and ears.
  * Study comparing reflexology to nonspecific foot massage reported a reduction in symptoms in both groups, but there was no significant difference between the groups.

- Acupuncture
  * Evidence is conflicting.
  * Systematic review failed to show beneficial effects of acupuncture over 'placebo'.
- Magnetism
  * Various forms such as bracelets and insoles. There is no known mechanism of action for magnet therapies for the treatment of hot flushes. There is no evidence of benefit at present.

HRT after cancer

- **Endometrial** – no increased risk of recurrence or a reduced recurrence rate with an increased disease-free interval. Most of these studies have been on early stage disease and the findings may be different in advanced cancer where there may be microscopic metastatic deposits. Local endometrial sarcomas are oestrogen sensitive and are a contraindication to HRT.
- **Ovarian cancer** – there is no evidence that oestrogen therapy following treatment for ovarian cancer will adversely affect the prognosis. Studies have shown either no difference in survival rate or an improvement in survival rate with the use of HRT in women with epithelial ovarian cancer. There is no evidence of an adverse effect of HRT on women with germ cell tumours. There are no data on the use of HRT following granulosa cell tumours, although HRT should be avoided in this situation largely on theoretical grounds.
- **Cervical** – no association between cervical cancer and HRT. HRT is not contraindicated after treatment for squamous cell carcinoma or adenocarcinoma of the cervix.
- **Vulval** – systemic and topical oestrogen can be used following vulval carcinoma. There is no evidence of an adverse effect with regard to recurrence of vulval disease.

Sexual function/androgens

Women with distressing low sexual desire and tiredness:

- Androgen supplementation – testosterone gels licensed for male use are available in 50 mg, 5ml sachets or tubes. Unlicensed prescribing by specialists is an option for female androgen replacement, at a reduced dosage of 0.5–1.0 mL/day or a quarter-sachet/tube on alternate days. Androgenic side effects and risks are minimal and reversible if testosterone levels are maintained within the female physiological range.
- Tibolone has a weak androgenic effect, which can have a beneficial effect on mood and libido.
- DHEA – further research is needed to confirm efficacy and safety.

Women requiring surgery

- Each woman requires an individual assessment of the risks and benefits of stopping HRT before elective surgery.
- Consider stopping HRT four weeks before elective surgery; this may not be necessary if appropriate thromboprophylaxis is used.

Risks of HRT

Outcome	HRT versus placebo per 10,000 person–years
Cardiovascular disease	+ 7 (37 vs 30 cases)
Stroke	+ 8 (29 vs 21 cases)
DVT/PE	+ 18 (34 vs 16 cases)
Breast cancer	+ 8 (38 vs 30 cases)
Colon cancer	– 6 (10 vs 16 cases)
Hip fracture	– 5 (10 vs 15 cases)

1. *Venous Thromboembolism and Hormone Replacement Therapy.* RCOG Green-top Guideline No. 19, 3rd edition, May 2011.
2. *Menopause and Osteoporosis.* SOGC, Update 2009.
3. *Alternatives to HRT for the Management of Symptoms of the Menopause.* Scientific Advisory Committee Opinion Paper 6, 2nd edition, September 2010.
4. *Clinical Knowledge Summaries.* http://www.cks.nhs.uk/menopause.
5. Marsden J. Hormone replacement therapy and breast disease. *The Obstetrician and Gynaecologist* 2010;12:155–163.
6. *MHRA's Drug Safety Update on HRT.* http://www.mhra.gov.uk/mhra/drugsafetyupdate.
7. Panay N, Hamoda H, Arya R, Savvas M. *The 2013 British Menopause Society and Women's Health Concern Recommendations on Hormone Replacement Therapy.* June 18, 2013.

CHAPTER 28 Epidemiology of cancer in females in the UK

Epidemiology of cancer in females in the UK, 2011

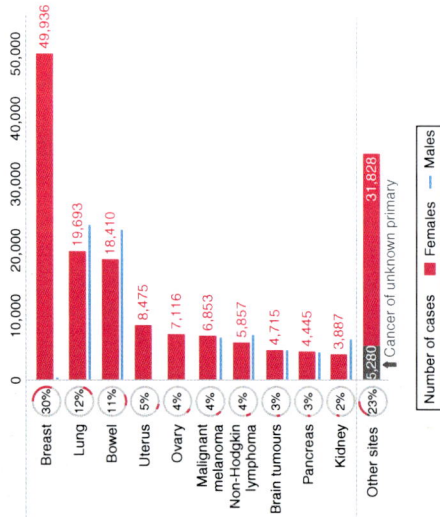

Female incidence
164,000 cases
UK, 2011

Breast 30%
Lung 12%
Bowel 11%
All other cancers 47%

Most common cancers in females, percentages of all cancer

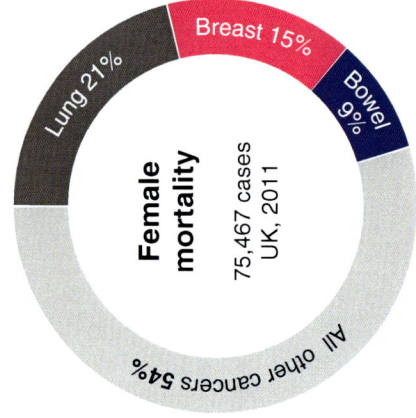

Female mortality
75,467 cases
UK, 2011

Breast 15%
Bowel 9%
Lung 21%
All other cancers 54%

Most common causes of cancer death, percentages of all cancer deaths

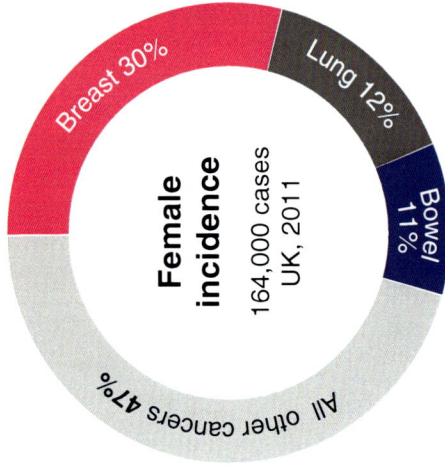

Breast 30% — 49,936
Lung 12% — 19,693
Bowel 11% — 18,410
Uterus 5% — 8,475
Ovary 4% — 7,116
Malignant melanoma 4% — 6,853
Non-Hodgkin lymphoma 4% — 5,857
Brain tumours 3% — 4,715
Pancreas 3% — 4,445
Kidney 2% — 3,887
Other sites 23% — 5,280 / 31,828

↑ Cancer of unknown primary

Number of cases ■ Females — Males

The 10 most common cancers

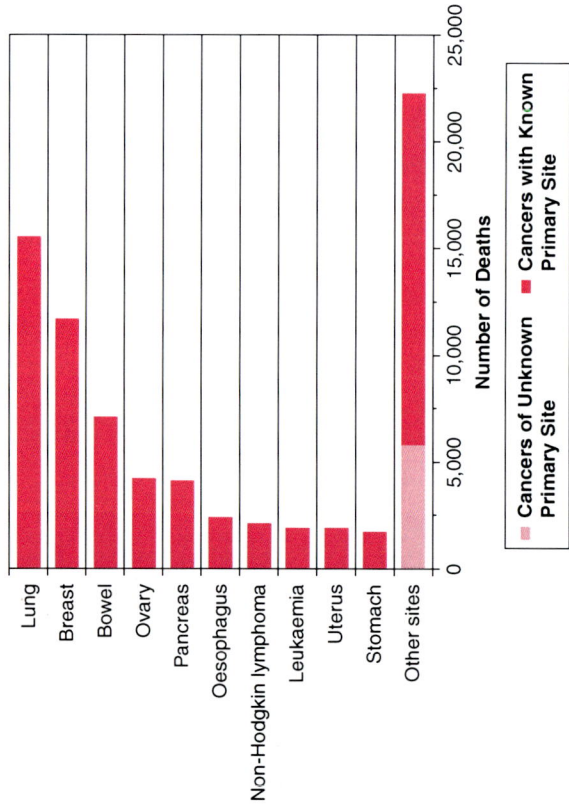

Number of Deaths

Lung
Breast
Bowel
Ovary
Pancreas
Oesophagus
Non-Hodgkin lymphoma
Leukaemia
Uterus
Stomach
Other sites

■ Cancers of Unknown Primary Site ■ Cancers with Known Primary Site

The 10 most common causes of cancer death

Epidemiology of gynaecological cancers in women in the UK – 2011

Gynaecological cancers	Numbers of new cases	European age-standardized (AS) incidence rates per 100,000, UK	Numbers of deaths	Age-standardized (AS) mortality and crude death rates per 100,000, UK
Vulva	1203	2.5	404	0.7
Vagina	256	0.6	91	0.2
Cervix	3064	8.7	972	2.4
Uterus	8475	20.4	1930	3.8
Ovary	7116	17.1	4272	9.0

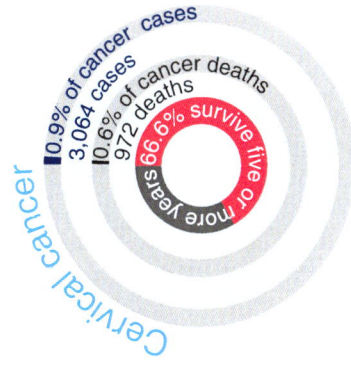

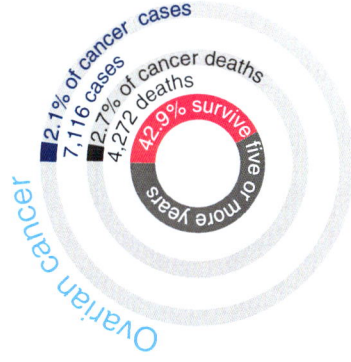

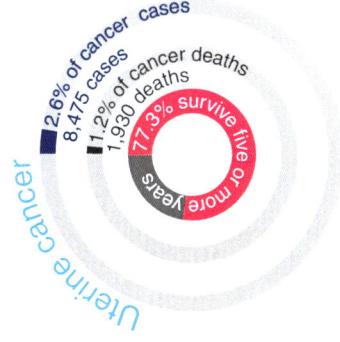

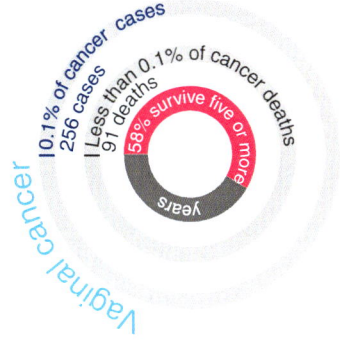

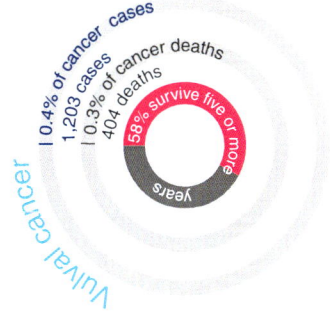

Cervical cancer
0.9% of cancer cases
3,064 cases
0.6% of cancer deaths
972 deaths
66.6% survive five or more years

Ovarian cancer
2.1% of cancer cases
7,116 cases
2.7% of cancer deaths
4,272 deaths
42.9% survive five or more years

Uterine cancer
2.6% of cancer cases
8,475 cases
1.2% of cancer deaths
1,930 deaths
77.3% survive five or more years

Vaginal cancer
0.1% of cancer cases
256 cases
Less than 0.1% of cancer deaths
91 deaths
58% survive five or more years

Vulval cancer
0.4% of cancer cases
1,203 cases
0.3% of cancer deaths
404 deaths
58% survive five or more years

1. http://guidance.nice.org.uk/CG122/Guidance
2. http://www.cancerresearchuk.org/cancer-info/cancerstats/incidence/commoncancers/july2014
3. http://www.cancerresearchuk.org/cancer-info/cancerstats/mortality/cancerdeaths/july2014
4. http://www.cancerresearchuk.org/cancer-info/cancerstats/types/cervix/july2014
5. http://www.cancerresearchuk.org/cancer-info/cancerstats/types/ovary/july2014
6. http://www.cancerresearchuk.org/cancer-info/cancerstats/types/uterus/july2014
7. http://www.cancerresearchuk.org/cancer-info/cancerstats/types/vagina/july2014
8. http://www.cancerresearchuk.org/cancer-info/cancerstats/types/vulva/july2014

CHAPTER 28 Epidemiology of cancer in females in the UK

Suspected gynaecological cancer – NICE recommendations for referral

If symptoms suggest gynaecological cancer, refer to a team specializing in the management of gynaecological cancer.

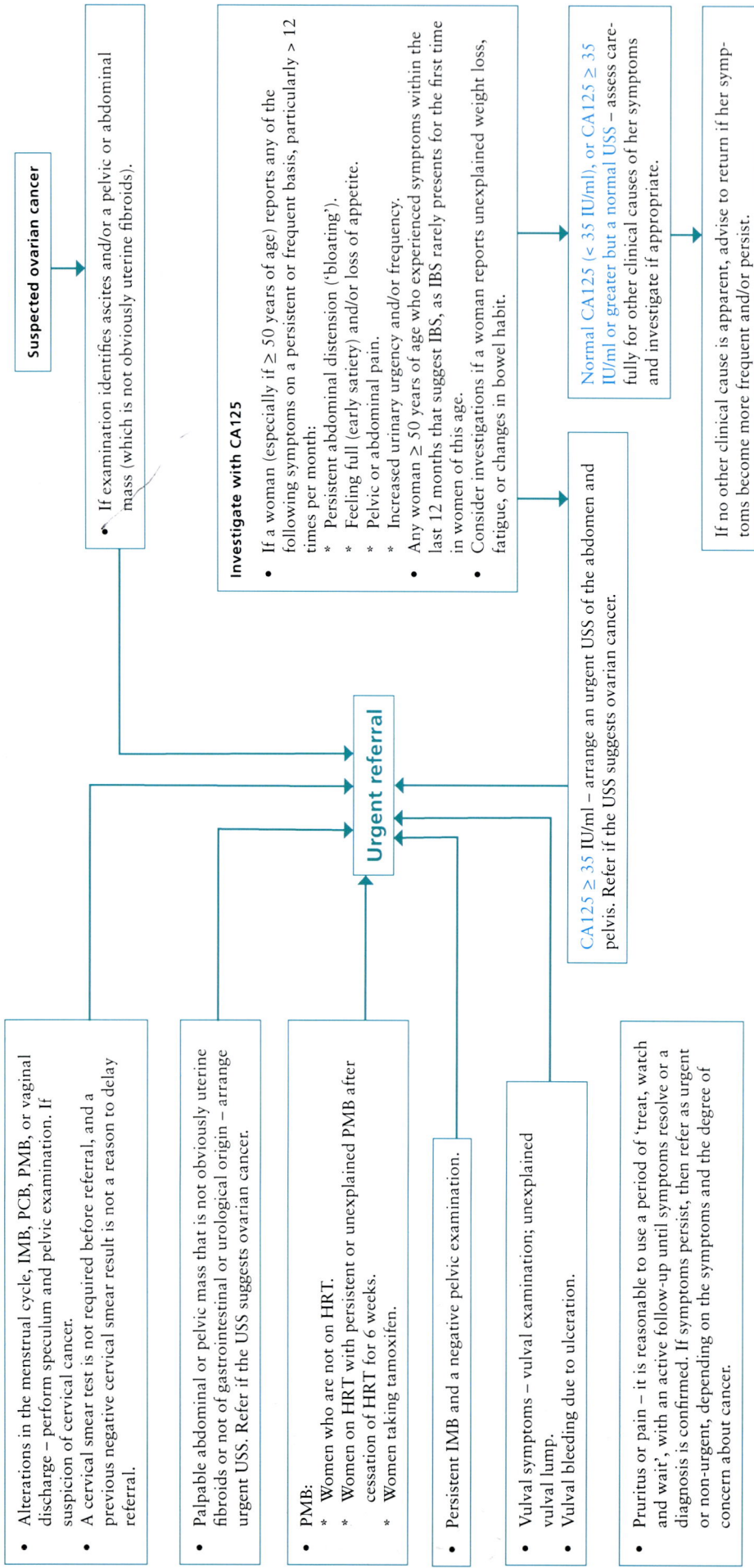

- Alterations in the menstrual cycle, IMB, PCB, PMB, or vaginal discharge – perform speculum and pelvic examination. If suspicion of cervical cancer.
- A cervical smear test is not required before referral, and a previous negative cervical smear result is not a reason to delay referral.

- Palpable abdominal or pelvic mass that is not obviously uterine fibroids or not of gastrointestinal or urological origin – arrange urgent USS. Refer if the USS suggests ovarian cancer.

- PMB:
  * Women who are not on HRT.
  * Women on HRT with persistent or unexplained PMB after cessation of HRT for 6 weeks.
  * Women taking tamoxifen.

- Persistent IMB and a negative pelvic examination.

- Vulval symptoms – vulval examination; unexplained vulval lump.
- Vulval bleeding due to ulceration.

- Pruritus or pain – it is reasonable to use a period of 'treat, watch and wait', with an active follow-up until symptoms resolve or a diagnosis is confirmed. If symptoms persist, then refer as urgent or non-urgent, depending on the symptoms and the degree of concern about cancer.

Urgent referral

Suspected ovarian cancer

- If examination identifies ascites and/or a pelvic or abdominal mass (which is not obviously uterine fibroids).

Investigate with CA125

- If a woman (especially if ≥ 50 years of age) reports any of the following symptoms on a persistent or frequent basis, particularly > 12 times per month:
  * Persistent abdominal distension ('bloating').
  * Feeling full (early satiety) and/or loss of appetite.
  * Pelvic or abdominal pain.
  * Increased urinary urgency and/or frequency.
- Any woman ≥ 50 years of age who experienced symptoms within the last 12 months that suggest IBS, as IBS rarely presents for the first time in women of this age.
- Consider investigations if a woman reports unexplained weight loss, fatigue, or changes in bowel habit.

CA125 ≥ 35 IU/ml – arrange an urgent USS of the abdomen and pelvis. Refer if the USS suggests ovarian cancer.

Normal CA125 (< 35 IU/ml), or CA125 ≥ 35 IU/ml or greater but a normal USS – assess carefully for other clinical causes of her symptoms and investigate if appropriate.

If no other clinical cause is apparent, advise to return if her symptoms become more frequent and/or persist.

ITCHING, PAIN, COLOUR, TEXTURE ~ other sites.
SMEARS, CANCER SPA.
9/0: IMMUNE (THYROID, DM, PERN
SMOKING
ATOPIC
HORMONAL (MEMORY
MEDS, INCONTINENCE

CHAPTER 29 Vulval dystrophy and vulvar intra-epithelial neoplasia

Background and prevalence

- Symptoms and signs of vulval skin disorders are common.
- Community-based surveys indicate that about one fifth of women have significant vulval symptoms.
- Lichen sclerosus accounts for at least 25% of the women seen in vulval clinics. Estimated incidence in patients referred to dermatology clinics is 1/300 to 1/1000.
- Specialist MDT and other services, such as a patch test clinic, psychosexual counsellors, or reconstructive surgeons, may be necessary for appropriate management.

History

- Nonspecific symptoms such as pruritus and pain; change in skin colour and texture.
- Explore symptoms at other skin sites.
- Past history of abnormal cervical cytology, smoking, and immune deficiency in women with suspected VIN.
- Personal or family history of:
  * Autoimmune conditions (thyroid disorders, alopecia areata, pernicious anaemia, type 1 diabetes) associated with lichen sclerosus and erosive lichen planus.
  * Atopic conditions (hay fever, asthma, eczema) associated with vulval dermatitis.
- Symptoms of urinary or faecal incontinence as dermatitis may be exacerbated by moisture, temperature, and friction.
- Medical and drug history – self-medication or previous inadequate or inappropriate treatments.
- Enquire about over-the-counter preparations that may aggravate skin conditions.
- Any potential allergens and irritants.

Examination

Systematic examination of the anogenital region and other skin and mucosal sites

- Systematically examine the vulva.
- Examine other lower genital tract sites including the vagina, cervix, and perianal skin.
- Examine the rest of the body including the mouth for signs of lichen planus, and the scalp, elbows, knees, and nails for psoriasis.
- Eczema may be seen at any site.

Differential diagnosis

DDx

- Dermatitis.
- Vulval candidiasis.
- Lichen simplex.
- Lichen sclerosus and lichen planus.
- Dermatoses.
- Infection.
- Contact dermatitis.
- Hormone deficiency.
- Systemic skin disorders.

Investigations

- Test for thyroid disease, diabetes, and STIs, if clinically indicated.
- Biopsy – not necessary when a clear diagnosis can be made on history and clinical examination.
  * Needed if the woman fails to respond to treatment or there is clinical suspicion of VIN or cancer.
  * Biopsy all atypical or suspicious areas to exclude invasive disease.
- Circulating autoantibodies – for other autoimmune conditions in women suspected of lichen sclerosus or lichen planus.
- Serum ferritin – in women with vulval dermatitis.
- Skin patch testing – for women with vulval dermatitis; 26–80% may have at least one positive result on patch testing.

Management

Rx

General advice

- Avoid any potential irritants.
- Emollients – protect the skin and restore skin barrier function.
- Avoid contact with soap, shampoo, and bubble bath. Use simple emollients as a soap substitute and general moisturizer.
- Avoid tight fitting garments that may irritate the area.
- Avoid use of spermicidally lubricated condoms.
- Provide a detailed explanation of the condition with an emphasis on the long-term implications.

VIN

Two types depending on its histopathological characteristics.

Differentiated type   *old ♀ ↑ to cancer*

- Rarer.
- Seen in older women, aged 55–85 years.
- Some cases are associated with lichen sclerosus.
- Linked to keratinizing squamous cell carcinomas of the vulva.
- Clinically (unifocal) in the form of an ulcer or plaque.
- Risk of progression appears to be higher than in usual type VIN.

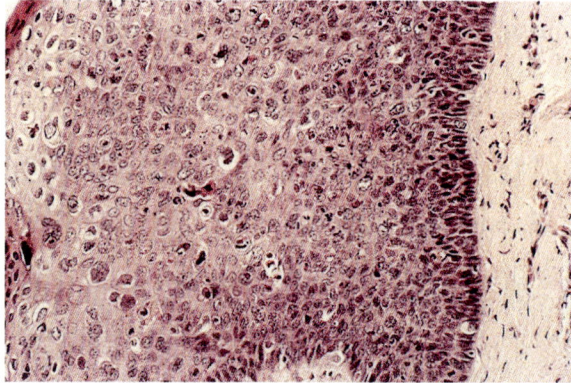

Usual type   *young ♀ → HPV - basaloid carcinoma*

- Warty, basaloid, and mixed.
- More common in women aged 35–55 years.
- Associated with HPV-16, CIN, VaIN, smoking, and chronic immunosuppression.
- May be multifocal and multicentric.
- Appearance varies widely: red, white, or pigmented; plaques, papules, or patches; erosions, nodules, warty or hyperkeratosis.
- Associated with warty or basaloid squamous cell carcinoma.

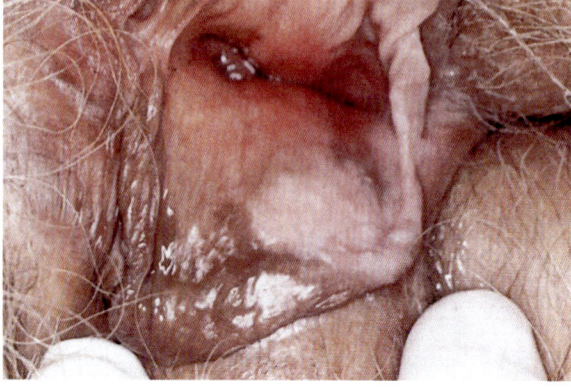

Management

(Rx symbol)

To relieve symptoms of severe pruritus, exclude invasive disease and reduce the risk of developing invasive cancer.

• Surgical management

- **Local excision** provides a specimen for histological diagnosis and is adequate, with the same recurrence rates as vulvectomy.
- **Simple vulvectomy and radical vulvectomy** are inappropriate owing to their adverse effects on sexual function and body image.
- 12–17% of women undergoing excision of VIN have clinically unrecognized invasion diagnosed on histology.
- Complete response rates are higher with excision than with ablative or medical treatment. Risk of recurrence is lower if surgical margins are free from disease. Even with clear surgical margins, there is still a residual risk of recurrence.
- Women undergoing surgical excision should have access to reconstructive surgery. With larger lesions, multifocal lesions, or certain anatomical sites, scarring and tension can result in pain and psychosexual morbidity.

Non-surgical management

- Women require regular, long-term follow-up.
- It avoids the complications of surgery and spares vulval anatomy.
- **Topical imiquimod cream** – 15–81% clinical and histological response rate; regimen used 2–3 times per week. Adverse effects include pain, erythema, and swelling, and can result in non-compliance.
- **Cidofovir** – has shown a clinical and histological response.
- **Laser ablation** – effective. Treatment failure rates are about 40%, but laser ablation is not suitable for hair-bearing skin owing to the involvement of skin appendages. Laser therapy is most useful where tissue conservation is important, such as in the glans and hood of the clitoris or when surgery is contraindicated.
- Small case series have evaluated the use of cavitron, ultrasonic surgical aspiration, photodynamic therapy, interferon, and therapeutic HPV vaccine, but there is insufficient evidence to recommend any of these for treatment in routine clinical care.

Surveillance

(grid illustration)

- Follow-up annually for vulvoscopy, or careful clinical assessment and biopsy of any suspicious areas.
- Risk of cancer developing within 8 years of diagnosis is 10–60%.
- Women treated surgically for VIN still have a residual risk of developing invasive cancer (4%)
- 4% of women diagnosed with VIN will have intra-epithelial neoplasia at other lower genital tract sites. Perform colposcopy at other lower genital tract sites. Women with usual type VIN with multifocal/multicentric disease are at higher risk of recurrence. Follow-up with specialist colposcopy service to ensure inspection of other lower genital tract sites, including the cervix, vagina, and vulval and perianal skin.

Lichen sclerosus

- Accounts for at least 25% of the women seen in vulval clinics, and one in 300–1000 of all patients referred to dermatology clinics.
- Can present at any age, but is more commonly seen in post-menopausal women.
- It is an autoimmune condition, with around 40% having another autoimmune condition.

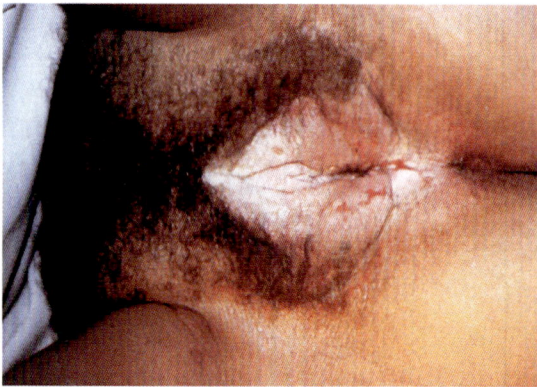

Symptoms

- Severe pruritus, which may be worse at night.
- Uncontrollable scratching may cause trauma with bleeding and skin splitting, and symptoms of discomfort, pain, and dyspareunia.
- Occasionally, the labia minora fuse together medially, which also restricts the vaginal opening and can cause difficulty with micturition, and even urinary retention.

Examination

- Whole vulval perianal area may be affected in a figure-of-eight distribution.
- Active inflammation with erythema and keratinization of the vulval skin.
- Hyperkeratosis can be marked with thickened white skin.
- Skin is often atrophic, with subepithelial haemorrhages, and it may split easily.
- Continuing inflammation results in inflammatory adhesions. Lateral fusion of the labia minora, which become adherent and eventually are completely reabsorbed. The hood of the clitoris and its lateral margins may fuse, burying the clitoris. Midline fusion can produce skin bridges at the fourchette and narrowing of the introitus.

Medical management – ultra-potent steroids

- Anti-inflammatory and immunosuppressive properties by altering lymphocyte differentiation and function.
- Clobetasol propionate is the most potent topical corticosteroid.
- Complete or partial resolution of symptoms in 54–96% of women.
- Probability of remission is significantly associated with age. Women under the age of 50 years have the highest response rates.
- Relapse 84% of women experience a relapse within 4 years.

- Various regimens are used; one of the most common is daily use for 1 month, alternate days for 1 month, twice weekly for 1 month, with review at 2–3 months. There is no evidence on the optimal regimen. Maintenance treatment may be required and can be either with weaker steroid preparations or less frequent use of very potent steroids.
- 30 g of very potent steroid lasts at least 3 months.
- Ointment bases are less allergenic but the choice of base will depend on patient tolerability.

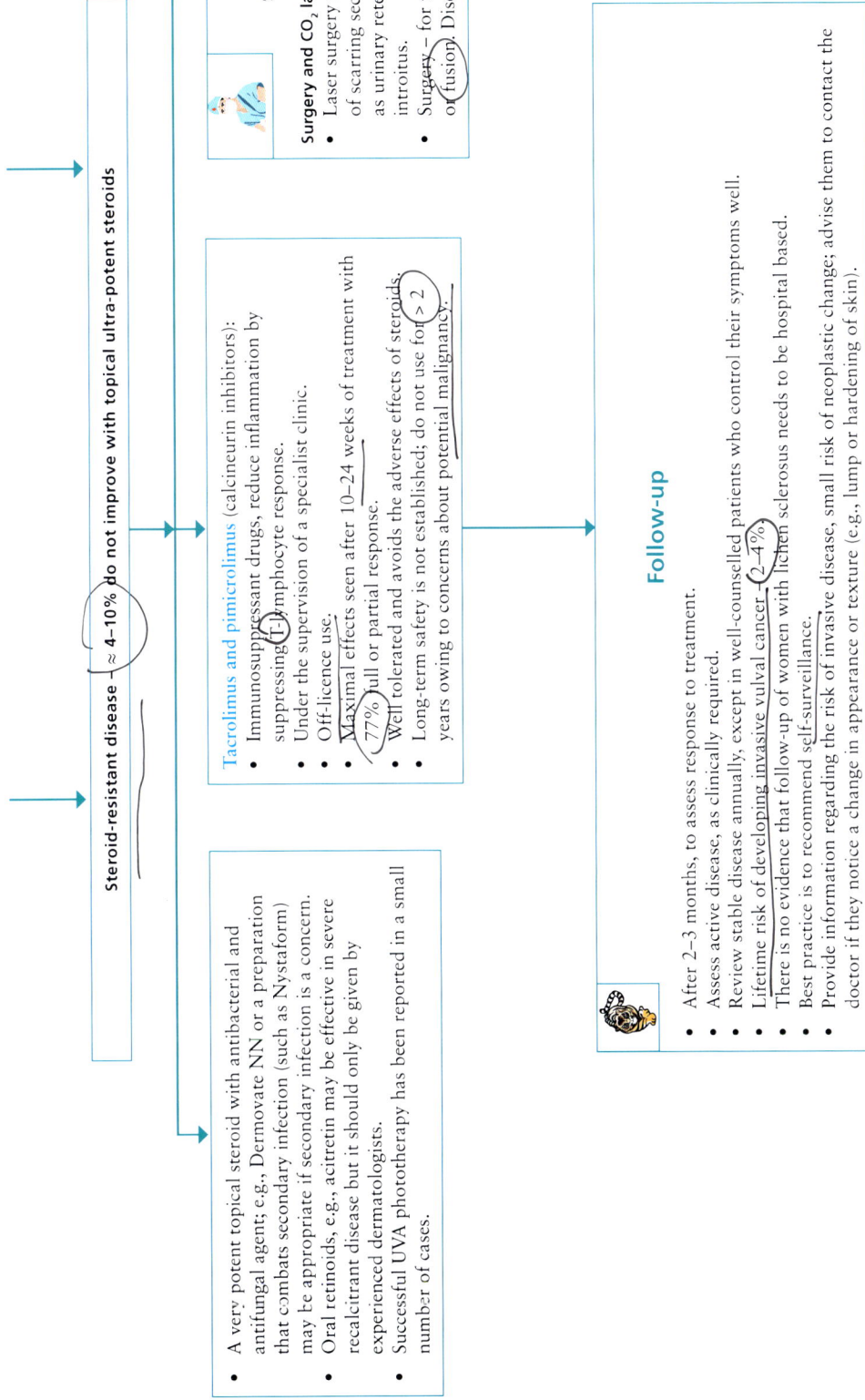

Steroid-resistant disease – ≈ 4–10% do not improve with topical ultra-potent steroids

- A very potent topical steroid with antibacterial and antifungal agent; e.g., Dermovate NN or a preparation that combats secondary infection (such as Nystaform) may be appropriate if secondary infection is a concern.
- Oral retinoids, e.g., acitretin may be effective in severe recalcitrant disease but it should only be given by experienced dermatologists.
- Successful UVA phototherapy has been reported in a small number of cases.

Tacrolimus and pimicrolimus (calcineurin inhibitors):
- Immunosuppressant drugs, reduce inflammation by suppressing T lymphocyte response.
- Under the supervision of a specialist clinic.
- Off-licence use.
- Maximal effects seen after 10–24 weeks of treatment with 77% full or partial response.
- Well tolerated and avoids the adverse effects of steroids.
- Long-term safety is not established; do not use for > 2 years owing to concerns about potential malignancy.

Surgical management

Surgery and CO$_2$ laser vaporization – not recommended.
- Laser surgery may be useful in treating the sequelae of scarring secondary to lichen sclerosus, such as urinary retention or narrowing of the vaginal introitus.
- Surgery – for the treatment of coexistent VIN/SCC or fusion. Disease tends to recur around the scar.

Follow-up

- After 2–3 months, to assess response to treatment.
- Assess active disease, as clinically required.
- Review stable disease annually, except in well-counselled patients who control their symptoms well.
- Lifetime risk of developing invasive vulval cancer – 2–4%.
- There is no evidence that follow-up of women with lichen sclerosus needs to be hospital based.
- Best practice is to recommend self-surveillance.
- Provide information regarding the risk of invasive disease, small risk of neoplastic change; advise them to contact the doctor if they notice a change in appearance or texture (e.g., lump or hardening of skin).

Other vulval skin conditions

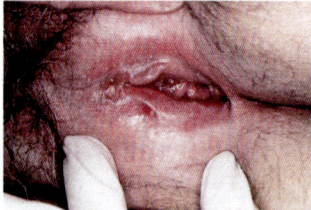

Lichen planus

- May affect skin anywhere on the body.
- Usually affects mucosal surfaces and is more commonly seen in oral mucosa.
- Polygonal flat-topped violaceous purpuric plaques and papules with a fine white reticular pattern (Wickham striae).
- In the mouth and genital region, it can be erosive and is more commonly associated with pain than with pruritus.
- Erosive lichen planus appears as a well-demarcated glazed erythema around the introitus.
- Aetiology is unknown; may be an autoimmune condition.

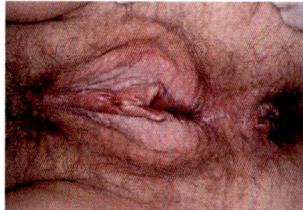

Lichen simplex chronic or chronicus vulval dermatitis

- Severe intractable pruritus, especially at night.
- Nonspecific inflammation often involves the labia majora but can extend to the mons pubis and inner thighs.
- There may be erythema and swelling with discrete areas of thickening and lichenification.
- Symptoms can be exacerbated by chemical or contact dermatitis, and are sometimes linked to stress or low body iron stores.
- Treatment – general care of the vulva; avoid potential irritants and use emollients and soap substitutes.
  * Antihistamines or anti-pruritics, especially if sleep is disturbed.
  * Moderate or ultra-potent topical steroids may be necessary to break the itch–scratch cycle.

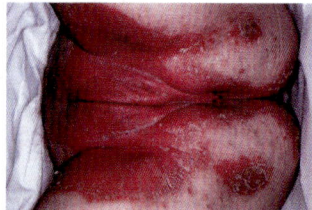

Vulval psoriasis

- Can involve the skin of the vulva but not vaginal mucosa.
- Appearance of vulval psoriasis differs from the typical scale of non-genital sites; it often appears as smooth, non-scaly red or pink discrete lesions.
- Examine other sites including nails and scalp.
- Emollients, soap substitutes, topical steroids, and calcipotriene.
- Do not use cold tar preparations in genital sites.

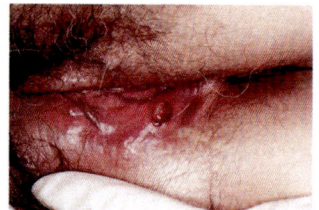

Behçet's disease

- A chronic multisystem disease characterized by recurrent oral and genital ulcers.
- Ulcers can involve cervix, vulva, or vagina.
- Ulcers are usually recurrent and painful and can leave scarring.
- Topical or systemic immunosuppressants.

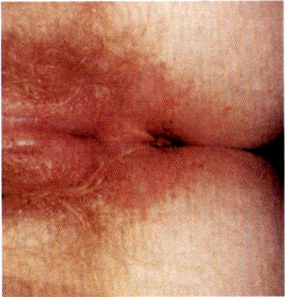

Vulval candidiasis

- Irritation and soreness of the vulva and anus rather than discharge.
- Diabetes, obesity, and antibiotic use may be contributory.
- May become chronic, with a leading edge of inflammation with satellite lesions extending out from the labia majora to the inner thighs or mons pubis.
- Prolonged topical antifungal therapy with oral or topical preparations.

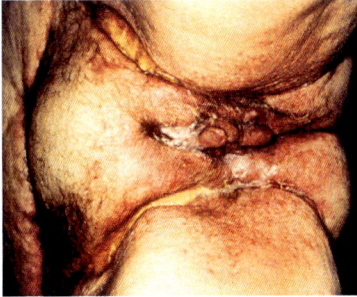

Vulval Crohn's disease

- Can involve the vulva by direct extension from involved bowel or 'metastatic' granulomas.
- Rarely, seen without known bowel disease or preceding the presentation of bowel disease.
- Vulva is often swollen and oedematous with granulomas, abscesses, draining sinuses, and ulceration.
- Avoid surgery as it can result in sinus and fistula formation and tissue breakdown.
- Treatments include metronidazole and oral immunomodulators.

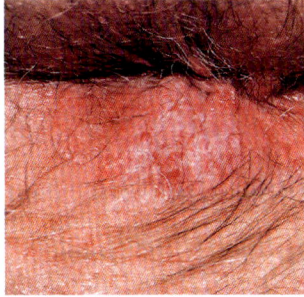

Paget's disease

- Rare vulval condition seen in post-menopausal women.
- Main symptom is pruritus.
- Lesions have a florid eczematous appearance with lichenification, erythema, and excoriation.
- Can be associated with an underlying adenocarcinoma.
- Check the gastrointestinal tract, urinary tract, and breasts.
- Surgical excision to exclude adenocarcinoma of a skin appendage. Surgical margins are difficult to achieve owing to subclinical disease, and recurrence is common.

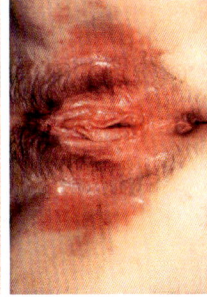

Seborrhoeic dermatitis

- Most common signs are scaling and erythema.
- Extra-genital areas are usually involved – eyebrows, nasolabial folds, peri-auricular, posterior hairline, and axilla.
- Short hyphae and spores of Tinea versicolor may be seen on the potassium hydroxide preparation of the lesional scales.
- Treatment is with topical keratolytic agents and/or 1% hydrocortisone preparation.

1. *The Management of Vulval Skin Disorders*. RCOG Green-top Guideline No. 58, February 2011.
2. British Association for Sexual Health and HIV, UK National Guideline on the Management of Vulval Conditions Clinical Effectiveness Group, 2007.
3. Black M, McKay M, Braude P, Vaughan-Jones S, Margesson L. *Obstetric and Gynecologic Dermatology, Second edition*. Saunders, 2008.

CHAPTER 30 Vulval cancer

Prevalence and incidence

- Cancer of the vulva and vagina accounts for < 1% of all cancer cases and 8% of gynaecological cancers diagnosed in women in the UK.
- The 20th most common cancer among women.
- UK (2010) – 1172 women diagnosed and 410 died from vulval cancer. Crude incidence rate is 1.7/100,000 women and a death rate is 1.2/100,000 women.
- Vulval cancer is a disease of elderly women in their 70s and 80s; incidence increases with age peaking in women aged 85 years or more; 80% occur among women > 60 years of age.
- Lifetime risk of developing vulval cancer is around 1/293 for women in the UK.

Risk factors

- Lichen sclerosus (4–7%), vulval intra-epithelial neoplasia (VIN) and multifocal disease (5–90%), Paget's disease, and melanoma *in situ*.
- Lichen sclerosus is relatively common and it is not practical to follow-up all women once their symptoms are controlled. Review urgently if persistent ulceration or new growth.
- High-grade VIN, VIN with high-grade multicentric disease, VIN in the immunosuppressed and those with Paget's disease or melanoma *in situ* probably pose higher risks for progression, therefore follow them up at least annually.
- HPV (types 16, 18, and 31) is associated with approximately 30–40% of cases and 80% of VIN.
- Previous cervical cancer or CIN increases risk of vulval cancer.
- Infection with HSV type 2 may increase the risk of vulval cancer. This virus may interact with HPV to cause vulval and other cancers in the genital and anal area.
- Women who have had radiotherapy treatment for uterine cancer have an increased risk of vulval cancer some years later.

History

- History – pruritus, discomfort, pain, visible or palpable lesion, ulceration, bleeding, dysuria or vaginal discharge. Skin showing colour changes, elevation or irregularity of surface.
- Post-menopausal woman presenting for the first time with lesions assumed to be vulval condyloma – get a biopsy for histological confirmation as newly acquired condylomas are unusual in this age group.
- Unexplained vulval lump/mass – refer urgently.
- Vulval bleeding, pruritus, pain, and ulceration – it is reasonable to use a period of 'treat, watch, and wait' with active follow-up until these symptoms resolve or a diagnosis is confirmed. If symptoms persist refer to secondary care.

Examination

- Inspection – 90% of women have a visible tumour. Assess the size and location. Assess involvement of the vagina, urethra, base of bladder, and anus.
- Palpate to assess whether the tumour is infiltrating deep to the pubic and ischial bones.
- EUA may be necessary because of the pain often associated with large tumours.
- Assess groin lymphadenopathy.

Screening

There is no screening procedure for vulval cancer.

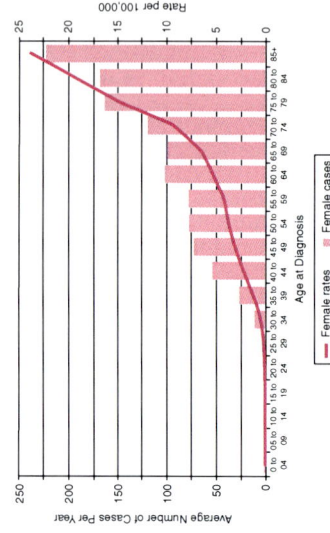

New cases per year and age-specific incidence rates, females, UK, 2009–2011

- For small suspicious lesions, refer women to a gynaecological cancer centre, to be seen within 2 weeks.
- Manage vulval cancer in gynaecological cancer centre by MDT (including gynaecological oncologist and clinical oncologist).
- If a surgical approach is not an option, manage by a clinical oncologist with an appointment within 2 weeks.
- Commence surgical treatment within 4 weeks of diagnosis.
- Commence radiotherapy within 4 weeks of the decision to treat.

- Histology:
  * Squamous cell carcinomas – 90%.
  * Melanoma, Paget's disease, Bartholin's gland tumours, adenocarcinoma, and basal cell carcinoma – 10%.
- Tumours most commonly occur on the labia majora, but are also found on the labia minora, clitoris, and perineum; melanomas are more likely to affect the clitoris or labia minora.

Representative biopsy

- Include the area of epithelium where there is a transition of normal to malignant tissue; of sufficient size (> 1 mm depth to allow differentiation between superficially invasive and frankly invasive tumours) and orientated to allow pathological interpretation.
- In cases of elderly woman with major medical problems and a severely symptomatic lesion, a small punch biopsy under LA may be adequate.
- In cases where the clinical diagnosis is apparent and the patient is very symptomatic, i.e., heavy bleeding or pain, definitive surgery to the vulval lesion may be performed but take biopsy (with frozen section) prior to any radical procedure.
- Consider excisional biopsy only in small lesions where a wide margin of normal tissue can also be excised.
- Do not undertake radical treatment without prior biopsy confirmation of malignancy.

Investigations

Once the diagnosis is confirmed, to determine the extent of the disease and suitability for treatment:

- Full blood count. • Biochemical profile. • Chest X-ray. • Electrocardiogram.
- Cervical smear if normal cervical smear is overdue.
- For tumour > 2 cm in diameter, perform CT of the chest, abdomen, and pelvis to detect disease above the inguinal ligament.
- Take a fine-needle aspirate of any clinically suspicious nodes or other metastases where the result will alter management.
- A preoperative vulvoscopy may help in the planning of surgery.

FIGO Staging, 2009

Stage I – tumour confined to vulva or vulva and perineum, greatest dimension ≤ 2 cm.

Stage II – tumour of any size with extension to adjacent per-ineal structures (lower third of urethra, lower third of vagina, anus), with negative LNs.

Stage III – tumour of any size with or without extension into adjacent perineal structures, with positive inguinofemoral LNs.

Stage IV

- IA – tumour confined to vulva or vulva and perineum, greatest dimension ≤ 2 cm, stromal invasion of ≤ 1.0 mm.
- IB – tumour confined to vulva or vulva and perineum, greatest dimension < 2 cm, stromal invasion > 1.0 mm with negative LNs.
- 5-year survival – 79%.

- 5-year survival – 59%.

- IIIA – with 1 LN metastasis, any size, or 2 LN metastases < 5 mm.
- IIIB – with ≥ 2 LN metastases > 5 mm or ≥ 3 LN metastases < 5 mm.
- IIIC – positive LNs with extracapsular spread.
- 5-year survival – 43%.

- IVA – tumour invades any of the following: * Bladder mucosa. * Rectal mucosa. * Upper urethral mucosa or is fixed to bone and/or bilateral regional LN metastases.
- IVB – any distant metastasis including pelvic LNs.
- 5-year survival – 13%.

Prognostic factors

- Histology represents a variable in determining the likelihood of LN involvement.
- Presence of infiltrative growth patterns, compared with a pushing pattern and LVSI, is associated with a higher local recurrence rate. Both are markers of poor prognosis but they do not indicate the need for adjuvant treatment.
- LVSI has not been associated with an increased risk of groin node metastasis.
- About 30% of women with operable disease have nodal spread.
- Nodal status, site, and size of the primary lesion are the main variables associated with prognosis.
- The 5-year survival in cases with no LN involvement is 80%. This falls to < 50% if the inguinal nodes are involved and 10–15% if the iliac or other pelvic nodes are involved.

FIGO Classification - carcinoma of the vulva

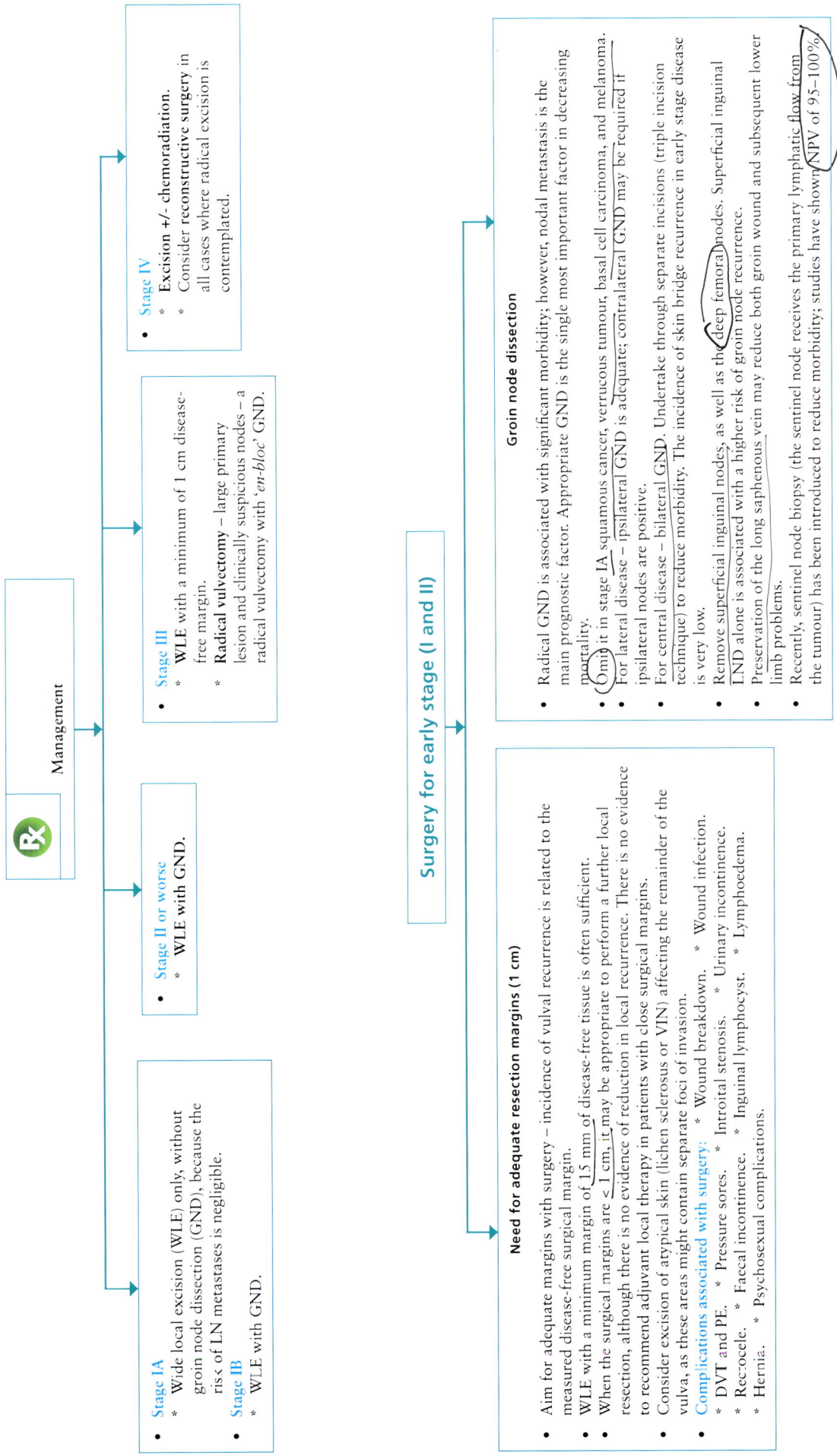

Management

- **Stage IA**
  * Wide local excision (WLE) only, without groin node dissection (GND), because the risk of LN metastases is negligible.
- **Stage IB**
  * WLE with GND.

- **Stage II or worse**
  * WLE with GND.

- **Stage III**
  * WLE with a minimum of 1 cm disease-free margin.
  * **Radical vulvectomy** – large primary lesion and clinically suspicious nodes – a radical vulvectomy with 'en-bloc' GND.

- **Stage IV**
  * Excision +/- chemoradiation.
  * Consider reconstructive surgery in all cases where radical excision is contemplated.

Surgery for early stage (I and II)

Need for adequate resection margins (1 cm)

- Aim for adequate margins with surgery – incidence of vulval recurrence is related to the measured disease-free surgical margin.
- WLE with a minimum margin of 15 mm of disease-free tissue is often sufficient.
- When the surgical margins are ≤ 1 cm, it may be appropriate to perform a further local resection, although there is no evidence of reduction in local recurrence. There is no evidence to recommend adjuvant local therapy in patients with close surgical margins.
- Consider excision of atypical skin (lichen sclerosus or VIN) affecting the remainder of the vulva, as these areas might contain separate foci of invasion.
- Complications associated with surgery: * Wound breakdown. * Wound infection. * DVT and PE. * Pressure sores. * Introital stenosis. * Urinary incontinence. * Rectocele. * Faecal incontinence. * Inguinal lymphocyst. * Lymphoedema. * Hernia. * Psychosexual complications.

Groin node dissection

- Radical GND is associated with significant morbidity; however, nodal metastasis is the main prognostic factor. Appropriate GND is the single most important factor in decreasing mortality.
- Omit it in stage IA squamous cancer, verrucous tumour, basal cell carcinoma, and melanoma.
- For lateral disease – ipsilateral GND is adequate; contralateral GND may be required if ipsilateral nodes are positive.
- For central disease – bilateral GND. Undertake through separate incisions (triple incision technique) to reduce morbidity. The incidence of skin bridge recurrence in early stage disease is very low.
- Remove superficial inguinal nodes, as well as the deep femoral nodes. Superficial inguinal LND alone is associated with a higher risk of groin node recurrence.
- Preservation of the long saphenous vein may reduce both groin wound and subsequent lower limb problems.
- Recently, sentinel node biopsy (the sentinel node receives the primary lymphatic flow from the tumour) has been introduced to reduce morbidity; studies have shown NPV of 95–100%.

Advanced vulval cancer (Stage III and IV) Multimodality treatment

Surgery – vulvectomy, GND

- Radical vulvectomy, anovulvectomy might be an option in selected cases.
- Skin-bridge recurrence is more likely to occur in patients with positive lymph nodes. An *en-bloc* dissection is advised if the nodes are known or suspected to be positive, to remove the tissue between the vulva and involved nodes.
- Reconstructive surgical techniques to enable primary surgical closure and to reduce morbidity due to scarring.
- GND – when there are clinically suspicious groin nodes.
- In cases with fixed or ulcerated groin nodes, consider surgery and/or RT. There are no data suggesting the superiority of one treatment over the other.

Radiotherapy

- RT allows for sphincter preserving surgery and as an alternative to surgery for GND.
- In the post-radiation setting, surgery can be more complicated and there is increased morbidity.

Primary radiotherapy

- Preoperative RT may allow for sphincter-preserving surgery.
- RT may also be used for histologically proven involved GLNs. It is unknown whether post-radiation GLN removal is advantageous in terms of outcome.
- Individual women who are not fit enough to withstand surgery can be treated with primary RT.

Adjuvant radiotherapy

- Factors influencing the need for RT are surgical margins and GLN positivity.
- Not enough evidence to recommend adjuvant local therapy in patients with close surgical margins.
- Adjuvant treatment for positive margins has an improved survival compared with observation.
- Consider adjuvant RT when:
  * Either groin has ≥ 2 LN involved with microscopic metastatic disease.
  * Or there is complete replacement.
  * And/or extra-capsular spread in any node.
- No evidence on whether adjuvant RT should be given to both sides or to the involved side only.
- Treat both groin and the pelvic nodes.

Chemotherapy

- Can be used:
  * As an adjuvant postoperatively, concomitant with RT for node-positive disease.
  * Concomitantly with pelvic RT for management of inoperable/unresectable disease.
  * Neoadjuvantly to 'downstage' tumours and to render them more suitable for either delayed primary surgery or RT.
  * Either alone or concomitant with RT for the management of relapsed disease.

Follow-up

- Long-term review is recommended, as these patients remain at an increased risk of developing carcinomas elsewhere in the genital tract and pelvis, even though routine follow-up does not offer early detection or survival advantage.
- Follow-up intervals are arbitrary and the following schedule is suggested:
  * 3-monthly in first year.
  * 6-monthly in second and third years.
  * Annual review thereafter.
- Women with carcinoma of the vulva are at an increased risk of developing other genital cancers, particularly cervical cancer.

Vulval cancer – 5 year survival rate %

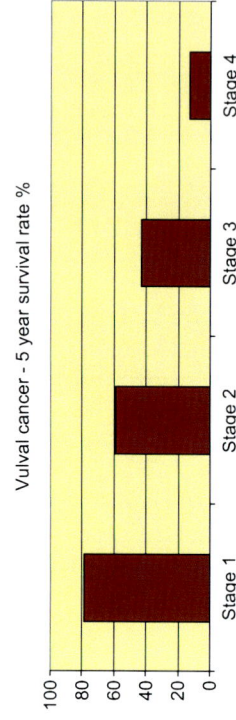

Recurrent disease

- Recurrence rate 15–33%. The most common site of recurrence is the vulva in 70%, the groin nodes in 24%, the pelvis in 16%, and distant metastases in 19% of cases.
- Treatment and outcome depend on the site and extent of the recurrence.
- Local recurrence – WLE can result in a 5-year survival rate of 56% when the inguinal nodes are negative.
- If excision would impair sphincter function, consider RT as the first choice. If RT has already been given to maximum dose, then consider excision.
- Groin recurrence has a much poorer prognosis and is difficult to manage. In women who have not been treated previously with groin RT, RT (with or without additional surgery) would be the preferred option. The options are much more limited in those who have already been irradiated; consider palliation, which may include surgery.
- Chemotherapy for relapsed disease may be determined by what previous treatments have been offered and also by the age, performance status, and renal function of the patient.

1. *Management of Vulval Cancer.* RCOG, 2006.
2. http://www.cancerresearchuk.org/cancer-info/cancerstats/types/vulva/incidence/july2014.
3. Edey K, Murdoch J. FIGO staging in vulval and endometrial cancer. *The Obstetrician and Gynaecologist* 2010;12:245–249.
4. http://www.imaios.com/e-Cases/Channels/Radiology/Radiological-classifications-commonly-used-on-medical-imaging/Carcinoma-of-the-vulva.

CHAPTER 31 Cervical intra-epithelial neoplasia and colposcopy

Background and pathogenesis

- CIN is the pre-invasive stage of cervical cancer. It denotes atypical changes in the transformation zone of the cervix. Time taken from development of cytological abnormality to invasive cancer could be up to 15–20 years. Most cases of CIN remain stable, or are eliminated by the host's immune system without intervention. However, a small percentage of cases progress to cervical cancer if left untreated. Roughly one third of early CIN lesions disappear spontaneously, one third persist, and one third progress to CIN 3 or invasive cancer.

- Regression rate depends mainly on the grade of CIN and the age of the woman. Regression is more common in women younger than 30 years. High-grade lesions of CIN 2 and CIN 3 have higher risk of progression to invasive cancer. Women who are immunocompromised are also at higher risk of progression.

- Cervical screening is a method of preventing cancer by detecting and treating early abnormalities which, if left untreated, could lead to cervical cancer.

- Since the start of NHS Cervical Screening Programme (NHSCSP), cervical cancer incidence rates have almost halved (16/100,000 women in 1986–1988 to 8.5/100,000 women in 2006–2008).

- Cervical screening saves approximately 4500 lives per year in England and prevents up to 3900 cases of cervical cancer per year in the UK. It can prevent around 75% of cancer cases in women who attend regularly.

HPV – HPV testing as a form of risk assessment

HPV – triage of low-grade abnormalities and test of cure – advantage is rapid diagnosis and, providing there is no abnormality, a rapid return to normal recall.

HPV testing for follow-up of treated CIN – there is some evidence to suggest that all women who have had treatment for CIN should have an HPV (Hybrid Capture or HC2) test and a cervical cytology after 6 months and HPV test after 12–18 months. If all three of these tests are negative, the patient can be returned to routine screening at 3- (for those < 49 years of age) or 5-yearly intervals (for those aged 50–64 years). If both cytology and HPV testing are negative at six months, then the risk of CIN 2+ over the next two years is less than 0.5%. Returning these women to normal recall after six months would prevent the need for 10 annual cytology tests as currently recommended.

Population screening with HPV testing – primary screening with high-risk HPV DNA testing generally detects more than 90% of all CIN 2/3 or cancer cases, and is ≈ 25% more sensitive than cytology at a cut-off of borderline dyskaryosis or worse. However, it is about 6% less specific. HPV testing is not currently recommended for routine use.

Offer routine screening for women – The NHS Cervical Screening Programme

- The first stage in cervical screening is taking a sample using liquid-based cytology (LBC).

Age of referral and smear intervals

- 3-year interval for women aged 25–49 years and 5 years for women 50–64 years of age. 3-yearly screening offers protection of 84% compared to 5-yearly screening (73%) for cervical cancer at ages 40–54 years, but is almost as good as annual screening (88%).

- Starting age of screening is 25 years old. Screening women under the age of 25 years may do more harm than good. In 2007, 56 cases of cervical cancer were registered among women aged 15–24 years in England and Wales and a total of 3 deaths were reported. The incidence of cervical cancer in the < 25-year age group is low and the prevalence of transient HPV infection is high. Much of the low-grade disease would resolve spontaneously. Screening may thus lead to unnecessary attendances at colposcopy, with the possibility of increased anxiety, overtreatment, and potentially negative consequences. Screening has not been shown to be effective at reducing the incidence of invasive cancer in women under the age of 25 years.

- Routine screening ends at the age of 65 years. Although it may possibly be safe to withdraw well-screened women with 3 consecutive negative cervical samples from the screening programme at age 50 years, at present there is insufficient evidence to warrant this.

- Additional cervical screening is not justified in any of the following situations, providing the woman is in the age group to be screened and has undergone screening within the previous 3–5 years:
  * On taking or starting to take an oral contraceptive.
  * On insertion of an IUCD.
  * On taking or starting to take HRT.
  * In association with pregnancy – either antenatally or postnatally, or after termination, unless a previous screening test was abnormal.
  * In women with genital warts.
  * In women with vaginal discharge.
  * In women with pelvic infection.
  * In women who have had multiple sexual partners.
  * In women who are heavy cigarette smokers.

Dyskaryosis – cytology findings

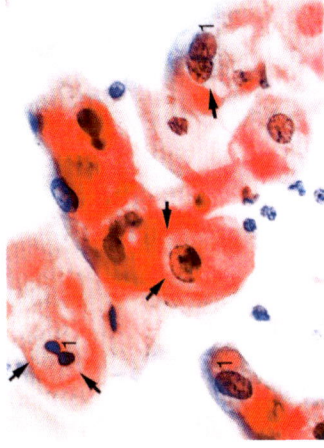

Severe dyskaryosis

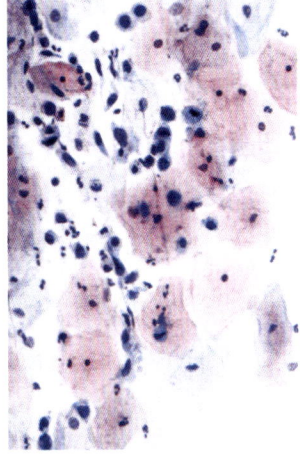

Mild dyskaryosis

- **Dyskaryosis** – a disproportionate nuclear enlargement in comparison to the amount of cytoplasm present in the cell. These cells have abnormal chromatin content and distribution and abnormal nuclear shape. These are precursors to cancer.
- **Mild dyskaryosis** – typical koilocytes – cells showing perinuclear clearing of the cytoplasm with a hard margin to the vacuole (arrowed) with features of mild dyskaryosis.
- **Moderate dyskaryosis** – intermediate squamous cells with dyskaryotic nuclei, with some binucleation and koilocytosis.
- **Severe dyskaryosis** – nuclei enlarged, with variation in shape and size, and hyperchromasia and irregular nuclear outline.

Refer to colposcopy – cervical screening showing:

- 3 consecutive inadequate samples (within 8 weeks).
- 3 borderline nuclear change in squamous cells in a series (within 8 weeks).
- 1 borderline nuclear change in endocervical cells (within 8 weeks).
- 3 abnormal tests at any grade in a 10-year period (within 8 weeks).
- Ideally, 1 mild dyskaryosis, but it remains acceptable to repeat the test. Women must be referred after 2 mild dyskaryosis results (within 8 weeks).
- 1 mocerate dyskaryosis (within 4 weeks).
- 1 severe dyskaryosis (within 4 weeks).
- 1 possible invasion (within 2 weeks).
- 1 possible glandular neoplasia (within 2 weeks).
- Women who have been treated for CIN and have not been returned to routine recall, and a subsequent test is reported as mild dyskaryosis or worse.

Gynaecological examination and onward referral for colposcopy if cancer is suspected for:

- Women with an abnormal cervix (within 2 weeks).
- Women presenting with symptoms of cervical cancer – such as PCB (particularly in women > 40 years of age), IMB, and persistent vaginal discharge.
- Contact bleeding at the time of cervical sampling may often occur and is not an indication for referral for colposcopy in the absence of other symptoms or an abnormal result.

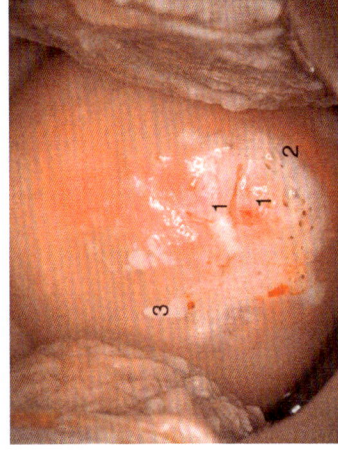

High-grade lesion

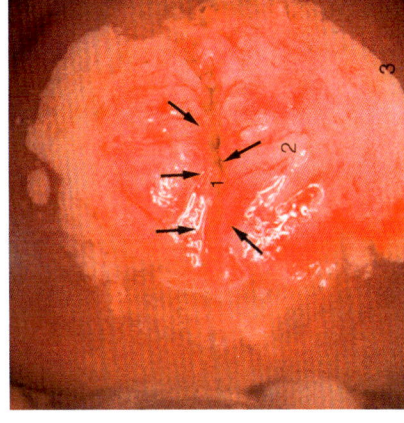

Low-grade lesion

Colposcopy

- Naked eye visualization of the cervix can only detect invasive disease but cannot differentiate pre-invasive disease from normal cervix. Colposcopic examination helps to identify these lesions. This allows clinical verification of cytology report.
- Colposcope provides illumination and magnification (6–40 fold) of the cervix.
- It is not diagnostic in itself, it helps to evaluate the abnormal cytology as an aid to diagnosis to guide further management.
- Consider colposcopic screening in addition to cytology for routine cervical screening in very high-risk groups of women who are at increased risk of CIN; they include immunosuppressed women, such as transplant recipients or patients with renal failure requiring dialysis.
- Take a history prior to examination – menstrual cycles/LMP, contraception, pregnancy, smoking, previous cytology/previous treatment if any.
- Saline, acetic acid and Lugol's iodine are used sequentially and changes on the cervix are noted as benign, low-grade CIN, high-risk CIN, or invasive changes.
- Record the following data at the colposcopic examination: * Reason for referral: * Grade of cytological abnormality. * Whether the examination is satisfactory (this is defined as the entire squamocolumnar junction having been seen and the upper limit of any cervical lesion also being seen). * Presence or absence of vaginal and/or endocervical extension. * Colposcopic features. * Colposcopic impression of lesion grade.

Women referred with mild dyskaryosis or less:

- Normal and satisfactory colposcopy – at low risk of developing cervical cancer. Repeat cytology in 6 months.
  * If this is normal, they can be returned to recall.
  * If this is borderline, repeat test in 12 months.
  * If this is mild dyskaryosis, repeat colposcopy with another cytology within 12 months.
  * Any other cytology result warrants further colposcopy with or without biopsies.
- Colposcopically directed punch biopsy from a normal transformation zone is of no benefit following a low-grade referral.
- Colposcopic low-grade lesion – may be treated or followed up at 6–12 months in the colposcopy clinic or by the GP. Colposcopic biopsy at initial assessment is not essential. If the lesion has not resolved within 2 years, take a biopsy. In practice, many women are offered treatment at this point as persistent surveillance risks default.

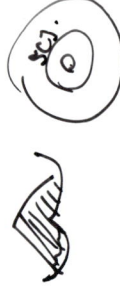

Women referred with moderate or severe dyskaryosis (high-grade):

- Normal colposcopy – these women are at significant risk of CIN 2 or 3 even in the presence of normal colposcopy. Take a biopsy. If treatment is not undertaken, keep a close surveillance with colposcopy and cytology every 6 months. If, at follow-up, a high-grade cytological abnormality persists, undertake an excisional treatment.
- Colposcopically low-grade lesion – with satisfactory colposcopy, take multiple biopsies as the likelihood of an underlying high-grade lesion in this situation is extremely high. If CIN 1 or less is confirmed, provide close colposcopic and cytological follow-up:

Excisional biopsy

- Undertake excisional biopsy only when:
  * Most of the ectocervix is replaced with high-grade abnormality.
  * Low-grade colposcopic change is associated with severe dyskaryosis or worse.
  * A lesion extends into the canal. Sufficient canal must be removed with endocervical extension of abnormality.
- Options are: knife cone biopsy, laser conization, large loop excision of the transformation zone (LLETZ), laser ablation, cryocautery, cold coagulation, and radical diathermy.
- Use cryocautery only for low-grade CIN with a double freeze–thaw–freeze technique. The rate of clearance of CIN 3 is poor. The double freeze technique has a lower incidence of residual disease compared with a single freeze technique.

Directed biopsy

- Unless an excisional treatment is planned, take a biopsy when the cytology indicates moderate dyskaryosis or worse, and always when a recognizably atypical transformation zone is present. Pregnancy is an exception.
- If colposcopically directed biopsy is reported as inadequate for histological interpretation, repeat it if there is a residual colposcopic lesion.
- All women must have histological diagnosis established before destructive therapy.

Ablative techniques are only suitable when:

- Entire transformation zone is visualized.
- There is no evidence of glandular abnormality.
- There is no evidence of invasive disease.
- There is no major discrepancy between cytology and histology. Only in exceptional circumstances should ablative treatment be considered for women over 50 years of age.

CIN in histology findings

CIN 1 features – abundant koilocytosis; the atypical cells extend through the epithelium with some differentiation in the middle and upper thirds and atypical basal changes.

CIN 2 – an increase in atypical supra-basal cells that extend through about half the epithelial thickness. Nuclear atypia and hyperchromasia are present, multinucleated cells are common, mitotic figures can be seen extending into the middle part of the epithelium.

CIN 3 – full thickness atypia with proliferation of supra-basal cells exhibiting hyperchromasia: hardly detectable surface differentiation with mitosis present close to the surface.

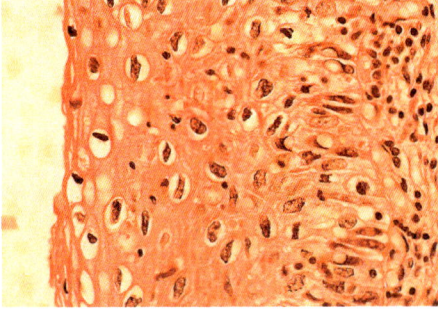

CIN 1

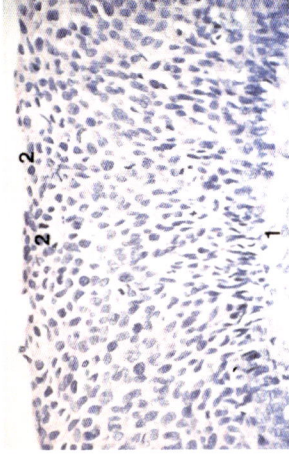

CIN 3

Repeat excision

- CIN 3 extending to the lateral or deep margins of excision (or uncertain margin status) results in a higher incidence of recurrence, but routine repeat excision is not needed provided:
  * There is no evidence of glandular abnormality.   *   There is no evidence of invasive disease.   *   The woman is <50 years of age.
- Repeat excision to try to obtain clear margins in all women >50 years old, who have CIN 3 at the lateral or deep margins, and in whom satisfactory cytology and colposcopy cannot be guaranteed.
- Women with adenocarcinoma *in situ* or cGIN who wish to retain fertility can be managed by local excision. Incomplete excision at the lateral or deep margins requires a further excision to obtain clear margins and exclude occult invasive disease.
- Micro-invasive squamous cancer FIGO stage IA 1 can be managed by local excisional techniques if the excision margins are free of both CIN and invasive disease. If the invasive lesion is excised but CIN extends to the excision margin, then a repeat excision to confirm excision of the CIN and to exclude further invasive disease is required. This should be performed, even in those cases planned for hysterectomy, to exclude an occult invasive lesion requiring radical surgery.

Follow-up with cytology at six months

- Women who do not have negative test results after treatment – re-colposcope at least once within 12 months.
- Women treated for high-grade disease (CIN 2, CIN 3, cGIN) require 6- and 12-month follow-up cytology and annual cytology for the subsequent 9 years (high-risk follow-up).
- Women treated for low-grade disease require 6-, 12-, and 24-month follow-up cytology. If all results are negative, then each woman may be returned to screening at the routine interval (low-risk follow-up).
- If a woman has not attended for all the specified cytology for her high-risk follow-up, allow her to return to routine screening provided her samples are normal at least 10 years after treatment.
- Women treated for cervical glandular intra-epithelial neoplasia (cGIN) are at somewhat higher risk of developing recurrent disease than those with high-grade CIN. In addition, recurrent disease is more difficult to detect cytologically in women with cGIN. Ideally, take 6-monthly samples for 5 years, followed by annual samples for a further 5 years.

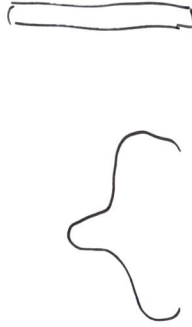

In women with severe cervical stenosis, it may not be possible to obtain a cytological sample that is representative of the whole transformation zone. The options are:

- Hysterectomy.
- Cervical dilatation.
- Withdrawal from further recall in the NHSCSP.

Consider cervical dilatation in all cases. Cervical dilatation or hysterectomy is recommended for women with a history of high-grade CIN, cGIN, or unexplained high-grade cytology.

Women who have had a hysterectomy with CIN

- These women are at risk of developing vaginal intra-epithelial neoplasia (VaIN) and invasive vaginal disease.
- For women on routine recall and with no CIN in their hysterectomy specimen, no further vaginal vault cytology is required.
- Women not on routine recall and with no CIN in their hysterectomy specimen – vaginal vault cytology at 6 months following hysterectomy.
- Women who undergo hysterectomy and have completely excised CIN – vaginal vault cytology at 6 and 18 months following hysterectomy.
- For women who undergo hysterectomy and have incompletely excised CIN (or uncertain excision), follow as if their cervix remained *in situ*:
  * CIN 1: vault cytology at 6, 12, and 24 months.
  * CIN 2/3: vault cytology at 6 and 12 months, followed by 9 annual cytology samples.
  * Follow-up for incompletely excised CIN continues to 65 years of age or until 10 years after surgery (whichever is later).

- There is evidence of a higher prevalence of benign endometrial cells in cervical samples taken using LBC.
- In women < 40 years of age, their presence has no significance; do not report or act upon them.
- In women > 40 years of age, their significance varies with the phase of the menstrual cycle, the use of some hormones, and the patient's clinical history. After the 14th day of the menstrual cycle, the presence of normal endometrial cells in a cervical sample may indicate endometrial pathology except in women who are receiving COCs, HRT, tamoxifen, or are fitted with an IUCD. In these women, provided there are no other clinical symptoms to suggest endometrial disease, no further clinical action is required. In the remaining women, such cells may be associated with endometrial pathology, particularly if out of phase or after the menopause. Refer for a gynaecological opinion.

Actinomyces-like organisms

- Usually seen in patients using an IUCD (including the Mirena IUS).
- If asymptomatic:
  * Do not remove the coil and do not offer antibiotics.
  * Perform an abdominal and pelvic examination.
  * Warn regarding the small possibility of developing pelvic actinomycosis and advise to return if she develops any symptoms.
- Do not repeat cytology unless the cervical cytology sample was inadequate or abnormal and is due for an early repeat.
  * If the asymptomatic patient wishes the device to be removed or it is due for removal, then send it for culture.
  * No follow-up is required.
- If the patient complains of specific symptoms – remove the device after ensuring that she has not had sexual intercourse in the preceding 5 days. These symptoms include:
  * Pelvic pain. * Deep dyspareunia. * Inter-menstrual bleeding (after 6 months of a device being *in situ*). * Vaginal discharge, dysuria, or significant pelvic tenderness.
  * Send the device for culture and advise alternative contraception. * Prescribe a course of antibiotics (amoxicillin 250 mg TDS for two weeks, or erythromycin 500 mg TDS for two weeks in penicillin-sensitive patients) and arrange gynaecological follow-up to ensure that the symptoms or signs have resolved.

What not to do

- Additional cervical screening is not justified in any of the following situations, providing the woman is in the age group to be screened and has undergone screening within the previous 3–5 years:
  * On taking or starting to take an oral contraceptive.
  * On insertion of an IUCD.
  * On taking or starting to take HRT.
  * In association with pregnancy – either antenatally or postnatally, or after termination, unless a previous screening test was abnormal.
  * In women with genital warts.
  * In women with vaginal discharge.
  * In women with pelvic infection.
  * In women who have had multiple sexual partners.
  * In women who are heavy cigarette smokers.

Prevalence and incidence

- Cervical cancer is the second most common cancer in women worldwide. The mortality is 10 times higher in developing countries, where > 80% of new cases occur.
- It is the 19th most common cancer in the UK and constitutes 2% of all cancers in women.
- In 2010, 2851 women were diagnosed and 936 died from cervical cancer in the UK.
- Crude incidence rate – 11 new cases per 100,000 women in the UK.
- The lifetime risk of developing cervical cancer in the UK is 1/134.
- The most common cancer in women < 35 years old.
- **Age-specific incidence rates – two peaks:** first in women aged 30–34 years (21/100,000 women) and the second in women aged 80–84 years (14/100,000 women). The earlier peak is related to women becoming sexually active with an increase of HPV; the second peak is due to increasing cancer incidence with age. In the UK, about 21% of new cases were in people aged ≥ 65 years.
- Cervical cancer mortality rates generally increase with age, with the highest number of deaths occurring in women in their late 70s.
- Survival rate – 84% of women survive for at least one year, falling to 67% surviving five years or more, to 63% at 10 years or more. Relative survival is higher in younger women – five-year relative survival ranges from 89% in 15–39 year olds to 22% in 80–99 year olds.

Risk factors

- Persistent infection with high-risk HPV is responsible for virtually all cases of cervical cancer. About 15 types of HPV are high risk for cervical cancer; HPV-16 and HPV-18 are the most prevalent. These two types cause about 70% of cervical cancers.
- Early age at first sexual intercourse and multiple sexual partners – higher risk of acquiring high-risk HPV.
- Other STIs – risk of squamous cell carcinoma (SCC) increases by about 80% in women with both HPV and Chlamydia infections and the risk is doubled in women with both herpes and HPV infections.
- Risk of SCC is increased by 50% in women who smoke.
- Immunocompromised states – risk is higher than average. Women with HIV, AIDS, or on immunosuppressants are at higher risk if they also have HPV infection.
- Risk is doubled in women who have taken the pill for at least 5 years. However, this is still a small risk and the pill has a protective effect against endometrial and ovarian cancers. The increased risk of cervical cancer begins to drop as soon as the pill is stopped and the risk is the same as background risk after 10 years.
- Women with partners who have been circumcised are at lower risk.
- No evidence that pregnancy increases the risk. The risk of SCC doubles with three or more children, compared to no children and risk of adenocarcinoma increases by 50%. Having the first baby early, before 17 years old, also doubles the risk compared to having the first baby at 25 years of age or older.
- Black women with HPV may have a higher risk than white women with HPV.
- Women with a first-degree relative with cervical cancer have double the risk of cervical cancer, compared to women without a family history.
- Occupation – exposure to tetrachloroethylene used in dry cleaning and metal degreasing.
- About 1% of cervical cancers in the UK are thought to be linked to this.
- Risk is higher in women with low socioeconomic background.
- Daughters of women who took diethylstilboestrol during pregnancy are more at risk of developing cervical cancer (clear cell adenocarcinoma).

Clinical features

- PCB, IMB, persistent/irregular vaginal bleeding, PMB.
- Abnormal and offensive vaginal discharge.
- Cervix looks or feels abnormal.

Referral to colposcopy

- Diagnosis is based on a surgical biopsy.
- If the lesion is large and clinically highly suspicious – take a directed biopsy.
- In smaller lesions – include whole lesion in the biopsy with a cone biopsy or a LLETZ.

Screening

See Chapter 31.

Examination/investigations for staging

- FIGO – staging is based on clinical examination. EUA with bimanual rectovaginal palpation.
- FBC, U&E, LFTs.
- Endocervical curettage, hysteroscopy, cystoscopy, proctoscopy.
- Chest X-ray and intravenous pyelogram.
- MRI abdomen and pelvis – superior to CT scan for tumour extension assessment.
- CT scan and MRI – pelvic and para-aortic nodal involvement.
- PET – has sensitivity and specificity of 100% and 99%, respectively. It is still under evaluation.
- Chest X-ray or thoracic CT scan for metastasis assessment.

Staging - FIGO classification

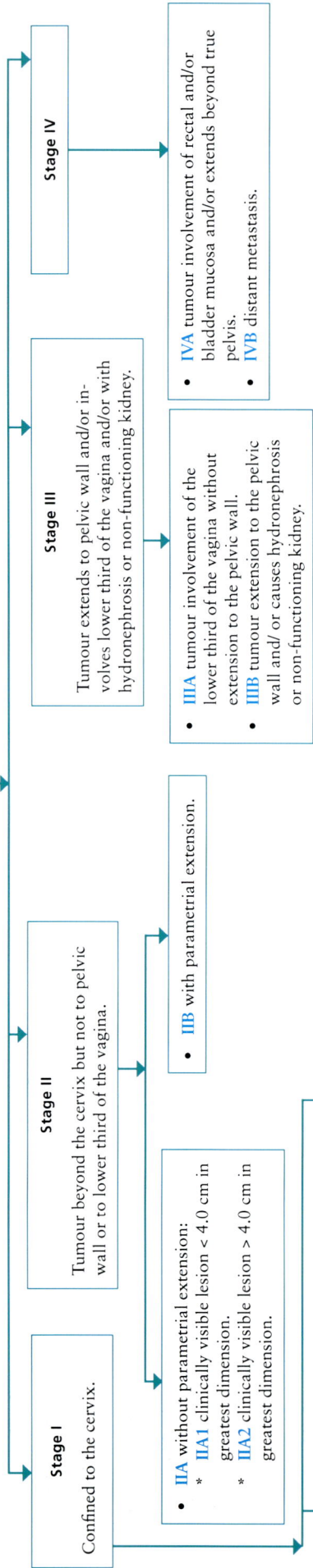

Stage I

Confined to the cervix.

- **IA:**
  - * **IA1** stromal invasion ≤ 3.0 mm in depth and ≤ 7.0 mm in horizontal spread.
    Risk of positive LNs – 1%.
  - * **IA2** stromal invasion > 3.0 mm and ≤ 5.0 mm with a horizontal spread of ≤ 7.0 mm.
    Risk of positive LNs – 4%.

- **IB:**
  Clinically visible lesion confined to cervix or microscopic lesion > IA2.
  - * **IB1** clinically visible lesion ≤ 4.0 cm in greatest dimension.
  - * **IB2** clinically visible lesion > 4.0 cm in greatest dimension.

Stage II

Tumour beyond the cervix but not to pelvic wall or to lower third of the vagina.

- **IIA** without parametrial extension:
  - * **IIA1** clinically visible lesion < 4.0 cm in greatest dimension.
  - * **IIA2** clinically visible lesion > 4.0 cm in greatest dimension.

- **IIB** with parametrial extension.

Stage III

Tumour extends to pelvic wall and/or involves lower third of the vagina and/or with hydronephrosis or non-functioning kidney.

- **IIIA** tumour involvement of the lower third of the vagina without extension to the pelvic wall.
- **IIIB** tumour extension to the pelvic wall and/ or causes hydronephrosis or non-functioning kidney.

Stage IV

- **IVA** tumour involvement of rectal and/or bladder mucosa and/or extends beyond true pelvis.
- **IVB** distant metastasis.

FIGO Classification – Carcinoma of the cervix uteri

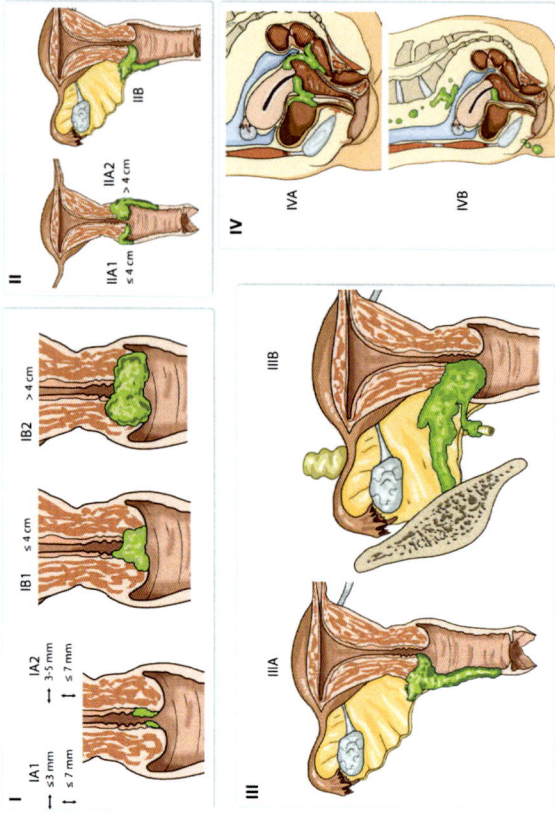

- Histological type – around two thirds of cervical cancers are SCC and around 15% are adenocarcinoma; the remainder of cases are poorly specified.
- There is an increase in relative distribution of adenocarcinoma in developed countries owing to the cervical screening programme.
- Adenocarcinoma has significantly lower survival rates compared with SCC.
- **Prognostic variables – tumour size, stage, nodal involvement, lymphovascular space involvement (LVSI), and histological subtype.**
- Presence of positive pelvic lymph nodes reduces the survival rate by 50%, stage for stage, whereas involvement of para-aortic lymph nodes reduces the survival by 75%.

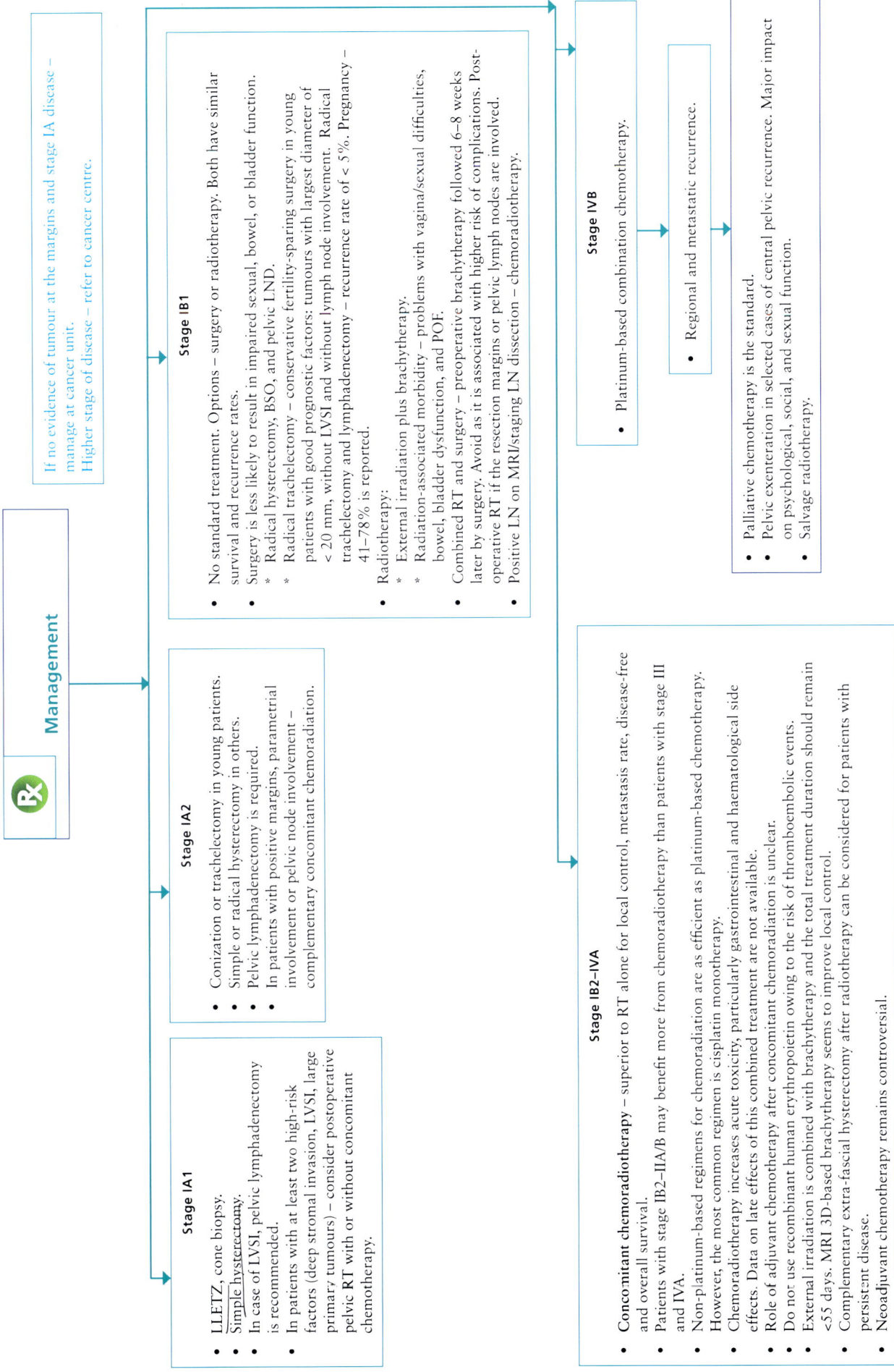

Rx

Management

If no evidence of tumour at the margins and stage IA disease – manage at cancer unit.
Higher stage of disease – refer to cancer centre.

Stage IA1

- LLETZ, cone biopsy.
- Simple hysterectomy.
- In case of LVSI, pelvic lymphadenectomy is recommended.
- In patients with at least two high-risk factors (deep stromal invasion, LVSI, large primary tumours) – consider postoperative pelvic RT with or without concomitant chemotherapy.

Stage IA2

- Conization or trachelectomy in young patients.
- Simple or radical hysterectomy in others.
- Pelvic lymphadenectomy is required.
- In patients with positive margins, parametrial involvement or pelvic node involvement – complementary concomitant chemoradiation.

Stage IB1

- No standard treatment. Options – surgery or radiotherapy. Both have similar survival and recurrence rates.
- Surgery is less likely to result in impaired sexual, bowel, or bladder function.
  * Radical hysterectomy, BSO, and pelvic LND.
  * Radical trachelectomy – conservative fertility-sparing surgery in young patients with good prognostic factors: tumours with largest diameter of < 20 mm, without LVSI and without lymph node involvement. Radical trachelectomy and lymphadenectomy – recurrence rate of < 5%. Pregnancy – 41–78% is reported.
- Radiotherapy:
  * External irradiation plus brachytherapy.
  * Radiation-associated morbidity – problems with vagina/sexual difficulties, bowel, bladder dysfunction, and POF.
- Combined RT and surgery – preoperative brachytherapy followed 6–8 weeks later by surgery. Avoid as it is associated with higher risk of complications. Post-operative RT if the resection margins or pelvic lymph nodes are involved.
- Positive LN on MRI/staging LN dissection – chemoradiotherapy.

Stage IB2–IVA

- **Concomitant chemoradiotherapy – superior to RT alone for local control, metastasis rate, disease-free and overall survival.**
- Patients with stage IB2–IIA/B may benefit more from chemoradiotherapy than patients with stage III and IVA.
- Non-platinum-based regimens for chemoradiation are as efficient as platinum-based chemotherapy. However, the most common regimen is cisplatin monotherapy.
- Chemoradiotherapy increases acute toxicity, particularly gastrointestinal and haematological side effects. Data on late effects of this combined treatment are not available.
- Role of adjuvant chemotherapy after concomitant chemoradiation is unclear.
- Do not use recombinant human erythropoietin owing to the risk of thromboembolic events.
- External irradiation is combined with brachytherapy and the total treatment duration should remain <55 days. MRI 3D-based brachytherapy seems to improve local control.
- Complementary extra-fascial hysterectomy after radiotherapy can be considered for patients with persistent disease.
- Neoadjuvant chemotherapy remains controversial.

Stage IVB

- Platinum-based combination chemotherapy.

- Regional and metastatic recurrence.

- Palliative chemotherapy is the standard.
- Pelvic exenteration in selected cases of central pelvic recurrence. Major impact on psychological, social, and sexual function.
- Salvage radiotherapy.

CHAPTER 32   Cervical cancer

Follow-up strategy – unclear

- Every 3 months for the first 2 years; every 6 months for the next 3 years, and yearly thereafter.
- Clinical examination (speculum and bimanual examination) including PAP smear.
- Suspected recurrence – EUA, biopsy, MRI, PET/CT might have a role in early local recurrence and metastasis detection.
- UK – majority of the patients are followed up for up to 5 years and then discharged.
- Cervical cytology – if there is high suspicion of residual VaIN.

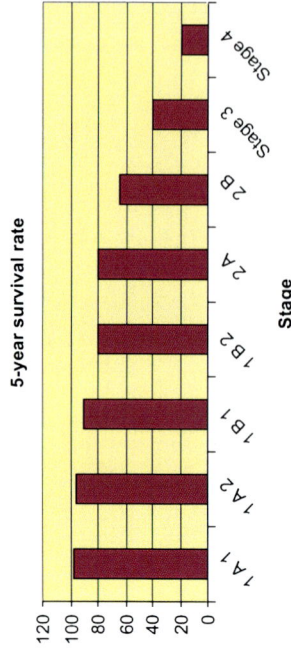

5-year survival rate

Bar chart of 5-year survival rate (%) by stage. Y-axis from 0 to 120. X-axis (Stage): 1A1, 1A2, 1B1, 1B2, 2A, 2B, Stage 3, Stage 4.

Stage

What will you do?
Cervical cancer in pregnancy

- Women usually present with vaginal bleeding – speculum examination is mandated to rule out cervical cancer.
- Biopsy may be associated with severe bleeding.
- Colposcopic appearance may be atypical, therefore refer to experienced colposcopist.
- MRI to assess the extent.
- Pregnancy does not adversely affect the outcome of cervical cancer.
- Treatment – same as in non-pregnant women.
- **Viable fetus** – radical hysterectomy can be performed at the time of Caesarean section.
- **At < 20 weeks** – radical hysterectomy could be performed without prior induction of abortion.

1. Haie-Meder C, Morice P, Castiglione M, for ESMO Guidelines Working Group. Cervical Cancer: ESMO Clinical Practice Guidelines for diagnosis, treatment and follow-up. *Ann Oncol* 2010;21(5):v37–v40. DOI:10.1093/annonc/mdq162.
2. Cancerresearch.org.uk.
3. WHO cancer cervix facts. http://www.who.int/reproductivehealth/topics/cancers/en/index.html.
4. http://www.imaios.com/e-Cases/Channels/Radiology/Radiological-classifications-commonly-used-on-medical-imaging/Carcinoma-of-the-cervix-uteri.

Background and pathogenesis

- Excessive cellular proliferation leads to an increased volume of endometrial tissue, where an increase of endometrial glands to stroma is seen at a ratio of > 1:1.
- There is risk of progression to endometrial carcinoma when hyperplasia is associated with cytological atypia.
- Majority of endometrial cancers (except serous, clear cell, and some endometrioid-type adenocarcinomas) follow a continuum from endometrial hyperplasia without atypia, to endometrial hyperplasia with atypia, to well-differentiated endometrial carcinoma.
- Categorized into simple and complex, based on the complexity and crowding of the glandular architecture.
- Some cases regress spontaneously.
- Most hyperplasias without atypia represent early, highly reversible lesions, and atypical endometrial hyperplasia is a precursor of endometrioid endometrial cancer.
- Atypical endometrial hyperplasia is considered as a pre-malignant lesion of the endometrium and redefined as endometrial intra-epithelial neoplasia (EIN).
- EIN lesions have an increased risk of developing carcinoma and require treatment.
  EIN classification:
  - * Simple (cystic) and complex (adenomatous) endometrial hyperplasia without atypia – endometrial hyperplasia
  - * Atypical endometrial hyperplasia – EIN.

Risk factors

- A relative excess of oestrogen, exogenous or endogenous, compared with progesterone.
- Seen in both pre-menopausal and post-menopausal women (approximately 15% of cases of women presenting with PMB).
- Post-menopausal women treated with supplemental oestrogens are at increased risk if a progestin is not used to oppose the proliferative actions of oestrogen on the endometrium. The risk increases with dose and duration of treatment with a 10-fold increased risk associated with each decade of use.
- Other risk factors – obesity, nulliparity, diabetes, and hypertension.
- PCOS – owing to unopposed oestrogenic stimulation secondary to anovulation.
- Women with hereditary non-polyposis colonic cancer (HNPCC) develop complex atypical endometrial hyperplasia at an earlier age.
- Peripheral conversion of androgens to oestrogens in androgen-secreting tumours of the adrenal cortex (rare).
- Tamoxifen has a partial agonist effect and can induce a proliferative effect on the endometrium, the increased risk persisting after cessation of treatment; 16% of women treated with tamoxifen developed atypical hyperplasia and 39% developed abnormal endometrial histology.

Routine screening for women at high risk of endometrial hyperplasia has not proven efficacious or cost-effective.

Clinical features

- Abnormal uterine bleeding – menorrhagia, IMB, PMB, irregular bleeding on HRT or tamox fen.
- Asymptomatic.

Investigations (See Chapter 35)

- **Blind endometrial biopsy** using the Pipelle, Vabra aspirator, and endometrial lavage:
  - * Pipelle biopsy – highest sensitivity (81%), sensitivity of Vabra (67%) and endometrial lavage (53%).
  - * Specificity of all three is high (>98%).
  - * Failure rate of 3% and an inadequate specimen rate of 1.5%.
- **Pipelle vs curette** – both are blind techniques and they do not sample the whole surface of the endometrium to be visualized, but performed alone has a high false-positive rate. Hysteroscopy with targeted biopsy has best sensitivity and specificity and is superior to hysteroscopy, dilatation and curettage, or endometrial biopsy performed alone.
- **Hysteroscopy – gold standard.** It allows the whole surface of the endometrium to be visualized. Associated with 96% agreement between biopsy pathology and final diagnosis for both procedures.
- **TVS** – see Chapter 35.
- **Sonohysterography and Pipelle biopsy** – sensitivity (94%) comparable to those of hysteroscopy and dilatation and curettage.

Rx **Management**

```
Simple hyperplasia          Complex hyperplasia          Complex atypical hyperplasia
```

Risk of progression

Simple hyperplasia

- Majority spontaneously regress.
- 18% persist.
- 3% progress to complex atypical hyperplasia.
- 1% progress to endometrial adenocarcinoma.

Complex hyperplasia

- Majority regress spontaneously.
- 22% persist.
- 4% progress to endometrial carcinoma.
- Mean duration to progression of approximately 10 years.

Complex atypical hyperplasia

- Progress in 29% of cases, with a mean duration to progression of 4 years.
- Risk of concomitant carcinoma is reported as up to 50% in recent studies.
- Endometrial carcinomas with concomitant hyperplasia are thought to be associated with less aggressive disease, tending to be of lower grade and stage with significantly lower recurrence risk and higher 5-year survival rates.
- However, a study reported – 37.5% of women with concomitant atypical hyperplasia had endometrial carcinoma with FIGO stage IB or higher.

Treatment

Conservative – persistent or ✓ progressive disease is seen in one third of conservatively managed cases.

Progestogens:
* Have both indirect anti-oestrogenic and direct antiproliferative effects on the endometrium.
* Route – systemically, either alone or in combination with oestrogen (COC or HRT), or locally in the form of LNG-IUS. Both routes have a 75–90% and 90–100% conversion rate of non-atypical endometrial hyperplasia to normal endometrium, respectively.

Surgical:
* In the presence of persistent symptoms or non-regressive disease, hysterectomy is appropriate.

Progestogen:
* In women (< 40 years – 94% success rate with 3–18 months of therapy; subsequent successful pregnancies are reported.
* In post-menopausal women, a 25% risk of progression to carcinoma is reported in those treated with MPA.
* Re-sample the endometrium after suitable therapeutic intervals (3–6 months) to ensure that hormonal ablation has occurred.

Surgical:
* Where fertility or significant surgical risk is not an issue – hysterectomy in view of the risk of coexisting malignancy or progression to cancer.
* Because of the risk of concomitant endometrial carcinoma and the possibility of it being of higher stage in some cases, evaluate women carefully for the possibility of more advanced disease prior to surgery.

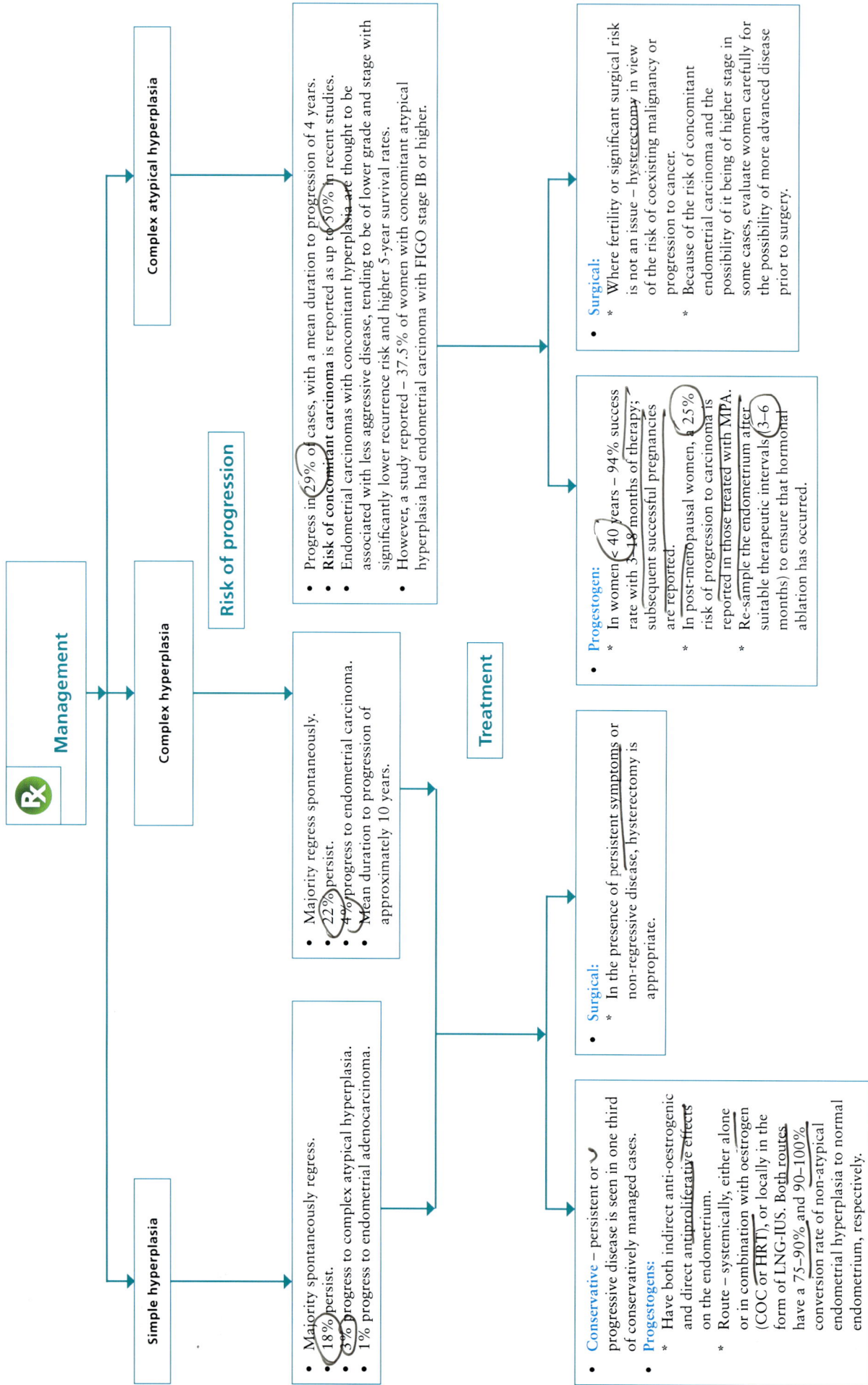

1. Palmer JE, Perunovic B, Tidy JA. Endometrial hyperplasia. *The Obstetrician and Gynaecologist* 2008;10:211–216.

Risk factors

Increase risk with:

- **Increased endogenous hormones:**
  * Excess exposure to oestrogen unopposed by progestogens.
  * Insulin and insulin-like growth factors increase the effect of oestrogen on uterine tissue.
  * PMW – high circulating levels of unopposed oestrogens and androgens.
  * Early menarche and late menopause owing to prolonged years of oestrogen exposure.
  * Amenorrhoea, infrequent or irregular periods (PCOS), anovulatory menstrual cycles.
- **Obesity** – risk is 2 to 3 times higher in overweight and obese women.
- **Exogenous hormones:**
  * UK Million Women study – increased risk of 50% among current users of oestrogen-only HRT and 80% in those using tibolone preparations.
  * Tamoxifen – trebles the risk of uterine cancer. This does not appear to be dose dependent, although the risk increases with duration of therapy. Excess deaths from uterine cancer among women taking tamoxifen are about 2/10,000 women each year.
- **Diabetes** – doubles the risk, with an independent effect owing to circulating insulin and free insulin-like growth factor 1.
- **Hereditary** – HNPCC accounts for < 5% of all endometrial cancer (See Chapter 37).

Reduced risk with:

- **COCs** – 6% reduction in risk for each year of use, due to fewer days of unopposed oestrogen exposure each month. The risk reduction persists for up to 20 years after stopping use. Women with high levels of sex hormone-binding globulin (which governs the bioavailability of oestrogens and androgens).
- **Pregnancy and parity** – reduces risk by 30% for a woman's first birth and by 25% for each successive birth. Older age at last birth has also been shown to reduce risk.
- **Physical activity** – most active women have a 23% reduction in risk.
- **Aspirin** – a meta-analysis reported a 13% risk reduction for any aspirin use with a stronger association for women who are obese (28% risk reduction); it may not benefit women who have a healthy weight.

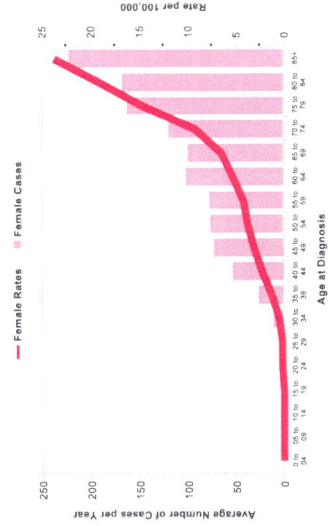

New cases per year and age-specific incidence rates, UK, 2009–2011

Prevalence and incidence

- Most common gynaecological malignancy in the developed world/UK.
- UK 2010 – 8288 women were diagnosed and 1937 died from uterine cancer.
- The 4th most common cancer in women in the UK (5% of all female cancers).
- Lifetime risk of developing uterine cancer in the UK – 1/46 women.
- **Age** – more common in post-menopausal women (PMW). Median age of occurrence is 63 years; > 90% of women are older than 50 years.
- Incidence rises from 2/100,000 women/year in women < 40 years of age to 40–50/100,000 among women aged 60–89 years.
- **Survival rate** – 90% of women survive for at least 1 year; 77% survive 5 years or more; 75% survive up to 10 years.
- **Stage** – 5-year survival is around 85% for stage I tumours, compared with 25% for stage IV.
- **Grade** – 81% 5-year survival in grade 1, stage IC tumours compared with 42% for grade 3 tumours of the same stage.

History

- Post-menopausal women – PMB, persistent/abnormal vaginal discharge.
- 25% of cases present in peri-menopausal women – irregular bleeding, IMB, PCB.
- Examination, investigations, and referral for PMB/abnormal bleeding in peri-menopausal women – see Chapter 35.
- **Refer all PMB and women aged > 45 years with abnormal uterine bleeding for assessment at a local cancer unit. (NICE)**

Investigations – preoperative evaluation for staging

- History, clinical examination, and endometrial biopsy.
- FBC, RFT, LFT, chest X-ray, ECG.
- TVS has sensitivity of 66–86% and specificity of 83–90% to detect tumour invasion extending through > half of myometrium.
- MRI best for defining myometrial spread. Absence of MRI evidence of deep myometrial penetration has a high NPV, but presence of MRI evidence of deep penetration has a lower PPV.
- If cervical involvement is suspected – contrast-enhanced dynamic MRI.
- CT of the chest, abdomen, and pelvis – for extra-uterine and extra-pelvic spread.
- PET to determine location of disease recurrence.

Screening

There is no screening test that is accurate and reliable enough to detect uterine cancer in the general population.

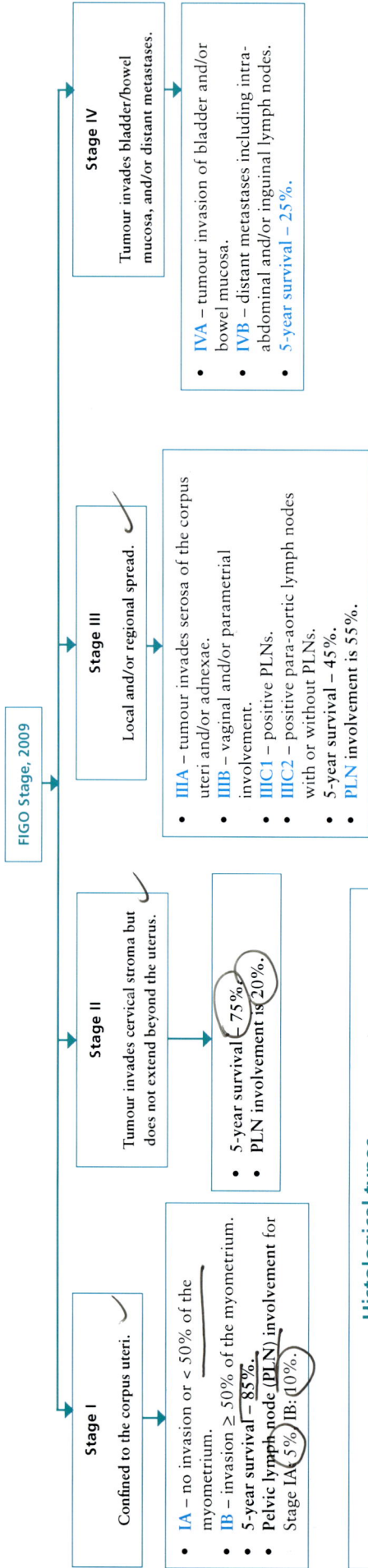

FIGO Stage, 2009

Stage I

Confined to the corpus uteri.

- IA – no invasion or < 50% of the myometrium.
- IB – invasion ≥ 50% of the myometrium.
- 5-year survival – 85%.
- Pelvic lymph node (PLN) involvement for Stage IA (5%) IB (10%).

Stage II

Tumour invades cervical stroma but does not extend beyond the uterus.

- 5-year survival – 75%
- PLN involvement is 20%.

Stage III

Local and/or regional spread.

- IIIA – tumour invades serosa of the corpus uteri and/or adnexae.
- IIIB – vaginal and/or parametrial involvement.
- IIIC1 – positive PLNs.
- IIIC2 – positive para-aortic lymph nodes with or without PLNs.
- 5-year survival – 45%.
- PLN involvement is 55%.

Stage IV

Tumour invades bladder/bowel mucosa, and/or distant metastases.

- IVA – tumour invasion of bladder and/or bowel mucosa.
- IVB – distant metastases including intra-abdominal and/or inguinal lymph nodes.
- 5-year survival – 25%.

Histological types

- Endometrioid (75%) – most common, composed of malignant glandular epithelial elements.
- Adenocarcinoma with squamous differentiation.
- Adenoacanthoma (benign squamous component).
- Adenosquamous (malignant squamous component).
- Uterine papillary serous (5%–10%).
- Clear cell (1%–5%).
- Malignant mixed Müllerian tumours or carcinosarcomas (1–2%).
- Uterine sarcomas (leiomyosarcoma, undifferentiated) (3%).
- Mucinous (1%).
- Undifferentiated.

Type 1 and Type 2 categories

Based on histopathology, molecular profile, and clinical course, endometrial cancers are divided into two categories.

- Type 1 – a slow-growing, low-grade (I–II) adenocarcinoma linked to oestrogen and obesity through the peripheral conversion of androstenedione to oestrone in body fat. * Diagnosed early and has a favourable prognosis. * Accounts for 80% of cases. * Usually grade I endometrioid adenocarcinomas, papillary serous and clear cell carcinomas, and carcinosarcomas.
- Type 2 – more aggressive, faster growing, unrelated to oestrogen. * Approximately 10% of cases. * They have p53 mutations and loss of heterozygosity at several chromosomal loci. * Prognosis is less favourable and presentation can occur at a more advanced stage.
- Endometrioid carcinoma is thought to progress through a pre-malignant stage of complex atypical hyperplasia in most cases, whereas papillary serous and clear-cell carcinomas arise as a result of a sequence of genetic mutations.

FIGO Classification - Carcinoma of the endometrium

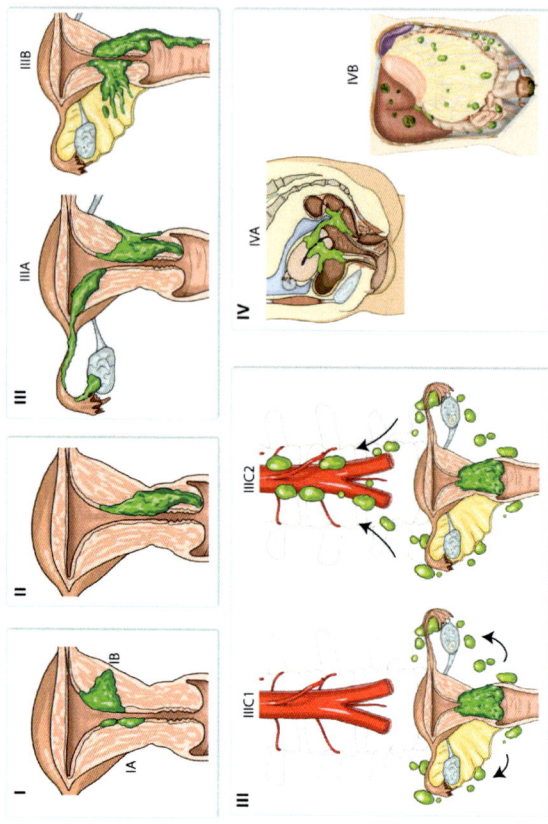

Used with permission from e-anatomy, Micheau A. Hoo D, www.imaios.com (http//www.imaios.com)

Management

- **Women with stage IA, Grade 1 or 2 (40% of cases) – treat at the cancer unit.**
- **Women with more advanced or high-risk cancers (stage I, Grade 3, stage IB, or higher), or those with morphological or other features associated with poor prognosis – treat at cancer centres.**

Stage I

- **TAH/BSO** – open or laparoscopic.
- Inspect and palpate liver, diaphragm, omentum, and peritoneal surfaces. Take peritoneal washings.
- A pelvic/para-aortic lymph node dissection (LND):
  * Ongoing debate. It may increase the risk of lymphoedema without a clear benefit.
  * RCT of LND and adjuvant external beam radiotherapy (MRC, NCRI, UK) – no evidence of benefit on overall survival or recurrence-free survival for pelvic LND in women with early endometrial cancer, and it is not recommended.

Stage II

- Suspected cervical involvement (MRI or cervical biopsy) – radical TAH/ BSO and consider pelvic/para-aortic lymph node dissection (LND). If adequate surgical margins are achieved and the nodes are free of disease – adjuvant RT is not indicated.
- Medically inoperable stage I/II (co-morbidities such as obesity, cardiac morbidity, diabetes) – may be treated by external beam radiotherapy (RT) and/or brachytherapy (BT).

Intra-abdominal disease

- Intra-abdominal disease (omental, nodal, ovarian, peritoneal involvement, ascites) – TAH/BSO and consider maximal surgical debulking.

Distant metastatic disease

- Distant metastatic disease (e.g., liver, lung) – consider palliative hysterectomy depending on patient's status, expected benefits, and MDT decision. Surgery may be followed by pelvic RT and/or chemotherapy.

Adjuvant treatment – controversial, with lack of clear evidence

Stage I

- **Stage IA, G1–2**
  * Observation.
- **Stage IA, G3**
  * Consider vaginal BT, depending on coexisting risk factors.
  * If LVSI and positive LN/no LND – consider pelvic RT.

- **Stage IB, G1–2**
  * Observation or vaginal BT.
  * Pelvic RT as in Stage IA, G3.
- **Stage IB, G3**
  * Vaginal BT alone.
  * Or pelvic RT as in Stage IA, G3.
  * Consider chemotherapy for high-grade cases.

Stage II

- Consider both pelvic RT and vaginal BT.
- G1 tumour – without LVSI and/or negative pelvic nodes after LND – vaginal BT alone.
- High-grade (G3) – adjuvant chemotherapy may reduce the rate of distant recurrences. Therefore, consider chemotherapy.

Stage III and IV

- Maximal surgical cytoreduction for patients without co-morbidities.
- **Approach Stage III with curative intent.**
  * Observation only could be an option for non-invasive grade 1–2, confined to the fundus with only positive cytology (stage IIIA with the old staging).
  * All other stage III tumours – pelvic RT with vaginal BT. Adjuvant chemotherapy may reduce the distant recurrences. Therefore, consider chemotherapy for stage III high-grade tumours, particularly those with PLN disease.
- Neoadjuvant chemotherapy can be considered for advanced tumours, followed by surgery.
- Consider pelvic RT either to palliate symptoms or as a high-dose palliative RT if it could offer a longer symptom-free interval.

Follow-up for recurrence

- Overall recurrence rate is 7–18%.
- There is lack of evidence for clear benefit and follow-up schedules. For the first 3 years, patients can be seen 3–4 times monthly. For the next 2 years, 6-monthly appointments are recommended.
- Assess – history, physical and vaginal examination.
- Symptoms of recurrence include vaginal bleeding, discharge, pressure symptoms.
- Investigate further (CT, MRI, blood tests, EUA) if clinically indicated.
- Management of recurrence depends on the sites of recurrence and previous treatment.
- Pelvic recurrence for RT–treated women who have not been exposed to previous radiation with RT. Surgery is an option for previously irradiated women with vaginal vault recurrence.
- During this surveillance, take into account the increased risk of cancers of the breast, ovary, and colon in patients with endometrial cancer.

- Hormonal treatment with high-dose oral progestogens is the main treatment in cases of multiple or distant recurrences.
- GnRH analogue is an option in progesterone refractory cases.
- Chemotherapy may be used with palliative intent.

Uterine cancer

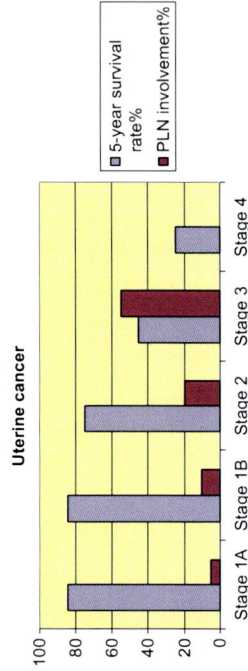

Legend: 5-year survival rate%; PLN involvement%

X-axis: Stage 1A, Stage 1B, Stage 2, Stage 3, Stage 4
Y-axis: 0 to 100

Papillary serous and clear cell carcinomas

- No definite evidence.
- Adjuvant therapy recommendations:
  * Stage IA – observation or chemotherapy or pelvic RT.
  * Stage IB II – chemotherapy with or without pelvic RT, with or without vaginal BT (especially in cervical stromal invasion).
  * Stage III IV – adequately debulked: chemotherapy and pelvic RT with or without vaginal BT (especially if there is cervical stromal invasion). Consider chemotherapy in inadequately debulked stage III or IV patients.

What not to do

- Pelvic/para-aortic LND in women with early endometrial cancer.
- Adjuvant progestogens.

1. Plataniotis G, Castiglione M, for the ESMO Guidelines Working Group. Endometrial cancer: ESMO Clinical Practice Guidelines for diagnosis, treatment, and follow-up. *Ann Oncol* 2010;21(5):v41–v45. DOI:10.1093/annonc/mdq245.
2. Holland CM. The role of pelvic and para-aortic lymph node dissection in the surgical treatment of endometrial cancer: a view from the UK. *The Obstetrician and Gynaecologist* 2009;11:205–209.
3. Mariani A, Dowdy S, Podratz K. The role of pelvic and para-aortic lymph node dissection in the surgical treatment of endometrial cancer: a view from the USA. *The Obstetrician and Gynaecologist* 2009;11:199–204.
4. Edey K, Murdoch J. FIGO staging in vulval and endometrial cancer. *The Obstetrician and Gynaecologist* 2010;12:245–249.
5. http://www.cancerresearchuk.org/cancer-info/cancerstats/types/uterus/incidence/july2014.
6. http://www.imaios.com/e-Cases/Channels/Radiology/Radiological-classifications-commonly-used-on-medical-imaging/Carcinoma-of-the-endometrium.

Background and incidence

- Episode of bleeding 12 months or more after the last period.
- Incidence – 14.3/1000 post-menopausal women (PMW).
- Endometrial cancer is present in approximately 10% of PMB.
- Other causes of PMB – cervical cancer, endometrial polyp, benign conditions of vulva and vagina.

Age

- Incidence of PMB decreases with age, but the probability of endometrial cancer increases.
- Risk of endometrial cancer:
  * Women up to 60 years – 10%.
  * Women > 60 years – 13%.

Hereditary non-polyposis colorectal cancer (HNPCC)

- Autosomal dominant.
- Familial aggregation of colorectal cancer and extra-colonic cancers of which endometrial cancer is the most common.
- Lifetime risk of endometrial cancer is 42–60%.
- Usually develops pre-menopausally.

History/risk factors

Single/multiple episodes of bleeding – no evidence of whether different patterns of PMB are more or less likely to be associated with endometrial cancer.

Tamoxifen

- Probability of endometrial cancer is substantially greater than 10%. They have a 3–6-fold greater incidence of endometrial cancer.
- Risk rises with both the use of higher doses and increasing duration of tamoxifen.
- Use beyond 5 years increases risk by at least 4-fold.
- Endometrial cancer in long-term users of tamoxifen has a poorer prognosis (due to less favourable histology and higher stage).

HRT

- PMB in HRT users is less likely to be associated with endometrial cancer than in non-HRT users.
- Non-users of HRT – risk of endometrial cancer is 6–12%.
- Users of HRT (combined) – risk of endometrial cancer is 1%.
- HRT with unopposed oestrogen increases the RR of endometrial cancer 6 times after 5 years of use.
- Risk for women on continuous combined HRT is similar to those not on HRT.
- Women on sequential HRT tend to have a thicker endometrium; thus a higher threshold needs to be used for identifying those with a significant probability of cancer.

Others – current evidence is insufficient to quantify the risk in:
- Obese patients with diabetes.
- Women with HT.
- Past history of hyper-oestrogenism (endogenous or exogenous) such as women with early menarche and late menopause.

Examination

Full pelvic examination and speculum examination of the cervix to rule out any local pathology. (NICE)

Refer urgently to secondary care – women with PMB who are:
- Not on HRT.
- On HRT with persistent or unexplained PMB after cessation of HRT for 6/52.
- Taking tamoxifen. (NICE)

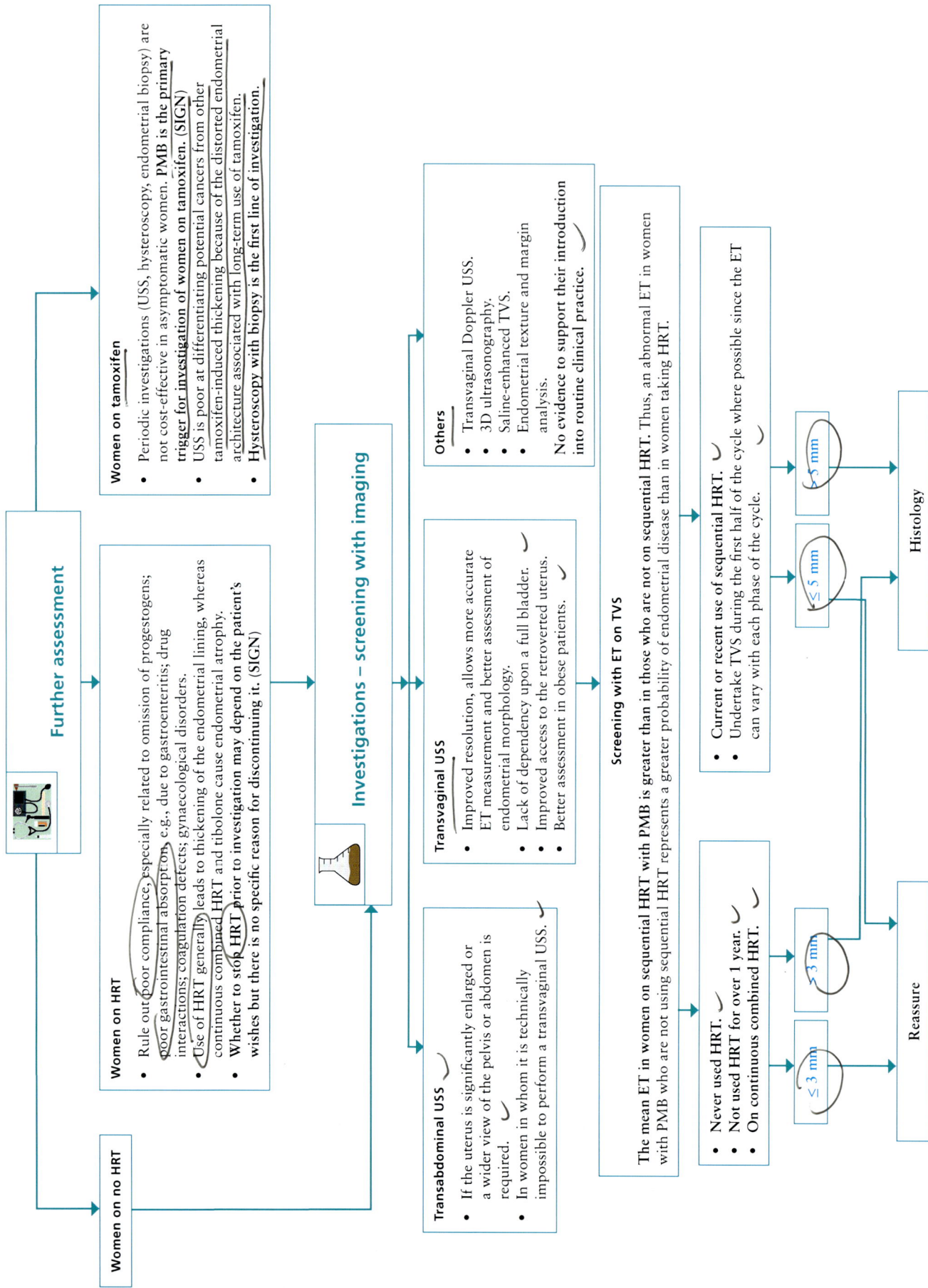

Further assessment

Women on no HRT

Women on HRT

- Rule out poor compliance, especially related to omission of progestogens; poor gastrointestinal absorption, e.g., due to gastroenteritis; drug interactions; coagulation defects; gynaecological disorders.
- Use of HRT generally leads to thickening of the endometrial lining, whereas continuous combined HRT and tibolone cause endometrial atrophy.
- Whether to stop HRT prior to investigation may depend on the patient's wishes but there is no specific reason for discontinuing it. (SIGN)

Women on tamoxifen

- Periodic investigations (USS, hysteroscopy, endometrial biopsy) are not cost-effective in asymptomatic women. **PMB is the primary trigger for investigation of women on tamoxifen.** (SIGN)
- USS is poor at differentiating potential cancers from other tamoxifen-induced thickening because of the distorted endometrial architecture associated with long-term use of tamoxifen.
- Hysteroscopy with biopsy is the first line of investigation.

Investigations – screening with imaging

Transabdominal USS

- If the uterus is significantly enlarged or a wider view of the pelvis or abdomen is required.
- In women in whom it is technically impossible to perform a transvaginal USS.

Transvaginal USS

- Improved resolution, allows more accurate ET measurement and better assessment of endometrial morphology.
- Lack of dependency upon a full bladder.
- Improved access to the retroverted uterus.
- Better assessment in obese patients.

Others

- Transvaginal Doppler USS.
- 3D ultrasonography.
- Saline-enhanced TVS.
- Endometrial texture and margin analysis.
- No evidence to support their introduction into routine clinical practice.

Screening with ET on TVS

The mean ET in women on sequential HRT with PMB is greater than in those who are not on sequential HRT. Thus, an abnormal ET in women with PMB who are not using sequential HRT represents a greater probability of endometrial disease than in women taking HRT.

- Current or recent use of sequential HRT.
- Undertake TVS during the first half of the cycle where possible since the ET can vary with each phase of the cycle.

- Never used HRT.
- Not used HRT for over 1 year.
- On continuous combined HRT.

> 5 mm

≤ 5 mm

> 3 mm

≤ 3 mm

Histology

Reassure

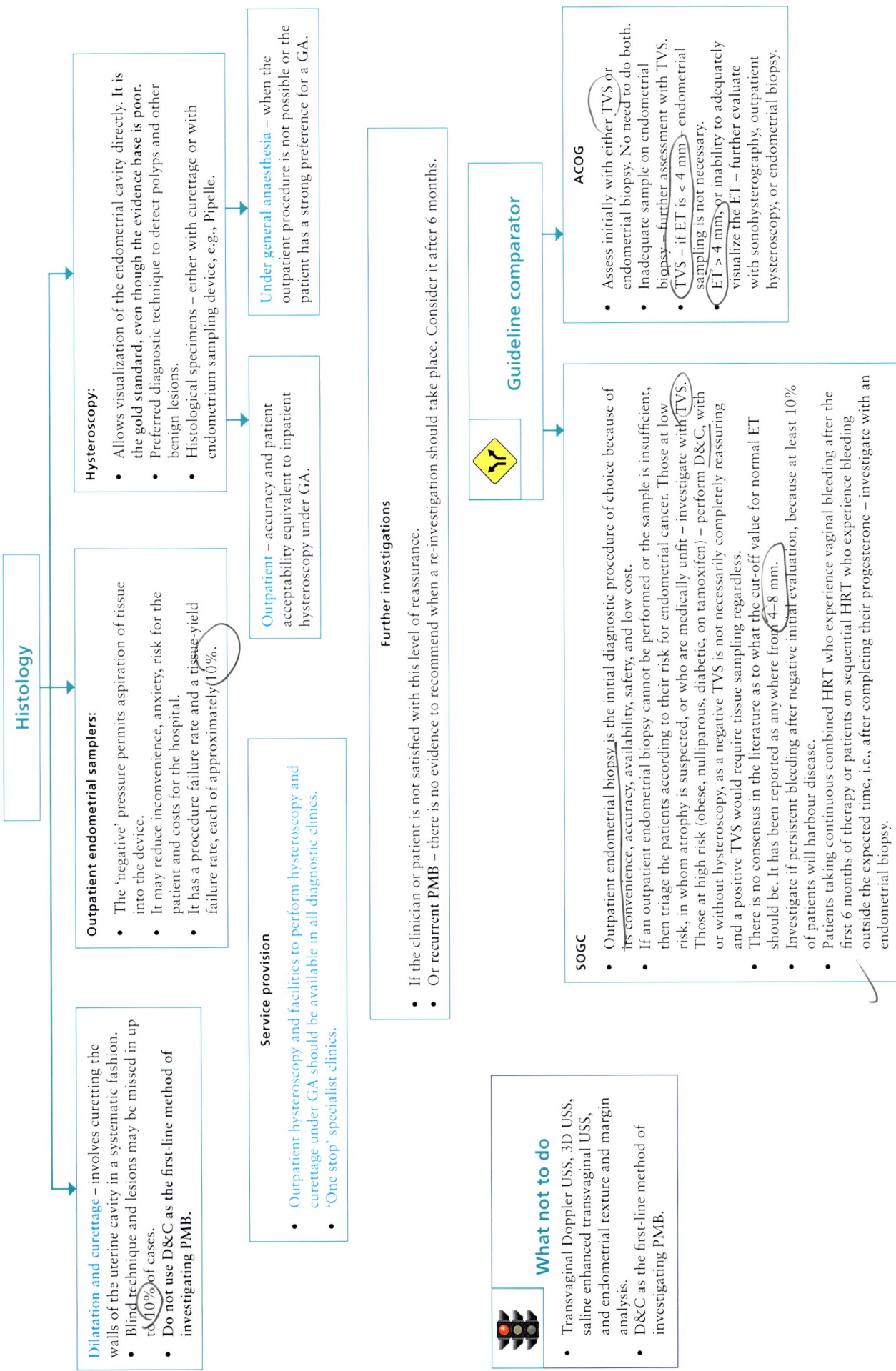

Histology

Dilatation and curettage – involves curetting the walls of the uterine cavity in a systematic fashion.

- Blind technique and lesions may be missed in up to 10% of cases.
- Do not use D&C as the first-line method of investigating PMB.

Outpatient endometrial samplers:

- The 'negative' pressure permits aspiration of tissue into the device.
- It may reduce inconvenience, anxiety, risk for the patient and costs for the hospital.
- It has a procedure failure rate and a tissue-yield failure rate, each of approximately 10%.

Hysteroscopy:

- Allows visualization of the endometrial cavity directly. It is the gold standard, even though the evidence base is poor.
- Preferred diagnostic technique to detect polyps and other benign lesions.
- Histological specimens – either with curettage or with endometrium sampling device, e.g., Pipelle.

Under general anaesthesia – when the outpatient procedure is not possible or the patient has a strong preference for a GA.

Outpatient – accuracy and patient acceptability equivalent to inpatient hysteroscopy under GA.

Service provision

- Outpatient hysteroscopy and facilities to perform hysteroscopy and curettage under GA should be available in all diagnostic clinics.
- 'One stop' specialist clinics.

Further investigations

- If the clinician or patient is not satisfied with this level of reassurance.
- Or **recurrent PMB** – there is no evidence to recommend when a re-investigation should take place. Consider it after 6 months.

Guideline comparator

ACOG

- Assess initially with either TVS or endometrial biopsy. No need to do both.
- Inadequate sample on endometrial biopsy – further assessment with TVS.
- TVS – if ET is < 4 mm – endometrial sampling is not necessary.
- ET > 4 mm, or inability to adequately visualize the ET – further evaluate with sonohysterography, outpatient hysteroscopy, or endometrial biopsy.

SOGC

- Outpatient endometrial biopsy is the initial diagnostic procedure of choice because of its convenience, accuracy, availability, safety, and low cost.
- If an outpatient endometrial biopsy cannot be performed or the sample is insufficient, then triage the patients according to their risk for endometrial cancer. Those at low risk, in whom atrophy is suspected, or who are medically unfit – investigate with TVS. Those at high risk (obese, nulliparous, diabetic, on tamoxifen) – perform D&C, with or without hysteroscopy, as a negative TVS is not necessarily completely reassuring and a positive TVS would require tissue sampling regardless.
- There is no consensus in the literature as to what the cut-off value for normal ET should be. It has been reported as anywhere from 4–8 mm.
- Investigate if persistent bleeding after negative initial evaluation, because at least 10% of patients will harbour disease.
- Patients taking continuous combined HRT who experience vaginal bleeding after the first 6 months of therapy or patients on sequential HRT who experience bleeding outside the expected time, i.e., after completing their progesterone – investigate with an endometrial biopsy.

What not to do

- Transvaginal Doppler USS, 3D USS, saline enhanced transvaginal USS, and endometrial texture and margin analysis.
- D&C as the first-line method of investigating PMB.

Asymptomatic endometrial thickening in post-menopausal women (SOGC)

What to do

- A woman who has increased ET and other positive findings on TVS, such as increased vascularity, heterogeneity of endometrium, particulate fluid, or thickened endometrium > 11 mm, investigate further.
- Decide about further investigations on an individual basis in asymptomatic women with increased ET and risk factors for endometrial cancer such as obesity, hypertension, and late menopause.
- Not all PMW who have asymptomatic endometrial polyps require surgery. Triage these women found to have asymptomatic polyps on USS for intervention according to size of the polyp, age, and other risk factors.

What not to do

- Do not use TVS as screening tool for endometrial cancer.
- Do not routinely perform endometrial sampling in a PMW without bleeding.
- Indications for tissue sampling of the endometrium in bleeding PMW with an ET of > 4–5 mm should not be extrapolated to asymptomatic women.
- In asymptomatic women on tamoxifen, do not perform a routine USS for ET.
- Significance of raised ET in asymptomatic PMW is not established; do not routinely start investigation. (ACOG)

1. *Investigation of Post-Menopausal Bleeding.* Scottish Intercollegiate Guidelines Network: A National Clinical Guideline, 2002.
2. NICE Referral Guidelines for Suspected Cancer, 2005.
3. *Diagnosis of Endometrial Cancer in Women with Abnormal Vaginal Bleeding.* SOGC Clinical Practice Guidelines No. 86, February 2000.
4. *The Role of Transvaginal Ultrasonography in the Evaluation of Postmenopausal Bleeding.* ACOG Committee Opinion, February 2009.
5. *Asymptomatic Endometrial Thickening.* SOGC Clinical Practice Guidelines No. 249, October 2010.

Background and prevalence

- Ovarian cysts are fluid-containing structures more than 30 mm in diameter.
- Up to 4% of women (median age 26 years), have an ovarian cyst > 30 mm in diameter in the luteal phase.
- Risk of malignancy increases with increasing tumour size and increasing age.
- Up to 10% of women have some form of surgery during their lifetime for an ovarian mass.
- In pre-menopausal women, almost all ovarian masses and cysts are benign.
- Overall incidence of a symptomatic ovarian cyst in a pre-menopausal women being malignant is approximately 1/1000, increasing to 3/1000 by the age of 50 years.
- Incidence of malignant ovarian cysts in the reproductive age group is 0.4–9/100,000 women; and in women aged 60–80 years is 60/100,000.
- In post-menopausal women, 21% of the cysts have abnormal ovarian morphology, either simple or complex.

History

- Take a detailed history along with risk factors or protective factors for ovarian malignancy and a family history of ovarian or breast cancer.
- Symptoms suggestive of endometriosis.
- Symptoms suggestive of ovarian malignancy – abdominal distension, appetite change including increased satiety, pelvic or abdominal pain, increased urinary urgency and/or frequency.
- Acute pain – consider ovarian accident (torsion, rupture, haemorrhage).

Examination

- Abdominal and vaginal examination – a large ovarian cyst may be palpable as a mass arising from the pelvis, separate from the uterus. Small cysts are often missed. Although clinica examination has poor sensitivity in the detection of ovarian masses (15–51%) it helps to evaluate mass tenderness, mobility, nodularity, and ascites.
- Assess for local lymphadenopathy and ascites.

- Evaluation of ovarian masses – to exclude malignancy and to decide when to refer to a gynaecological oncologist.
- General presentation
  Peri-menopausal woman:
  * Incidental finding.
  * Acute presentation with pain.
  * Symptoms of endometriosis.
  Post-menopausal women:
  * Result of screening.
  * Investigations for a suspected pelvic mass.
  * Incidental finding.

Differential diagnosis – adnexal masses

DDx

- Benign ovarian mass – functional cysts, endometriomas, benign tumours.
- Benign non-ovarian mass – paratubal cyst, hydrosalpinges, tubo-ovarian abscess, peritoneal pseudocysts, appendiceal abscess, diverticular abscess, pelvic kidney.
- Primary malignant ovarian tumour.
- Secondary malignant ovarian tumour – breast and gastrointestinal carcinoma.

Investigations

MRI, CT

- MRI, CT, PET) – role yet to be established.
- MRI may be superior to CT and USS in diagnosis and staging of ovarian mass.
- TVS has greater sensitivity than either MRI or PET in distinguishing benign from malignant disease, at the expense of some specificity.
- Owing to the lack of clear evidence of benefit, the relative expense, and limited availability of these modalities, their routine use is not recommended.

Ultrasound scan

- TVS – greater sensitivity and provides more details than TAS. Larger masses may need to be assessed by TAS as well.
- Sonographic features suggestive of ovarian malignancy include larger size, presence of septations, papillary formations, echogenic solid areas, and free fluid in the pouch of Douglas.
- TVS – a sensitivity of 89% and specificity of 73% with the use of morphology index. However, specificity of TVS for the detection of malignancy is not sufficiently high for it to be used alone as a screening test.
- Use of colour flow Doppler does not significantly improve diagnostic accuracy but the combined use of TVS with colour flow mapping and 3D imaging may improve sensitivity.
- Doppler ultrasound assessment of cyst wall blood flow does not differentiate between benign and malignant ovarian cysts. This is probably because of the presence of neoangiogenesis in both malignant and functional tumours.
- No single ultrasound finding differentiates categorically between benign and malignant ovarian masses.

Tumour markers

Serum CA125

- It is raised in > 80% of ovarian cancer cases (epithelial cancer). However, it is raised in only 50% of stage I cases.
- With a cut-off of 30 units/ml, it has sensitivity of 81% and specificity of 75%.
- It is not specific for ovarian cancer as it may also be raised in benign conditions – fibroids, endometriosis, adenomyosis, benign cysts, and in many other malignancies.
- It is unreliable in differentiating benign from malignant ovarian masses in pre-menopausal women because of the increased rate of false positives and reduced specificity.

Serum CA125 in peri-menopausal women

- Do not request when a clear USS diagnosis of a simple ovarian cyst has been made.
- Raised and < 200 units/ml – further investigation may be appropriate to exclude/treat the common differential diagnoses.
- Raised – serial monitoring of CA125 may be helpful as rapidly rising levels are more likely to be associated with malignancy.
- > 200 units/ml – discuss with a gynaecological oncologist.

Lactate dehydrogenase (LDH), -AFP, and hCG

In all women under age of 40 years with a complex ovarian mass because of the possibility of germ cell tumours.

Estimate the risk of malignancy

International Ovarian Tumor Analysis (IOTA) Group

- To estimate risk of malignancy in pre-menopausal women without using CA125. The use of specific ultrasound morphological findings without CA125 has high sensitivity, specificity, and likelihood ratios.
- **B-rules** – unilocular cysts, presence of solid components where the largest solid component < 7 mm, presence of acoustic shadows, smooth multi-locular tumour with a largest diameter < 100 mm, no blood flow. Classify masses as benign (B-rules) or malignant (M-rules).
- **M-rules** – irregular solid tumour, ascites, at least four papillary structures, irregular multi-locular solid tumour with largest diameter ≥100 mm, very strong blood flow.
- Using these rules, the sensitivity is 95%, specificity 91%, positive likelihood ratio 10, and negative likelihood ratio 0.06.
- Refer women with an ovarian mass with any of the M-rules ultrasound findings to a gynaecological oncologist.

Risk of malignancy index (RMI)

- Combines sonographic findings, menopausal status, and serum CA125 levels to provide an estimate of the risk of malignancy.
- With a cut-off point of 250 units/ml, sensitivity is 70% and specificity is 90%.
- RMI = U × M × CA125.
- U = 0 (USS score of 0), U = 1 (USS score of 1), U = 3 (USS score of 2–5).
- USS are scored one point for each of the following characteristics: multilocular cyst, evidence of solid areas, evidence of metastases, presence of ascites, bilateral lesions.
- M = 3 for all post-menopausal women, 1 for pre-menopausal women.
- CA125 is serum CA125 measurement in units/ml.

℞ Management in post-menopausal women – based on RMI

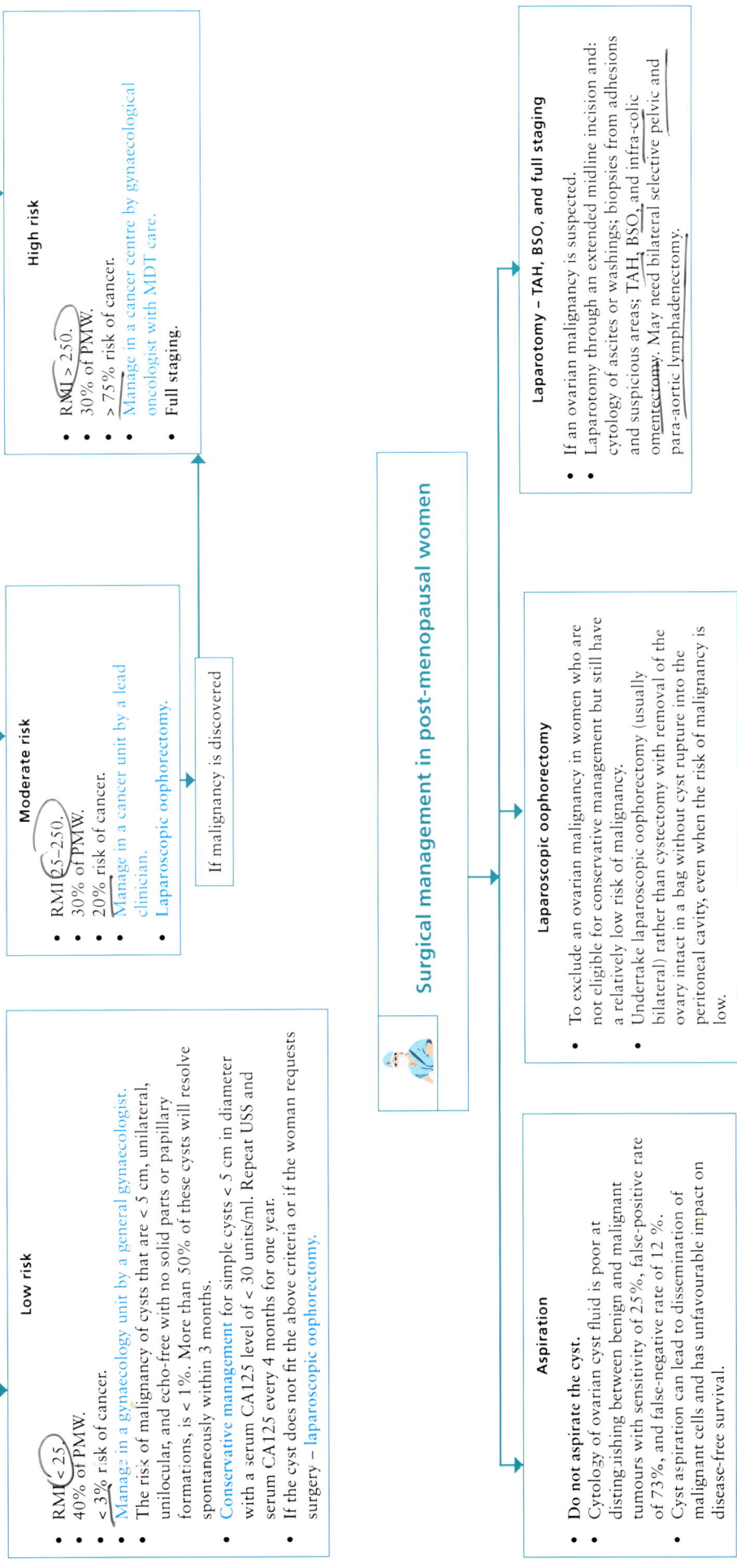

Low risk

- RMI <25.
- 40% of PMW.
- < 3% risk of cancer.
- Manage in a gynaecology unit by a general gynaecologist.
- The risk of malignancy of cysts that are < 5 cm, unilateral, unilocular, and echo-free with no solid parts or papillary formations, is < 1%. More than 50% of these cysts will resolve spontaneously within 3 months.
- Conservative management for simple cysts < 5 cm in diameter with a serum CA125 level of < 30 units/ml. Repeat USS and serum CA125 every 4 months for one year.
- If the cyst does not fit the above criteria or if the woman requests surgery – laparoscopic oophorectomy.

Moderate risk

- RMI 25–250.
- 30% of PMW.
- 20% risk of cancer.
- Manage in a cancer unit by a lead clinician.
- Laparoscopic oophorectomy.

If malignancy is discovered

High risk

- RMI > 250.
- 30% of PMW.
- > 75% risk of cancer.
- Manage in a cancer centre by gynaecological oncologist with MDT care.
- Full staging.

Surgical management in post-menopausal women

Aspiration

- **Do not aspirate the cyst.**
- Cytology of ovarian cyst fluid is poor at distinguishing between benign and malignant tumours with sensitivity of 25%, false-positive rate of 73%, and false-negative rate of 12 %.
- Cyst aspiration can lead to dissemination of malignant cells and has unfavourable impact on disease-free survival.

Laparoscopic oophorectomy

- To exclude an ovarian malignancy in women who are not eligible for conservative management but still have a relatively low risk of malignancy.
- Undertake laparoscopic oophorectomy (usually bilateral) rather than cystectomy with removal of the ovary intact in a bag without cyst rupture into the peritoneal cavity, even when the risk of malignancy is low.

Laparotomy – TAH, BSO, and full staging

- If an ovarian malignancy is suspected.
- Laparotomy through an extended midline incision and: cytology of ascites or washings; biopsies from adhesions and suspicious areas; TAH, BSO, and infra-colic omentectomy. May need bilateral selective pelvic and para-aortic lymphadenectomy.

If a malignancy is revealed – refer urgently to a cancer centre for further management.

See Chapter 37.

℞ Management in pre-menopausal women

Expectant

- Small (< 50 mm diameter) simple ovarian cysts – do not require follow-up as these cysts are very likely to be physiological and almost always resolve within 3 menstrual cycles.
- Simple ovarian cysts of 50–70 mm in diameter – follow-up yearly with USS.

Medical management

- Cochrane review – use of the COCs does **not promote the resolution of functional ovarian cysts.**
- Hormonal suppression, with the COCs, may be useful in young women who develop recurrent painful functional cysts in the ovaries.

Surgical management

- **Simple ovarian cysts of > 70 mm in diameter** – consider for either further imaging (MRI) or surgical intervention, owing to difficulties in examining the entire cyst adequately with USS.
- Surgically manage ovarian cysts that persist or increase in size as they are unlikely to be functional. There is no consensus on the size above which surgery is indicated. Most studies have used an arbitrary maximum diameter of 50–60 mm to offer conservative management.
- Appropriate route for the surgical management depends on – the woman (suitability for laparoscopy and her wishes), the mass (size, complexity, likely nature), and the setting (surgeon's skills and equipment).

Cyst aspiration

- Transvaginal USS-guided or laparoscopic.
- **It is associated with a high rate of recurrence of 53%–84%.**
- Aspiration is not superior to regular observation.
- Consider cyst aspiration:
  * Treatment of a simple cyst during ovulation induction for treatment of infertility.
  * In women with symptomatic cysts who are at high risk of medical complications of anaesthesia.

Cystotomy

- Cystotomy and stripping of cyst wall – the cyst is opened and the internal cyst wall is stripped away from the underlying stroma. There is a higher chance of bleeding from the stripped site and damage to adjacent primordial follicles with possible compromise of ovarian function and higher incidence of adhesion formation.
- Cystotomy and ablation of cyst wall – the cyst is first aspirated then opened sufficiently to admit a diathermy or laser. The cyst wall is then destroyed. A proportion of ovarian follicles will be lost due to thermal injury. Consider this if the cyst lining seems more adherent and vascular.

Cystectomy

- Removal of the cyst intact. The resulting defect may either be closed with sutures, treated with bipolar cautery, or left open to heal. No method is superior in terms of healing and postoperative adhesion formation.
- It is the preferred method of treatment of:
  * Dermoid cysts, in order to avoid intraperitoneal spillage of cyst content.
  * If there is a low but possible chance of malignancy in a young woman wishing to preserve her fertility.

Oophorectomy

- Preoperatively discuss the possibility of removing the ovary.
- Oophorectomy may be necessary if the ovary is grossly distorted with multiple endometriomas with complete loss of normal ovarian tissue.

Surgical management (contd.)

Laparotomy and staging

- In presence of large masses with solid components, laparotomy may be appropriate. Also indicated:
  * If there is suspicion of malignancy.
  * If the patient is unfit for laparoscopy because of obesity or extensive abdominal scarring following previous surgery.
- Maximum cyst size above which laparotomy should be considered is controversial. Cyst rupture is reported more often in the laparoscopy group in women with cysts > 70 mm. It is likely that drainage or removal of large ovarian cysts will require significant extension of the laparoscopic port incision, in which case the advantages of laparoscopic approach would be reduced.

Laparoscopy

- It is associated with lower postoperative pain, fewer postoperative complications, and shorter recovery time. It is preferred to laparotomy in suitable patients. It is also cost-effective because of earlier discharge and return to work.
- Avoid unplanned rupture of the cyst to avoid spillage of cyst contents because:
  * The apparently benign characteristics of a cyst on preoperative and intraoperative assessment cannot absolutely preclude malignancy.
  * Chemical peritonitis owing to spillage of dermoid cyst contents occurs in < 0.2% of cases.
- Consider using a tissue bag to avoid peritoneal spill of cystic contents.
- If inadvertent spillage does occur, lavage the peritoneal cavity meticulously. Remove any solid content using an appropriate bag.
- RCOG – in case of endometrioma, obtain histology to exclude rare cases of malignancy. Obtaining such histology using the standard surgical technique will inevitably cause peritoneal spill of cyst contents. There is a risk of inadvertently upstaging a tumour if the suspected endometrioma is actually a malignant tumour. As there is no effective preoperative discriminator between an endometrioma and some rare cases of ovarian cancer, such upstaging may be inevitable. This is rare: in one series, no cases of malignancy in 814 women were reported with endometriomas of > 30 mm in diameter.
- Try to remove benign ovarian masses via the umbilical port. This results in less postoperative pain and a quicker retrieval time than when using lateral ports of the same size.
- Avoidance of extending accessory ports reduces postoperative pain, incidence of incisional hernia, and epigastric vessel injury. It also has better cosmesis.

What not to do

- CA125, when a clear USS diagnosis of a simple ovarian cyst has been made.
- Routine use of CT, MRI.
- Aspiration of ovarian cyst.
- Spillage of cyst contents.
- Follow-up for women with small (< 50 mm diameter) simple ovarian cysts.

1. *Management of Suspected Ovarian Masses in Premenopausal Women.* Joint RCOG/BSGE Green-top Guideline No. 62, 2011.
2. *Ovarian Cysts in Postmenopausal Women.* RCOG Guideline No. 34, October 2003.
3. *Initial Evaluation and Referral Guidelines for Management of Pelvic/Ovarian Masses.* Joint SOGC/GOC/SCC Clinical Practice Guideline No 230, July 2009.
4. American College of Obstetricians and Gynecologists. *Management of Adnexal Masses.* ACOG Practice Bulletin No. 83. 2007.
5. Hart FJ, Hickey M, Maouris P, Buckett W. Excisional surgery versus ablative surgery for ovarian endometriomata. *Cochrane Database Syst Rev* 2008;2:CD004992.

CHAPTER 37 Ovarian cancer

Prevalence and incidence

In the UK

- Ovarian cancer is the 5th most common cancer in women and the second most common gynaecological cancer.
- There are 7000 (20.9/100,000 women) new cases per year.
- Lifetime risk of ovarian cancer is 1/54.
- ≈4300 women die of ovarian cancer every year.
- 6% of all cancer deaths in women. Ovarian cancer accounts for more deaths than all the other gynaecological cancers combined.
- 72% of women survive for at least one year, falling to 43% by 5 years or more.

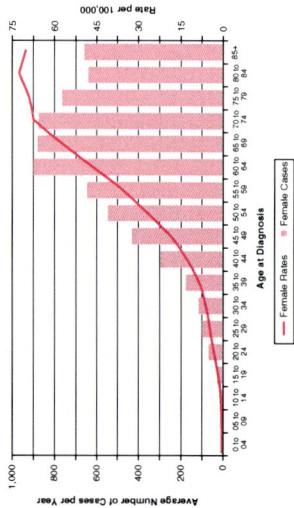

New cases per year and age-specific incidence rates, UK, 2009–2011

History

- Any of the following symptoms, which are persistent or frequent particularly for more than 12 times/month (especially in women ≥ 50 years of age):
  * Persistent abdominal distension ('bloating').
  * Feeling full (early satiety) and/or loss of appetite.
  * Pelvic or abdominal pain.
  * Increased urinary urgency and/or frequency.
- Symptoms within the last 12 months that suggest IBS, as IBS rarely presents for the first time in women of this age.
- Unexplained weight loss, fatigue, changes in bowel habit.
- PMB.

Examination

- A pelvic or abdominal mass. • Ascites.

Risk factors

- Age – disease of older, post-menopausal women with over 80% of cases being diagnosed in women aged over 50 years. There is a steep increase in incidence after the usual age of the menopause. The highest age-specific incidence rates are seen for women aged 80–84 years (69/100,000), dropping to 64/100,000 in women aged ≥ 85 years.
- Ethnicity – higher in whites compared with Asians and blacks.
- Family history – women with no family history have 1.5% lifetime risk; those with one affected first-degree relative have 5% lifetime risk; and those with two first-degree relatives have a 7% lifetime risk.
- Genetics – approximately 5–10% of cases are a result of BRCA1 and BRCA2 mutations. Lifetime risk with BRCA mutations ≤ 15–60%. Associated with multiple primary cancers or early onset cancers in a family tree (breast/ovary/colorectal).
- Risk tends to be reduced by factors that interrupt ovulation such as pregnancy, breastfeeding and oral contraceptive use. While prolonged exposure to ovulation such as nulliparity and infertility increase risk. Women who have given birth have a lower risk of ovarian cancer than women who have not.
- HRT – 5 years of use of oestrogen-only HRT increased the risk by 22%, significantly more than the 10% risk increase with use of oestrogen–progestin HRT. The risk is increased for current users of HRT and the risk increases with duration of use, becoming significant after 7 or more years of use. Past or short-term use of HRT is unlikely to increase the risk of ovarian cancer.
- Smoking increases risk of ovarian cancer, doubling risk of mucinous tumours.

Screening

Low-risk women

- CA125 – low sensitivity and specificity.
  * Only about 85% of women with ovarian cancer have raised CA125.
  * Only 50% of women with early stage ovarian cancer have raised CA125.
  * Women with other conditions can also have raised CA125.
- TVS – low specificity.
- UKCTOCS – investigates ovarian cancer screening in women in the general population between the ages of 50 and 74 years, with CA125 and TVS. Early results suggest that CA125 and TVS can be used on a large scale to successfully identify ovarian cancers. Over the next 5 years, the study will be looking at whether an ovarian screening programme using these tests could help to reduce deaths in the UK from ovarian cancer.

High-risk women

Women with ≥ 2 relatives on the same side of the family diagnosed with ovarian cancer or breast cancer at a young age (strong family history or inheritance of a particular faulty gene). (Cancerresearch.org.uk, nhs.uk)
- If at higher risk, women can be screened for breast cancer from 35 years old onwards or from 5 years before the age at which the youngest relative was diagnosed.
  * Screening will then carry on yearly for the rest of life.
- The UK Familial Ovarian Cancer Screening Study (UKFOCSS) study – screening women who are at a high risk of developing ovarian cancer because of a family history of cancer of the ovary or breast, or they have family members with a known genetic fault (such as BRCA1 or BRCA2). Results awaited.

Investigations

NICE referral pathway
Primary healthcare – GP

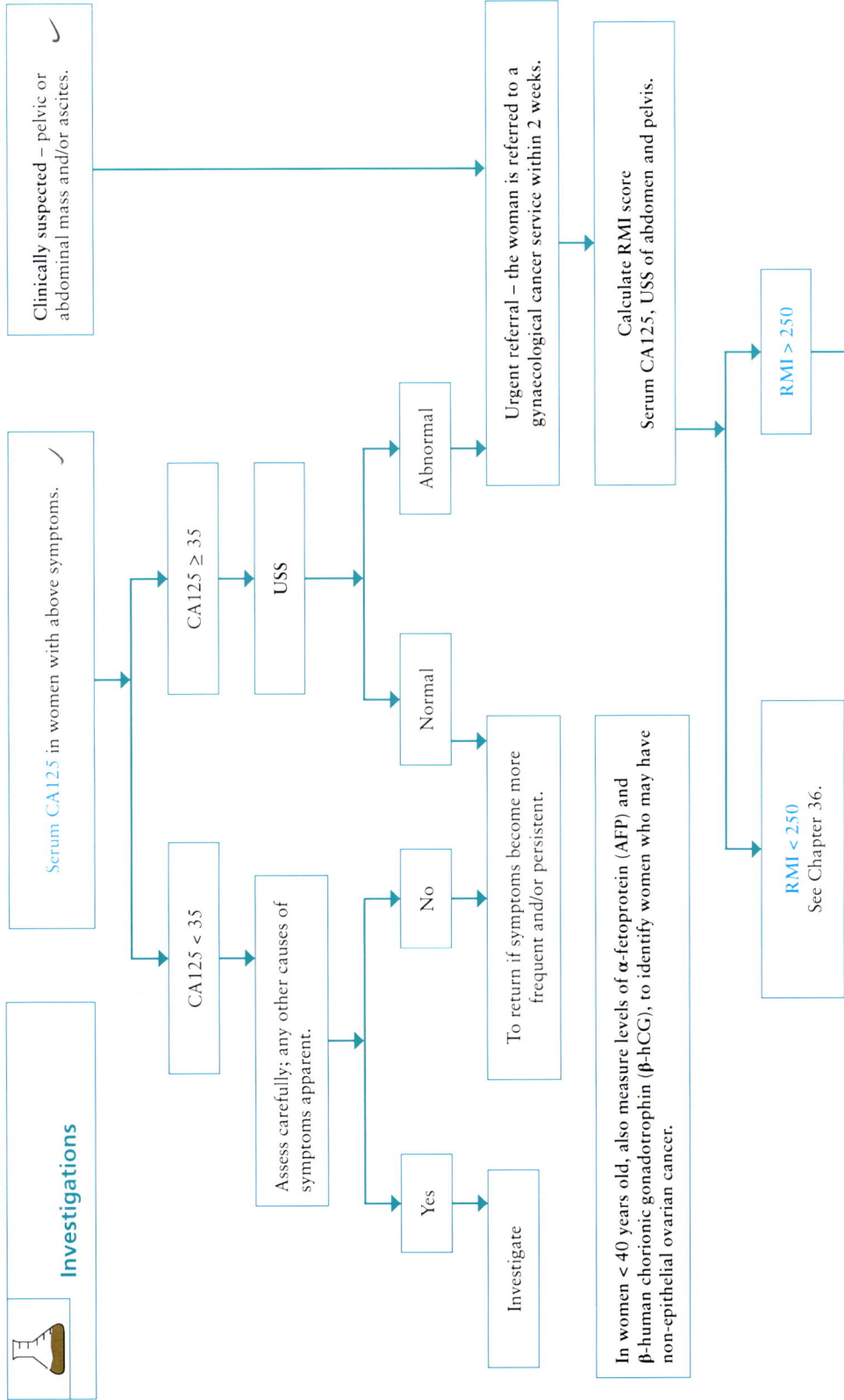

Serum CA125 in women with above symptoms.

Clinically suspected – pelvic or abdominal mass and/or ascites.

CA125 < 35

Assess carefully; any other causes of symptoms apparent.

- **Yes** → Investigate
- **No** → To return if symptoms become more frequent and/or persistent.

CA125 ≥ 35 → **USS**

- **Normal** → To return if symptoms become more frequent and/or persistent.
- **Abnormal** → Urgent referral – the woman is referred to a gynaecological cancer service within 2 weeks.

Calculate RMI score
Serum CA125, USS of abdomen and pelvis.

- **RMI < 250** See Chapter 36.
- **RMI > 250** → **Referral to gynaecology oncology centre for MDT** (gynaecological oncologists, medical oncologists, pathologists, radiologists, and nurses).
  - **CT scan** of the pelvis and abdomen (thorax if clinically indicated).
  - Chest X-ray, FBC, renal and LFT before surgery/chemotherapy.
  - Offer information, including psychosocial and psychosexual issues.
  - **Surgical staging or tissue diagnosis** by histology or cytology.

In women < 40 years old, also measure levels of α-fetoprotein (AFP) and β-human chorionic gonadotrophin (β-hCG), to identify women who may have non-epithelial ovarian cancer.

RMI = USS score (U) × menopausal status (M) × CA125 level.
USS = 1 point for each: multilocular cysts, solid areas, metastases, ascites, bilateral lesions. U = 0 for a USS score of 0 points, U = 1 for an USS score of 1 point, U = 3 for an USS score of 2–5 points.
Menopausal status is scored as 1 = pre-menopausal and 3 = post-menopausal.

CHAPTER 37 Ovarian cancer

Staging

FIGO and American Joint Committee on Cancer (AJCC)

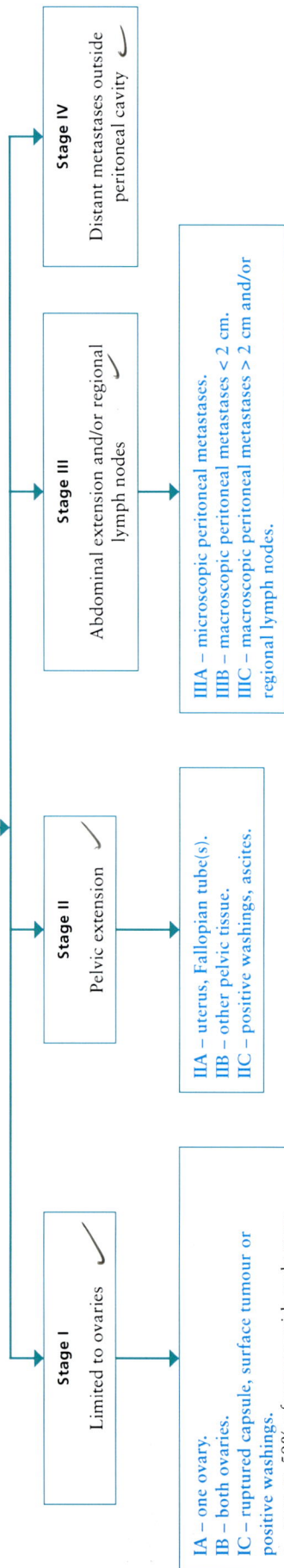

Stage I	**Stage II**	**Stage III**	**Stage IV**
Limited to ovaries	Pelvic extension	Abdominal extension and/or regional lymph nodes	Distant metastases outside peritoneal cavity

IA – one ovary.
IB – both ovaries.
IC – ruptured capsule, surface tumour or positive washings.

- ≈ up to 50% of women with early stage cancer will develop a recurrence and 20–30% will die from the disease.
- Women with stage I disease tend to be younger; 50% will have a normal serum CA125 level; USS features can appear benign.
- ≈ 25% of women with apparent early stage will have more advanced disease.

IIA – uterus, Fallopian tube(s).
IIB – other pelvic tissue.
IIC – positive washings, ascites.

Stage I tumours with dense adhesions to other pelvic structures should be 'upstaged' and treated as stage II tumours, as the relapse rate appears to be similar.

IIIA – microscopic peritoneal metastases.
IIIB – macroscopic peritoneal metastases < 2 cm.
IIIC – macroscopic peritoneal metastases > 2 cm and/or regional lymph nodes.

- Type of surgery and postoperative chemotherapy depends upon the stage and other clinicopathological prognostic factors.
  Favourable prognostic factors:
  * Surgical stage. * Small tumour volume (before and after surgery). * Younger age.
  * Good performance status. * Cell type other than mucinous or clear cell.
  * Well-differentiated tumour. * Absence of ascites.
- Good prognostic factors for patients with stage I disease: * Low grade.
  * Absence of dense adhesions. * Minimal ascites. * Subgroups A/B vs C.
  * Cell type other than clear cell.

Epithelial ovarian cancer subtypes – serous, mucinous, endometrioid, clear cell, transitional cell, mixed, and undifferentiated carcinomas.

FIGO Classification – Ovary

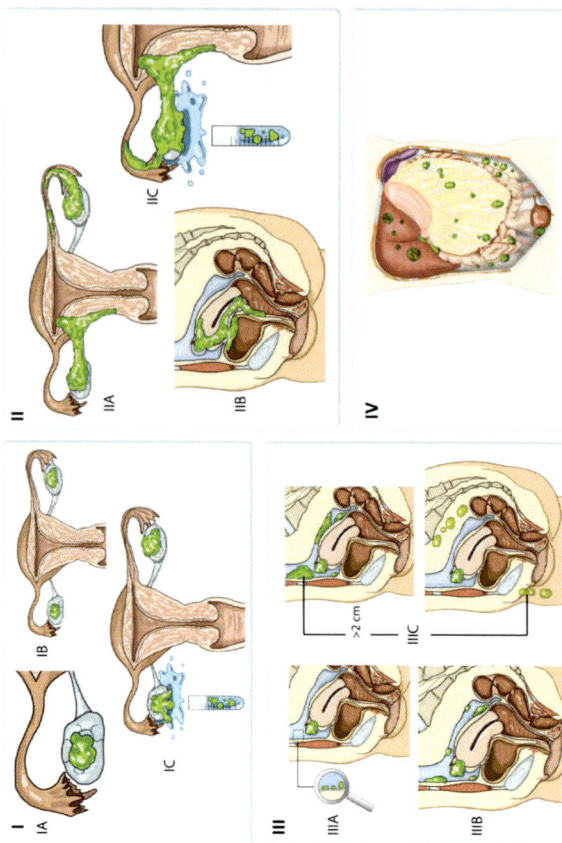

Used with permission from e-anatomy, Micheav A. Hoo D, www.imaios.com (http//www.imaios.com)

Management

Early stage disease, FIGO stage I and IIA

- **Optimal surgery** – midline laparotomy, TAH, BSO, infracolic omentectomy; biopsies of any peritoneal deposits; random biopsies of the pelvic and abdominal peritoneum; and retroperitoneal lymph node assessment.
- **Retroperitoneal lymph node assessment** – sampling of retroperitoneal lymphatic tissue from the para-aortic area and pelvic side walls if there is a palpable abnormality, or random sampling if there is no palpable abnormality.
- Do not perform **systematic retroperitoneal lymphadenectomy** (SRL – block dissection of lymph nodes from the pelvic side walls to the level of the renal veins) as part of standard surgical treatment.

- Younger patients with localized, unilateral tumours and favourable histology, who wish to conserve fertility, unilateral salpingo-oophorectomy may be sufficient. Wedge biopsy of the contralateral ovary – if the contralateral ovary is not normal on inspection.

- Stage IA/B, well-differentiated, non-clear cell histology – optimal surgery alone is adequate.
- Do not offer adjuvant chemotherapy to women who have had optimal surgical staging and have low-risk stage I disease (grade 1 or 2, stage IA or IB).

Role of systematic retroperitoneal lymphadenectomy (SRL)

- Around 22% of women considered to have stage I ovarian cancer will have occult retroperitoneal lymph node metastases, which can only be identified by removing affected nodes. Current surgical staging guidelines recommend only sampling a number of pelvic and/or para-aortic nodes, whereas SRL aims to remove all pelvic and para-aortic lymph nodes up to the renal vessels as a block dissection on both sides.
- SRL is a major surgical procedure with potential risks of prolonged anaesthesia and surgical complications such as increased blood loss and transfusion, ureteric injury, lymphoedema, lymphocysts, damage to nerves and major vessels.
- No international agreement on whether the potential survival benefits of SRL outweigh the risks.
- Use of perioperative frozen section might be a way of selecting patients who need SRL.

Advanced disease, FIGO stage IIB and above

See next page.

- Stage IA/B poorly differentiated, densely adherent, clear cell histology and all grades, stage IC and IIA – optimal surgery, staging, and adjuvant chemotherapy. Women with high-risk stage I disease (grade 3 or stage IC) – adjuvant chemotherapy with 6 cycles of carboplatin.

Role of adjuvant systemic chemotherapy

- In women with apparent stage I disease, chemotherapy can be given in certain circumstances, such as poorly differentiated tumours and in certain histological subtypes (for example, clear cell carcinomas). This is done to treat residual disease that is suspected but may not, in fact, exist. Therefore, some women without residual disease will receive chemotherapy with its associated risks.
- Cochrane review – women receiving adjuvant therapy have a considerable advantage in overall survival and progression-free survival. In particular, those women who have been inadequately staged gain survival advantage from immediate adjuvant chemotherapy.

Advanced disease, FIGO stage IIB–IIIC

Maximal cytoreduction + chemotherapy

- Surgery – TAH, BSO, omentectomy with staging biopsies. Maximal cytoreduction with the objective of complete resection of all macroscopic disease.
- If initial maximal cytoreduction is not performed, consider **interval debulking surgery (IDS)** in patients responding to chemotherapy, or showing stable disease.
- IDS should ideally be performed after 3 cycles of chemotherapy, followed by 3 further cycles of chemotherapy.

- There is no evidence of a survival benefit for 'second-look' surgery following completion of chemotherapy in patients whose disease appears to be in complete remission.
- Value of secondary tumour reduction at the time of second-look laparotomy is not clear.

- **First-line chemotherapy** (usually following surgery).
  * Paclitaxel in combination with a platinum-based compound (PBC).
  * Or platinum-based therapy (PBT) alone (cisplatin or carboplatin).
- Do not offer intraperitoneal chemotherapy, except as part of a clinical trial. (NICE)
- **Consider neoadjuvant chemotherapy** for patients considered initially not optimally resectable. The survival outcome may be inferior to that from successful primary surgery followed by chemotherapy.

Advanced disease, FIGO stage IV

Maximal cytoreduction/tissue biopsy + chemotherapy

- Patients may obtain a survival advantage from having **maximal surgically cytoreduction** at initial laparotomy.
- Younger patients with good performance status, pleural effusion as the only site of disease outside the abdominal cavity, small volume metastases, and no major organ dysfunction should be considered for **surgery as for stage IIB–III disease.**
- If surgery is not planned, the diagnosis should be confirmed by biopsy and **chemotherapy** administered as recommended for stage IIB–IIIC disease.

- **Tissue diagnosis** – obtain a tissue diagnosis by histology (or cytology) in all but exceptional cases prior to chemotherapy.
- Offer chemotherapy without a tissue diagnosis (histology or cytology), only:
  * In exceptional cases, after discussion with the MDT.
  * After discussion with the woman regarding the possible benefits and risks.
- If surgery has not been performed, use histology rather than cytology to obtain a tissue diagnosis by:
  * Percutaneous image-guided biopsy.
  * Consider laparoscopic biopsy if percutaneous image-guided biopsy is not feasible or has not produced an adequate sample.
  * Use cytology if histology is not appropriate.

There is no evidence to support the use of adjuvant radiotherapy in epithelial ovarian cancer.

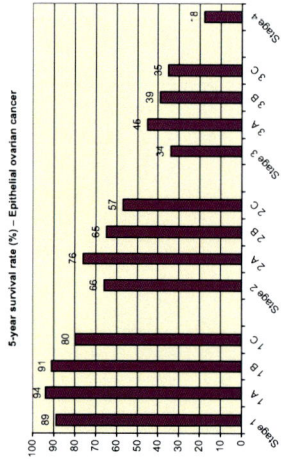

5-year survival rate (%) – Epithelial ovarian cancer

Next page

Evidence round-up

Advanced disease, FIGO stage II and above

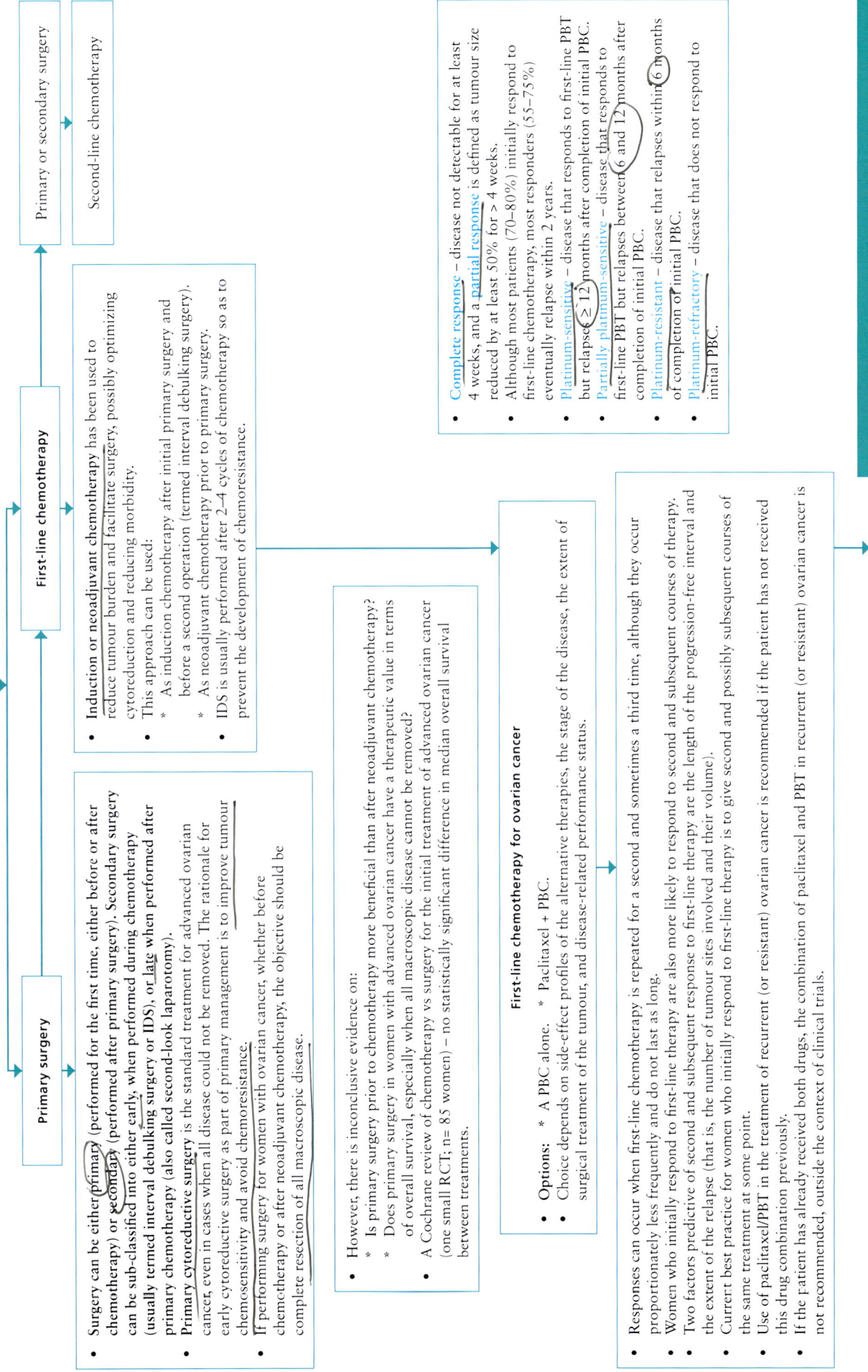

Primary surgery → **First-line chemotherapy** → **Primary or secondary surgery** → **Second-line chemotherapy**

- Surgery can be either (primary) (performed for the first time, either before or after chemotherapy) or (secondary) (performed after primary surgery). Secondary surgery can be sub-classified into either early, when performed during chemotherapy (usually termed interval debulking surgery or IDS), or late when performed after primary chemotherapy (also called second-look laparotomy).
- Primary cytoreductive surgery is the standard treatment for advanced ovarian cancer, even in cases when all disease could not be removed. The rationale for early cytoreductive surgery as part of primary management is to improve tumour chemosensitivity and avoid chemoresistance.
- If performing surgery for women with ovarian cancer, whether before chemotherapy or after neoadjuvant chemotherapy, the objective should be complete resection of all macroscopic disease.

- Induction or neoadjuvant chemotherapy has been used to reduce tumour burden and facilitate surgery, possibly optimizing cytoreduction and reducing morbidity.
- This approach can be used:
  * As induction chemotherapy after initial primary surgery and before a second operation (termed interval debulking surgery).
  * As neoadjuvant chemotherapy prior to primary surgery.
  * IDS is usually performed after 2–4 cycles of chemotherapy so as to prevent the development of chemoresistance.

- However, there is inconclusive evidence on:
  * Is primary surgery prior to chemotherapy more beneficial than after neoadjuvant chemotherapy?
  * Does primary surgery in women with advanced ovarian cancer have a therapeutic value in terms of overall survival, especially when all macroscopic disease cannot be removed?
- A Cochrane review of chemotherapy vs surgery for the initial treatment of advanced ovarian cancer (one small RCT; n= 85 women) – no statistically significant difference in median overall survival between treatments.

First-line chemotherapy for ovarian cancer

- **Options:** * A PBC alone. * Paclitaxel + PBC.
- Choice depends on side-effect profiles of the alternative therapies, the stage of the disease, the extent of surgical treatment of the tumour, and disease-related performance status.

- Responses can occur when first-line chemotherapy is repeated for a second and sometimes a third time, although they occur proportionately less frequently and do not last as long.
- Women who initially respond to first-line therapy are also more likely to respond to second and subsequent courses of therapy.
- Two factors predictive of second and subsequent response to first-line therapy are the length of the progression-free interval and the extent of the relapse (that is, the number of tumour sites involved and their volume).
- Current best practice for women who initially respond to first-line therapy is to give second and possibly subsequent courses of the same treatment at some point.
- Use of paclitaxel/PBT in the treatment of recurrent (or resistant) ovarian cancer is recommended if the patient has not received this drug combination previously.
- If the patient has already received both drugs, the combination of paclitaxel and PBT in recurrent (or resistant) ovarian cancer is not recommended, outside the context of clinical trials.

- Complete response – disease not detectable for at least 4 weeks, and a partial response is defined as tumour size reduced by at least 50% for > 4 weeks.
- Although most patients (70–80%) initially respond to first-line chemotherapy, most responders (55–75%) eventually relapse within 2 years.
- Platinum-sensitive – disease that responds to first-line PBT but relapse ≥ 12 months after completion of initial PBC.
- Partially platinum-sensitive – disease that responds to first-line PBT but relapses between 6 and 12 months after completion of initial PBC.
- Platinum-resistant – disease that relapses within 6 months of completion of initial PBC.
- Platinum-refractory – disease that does not respond to initial PBC.

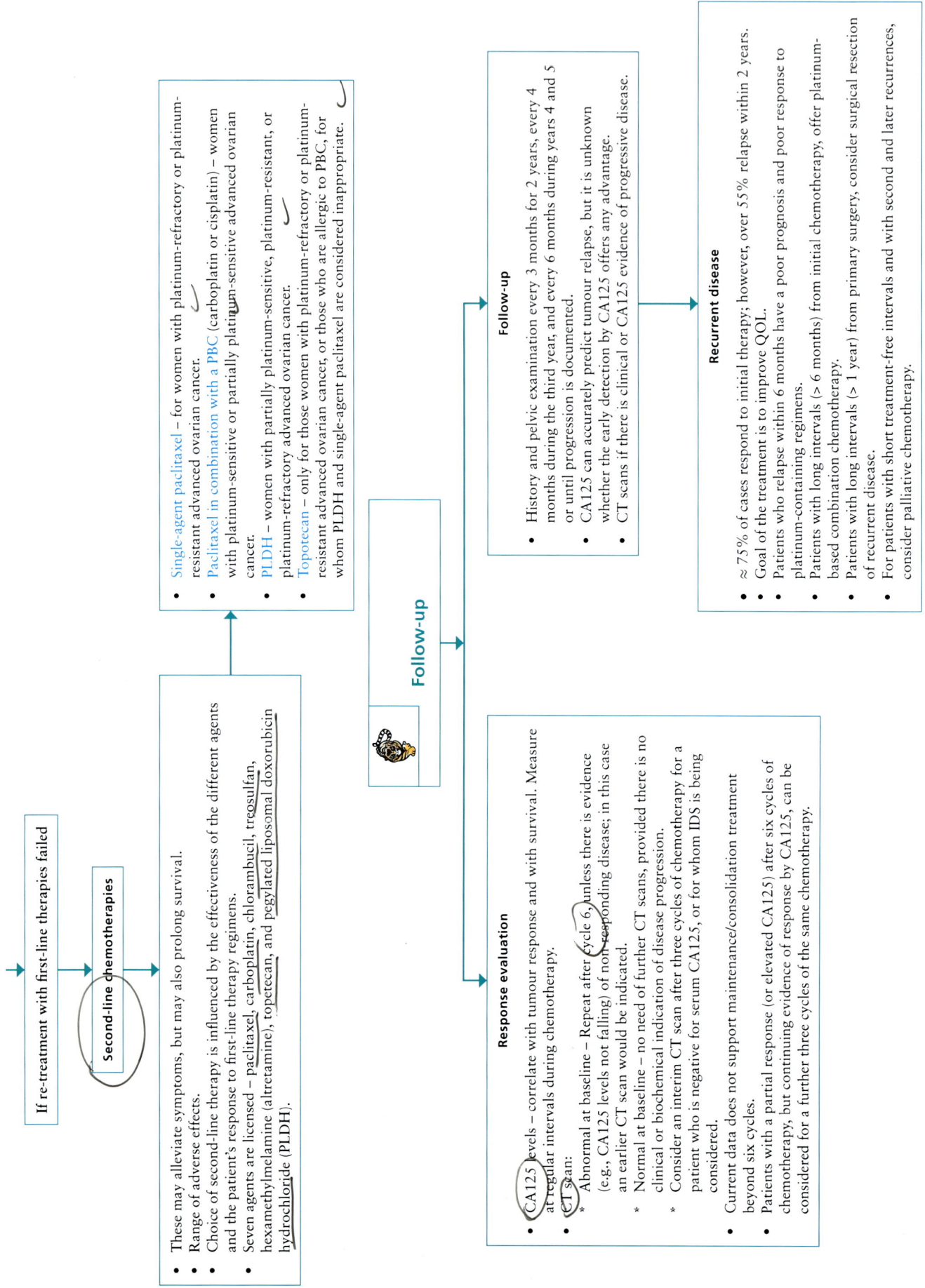

If re-treatment with first-line therapies failed

Second-line chemotherapies

- These may alleviate symptoms, but may also prolong survival.
- Range of adverse effects.
- Choice of second-line therapy is influenced by the effectiveness of the different agents and the patient's response to first-line therapy regimens.
- Seven agents are licensed – paclitaxel, carboplatin, chlorambucil, treosulfan, hexamethylmelamine (altretamine), topotecan, and pegylated liposomal doxorubicin hydrochloride (PLDH).

- Single-agent paclitaxel – for women with platinum-refractory or platinum-resistant advanced ovarian cancer.
- Paclitaxel in combination with a PBC (carboplatin or cisplatin) – women with platinum-sensitive or partially platinum-sensitive advanced ovarian cancer.
- PLDH – women with partially platinum-sensitive, platinum-resistant, or platinum-refractory advanced ovarian cancer.
- Topotecan – only for those women with platinum-refractory or platinum-resistant advanced ovarian cancer, or those who are allergic to PBC, for whom PLDH and single-agent paclitaxel are considered inappropriate.

Follow-up

Response evaluation

- CA125 levels – correlate with tumour response and with survival. Measure at regular intervals during chemotherapy.
- CT scan:
  * Abnormal at baseline – Repeat after cycle 6, unless there is evidence (e.g., CA125 levels not falling) of non-responding disease; in this case an earlier CT scan would be indicated.
  * Normal at baseline – no need of further CT scans, provided there is no clinical or biochemical indication of disease progression.
  * Consider an interim CT scan after three cycles of chemotherapy for a patient who is negative for serum CA125, or for whom IDS is being considered.
- Current data does not support maintenance/consolidation treatment beyond six cycles.
- Patients with a partial response (or elevated CA125) after six cycles of chemotherapy, but continuing evidence of response by CA125, can be considered for a further three cycles of the same chemotherapy.

Follow-up

- History and pelvic examination every 3 months for 2 years, every 4 months during the third year, and every 6 months during years 4 and 5 or until progression is documented.
- CA125 can accurately predict tumour relapse, but it is unknown whether the early detection by CA125 offers any advantage.
- CT scans if there is clinical or CA125 evidence of progressive disease.

Recurrent disease

- ≈ 75% of cases respond to initial therapy; however, over 55% relapse within 2 years.
- Goal of the treatment is to improve QOL.
- Patients who relapse within 6 months have a poor prognosis and poor response to platinum-containing regimens.
- Patients with long intervals (> 6 months) from initial chemotherapy, offer platinum-based combination chemotherapy.
- Patients with long intervals (> 1 year) from primary surgery, consider surgical resection of recurrent disease.
- For patients with short treatment-free intervals and with second and later recurrences, consider palliative chemotherapy.

What will you do?
Role of laparoscopy in ovarian cancer

Laparoscopy for early ovarian cancer

Suspected malignant cyst:

* Obtain pelvic washings at the beginning of the procedure.
* Avoid intentional rupture or open aspiration of any cyst.
* Aspirate cysts within an endoscopic bag to facilitate removal.

Ovarian cancer:

* Role of laparoscopic approach is unclear.
* Obvious spread of disease beyond the ovaries (FIGO stages II–IV) should prompt conversion to a full staging laparotomy.
* One may abandon the operation after performing a biopsy and refer the woman to a gynaecological oncology centre.
* Potential risks of laparoscopic surgery for stage I cancer include under-staging and dissemination of the malignancy.
* Port site metastases have been reported in 1–20% of women with ovarian cancer and in women with advanced disease; it seems unlikely that women with unruptured stage I disease with negative washings are at significant risk.

What will you do?
Young women with ovarian cancer

Fertility-sparing surgery for early ovarian cancer

* The chance that an ovarian cyst is malignant or borderline in a woman < 40 years of age is around 10%.
* In women with a suspicious complex ovarian cyst or mass who wish to conserve their fertility, it would be reasonable to offer a unilateral oophorectomy combined with surgical staging.
* Microscopic involvement of a normal-looking contralateral ovary is rare in stage I ovarian cancer, with a reported frequency of 2.5%.
* Frozen section analysis of abnormal ovarian lesions can avoid unnecessary staging surgery in 99% of women with benign lesions but should identify 90% of women who would benefit.
* A unilateral oophorectomy combined with surgical staging is an optimal primary treatment for borderline or germ cell tumours.
* Effect on fertility of chemotherapy drugs such as platinum agents and taxanes is not well established. The fertility effect of alkylating agents in breast cancer is age-dependent and this suggests that the degree of ovarian reserve is important.
* Women should be fully aware that declining adjuvant treatment can affect their prognosis but they may wish to accept this risk to conserve their fertility. Evidence is limited on this subject.

What not to do

* Screening of low-risk or high-risk women.
* Use of MRI routinely. (NICE)
* Stage I – systematic retroperitoneal lymphadenectomy.
* Stage II and III – intraperitoneal chemotherapy, except as part of a clinical trial. (NICE)
* Adjuvant radiotherapy in epithelial ovarian cancer.
* Maintenance/consolidation treatment beyond 6 cycles.
* Intentional rupture or open aspiration of any cyst at the time of laparoscopy.

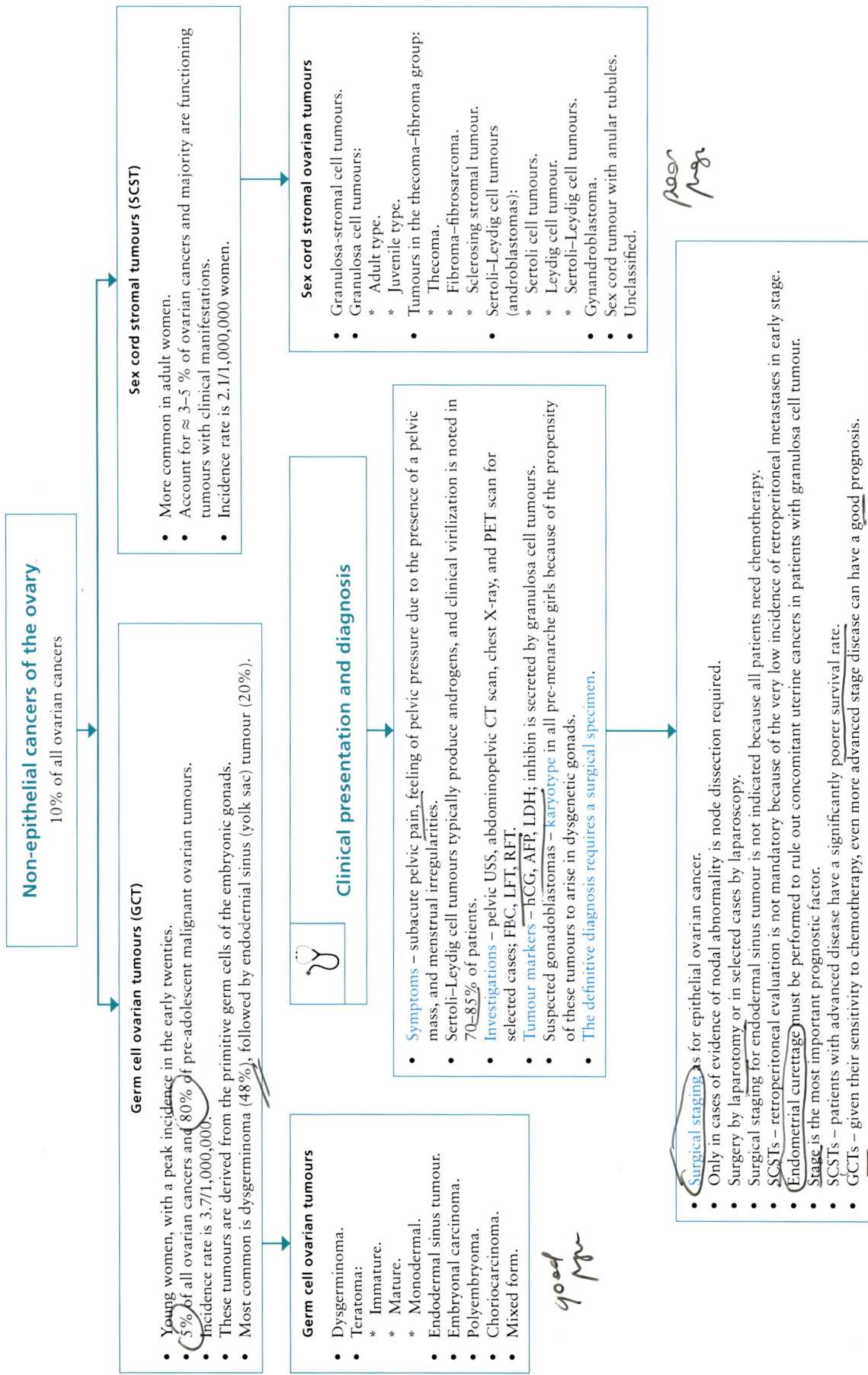

Non-epithelial cancers of the ovary

10% of all ovarian cancers

Germ cell ovarian tumours (GCT)

- Young women, with a peak incidence in the early twenties.
- 5% of all ovarian cancers and 80% of pre-adolescent malignant ovarian tumours.
- Incidence rate is 3.7/1,000,000.
- These tumours are derived from the primitive germ cells of the embryonic gonads.
- Most common is dysgerminoma (48%), followed by endodermal sinus (yolk sac) tumour (20%).

Germ cell ovarian tumours

- Dysgerminoma.
- Teratoma:
  * Immature.
  * Mature.
  * Monodermal.
- Endodermal sinus tumour.
- Embryonal carcinoma.
- Polyembryoma.
- Choriocarcinoma.
- Mixed form.

good
Mo

Sex cord stromal tumours (SCST)

- More common in adult women.
- Account for ≈ 3–5 % of ovarian cancers and majority are functioning tumours with clinical manifestations.
- Incidence rate is 2.1/1,000,000 women.

Sex cord stromal ovarian tumours

- Granulosa-stromal cell tumours.
- Granulosa cell tumours:
  * Adult type.
  * Juvenile type.
- Tumours in the thecoma–fibroma group:
  * Thecoma.
  * Fibroma–fibrosarcoma.
  * Sclerosing stromal tumour.
- Sertoli–Leydig cell tumours (androblastomas):
  * Sertoli cell tumours.
  * Leydig cell tumour.
  * Sertoli–Leydig cell tumours.
- Gynandroblastoma.
- Sex cord tumour with anular tubules.
- Unclassified.

poor
Mo

Clinical presentation and diagnosis

- Symptoms – subacute pelvic pain, feeling of pelvic pressure due to the presence of a pelvic mass, and menstrual irregularities.
- Sertoli–Leydig cell tumours typically produce androgens, and clinical virilization is noted in 70–85% of patients.
- Investigations – pelvic USS, abdominopelvic CT scan, chest X-ray, and PET scan for selected cases; FBC, LFT, RFT.
- Tumour markers – hCG, AFP, LDH; inhibin is secreted by granulosa cell tumours.
- Suspected gonadoblastomas – karyotype in all pre-menarche girls because of the propensity of these tumours to arise in dysgenetic gonads.
- The definitive diagnosis requires a surgical specimen.

- Surgical staging is for epithelial ovarian cancer.
- Only in cases of evidence of nodal abnormality is node dissection required.
- Surgery by laparotomy or in selected cases by laparoscopy.
- Surgical staging for endodermal sinus tumour is not indicated because all patients need chemotherapy.
- SCSTs – retroperitoneal evaluation is not mandatory because of the very low incidence of retroperitoneal metastases in early stage.
- Endometrial curettage must be performed to rule out concomitant uterine cancers in patients with granulosa cell tumour.
- Stage is the most important prognostic factor.
- SCSTs – patients with advanced disease have a significantly poorer survival rate.
- GCTs – given their sensitivity to chemotherapy, even more advanced stage disease can have a good prognosis.

Management

Germ cell tumours

- Unilateral salpingo-oophorectomy with preservation of the contralateral ovary and the uterus is possible, even in advanced stages, owing to the sensitivity of the tumour to chemotherapy.
- No systematic ovarian biopsy need be performed where the contralateral ovary is macroscopically normal.

Early stage disease, Stage I–IIA

- 60–70% are diagnosed at an early stage.
- Stage I has long-term disease-free status of 90%.
- After adequate surgical staging, further adjuvant treatment is not required.
- Stage IA immature teratoma or stage I pure dysgerminoma can be treated with surgery only.
- All patients with stage I endodermal sinus are treated with adjuvant combination chemotherapy of bleomycin, etoposide, and cisplatin (BEP).

Advanced disease, Stage IIB–IV

- Debulking surgery, but without major extensive procedures given the high chemosensitivity.
- Platinum-based regimens are the treatment of choice (BEP).
- Optimal duration of therapy is debatable, but three cycles of BEP with completely resected disease and four cycles for patients with macroscopic residual disease seem appropriate.
- Even though dysgerminomas are very sensitive to radiation therapy, there is no evidence to support the use of adjuvant radiation therapy for advanced stage GCTs.

Sex cord stromal tumours

- Conservative surgery in young patients at stage I.
- Post-menopausal women and in patients with advanced stage disease or with bilateral ovarian involvement – TAH and BSO with surgical staging.

Early stage disease, Stage I–IIA

- 60–95% are at stage I at the time of diagnosis.
- Stage I has long-term disease-free status is 90% of the cases.
- Any postoperative treatment is controversial.
- Some authors suggest adjuvant therapy for stage IC patients with high mitotic index. In this case, platinum-based chemotherapy is the treatment of choice.

Advanced disease, Stage IIB–IV

- Debulking surgery.
- Platinum-based chemotherapy with an overall response rate of 63–80%.
- The BEP regimen for 3–6 cycles for adjuvant postoperative chemotherapy and for patients with recurrent SCSTs.
- Taxanes have a favourable toxicity profile.
- Taxane and platinum combination chemotherapy needs future trials.
- Little evidence exists for the use of hormonal or radiation therapy.

Follow-up

Response evaluation

- Serum tumour markers (hCG, AFP, LDH, CA125, and inhibin) can accurately correlate with tumour response during chemotherapy.
- CT scan of the abdomen, pelvis, and chest (in case of suspected lung metastases), and pelvic ultrasound to evaluate the response to chemotherapy in patients with measurable disease.

Follow-up

- **GCT** – ≈ 75% of recurrences occur within the first year after initial treatment; the most common site is the peritoneal cavity and more rarely the retroperitoneal lymph nodes.
- **SCST** – has indolent nature with a tendency to late recurrence (median time to relapse is 4–6 years), requires long-term surveillance. Common sites of recurrence are the upper abdomen (55–70%) and the pelvis (30–45%).

The follow-up visit:
- History, physical, and pelvic examination.
- Tumour markers every 3 months for the first 2 years, and every 6 months during years 3–5 or until progression is documented.
- Pelvic USS every 6 months in those patients who underwent fertility-sparing surgery, whereas CT scan of the abdomen and pelvic is usually performed yearly.

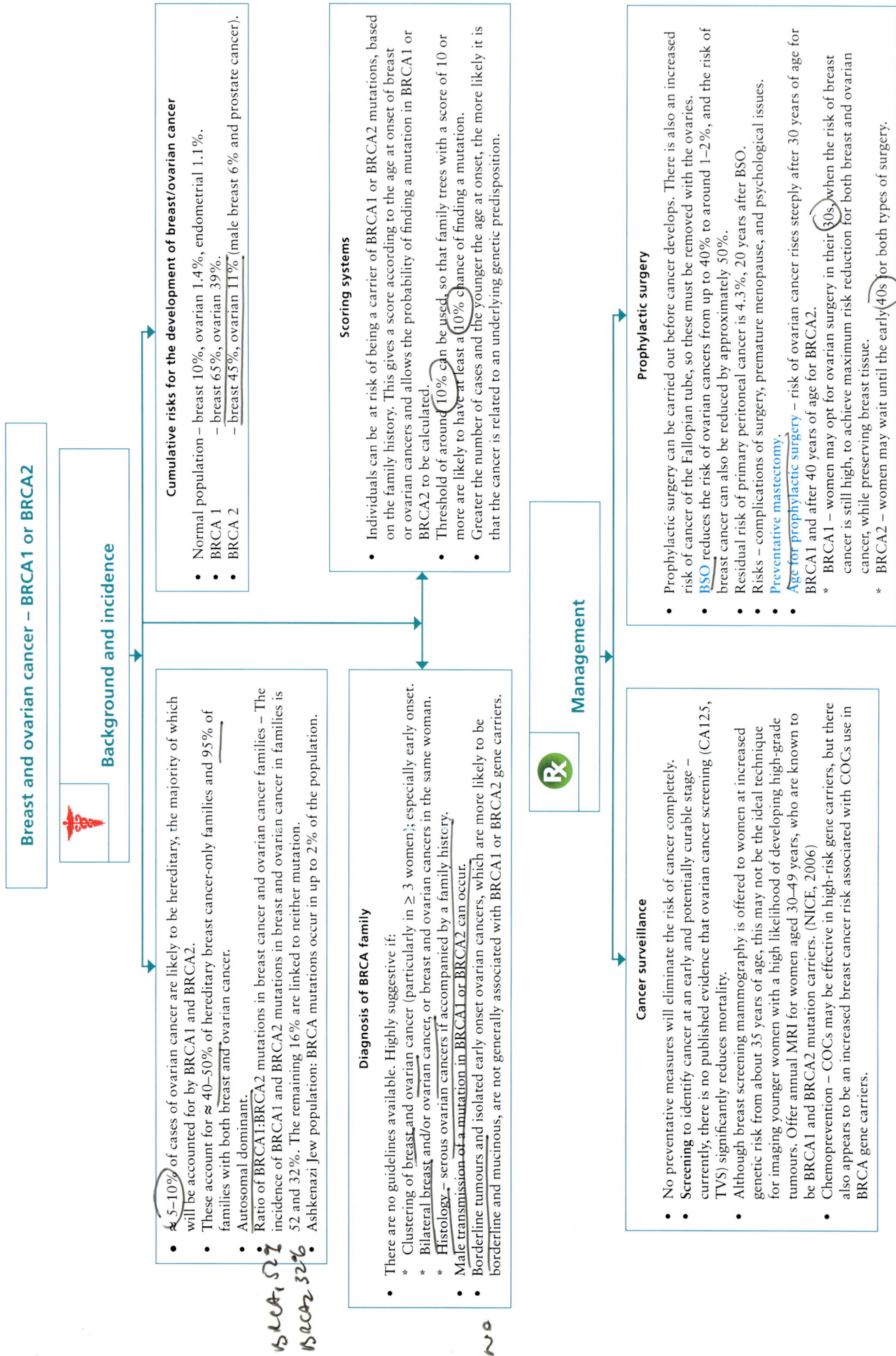

Breast and ovarian cancer – BRCA1 or BRCA2

Background and incidence

- ≈ 5–10% of cases of ovarian cancer are likely to be hereditary, the majority of which will be accounted for by BRCA1 and BRCA2.
- These account for ≈ 40–50% of hereditary breast cancer-only families and 95% of families with both breast and ovarian cancer.
- Autosomal dominant.
- Ratio of BRCA1:BRCA2 mutations in breast cancer and ovarian cancer families – The incidence of BRCA1 and BRCA2 mutations in breast and ovarian cancer in families is 52 and 32%. The remaining 16% are linked to neither mutation.
- Ashkenazi Jew population: BRCA mutations occur in up to 2% of the population.

(handwritten: BRCA₁ 5Z, BRCA₂ 32%)

Cumulative risks for the development of breast/ovarian cancer

- Normal population – breast 10%, ovarian 1.4%, endometrial 1.1%.
- BRCA 1 – breast 65%, ovarian 39%.
- BRCA 2 – breast 45%, ovarian 11% (male breast 6% and prostate cancer).

Diagnosis of BRCA family

- There are no guidelines available. Highly suggestive if:
- * Clustering of breast and ovarian cancer (particularly in ≥ 3 women); especially early onset.
- * Bilateral breast and/or ovarian cancer, or breast and ovarian cancers in the same woman.
- * Histology – serous ovarian cancers if accompanied by a family history.
- Male transmission of a mutation in BRCA1 or BRCA2 can occur.
- Borderline tumours and isolated early onset ovarian cancers, which are more likely to be borderline and mucinous, are not generally associated with BRCA1 or BRCA2 gene carriers.

(handwritten: ✓ a)

Scoring systems

- Individuals can be at risk of being a carrier of BRCA1 or BRCA2 mutations, based on the family history. This gives a score according to the age at onset of breast or ovarian cancers and allows the probability of finding a mutation in BRCA1 or BRCA2 to be calculated.
- Threshold of around 10% can be used, so that family trees with a score of 10 or more are likely to have at least a 10% chance of finding a mutation.
- Greater the number of cases and the younger the age at onset, the more likely it is that the cancer is related to an underlying genetic predisposition.

Management

Cancer surveillance

- No preventative measures will eliminate the risk of cancer completely.
- **Screening** to identify cancer at an early and potentially curable stage – currently, there is no published evidence that ovarian cancer screening (CA125, TVS) significantly reduces mortality.
- Although breast screening mammography is offered to women at increased genetic risk from about 35 years of age, this may not be the ideal technique for imaging younger women with a high likelihood of developing high-grade tumours. Offer annual MRI for women aged 30–49 years, who are known to be BRCA1 and BRCA2 mutation carriers. (NICE, 2006)
- **Chemoprevention** – COCs may be effective in high-risk gene carriers, but there also appears to be an increased breast cancer risk associated with COCs use in BRCA gene carriers.

Prophylactic surgery

- Prophylactic surgery can be carried out before cancer develops. There is also an increased risk of cancer of the Fallopian tube, so these must be removed with the ovaries.
- BSO reduces the risk of ovarian cancers from up to 40% to around 1–2%, and the risk of breast cancer can also be reduced by approximately 50%.
- Residual risk of primary peritoneal cancer is 4.3%, 20 years after BSO.
- Risks – complications of surgery, premature menopause, and psychological issues.
- Preventative mastectomy.
- Age for prophylactic surgery – risk of ovarian cancer rises steeply after 30 years of age for BRCA1 and after 40 years of age for BRCA2.
- * BRCA1 – women may opt for ovarian surgery in their 30s, when the risk of breast cancer is still high, to achieve maximum risk reduction for both breast and ovarian cancer, while preserving breast tissue.
- * BRCA2 – women may wait until the early 40s for both types of surgery.

Hereditary non-polyposis colorectal cancer syndrome (HNPCC)

Background and incidence

- Autosomal dominant.
- Mutations in mismatch repair genes MLH1, MSH2, and MSH6.
- Mutation carriers susceptible to colorectal cancer, endometrial and ovarian cancer, other gastrointestinal tract cancers, urothelial, and brain cancers.
- Smaller percentage of endometrial cancer is likely to be hereditary, with estimates of at least 1.8% of endometrial cancer attributed to HNPCC.

- Cumulative risks for the development of ovarian/endometrial cancer:
  * MLH1 – ovarian 3.4%, endometrial 27%.
  * MSH2 – ovarian 10.4%, endometrial 40%.
  * MSH6 – endometrial 71%.
- MSH2 has a higher risk than MLH1 mutation carriers and MLH1/MSH2 have a higher risk in comparison with MSH6.

Diagnosis of HNPCC family

- Diagnosis of HNPCC family is clinical.
- The Amsterdam criteria (1999) for HNPCC-associated cancers are frequently used to select families for molecular testing. Based on an early age of cancer onset, multiple cancers, and clustering of HNPCC-associated cancers in the family history –
  * There are at least three relatives with an HNPCC-associated cancer (large bowel, endometrium, small bowel, ureter, or renal pelvis; not including stomach, ovary, brain, bladder, or skin). * One affected person is a first-degree relative of the other two.
  * At least two successive generations are affected.
  * At least one person was diagnosed before the age of 50 years.
  * Familial adenomatous polyposis has been excluded.
  * Tumours have been verified by pathological examination.

- Prevalence of mismatch repair gene mutations in HNPCC families – 45% of the families meeting the Amsterdam criteria will have a mutation in MLH1/MSH2.
- MSH6 has a slightly different phenotype in comparison with these two genes, with a later onset of colorectal cancer and a propensity for endometrial cancer in females. The frequency of MSH6 mutations has been estimated to be approximately 10% of all mismatch repair mutations in HNPCC families.
- Up to 50% of HNPCC families do not have an identifiable mutation in any of the known mismatch repair genes.

Management

- Cancer surveillance – 2-yearly colonoscopy may reduce the incidence and mortality from colorectal cancer.
- No such evidence exists for endometrial and ovarian cancer screening.
- Prophylactic hysterectomy/oophorectomy is an option for carrier women, especially for those with a mutation in MSH6, but long-term follow-up is insufficient and further data are needed.
- Trials of ovarian cancer surveillance and IUCDs containing progestogens are ongoing.

1. Colombo N, Peiretti M, Castiglione M. for the ESMO Guidelines Working Group. Non-epithelial ovarian cancer: ESMO clinical recommendations for diagnosis, treatment, and follow-up. *Ann Oncol* 2009;20(4):24–26.
2. Aebi S, Castiglione M. for the ESMO Guidelines Working Group. Newly and relapsed epithelial ovarian carcinoma: ESMO clinical recommendations for diagnosis, treatment, and follow-up. *Ann Oncol* 2009;20(4):iv21–iv23. DOI:10/1093/annonc/mdp117.
3. *Ovarian Cancer: the Recognition and Initial Management of Ovarian Cancer.* NICE Clinical Guideline, April 2011.
4. Devlin LA, Morrison PJ. Inherited gynaecological cancer syndromes. *The Obstetrician and Gynaecologist* 2008;10:9–15.
5. Ali SN, Ledermann JA. Current practice and new developments in ovarian cancer chemotherapy. *The Obstetrician and Gynaecologist* 2007;9:265–269.
6. Images: National Cancer Institute at National Institute of Health.
7. http://www.cancerresearchuk.org/cancer-info/cancerstats/types/ovary/incidence/july2014.
8. *Guidance on the Use of Paclitaxel in the Treatment of Ovarian Cancer.* NICE Technology Appraisal Guidance, January 2003 (last modified, May 2005).
9. http://www.imaios.com/e-Cases/Channels/Radiology/Radiological-classifications-commonly-used-on-medical-imaging/Ovarian-cancer.

CHAPTER 37 Ovarian cancer

CHAPTER 38 Chronic pelvic pain (CPP)

Background and definition

- Definition – intermittent or constant pain in the lower abdomen or pelvis of at least 6 months' duration, not occurring exclusively with menstruation or intercourse and not associated with pregnancy.
- It may be associated with incomplete relief with most treatments; significantly impaired function at home or work; signs of depression, such as early awakening, weight loss, or anorexia; and may significantly impact on a woman's quality of life (QOL).
- Incidence – affects 1/6 of the adult female population.
- Issues – psychological and social issues such as depression and sleep disorders.
- Aetiology is unclear. CPP should be seen as a symptom with a number of contributory factors rather than as a diagnosis in itself.

History

- Pattern of the pain and its association with the menstrual cycle, aggravating and alleviating factors, and the effect of movement and posture on pain.
- Clinical measurement of pain level at each visit; e.g., 'on a scale of 0 to 10'.
- Bladder and bowel symptoms.
- Results of previous attempts at treatment and the amount of medication used.
- Daily pain diary for 2–3 menstrual cycles may be helpful in tracking symptoms or activities associated with the pain.
- Impact of pain on the patient's QOL; effect of pain on daily activities, work, relationships, sleep, or sexual functioning.
- Psychological assessment: symptoms such as sleep or appetite disturbance and tearfulness, current stress in life, etc.
- Main concern about the pain; understanding of pain and treatment expectations.
- Abuse history – past or present sexual assault, particularly intimate partner violence. Although abuse is rarely a cause of pelvic pain, a history of abuse often makes it more difficult for a woman to deal with pelvic pain.

Examination

Goal – to look for pathological conditions and to reproduce patient's usual pain to help identify physical contributors. Identifying a focal area of tenderness can help target specific therapy.

- **General** – demeanour, mobility, and posture, such as abnormal gait, guarding, and careful positioning.
- **Back** – for scoliosis, sacroiliac tenderness, trigger points, and pelvic asymmetry.
- **Abdomen** – for trigger points, head-raise test.
- **Vulva** – a cotton swab to perform a sensory examination and to identify areas of tenderness.
- Speculum examination – cervical lesions, infections, and endometriosis implants can be identified.
- Post-hysterectomy dyspareunia may arise from localized lesions or nerve entrapment at the vaginal vault: palpating the vault with a long cotton swab may assist in identifying focal source.
- **Pelvic examination:**
  * Tone and muscle control.   * Whether vaginismus is present.   * Cervical motion tenderness.
  * Uterine mobility.   * Uterine or adnexal tenderness and masses.
- Assess for any rectovaginal nodules, scarring, or tethering – a rectovaginal examination to determine its extent.

Differential diagnosis

DDx

Gynaecological – usually cyclical pain.
- Endometriosis, adenomyosis, fibroids. Pelvic venous congestion, chronic PID.
- Adhesions – dense vascular adhesions are likely to be a cause of CPP, as dividing them appears to relieve pain. However, adhesions may be asymptomatic. Adhesions may be caused by endometriosis, previous surgery, or previous infection.
- Two distinct forms of adhesive disease are recognized:
  * Residual ovary syndrome – a small amount of ovarian tissue inadvertently left behind following oophorectomy, which may become buried in adhesions.
  * Trapped ovary syndrome – a retained ovary becomes buried in dense adhesions following hysterectomy. Removal of all ovarian tissue or suppression using a GnRHa may relieve pain.

Non-gynaecological:
- Irritable bowel syndrome (IBS), constipations, inflammatory bowel disease.
- Interstitial cystitis, chronic UTI, urethral syndrome.
- Musculoskeletal pain, low back pain, disc disease.
- Nerve entrapment in scar tissue, fascia, or a narrow foramen – pain and dysfunction in the distribution of that nerve. The incidence of nerve entrapment defined as highly localized, sharp, stabbing, or aching pain, exacerbated by particular movements and persisting beyond 5 weeks, or occurring after a pain-free interval.
- Psychological.
- Sexual or physical abuse – child sexual abuse may initiate a cascade of events or reactions, which make an individual more vulnerable to the development of CPP as an adult. Women who continue to be abused are particularly at risk.

Service provision

- Discuss women's concerns and issues. When the patient feels that her experience of the pain is believed and that the clinician will do his/her best to help, there is better compliance with the proposed treatment plans. There is higher acceptance by the patient of more realistic goals of treatment, such as improved function and QOL, as opposed to complete resolution of pain.
- Discuss the multifactorial nature of CPP. The aim is to develop a partnership between the clinician and the woman to plan a management programme.
- CPP clinics with multidisciplinary approach – the integrated approach looking for organic, psychological, dietary, and environmental causes of the pain has been reported to be associated with significantly greater pain relief than the standard treatment.

Initial management at primary care

Many women with CPP can be managed in primary care by GPs.

'Red flag' symptoms and signs

- Bleeding per rectum. • PCB. • Excessive weight loss.
- New bowel symptoms in patients > 50 years of age.
- New pain after the menopause.
- Pelvic mass. • Suicidal ideation.
- Irregular vaginal bleeding in women > 40 years of age.

Investigations

- Screen for chlamydia and gonorrhoea, if there is any suspicion of PID.
- Offer screening for STIs for all sexually active women.

General

- Analgesics – regular NSAIDs with or without paracetamol or co-dydramol may be useful.
- Do not prescribe opioids for regular use.
- Amitriptyline or gabapentin may be useful for the treatment of neuropathic pain.
- Non-pharmacological modalities – TENS, acupuncture, acupressure, vitamin B1, magnesium supplementation, and other complementary therapies may be helpful.

Cyclical pain

- Therapeutic trial of ovarian suppression (COCs, progestogens, danazol, or GnRHa) for a period of 3–6 months. It can be an effective treatment for pain associated with endometriosis, and the response to ovarian suppression can therefore be a useful diagnostic tool.
- Where pain is strikingly cyclical and no abnormality is palpable at vaginal examination, a therapeutic trial of a GnRH agonist may be more helpful than a diagnostic laparoscopy.
- The LNG-IUS could be considered.
- Pelvic venous congestion also appears to be well controlled by ovarian suppression.

Referral

- When pain has not been explained to the woman's satisfaction or when pain is inadequately controlled.
- If the history suggests that there is a specific non-gynaecological component to the pain, refer to the relevant HCP – such as gastroenterologist, urologist, genitourinary medicine physician, physiotherapist, psychologist, or psychosexual counsellor.

Investigations at secondary level

Imaging

- TVS to screen and assess adnexal masses such as endometriomas, hydrosalpinges, or fibroids. Endometriomas can be accurately distinguished from other adnexal masses by TVS. It is of little value for the assessment of other causes of CPP, including peritoneal endometriosis. However, presence of soft markers such as tenderness or poor ovarian mobility can improve the pre-laparoscopy probability of identifying relevant pathology at laparoscopy from 58 to 73%. In the absence of soft markers, the pre-laparoscopy likelihood of pathology is 20%. TVS may therefore have a role in identifying those women who are less likely to obtain a positive diagnosis from a diagnostic laparoscopy.
- TVS and MRI are useful to diagnose adenomyosis. The sensitivity of MRI and TVS is comparable. Diagnostic accuracy of TVS for adenomyosis – sensitivity of 83% and specificity of 85%.
- Role of MRI in diagnosing small deposits of endometriosis is uncertain. It is useful in the assessment of palpable nodules in the pelvis or when symptoms suggest the presence of rectovaginal disease.

Diagnostic laparoscopy

- Diagnostic laparoscopy was regarded as the 'gold standard' in the diagnosis of CPP. It may be better seen as a second-line investigation if other therapeutic interventions fail. It is the only test capable of diagnosing peritoneal endometriosis and adhesions. Conditions such as IBS and adenomyosis are not visible at laparoscopy. A third to a half of diagnostic laparoscopies will be negative. The consequences of a negative laparoscopy have not been well studied. Much of the pathology identified is not necessarily the cause of pain.
- Often when the suspicion of adhesive disease or endometriosis requiring surgical intervention is high, or concerns such as the presence of endometriosis or adhesions potentially affecting fertility.
- Diagnostic laparoscopy may have a role in developing a woman's beliefs about her pain. A change in health beliefs as a result of having a laparoscopy both with positive or negative findings could help in improving pain scores.
- Micro-laparoscopy or 'conscious pain mapping' – The technique seems to provide an opportunity to confirm particular lesions as the source of the woman's pain; however, questions remain as to the acceptability, reproducibility, and validity of this technique.

Rx **Management**

Treat any positive diagnosis on laparoscopy

- Adhesions, ovarian remnant syndrome (ORS), pelvic congestion syndrome, residual ovary syndrome (ROS), post-hysterectomy CPP.
- Ovarian cysts (see Chapter 36) – chronic ovarian cysts do not usually produce pain.
- PID (see Chapter 39). * One of the long-term sequelae of PID is CPP. CPP has been reported to occur in 18–33% of women after an episode of PID. * Women with CPP are more likely to report a history of PID and a greater number of previous PID episodes.
- Endometriosis (see Chapter 12), adenomyosis (see Chapter 11), fibroids (see Chapter 10).
- Interstitial cystitis (IC); irritable bowel syndrome (IBS)

If negative laparoscopy

- Presacral neurectomy – limited efficacy. (ACOG)
- Laparoscopic uterosacral nerve ablation (LUNA) – ineffective. (RCOG)
- Sacral nerve stimulation may decrease pain in up to 60% of women. (ACOG)
- Injection of the trigger points of abdominal wall, vagina and sacrum with local anesthetic may provide temporary or prolonged relief. (ACOG)
- Antidepressants may be helpful. (ACOG)
- Even if no explanation for the pain can be found initially, treat the pain empirically and develop a management plan with the woman. If pain is not adequately controlled, refer to a pain management team or a specialist pelvic pain clinic.

Pelvic congestion syndrome

- Dilated pelvic veins have been observed in some women with CPP. Symptoms may include a dull aching pain as well as menstrual disorders. Vulval varicosities may be associated.
- Investigations – pelvic venography, Doppler USS, and MRI. In asymptomatic women undergoing MRI 38% incidence of pelvic congestion syndrome has been reported.
- Do not offer hysterectomy as a management option for pelvic congestion syndrome.
- Ovarian vein ligations and percutaneous embolizations have been reported, but no controlled clinical trials have evaluated the safety and long-term effectiveness of these approaches.
- Consider progestogens daily in high doses. (ACOG)

Post-hysterectomy CPP

- Hysterectomy is an effective treatment for CPP associated with reproductive symptoms and results in pain relief in 75–95% of women. (ACOG). CPP has been the principal indication for 10–12% of hysterectomies in the United States and Canada.
- Post-hysterectomy CPP – 22% of women with hysterectomy for CPP of unknown aetiology report persistent CPP and 5% report unchanged or increased pain. The probability of persistent pain is higher among women <30 years old, those with no identified pelvic disease, those who are economically disadvantaged, those with > 2 pregnancies, and those with a history of PID. For each of these subgroups, 30–40% continue to have CPP.
- Laparoscopic evaluation of women with CPP after hysterectomy and BSO may reveal adhesions, adnexal remnants, abnormal appendix, and abnormal peritoneum. Main biopsy findings are endometriosis and chronic inflammation.

Ovarian remnant syndrome (ORS)

- ORS arises from unintentional, incomplete dissection and removal of the ovary during a difficult or emergency oophorectomy or implantation and growth of displaced ovarian tissue in the abdomen or pelvic cavity during oophorectomy. Often seen in patients with severe endometriosis and pelvic adhesions.
- Incidence – 18% of women presenting with CPP. After removal of the ovarian remnants, 80% of women may report complete resolution of the CPP.
- Symptoms may present as CPP (sometimes cyclical), or as a pelvic mass with the absence of vasomotor symptoms.
- On vaginal examination, a tender lateral pelvic cyst may be palpable.
- Pre-menopausal levels of FSH and oestradiol; USS may show pelvic cystic structure.
- Treatment – GnRHa with add-back therapy; surgical excision of the ovarian remnant with a retroperitoneal; approach with wide local excision and lysis of adhesions.

Adhesions

- Caused mainly by surgery, endometriosis, and abdominal or pelvic infection.
- Adhesions are found in 25–50% of women with CPP, but their role as a cause of CPP remains controversial. A correlation between CPP and adhesions remains uncertain.
- Retrospective series reported 69–82% reduction of CPP after adhesiolysis.
- Adhesiolysis by laparotomy has no more benefit than the wait-and-see approach. Only the women with severe multiple vascularized adhesions involving the serosa of the small bowel or, to a lesser extent, the colon may benefit from adhesiolysis.
- Laparoscopic adhesiolysis vs diagnostic laparoscopy – similar number (27%) of patients in each group report resolution or substantial reduction of pain. There is higher risk of complications in operative laparoscopy compared to diagnostic laparoscopy (10% vs 0%).
- Adhesiolysis has not been shown to be effective in achieving pain control in RCTs. Current evidence does not support routine adhesiolysis for CPP.

Residual ovary syndrome

- Characterized by either recurrent pelvic pain or a persistent pelvic mass after hysterectomy. Incidence is 2.8% after hysterectomies with preservation of one or both ovaries.
- Indications for removal of the residual ovaries included CPP in 2.0%, persistent asymptomatic pelvic mass in 0.7%, and acute pelvic pain in 0.1% of patients. Ovarian malignancy is seen in 3.5/1000 cases.

Interstitial cystitis

Prevalence and incidence

- IC is a poorly understood chronic inflammatory condition of the bladder.
- Its causes are unknown, its pathophysiology remains uncertain, and the efficacy of treatment is questionable.
- Prevalence of IC in the United States is 10–67/100,000.
- Possible causes – infection, lymphatic or vascular obstruction, immunological deficiencies, glycosaminoglycan layer deficiency, presence of a toxic urogenous substance, neural factors, and primary mast cell disorder.

Clinical features

- Pelvic pain and irritative voiding symptoms, such as frequency, urgency, and nocturia.
- Frequency 8–15 times/day (average volume of 70–90 ml); once or twice per night.
- Pain can radiate to suprapubic area, perineum, vulva, vagina, low back, medial thighs.
- Pain can increase during or after sexual intercourse.
- Symptoms can fluctuate during the menstrual cycle, with a premenstrual flare in some cases.
- Examination may reveal pelvic, uterine, and bladder tenderness.

Investigations

- Diagnostic criteria and tests for IC are controversial. Symptom-based clinical diagnosis is recommended.
- Urinalysis and urine culture to rule out microscopic haematuria and infections.
- Cystoscopy – glomerulation, submucosal haemorrhage, and terminal haematuria may be found. Cystoscopic findings may help with prognosis, because patients with ulcers and significantly reduced bladder capacity do not respond favourably to treatment.
- Presence of IC does not necessarily correlate with the laparoscopic findings. It is, therefore, not possible to suggest that cystoscopy is necessary only if the results of laparoscopy are negative, or to suggest that cystoscopy is unnecessary if endometriosis or other pelvic disorders are found.
- The intra-vesical potassium chloride (KCl) sensitivity test is a minimally invasive diagnostic test. It may identify a subgroup of IC patients with epithelial permeability dysfunction and may predict the response to pentosan polysulphate sodium (Elmiron). False-positive results can occur with detrusor instability, radiation damage, and bacterial cystitis.

Management

- MDT – gynaecologists, urologists, and GPs.
- Pentosan polysulphate sodium – works by repairing the altered permeability of the bladder surface. Only 28–32% of patients will have improvement with this therapy.
- GnRHa or COCs – for patients with IC with pre-menstrual flare of symptoms. Symptoms are reduced during therapy but relapse is common.
- Hydro-distention at the time of cystoscopy is therapeutic in 20–30% of patients, who experience relief for 3–6 months.
- Consider IC in the differential diagnostic of CPP, especially in women presenting with bladder or pelvic pain or dyspareunia, even if the symptoms increase in the pre-menstrual period.
- IC is a common cause of CPP and often coexists with endometriosis.

Irritable bowel syndrome

Prevalence and incidence

- IBS affects up to 15% of adults, twice as common in women than men.
- Multifactorial pathophysiology – altered bowel motility, visceral hypersensitivity, and psychosocial factors.
- Symptoms suggesting IBS exist in 50–80% of patients presenting with CPP.
- In women referred to a gynaecology clinic, the prevalence of IBS – 37%.
- IBS can coexist with other pelvic diseases or be the sole cause of CPP in women.

Diagnosis – the Rome II criteria

- In the preceding year, the patient should have had > 12 weeks of abdominal discomfort or pain and at least two of the following:
  * Pain or discomfort that is relieved after defecation.
  * Association of the onset of pain or discomfort with a change in stool frequency, or stool appearance.
- In the presence of bloating or a feeling of abdominal distension, organic disease must be excluded.

History

- Abdominal pain and discomfort, bloating, and disturbed bowel habits (diarrhoea, constipation, or both). * Abnormal stool frequency (< 3 bowel movements per week or > 3 per day). * Abnormal stool form. * Abnormal stool passage (straining, urgency, feeling of incomplete evacuation). * Passage of mucus.
- It can be associated with dyspareunia, and bowel symptoms worsen during menstruation in 50% of women.
- Symptom-based diagnostic criteria – diagnosis of IBS with a PPV of 98%.

Investigations

- Initial investigations – FBC, TFT, and LFT.
- For patients < 40 years of age and a negative history, evaluation should include sigmoidoscopy.
- For patients > 45 years of age or with rectal bleeding, weight loss, anaemia, or a family history of colorectal cancer, colonoscopy or sigmoidoscopy with a barium enema should be performed.

Management of IBS

- Offer a trial of antispasmodics – smooth-muscle relaxants such as mebeverine.
- Efficacy of bulking agents has not been established but they are commonly used.
- Amending the diet to control symptoms – using an exclusion diet. 36% are able to identify one or more dietary components, the avoidance of which can lead to sustained improvement in symptoms. The most commonly implicated foods are dairy products and grains.

Lifestyle

- Dietary manipulation may be of benefit. Elimination of dietary lactose, sorbitol, and fructose may be of value. About 40% of patients with IBS have lactose intolerance.
- Caffeinated products, carbonated products, and gas-producing foods may contribute to bloating.
- Smoking and gum chewing lead to more swallowing of air and may increase gas or bloating.
- Excessive alcohol consumption may lead to increased rectal urgency.

Medical management

- Pain – antispasmodic agents or tricyclic compounds may be helpful.
- Constipation – increase dietary fibre along with osmotic laxatives. Discourage long-term use of stimulant laxatives.
- Diarrhoea – increase dietary fibre and antidiarrhoeal agents such as loperamide.
- Serotonin receptor agonists stimulate colonic motility and may diminish visceral hypersensitivity.
- Peppermint oil decreases abdominal distension, reduces stool frequency, decreases borborygmi, and reduces flatulence.
- GnRH analogues can result in a significant reduction in abdominal pain and nausea in pre-menopausal women with functional bowel disease.
- Combining psychological treatment with medical therapy improves the clinical response more than that with medical therapy only.

What not to do

- Routine adhesiolysis for CPP.
- MRI in diagnosing small deposits of endometriosis
- Diagnostic laparoscopy as first-line option for the diagnosis of CPP.
- Presacral neurectomy for treatment of CPP.
- Laparoscopic uterosacral nerve ablation (LUNA) for management of CPP.

Evidence round-up – systematic review

- Laparoscopic adhesiolysis or laparoscopic uterosacral nerve ablation do not improve pain scores more than diagnostic laparoscopy. The evidence to conclude that surgical intervention is either effective or ineffective or that one technique is superior to another is insufficient.
- RCTs comparing LUNA with no additional intervention – there is no significant difference between LUNA and No LUNA for the pain recorded over a 12-month period. LUNA does not result in improved CPP.
- Psychological therapies for chronic pelvic pain – the current evidence does not conclude whether psychological interventions have an effect on self-reported pain scores in women with CPP.

Consent – diagnostic laparoscopy

Discuss

- Explain the procedure: insertion of a laparoscope through a small incision to identify the problem.
- Intended benefits: to find the cause of symptoms. Occasionally, a minor laparoscopic procedure is appropriate to treat some of the identified causes or relieve the symptoms.
- Laparoscopy may not identify an obvious cause for the presenting complaint.
- Benefits and risks of any available alternative
- Treatments, including no treatment. Discuss the role of prior diagnostic imaging together with the option of no investigation.
- Form of anaesthesia.

Serious risks: 2/1000.
- Damage to bowel, bladder, uterus, or major blood vessels: 2.4/1000, which would require immediate repair by laparoscopy or laparotomy. However, up to 15% of bowel injuries might not be diagnosed at the time of laparoscopy.
- Failure to gain entry to abdominal cavity and to complete intended procedure.
- Hernia at site of entry.
- Death: 3–8/100,000 undergoing laparoscopy die as a result of complications.
- **Frequent risks:** wound bruising, shoulder-tip pain, wound gaping, wound infection.
- Women who are obese, who have significant pathology, who have had previous surgery, or who have pre-existing medical conditions – quoted risks for serious or frequent complications will be increased. The risk of serious complications at laparoscopy also increases if an additional therapeutic procedure is performed.

Extra procedures

- Any extra procedures which may become necessary:
  * Laparotomy.
  * Repair of damage to bowel, bladder, uterus, or blood vessels.
  * Blood transfusion.

Risks

Very common	1/1 to 1/10.
Common	1/10 to 1/100.
Uncommon	1/100 to 1/1000.
Rare	1/1000 to 1/10,000.

1. *The Initial Management Of Chronic Pelvic Pain.* RCOG Guideline No. 41, 2012.
2. Consensus Guidelines for the Management of Chronic Pelvic Pain SOGC Clinical Practice Guidelines No164. Part one of two, August 2005. *J Obstet Gynaecol Can* 2005;27(8):781–801
3. *Chronic Pelvic Pain: Clinical Management Guidelines for Obstetricians and Gynaecologists.* ACOG Practice Bulletin Number 51, 2004.
4. Yunker A, Sathe NA, Reynolds WS, Likis FE, Andrews J. Systematic review of therapies for noncyclic chronic pelvic pain in women. *Obstet Gynecol Surg.* 2012;67(7):417–425.
5. Champaneria R, Daniels JP, Raza A, Pattison HM, Khan KS. Psychological therapies for chronic pelvic pain: systematic review of randomized controlled trials. *Acta Obstet Gynecol Scand* 2012;91(3):281–286.
6. Daniels JP, Middleton L, Xiong T, et al. for International LUNA IPD Meta-analysis Collaborative Group. Individual patient data meta-analysis of randomized evidence to assess the effectiveness of laparoscopic uterosacral nerve ablation in chronic pelvic pain. *Hum Reprod Update* 2010;16(6):568–576.

CHAPTER 38 Chronic pelvic pain

CHAPTER 39 Acute pelvic inflammatory disease

Background and definition

- Ascending infection from the endocervix causing endometritis, salpingitis, parametritis, oophoritis, tubo-ovarian abscess, and/or pelvic peritonitis.
- Causative agents – STIs such as Chlamydia trachomatis, Neisseria gonorrhoeae, Mycoplasma genitalium, anaerobes, and other organisms.
- PID develops in 10–45% of women with endocervical gonorrhoeae and in 10–30% of women with endocervical Chlamydia infection.

Prevalence

- Incidence of PID is unknown because of the difficulty in making a clinical diagnosis, because it is often asymptomatic and can present atypically. Up to two thirds of cases remain unrecognized.
- PID is reported in 1.7% of GP attendances in women of 16–46 years of age.
- 10–15% of women of reproductive age have had one episode of PID.

Risk factors for PID

- Young age (< 25 years old). • Early age of first coitus.
- Multiple sexual partners.
- Recent new partner (within the previous 3 months).
- History of STI in the woman or her partner.
- Recent instrumentation of the uterus.

History

- Bilateral lower abdominal pain or pelvic pain.
- Deep dyspareunia particularly of recent onset.
- Abnormal vaginal or cervical discharge.
- Abnormal vaginal bleeding (IMB or PCB), which may be secondary to cervicitis and endometritis.
- Right upper quadrant pain owing to peri-hepatitis.
- Current and recent medication.

Examination

- Fever (> 38°C) – only one third of women with acute PID have a temperature of > 38°C.
- Abdominal examination – bilateral lower abdominal tenderness.
- Speculum examination – abnormal vaginal or cervical discharge.
- Vaginal examination – cervical motion tenderness, adnexal tenderness (with or without a palpable mass), and/or uterine tenderness.

Risks or complications

- Sequelae – delay of only a few days in receiving appropriate treatment markedly increases the risk of sequelae such as infertility, ectopic pregnancy, and chronic pelvic pain (CPP).
- Risk of infertility is related to the number of episodes of PID and their severity: 0.6% of women develop infertility after an episode of mild PID, and 21% of women after two episodes of PID.
- CPP or abdominal pain develops in 18% of women who had PID.
- About a third of women have repeated infections.
- Fitz–Hugh–Curtis syndrome: right upper quadrant pain associated with peri-hepatitis occurs in up to 10–20% of women with PID.

Differential diagnosis – lower abdominal pain in a young woman

- Ectopic pregnancy; miscarriage. Exclude pregnancy in all women suspected of having PID.
- Acute appendicitis – nausea and vomiting occurs in most patients with appendicitis but only 50% of those with PID. Cervical excitation may be present in about a quarter of women with appendicitis.
- Endometriosis.
- IBS (other gastrointestinal disorders). • UTI.
- Ovarian cyst complications such as rupture or torsion.
- Functional pain (pain of unknown physical origin).

Clinical symptoms and signs lack sensitivity and specificity. The PPV of a clinical diagnosis is 65–90% compared to laparoscopic diagnosis.

Keep a low threshold for empirical treatment because of the lack of definitive clinical diagnostic criteria and because the potential consequences of not treating PID are significant.

Investigations

- Urine pregnancy test to exclude ectopic pregnancy. When the risk of ectopic pregnancy is high, repeat it 21 days after the date of last UPSI.
- Urine analysis and culture to rule out UTI.
- Excess leucocytes on a wet-mount vaginal smear are associated with PID, but are also found in women with isolated lower genital tract infection. The absence of endocervical or vaginal pus cells on a wet-mount has a good NPV (95%) but their presence is nonspecific (poor PPV, 17%).
- Peripheral blood leucocytosis, elevated ESR, or CRP support the diagnosis and can provide a useful measure of disease severity but are nonspecific.
- TVS with power Doppler can identify inflamed and dilated Fallopian tubes, tubo-ovarian masses, ovarian cyst, and cyst accidents. It may differentiate PID from acute appendicitis in a minority of cases.
- CT and MRI can assist in making a diagnosis but the evidence is limited.
- Laparoscopy enables specimens to be taken from the Fallopian tubes and the pouch of Douglas and can provide information on the severity of the condition. It lacks sensitivity; 15–30% of suspected cases may have no laparoscopic evidence of acute infection despite organisms being identified from the Fallopian tubes. Do not perform routinely due to the cost, the potential difficulty in identifying mild intra-tubal inflammation or endometritis, and high rates of intra- and inter-observer variation in diagnosing PID.
- Endometrial biopsy: presence of histological endometritis is not associated with higher rates of infertility, CPP, or recurrent PID.

Microbiological investigations

- High vaginal swab for bacterial vaginosis and candidiasis.
- Test for gonorrhoea and chlamydia. A positive result gives support to the clinical diagnosis of PID; however, the absence of confirmed infection in the lower genital tract site does not exclude PID.
- Gonorrhoea – endocervical specimen culture, or by NAAT. If gonorrhoea is detected using a NAAT, take an additional endocervical swab for culture to report antibiotic sensitivities.
- Chlamydia – endocervical specimen, preferably using a NAAT.
- Urethral sample can increase the diagnostic yield for gonorrhoea and chlamydia but undertake it only if the more sensitive NAAT is not available.
- A first-catch urine sample or self-taken vulvovaginal swab sample provides an alternative sample for some NAATs.
- Other organisms including M. genitalium have been associated with PID, but do not screen routinely because of limited information on prevalence, natural history, treatment, and cost effectiveness.

Management

Currently limited evidence for the efficacy of antibiotic therapy in preventing the long-term complications of PID.

Medical management

Outpatient setting

- Provide appropriate analgesia.
- Commence antibiotic treatment as soon as the diagnosis is suspected. Broad-spectrum antibiotics to cover N. gonorrhoeae, C. trachomatis, and anaerobic infection.
- Review at 72 hours, particularly for those with a moderate or severe presentation.
- Advise to avoid UPSI until the patient and her partner(s) have completed treatment and follow-up.

- Recommended regimens:
  * IM ceftriaxone 250 mg stat or IM cefoxitin 2 g stat with oral probenecid 1 g followed by oral doxycycline 100 mg BD plus metronidazole 400 mg BD for 14 days.
  * Oral ofloxacin 400 mg BD plus oral metronidazole 400 mg BD for 14 days.
- In both regimens, metronidazole is included to improve coverage for anaerobic bacteria. Anaerobes are of relatively greater importance in patients with severe PID, and metronidazole may be discontinued in those patients with mild or moderate PID who are unable to tolerate it, as its addition provides uncertain additional efficacy.
  * Oral cefixime as a single dose (off-label use) can be used as an alternative to ceftriaxone.
- Avoid ofloxacin in patients who are at high risk of gonococcal PID because of increasing quinolone resistance in the UK.
- Alternative regime (evidence is less strong) – IM ceftriaxone followed by azithromycin 1 g/week for 2 weeks.

Admission to hospital

- **Indications:**
  - * Suspected ectopic pregnancy or appendicitis.
  - * Clinically severe disease with fever > 38°C.
  - * Tubo-ovarian abscess.
  - * Signs of pelvic peritonitis.
  - * PID in pregnancy.
  - * Lack of response or intolerance to oral therapy with outpatient setting.
- IV antibiotics until 24 hours after clinical improvement, followed by oral antibiotics.
- Choice of appropriate regimen is influenced by local antimicrobial sensitivity patterns, the local epidemiology of specific infections, cost, woman's preference and compliance, and severity of disease.
- No evidence of the superiority of any one of the suggested regimens over the others.

Regimens:

- * IV cefoxitin 2 g TDS plus IV/oral doxycycline 100 mg BD followed by oral doxycycline 100 mg BD plus oral metronidazole 400 mg BD for a total of 14 days.
- * IV clindamycin 900 mg TDS plus IV gentamicin (2 mg/kg loading dose followed by 1.5 mg/kg TID [a single daily dose of 7 mg/kg may be substituted]) followed by either oral clindamycin 450 mg QID for 14 days, or oral doxycycline 100 mg BD plus oral metronidazole 400 mg BD for 14 days.
- * Gentamicin levels need to be monitored if this regimen is used.

Alternative regimens

- * IV ofloxacin 400 mg BD plus IV metronidazole 500 mg TID for 14 days.
- * IV ciprofloxacin 200 mg BD plus IV/oral doxycycline 100 mg BD plus IV metronidazole 500 mg TID for 14 days.

Surgical management

- In severe cases or where there is clear evidence of a pelvic abscess – drain the abscess.
- Laparoscopic division of adhesions and drainage of pelvic abscesses may help early resolution of the disease.
- USS-guided drainage of pelvic fluid collections is less invasive and may be equally effective.
- Adhesiolysis in cases of peri-hepatitis – no evidence that this is superior to antibiotic therapy.

Provide information to woman

- Detailed explanation of the condition and long-term implications for her health and the health of her partner(s).
- Explanation of treatment and its possible adverse effects.
- That following treatment, fertility is usually maintained but there is a risk of future infertility, CPP, or ectopic pregnancy.
- Repeat episodes of PID are associated with an exponential increase in the risk of infertility.
- Discuss contraceptive options. Use of barrier contraception significantly reduces risk of PID.
- Need to screen sexual contacts to prevent her becoming re-infected.
- Clinically, more severe disease is associated with a greater risk of sequelae.
- The earlier treatment is given, the lower the risk of future fertility problems.

Follow-up

4–6 weeks follow-up

- **To assess:**
  - * Adequate clinical response.
  - * Compliance with oral antibiotics.
  - * Screen and treat sexual contacts.
- **Test of cure:**
  - * Repeat testing for gonorrhoea after treatment in cases initially found to be infected, unless sensitivity testing of the isolate confirms sensitivity to the prescribed antibiotic.
  - * Repeat testing for chlamydia and gonorrhoea in cases with persisting symptoms, poor compliance with antibiotics, and/or tracing of sexual contacts indicate the possibility of persisting or recurrent infection.

Contraception options

- Can use – COCs, POP, depot progestogen injection, progesterone implant.
- **COCs:** Screen women on hormonal contraception presenting with breakthrough bleeding for genital tract infection, especially C. trachomatis.
  - * Use of the COCs was regarded as protective against symptomatic PID. Recent studies, however, have shown an association with an increased incidence of asymptomatic cervical infection with C. trachomatis, with possible suggestion that the COCs may mask endometritis.
- **IUD and IUS:** For women with a history of PID, the relative risk of PID is increased 6-fold in the 20 days following insertion, but the absolute risk remains low (≈ 1%). After this time, the risk is the same as for the population without an IUD and remains low unless there is exposure to STI.
  - * There are significantly fewer removals for PID with LNG-IUS as compared to Cu IUD. If a woman is likely to be at risk of future PID and requests an IUD for contraception, the LNG-IUS would be the most appropriate choice.

Treatment of PID in specific circumstances

Pregnant women

- PID is rare in women with an IUP except in the case of septic abortion. In septic abortion, the infective organism is unlikely to be a sexually transmitted pathogen.
- In pregnancy, PID is associated with an increase in both maternal and fetal morbidity, therefore treat with parenteral therapy, although none of the regimens is of proven safety in this situation. (BASHH)
- The risk of giving any of the recommended antibiotic regimens in very early pregnancy is low, as significant drug toxicity results in failed implantation.
- Treatment regimens depend upon organisms isolated.
- Avoid drugs known to be toxic in pregnancy, e.g., terracyclines.
- A combination of cefotaxime, azithromycin, and metronidazole may be used.
- Risks associated with metronidazole are uncertain but no confirmed associations have been reported.

Woman with IUCD

- If symptoms have not resolved within 72 hours, consider removing the IUD.
- Removal of the IUD may be associated with better short-term clinical outcomes, but balance the decision to remove it against the risk of pregnancy in those who have had otherwise UPSI in the preceding days.
- Consider hormonal emergency contraception for women in this situation.

Management of sexual partner(s)

- Proven or suspected STI – refer index woman and her current sexual partner(s) to a GUM clinic for screening other STIs, treatment, and contact tracing.
- Contact tracing – trace sexual partners within a six-month period of the onset of symptoms.
- Advise to avoid intercourse until woman and her partner(s) have completed the treatment course.
- Empirically treat for chlamydia in all sexual partners, owing to the variable sensitivity of currently available diagnostic tests.
- Gonorrhoea diagnosed in the sexual partner – treat appropriately and concurrently with the index woman.
- If adequate screening for gonorrhoea and chlamydia in the sexual partner(s) is not possible, treat empirically for both gonorrhoea and chlamydia.

Women with HIV

- Manage in conjunction with the HIV physician.
- These women may have clinically more severe PID but respond equally well to treatment as women who are not infected. Therefore, treat with standard antibiotics.

Young women

- Women under the age of 25 years: keep a low threshold for diagnosis and treatment of PID, owing to the higher incidence of disease in this group and the potential impact on future fertility.
- Avoid ofloxacin, where possible, when bone development is still occurring.
- Doxycycline can safely be used in children over the age of 12 years.

What not to do

- Do not wait for swab results. Start empirical antibiotics as soon as a presumptive diagnosis of PID is made clinically.
- Combination of oral doxycycline and metronidazole (without ceftriaxone).
- Azithromycin monotherapy.
- Oral cephalosporin as part of the treatment regimen.
- Women who are at high risk of gonococcal PID – use of regimens containing ofloxacin or azithromycin alone.

1. *Management of Acute Pelvic Inflammatory Disease.* RCOG Green-top Guideline No. 32, November 2008.
2. Clinical Knowledge Summaries. http://www.cks.nhs.uk/pelvic_inflammatory_disease.
3. BASHH. *United Kingdom National Guideline for the Management of Pelvic Inflammatory Disease.* http://www.bashh.org/documents/118/118.pdf.
4. *Pelvic Inflammatory Disease. Canadian Guidelines on Sexually Transmitted Infections.* Public Health Agency of Canada, 2010.

CHAPTER 40　Vaginal discharge

Background

- Normal physiological discharge changes with the menstrual cycle.
- Abnormal vaginal discharge is characterized by a change of colour, consistency, volume, or odour, and may be associated with symptoms such as itch, soreness, dysuria, pelvic pain, or IMB/PCB.
- In women of reproductive age complaining of vaginal discharge, the most common cause is physiological, but exclude infective and other causes.

Differential diagnosis (see Table)

DDx

Physiological

- Commonest cause; diagnosis of exclusion.
- Cyclicity of the discharge – Prior to ovulation oestrogen concentration increases altering cervical mucus to fertile, clearer, wetter, stretchy, and slippery. After ovulation, progesterone concentration increases, altering cervical mucus to become thick and sticky.
- Vagina is colonized by lactobacilli and other bacteria from puberty. Lactobacilli metabolize glycogen in the vaginal epithelium to produce lactic acid, thus the vaginal environment is normally acidic (pH < 4.5).
- Some commensal organisms can constitute infection if they overgrow.

Infective

- **Vaginal infection:**
  * Non-STI – bacterial vaginosis (BV), vulvovaginal candidiasis (VVC).
  * STI – trichomoniasis (TV).
- **Endocervical infections** caused by chlamydia or gonorrhoea:
- PID.

Non-infective

- Foreign bodies (tampons).
- Cervical polyps and ectopy.
- Genital tract malignancy.
- Fistulae.
- Allergic reactions.
- Atrophic vaginitis in post-menopausal women.

History and assessment of risk for STIs

- Characteristics of the discharge – onset, duration, colour, odour, consistency, cyclicity, exacerbating factors.
- Associated symptoms – itch, superficial dyspareunia, dysuria.
- Symptoms indicative of upper reproductive tract infection – abdominal pain, fever, deep dyspareunia, abnormal bleeding.
- **Sexual history – high risk of STI if aged < 25 years, new partner or > 1 partner in the last year, previous STIs.**
- Obstetric history – pregnancy, postpartum, post-abortion, contraceptive use.
- History of uterine instrumentation (TOP, ERPC, HSG, hysteroscopy).
- Concurrent medications (antibiotics, corticosteroids); medical conditions (diabetes, immunocompromised state).
- Previous treatments used (prescription and over-the-counter).

Examination may be omitted with empirical treatment

- Women at low risk of STIs.
- No symptoms of other conditions causing vaginal discharge.
- No symptoms suggestive of upper reproductive tract infection.
- The woman can return for follow-up if symptoms do not resolve.
- Symptoms have not developed following a gynaecological procedure.
- **Characteristic symptoms of VVC; AND this is a first episode of suspected VVC, or if recurrent, recurrence is infrequent (< 4 times a year).**
- **Characteristic symptoms of BV; AND this is a first episode of suspected BV, or if recurrent, a previous episode of similar symptoms was confirmed to be BV.**

A previous diagnosis of BV can be assumed to be reliable if:
  * Characteristic symptoms and signs of BV were present.
  * Symptoms and signs of other conditions causing vaginal discharge were absent.
  * There was no microbiological evidence of presence of any other infection from swabs.
  * Symptoms and signs cleared following antibiotic treatment.

Empirical treatment

- **Swabs may be omitted with empirical treatment (HPA).**
- Non-offensive white discharge with an itch – VVC – treat with antifungals.
- Offensive discharge without itch – BV – treat with metronidazole.

Recurrent or failed treatment

Examine all other women

Cervicitis or PID

- Vaginal discharge associated with PCB/IMB, lower abdominal pain with or without fever, dysuria, deep dyspareunia.
- Cervicitis – inflamed cervix, which bleeds easily and may be associated with a mucopurulent discharge.
- Adnexal tenderness and cervical excitation on bimanual palpation.

Examine all other women (contd.)

- Local inspection – signs of vulval inflammation, excoriations, vulval satellite lesions of erythema.
- Speculum examination – signs of cervicitis, vaginitis, amount, consistency and colour of vaginal discharge, and any foreign body.
- Bimanual palpation – cervical motion tenderness, uterine tenderness, adnexal tenderness, and abnormal mass.
- pH testing of vaginal discharge with narrow-range pH paper to assess the probability of causes such as BV or TV (pH ≥ 4.5) or candida (pH < 4.5). It cannot help distinguish between BV and TV.

Investigations

Swabs may be omitted with empirical treatment (HPA)

- Combination of clinical features and a measurement of vaginal pH is a sensitive, although not very specific predictor of the cause of vaginal discharge. Using these criteria, the diagnosis is missed in only a few women with BV or VVC. However, a moderate number of women who do not have VVC or BV will be incorrectly diagnosed with these conditions.
- Specificity is significantly increased when results of endocervical swabs for chlamydia and gonorrhoea and HVS are available.

Swabs are recommended

- When clinical features are not clearly suggestive of either BV or VVC, or:
  * An increased risk of STI. * Cervicitis on examination.
  * Suspected PID. * A poor response to initial treatment.
  * Recurrent vaginal discharge. * Discharge of uncertain cause.
  * Discharge after a gynaecological procedure or childbirth.
  * Within 3 weeks of IUCD insertion. * Woman requests investigations.
- HVS from the lateral vaginal wall and posterior fornix:
  * Microscopy and dry Gram stain – BV (clue cells and proportions of lactobacilli and other organisms), candida (spores and pseudophytes).
  * Saline wet microscopy – TV (flagellate protozoa), candida (pseudohyphae).
  * Culture – candida, BV, chlamydia, gonorrhoea (chocolate agar media).
  * HVS for suspected TV should be examined in the laboratory within 6 hours. It is therefore recommended that these women are referred to GUM clinic.
- Endocervical swab for chlamydia and gonorrhoea.
- Swabs from other sites may be appropriate, based on clinical history (urethral, rectal, oropharyngeal).

Management

Empirically treat while awaiting swab results in cases of:

- Cervicitis – treat for chlamydia.
- Suspected PID (see Chapter 39).
- BV, VVC.
- Suspected TV – if referral to GUM is not feasible.

Refer:

- Urgent admission for women with PID who are pregnant, pyrexial and unwell, or unable to take oral fluids or medications.
- Suspected gynaecological cancer.
- Referral to a GUM clinic for women with:
  * Suspected TV.
  * For partner notification in cases of confirmed gonorrhoea, chlamydia, or TV.

	Candidiasis	BV	TV
Causative organism	Second most common cause of infective vaginal discharge. C. albicans is a vaginal commensal found in 10–20% of asymptomatic women. Acute vulvovaginal candidiasis (VVC) is caused by overgrowth of C. albicans (80–95% of cases) or C. glabrata (5%).	Most common cause of infective vaginal discharge. An overgrowth of anaerobic organisms (Gardnerella vaginalis, Prevotella species, Mycoplasma hominis, and Mobiluncus species) that replace normal lactobacilli.	Flagellated protozoan.
STI	Not STI.	Not STI.	STI.
Odour	Odourless discharge.	A fishy-smelling thin discharge.	A fishy-smelling discharge.
Itching	Associated with itching and superficial soreness.	Not associated with itching or soreness.	Associated with itching and soreness.
	Superficial dyspareunia, dysuria.		Dysuria due to urethral infection.
Discharge	Thick white curdy discharge.	White/grey homogeneous coating of vaginal walls and vulva.	Greenish-yellow frothy discharge.
Examination	Vulval and vaginal erythema, oedema, fissuring, satellite lesions of erythema.	No vulval inflammation.	Vulvitis, vaginitis, strawberry cervix.
Vaginal pH	Acidic pH.	Vaginal pH $\geq$ 4.5.	Vaginal pH of > 4.5.
		Amsel's criteria (3/4 present): • White discharge. • pH > 4.5. • Fishy odour (with addition of 10% KOH). • Clue cells (vaginal epithelial cells surrounded by bacteria).	
Investigation	HVS – microscopy and Gram stain.	HVS – microscopy and Gram stain.	HVS – microscopy and wet mount.
Treatment	Vaginal and oral antifungals (azoles) are equally effective.	Oral metronidazole (400–500 mg twice daily for 5–7 days, or a single 2 g dose).	Oral metronidazole (a single 2 g oral dose or 400 mg twice daily for 5–7 days).
Local treatment	Vulval antifungals can be used if women have vulval symptoms.	Metronidazole vaginal gel, oral clindamycin, or clindamycin cream.	
Sexual partners	Testing and treatment of male sexual partner(s) is not indicated.	Testing and treatment of the male sexual partner(s) is not indicated.	Notification and treatment for all partners in the last 6 months is recommended.
Contraception	Latex condoms, diaphragms, and cervical caps may be damaged by some vaginal/vulval antifungal treatments.	Women should use additional barrier contraceptive protection (e.g., condoms) during the antibiotic course and for 7 days afterwards.	

Vaginal discharge in pregnancy

Bacterial vaginosis

- Treat as for non-pregnant women.
- Although BV is associated with late miscarriage, preterm labour, premature rupture of membranes, low birth weight, and postpartum endometritis, routine screening for BV in pregnancy is not yet recommended.
- Current guidelines – screen for BV only for women with a previous preterm birth (< 28 weeks' gestation) or second-trimester miscarriage.

Vulvovaginal candidiasis

- VVC is common in pregnancy.
- Treatment is the same as for non-pregnant women but may need to be of longer duration (for up to 7 days).
- Cochrane review – vaginal imidazole more effective than nystatin.
- Avoid oral antifungals because of potential teratogenicity.

Trichomonas vaginalis

- There is no indication for routine screening in pregnancy.
- Treatment – oral metronidazole for 7 days.
- There is increasing evidence that TV may be associated with preterm delivery and low birth weight.

What not to do

- Routine screening for BV in pregnancy.
- Routine screening of TV in pregnancy.

Recurrent vaginal discharge

- Can result in psychosexual problems and depression. Provide appropriate counselling.
- Consider the diagnosis and treat acute infections.
- Investigate for potential underlying conditions (e.g., diabetes, immunosuppression, corticosteroid therapy, or concurrent antibiotic use).
- Advise to avoid use of douches, shower gels, antiseptic agents, and shampoo in the bath.

Bacterial vaginosis

- Despite high initial cure rates (70–80%), recurrence occurs within 3 months of treatment in 15–30% of women.
- Most relapses occur in the first year and are not thought to be due to drug resistance.
- Consider suppressive regimens, but evidence to support their effectiveness is limited.
* 5 g metronidazole intravaginal gel twice weekly for 4–6 months after an initial 10-day treatment.
* 40C mg metronidazole orally twice daily for 3 days at the start and end of menstruation.

Vulvovaginal candidiasis

- ≥ 4 episodes in 12 months; occurs in < 5% of women. Not clear whether it is a result of re-colonization or new growth.
- Induction and maintenance regimen may be used for 6 months.
- Induction – daily vaginal clotrimazole/oral fluconazole/itraconazole for 6–12 days.
- Maintenance – weekly or monthly treatments for 6 months (oral fluconazole 100 mg weekly, clotrimazole pessary 500 mg weekly, or oral itraconazole 400 mg).
- Relapse occurs in up to 50% of women after cessation of maintenance therapy. Induction and maintenance treatment may need to be restarted and continued for a longer period (12 months).

Trichomonas vaginalis

- Usually a result of re-infection, but consider the possibility of drug resistance.
- Treatment, education, and partner notification are required.

1. *The Management of Women of Reproductive Age Attending Non-Genitourinary Medicine Settings Complaining of Vaginal Discharge.* FFPRHC and BASHH Guidance, January 2006.
2. *Management of Abnormal Vaginal Discharge in Women. Quick Reference Guide for Primary Care for Consultation and Adaptation.* Health Protection Agency, 2007. http://www.hpa.org.uk.
3. *Clinical Knowledge Summaries – Vaginal Discharge.* http://www.cks.nhs.uk/vaginal_discharge

CHAPTER 41 Bacterial vaginosis

Background and prevalence

- Most common cause of abnormal discharge in women of reproductive age.
- Characterized by an overgrowth of anaerobic organisms (Gardnerella vaginalis, Prevotella species, Mycoplasma hominis, Mobiluncus species) in the vagina, leading to replacement of lactobacilli and an increase in pH from < 4.5 to as high as 7.0.
- Prevalence: 5–50%; 12% in pregnant women in the UK and 30% in women undergoing TOP.
- Prevalence is higher in sexually active women with early age at first intercourse, higher number of sexual partners, black women, smokers, and those with an IUCD.
- Spontaneous onset and remission of BV can occur.
- Not a sexually transmitted disease.

Risks or complications

- It may be associated with non-gonococcal urethritis (NGU) in male partners.
- Associated with increased incidence of vaginal cuff cellulitis and abscess formation following transvaginal hysterectomy.
- No studies regarding the possible role of BV in the onset of PID following insertion of an IUCD.
- PID – prevalence of BV is reported to be high in women with PID. It may be predictive of subsequent PID associated with gonorrhoea or chlamydia. However, there is no evidence on whether treating asymptomatic women with BV reduces their risk of developing PID subsequently.
- **Pregnancy** – BV is associated with late miscarriage, preterm birth, preterm premature rupture of membranes, and postpartum endometritis.
- BV is common in women undergoing elective TOP, and is associated with post-TOP endometritis and PID.

History and examination

- Approximately 50% are asymptomatic.
- Offensive fishy-smelling vaginal discharge.
- Not associated with soreness, itching, or irritation.
- Thin, white, homogeneous discharge coating the walls of the vagina and vestibule.

Diagnosis

- BASHH recommend using the Hay/Ison criteria.
- Isolation of Gardnerella vaginalis cannot be used to diagnose BV because it can be cultured from the vagina in > 50% of normal women.

- **Amsel criteria** – at least 3/4 criteria for the diagnosis:
  * Thin, white, homogeneous discharge.
  * Clue cells on microscopy of wet mount.
  * pH of vaginal fluid > 4.5.
  * Release of a fishy odour on adding alkali (10% KOH).

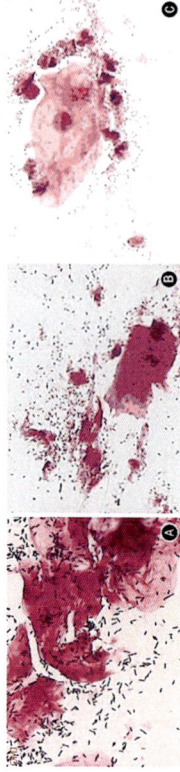

Fig. A   Fig. B   Fig. C

- **A Gram stained vaginal smear – the Hay/Ison criteria:**
  * Grade 1 (Fig. A: normal): lactobacilli predominate.
  * Grade 2 (Fig. B: intermediate): mixed flora with some lactobacilli, but Gardnerella or Mobiluncus is also present.
  * Grade 3 (Fig. C: BV): predominantly Gardnerella and/or Mobiluncus, few or absent lactobacilli.
- **The Nugent score** – estimate the relative proportions of bacterial morphotypes to give a score between 0 and 10. A score of < 4 is normal, 4–6 is intermediate, and > 6 is BV.

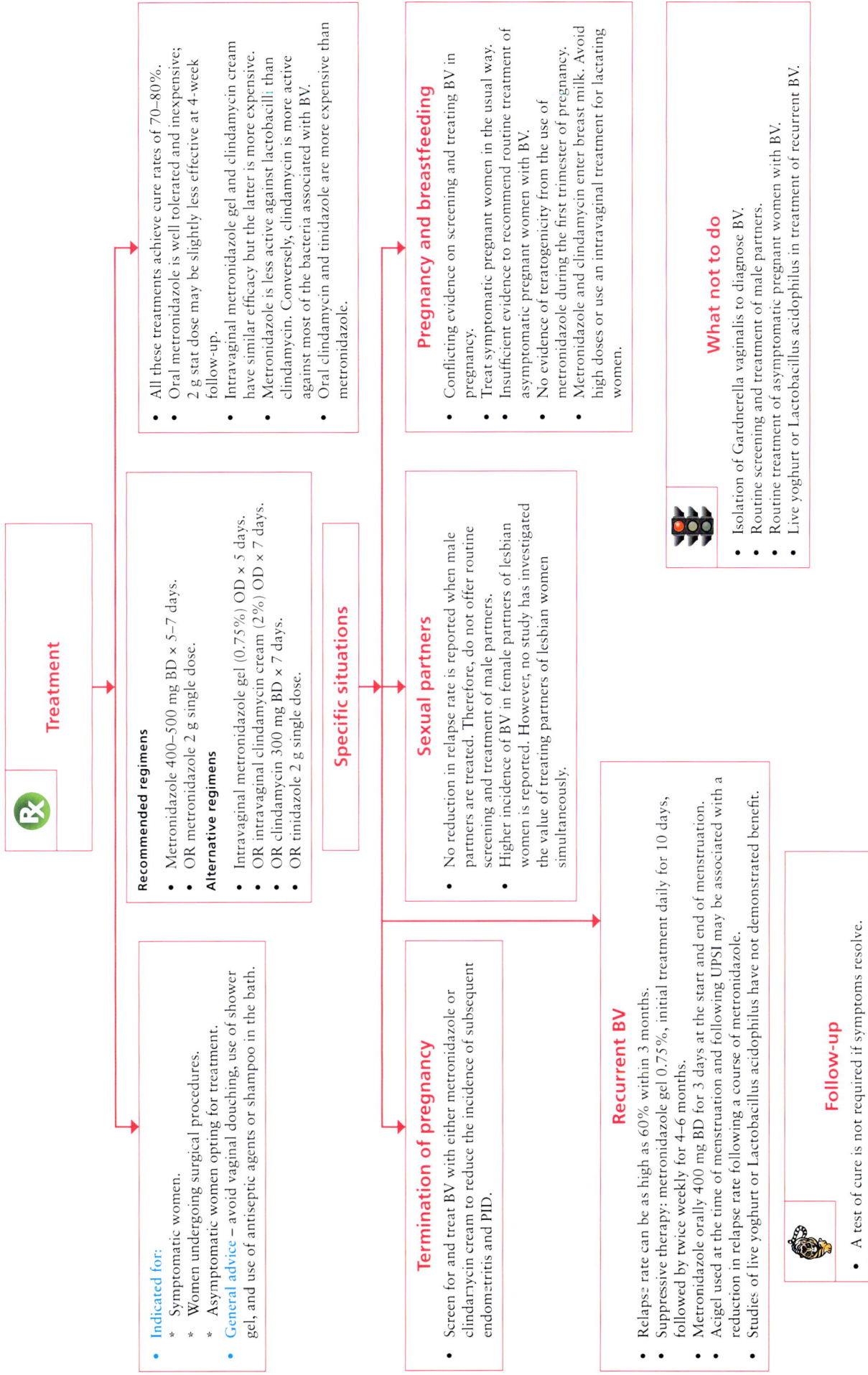

Treatment

Indicated for:
* Symptomatic women.
* Women undergoing surgical procedures.
* Asymptomatic women opting for treatment.
* General advice – avoid vaginal douching, use of shower gel, and use of antiseptic agents or shampoo in the bath.

Recommended regimens
* Metronidazole 400–500 mg BD × 5–7 days.
* OR metronidazole 2 g single dose.

Alternative regimens
* Intravaginal metronidazole gel (0.75%) OD × 5 days.
* OR intravaginal clindamycin cream (2%) OD × 7 days.
* OR clindamycin 300 mg BD × 7 days.
* OR tinidazole 2 g single dose.

* All these treatments achieve cure rates of 70–80%.
* Oral metronidazole is well tolerated and inexpensive; 2 g stat dose may be slightly less effective at 4-week follow-up.
* Intravaginal metronidazole gel and clindamycin cream have similar efficacy but the latter is more expensive.
* Metronidazole is less active against lactobacilli than clindamycin. Conversely, clindamycin is more active against most of the bacteria associated with BV.
* Oral clindamycin and tinidazole are more expensive than metronidazole.

Specific situations

Sexual partners
* No reduction in relapse rate is reported when male partners are treated. Therefore, do not offer routine screening and treatment of male partners.
* Higher incidence of BV in female partners of lesbian women is reported. However, no study has investigated the value of treating partners of lesbian women simultaneously.

Pregnancy and breastfeeding
* Conflicting evidence on screening and treating BV in pregnancy.
* Treat symptomatic pregnant women in the usual way.
* Insufficient evidence to recommend routine treatment of asymptomatic pregnant women with BV.
* No evidence of teratogenicity from the use of metronidazole during the first trimester of pregnancy.
* Metronidazole and clindamycin enter breast milk. Avoid high doses or use an intravaginal treatment for lactating women.

Termination of pregnancy
* Screen for and treat BV with either metronidazole or clindamycin cream to reduce the incidence of subsequent endometritis and PID.

Recurrent BV
* Relapse rate can be as high as 60% within 3 months.
* Suppressive therapy: metronidazole gel 0.75%, initial treatment daily for 10 days, followed by twice weekly for 4–6 months.
* Metronidazole orally 400 mg BD for 3 days at the start and end of menstruation. Acigel used at the time of menstruation and following UPSI may be associated with a reduction in relapse rate following a course of metronidazole.
* Studies of live yoghurt or Lactobacillus acidophilus have not demonstrated benefit.

Follow-up
* A test of cure is not required if symptoms resolve.

What not to do
* Isolation of Gardnerella vaginalis to diagnose BV.
* Routine screening and treatment of male partners.
* Routine treatment of asymptomatic pregnant women with BV.
* Live yoghurt or Lactobacillus acidophilus in treatment of recurrent BV.

1. Yan D, Lü Z, Su J. Comparison of main Lactobacillus species between healthy women and women with bacterial vaginosis. *Chinese Med J* 2009;122(22):2748–2751.

CHAPTER 41 Bacterial vaginosis

CHAPTER 42 Vulvovaginal candidiasis

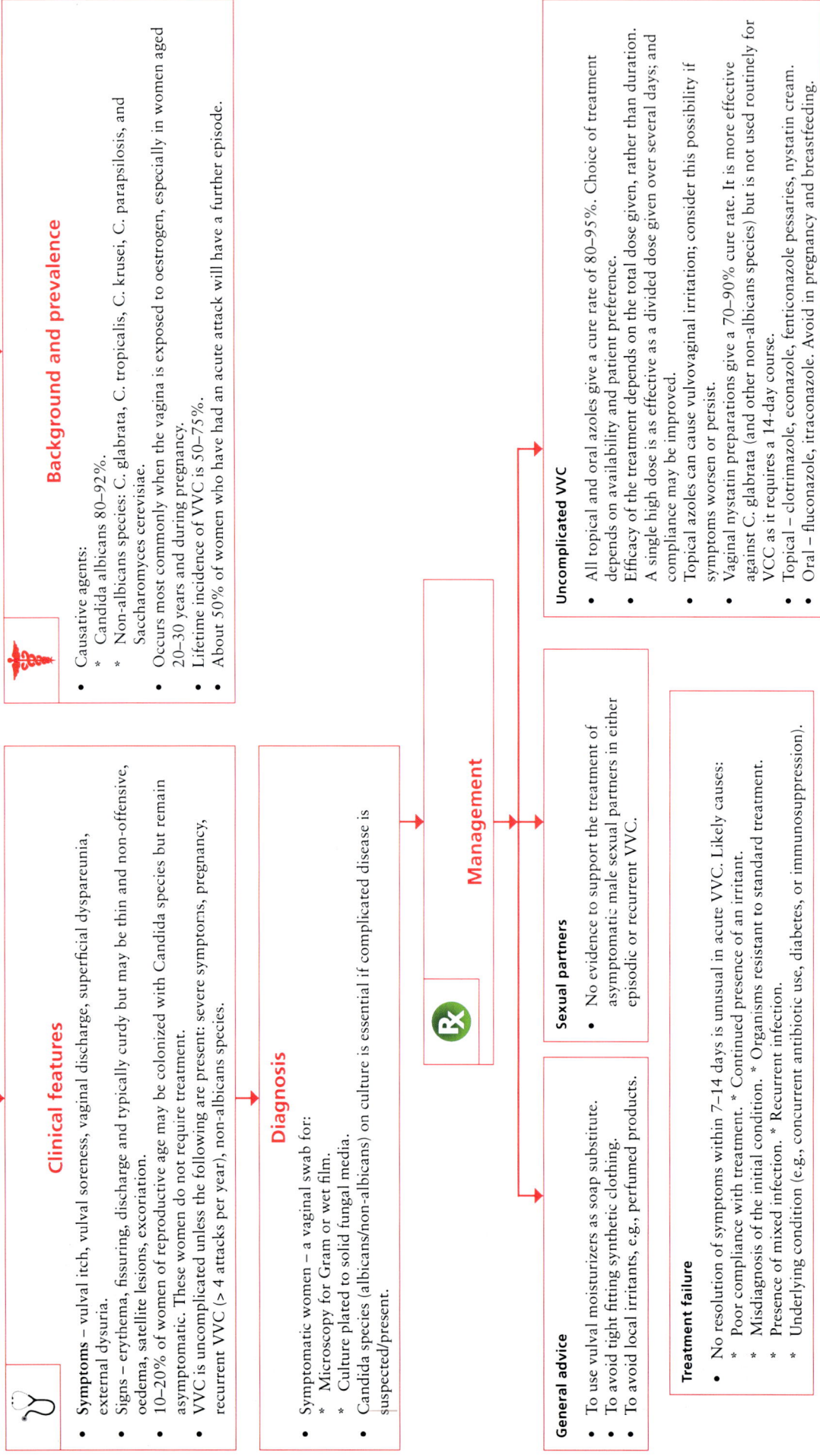

Background and prevalence

- Causative agents:
  * Candida albicans 80–92%.
  * Non-albicans species: C. glabrata, C. tropicalis, C. krusei, C. parapsilosis, and Saccharomyces cerevisiae.
- Occurs most commonly when the vagina is exposed to oestrogen, especially in women aged 20–30 years and during pregnancy.
- Lifetime incidence of VVC is 50–75%.
- About 50% of women who have had an acute attack will have a further episode.

Clinical features

- **Symptoms** – vulval itch, vulval soreness, vaginal discharge, superficial dyspareunia, external dysuria.
- Signs – erythema, fissuring, discharge and typically curdy but may be thin and non-offensive, oedema, satellite lesions, excoriation.
- 10–20% of women of reproductive age may be colonized with Candida species but remain asymptomatic. These women do not require treatment.
- VVC is uncomplicated unless the following are present: severe symptoms, pregnancy, recurrent VVC (> 4 attacks per year), non-albicans species.

Diagnosis

- Symptomatic women – a vaginal swab for:
  * Microscopy for Gram or wet film.
  * Culture plated to solid fungal media.
- Candida species (albicans/non-albicans) on culture is essential if complicated disease is suspected/present.

Management

Uncomplicated VVC

- All topical and oral azoles give a cure rate of 80–95%. Choice of treatment depends on availability and patient preference.
- Efficacy of the treatment depends on the total dose given, rather than duration. A single high dose is as effective as a divided dose given over several days; and compliance may be improved.
- Topical azoles can cause vulvovaginal irritation; consider this possibility if symptoms worsen or persist.
- Vaginal nystatin preparations give a 70–90% cure rate. It is more effective against C. glabrata (and other non-albicans species) but is not used routinely for VVC as it requires a 14-day course.
- Topical – clotrimazole, econazole, fenticonazole pessaries, nystatin cream.
- Oral – fluconazole, itraconazole. Avoid in pregnancy and breastfeeding.

General advice

- To use vulval moisturizers as soap substitute.
- To avoid tight fitting synthetic clothing.
- To avoid local irritants, e.g., perfumed products.

Sexual partners

- No evidence to support the treatment of asymptomatic male sexual partners in either episodic or recurrent VVC.

Treatment failure

- No resolution of symptoms within 7–14 days is unusual in acute VVC. Likely causes:
  * Poor compliance with treatment. * Continued presence of an irritant.
  * Misdiagnosis of the initial condition. * Organisms resistant to standard treatment.
  * Presence of mixed infection. * Recurrent infection.
  * Underlying condition (e.g., concurrent antibiotic use, diabetes, or immunosuppression).

Follow-up

- Unnecessary if symptoms resolve. Test of cure is unnecessary.

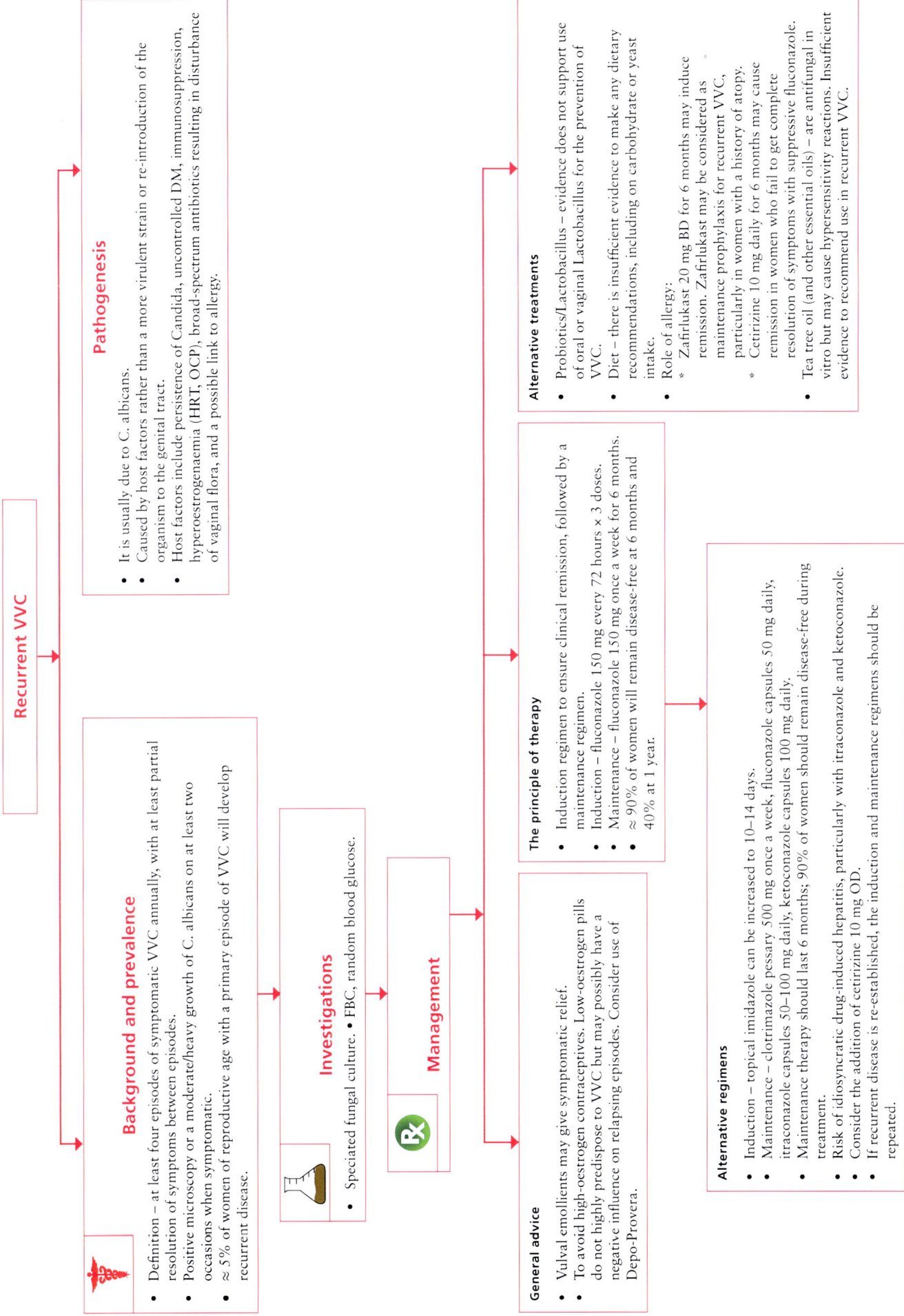

Recurrent VVC

Pathogenesis

- It is usually due to C. albicans.
- Caused by host factors rather than a more virulent strain or re-introduction of the organism to the genital tract.
- Host factors include persistence of Candida, uncontrolled DM, immunosuppression, hyperoestrogenaemia (HRT, OCP), broad-spectrum antibiotics resulting in disturbance of vaginal flora, and a possible link to allergy.

Background and prevalence

- Definition – at least four episodes of symptomatic VVC annually, with at least partial resolution of symptoms between episodes.
- Positive microscopy or a moderate/heavy growth of C. albicans on at least two occasions when symptomatic.
- ≈ 5% of women of reproductive age with a primary episode of VVC will develop recurrent disease.

Investigations

- Speciated fungal culture. • FBC, random blood glucose.

Management

General advice

- Vulval emollients may give symptomatic relief.
- To avoid high-oestrogen contraceptives. Low-oestrogen pills do not highly predispose to VVC but may possibly have a negative influence on relapsing episodes. Consider use of Depo-Provera.

The principle of therapy

- Induction regimen to ensure clinical remission, followed by a maintenance regimen.
- Induction – fluconazole 150 mg every 72 hours × 3 doses.
- Maintenance – fluconazole 150 mg once a week for 6 months.
- ≈ 90% of women will remain disease-free at 6 months and 40% at 1 year.

Alternative regimens

- Induction – topical imidazole can be increased to 10–14 days.
- Maintenance – clotrimazole pessary 500 mg once a week, fluconazole capsules 50 mg daily, itraconazole capsules 50–100 mg daily, ketoconazole capsules 100 mg daily.
- Maintenance therapy should last 6 months; 90% of women should remain disease-free during treatment.
- Risk of idiosyncratic drug-induced hepatitis, particularly with itraconazole and ketoconazole.
- Consider the addition of cetirizine 10 mg OD.
- If recurrent disease is re-established, the induction and maintenance regimens should be repeated.

Alternative treatments

- Probiotics/Lactobacillus – evidence does not support use of oral or vaginal Lactobacillus for the prevention of VVC.
- Diet – there is insufficient evidence to make any dietary recommendations, including on carbohydrate or yeast intake.
- Role of allergy:
  * Zafirlukast 20 mg BD for 6 months may induce remission. Zafirlukast may be considered as maintenance prophylaxis for recurrent VVC, particularly in women with a history of atopy.
  * Cetirizine 10 mg daily for 6 months may cause remission in women who fail to get complete resolution of symptoms with suppressive fluconazole.
- Tea tree oil (and other essential oils) – are antifungal in vitro but may cause hypersensitivity reactions. Insufficient evidence to recommend use in recurrent VVC.

VVC – specific conditions

Severe VVC

- Regardless of a history of recurrence, repeat fluconazole 150 mg after 3 days as this improves symptomatic response but not recurrence.
- There is no benefit of 7-day local treatment over a single oral dose of fluconazole. If oral treatment is contraindicated, repeat a single dose pessary after 3 days.
- Low-potency corticosteroids may improve symptomatic relief in conjunction with adequate antifungal therapy.

HIV infection

- VVC occurs more frequently and with greater persistence in HIV-infected women.
- Treatment – conventional methods including use of suppressive antifungal regimens if necessary.

Diabetes mellitus

- Symptomatic VVC is more prevalent in diabetics and most problematic in those with poor control.
- Increased prevalence of species other than C. albicans, in particular C. glabrata.
- Optimize glycaemic control.
- If C. albicans is isolated – single-dose fluconazole (150 mg) gives a similar response to that in non-diabetics.
- Symptomatic women with C. glabrata – boric acid 600 mg intravaginal suppository once a day for 14 days is as effective as fluconazole 150 mg stat.

Non-albicans species

- Majority are C. glabrata and are still susceptible to azoles. C. krusei is intrinsically resistant to fluconazole.
- Longer courses may be needed, although there are no data on optimum duration; 2 weeks is suggested.
- Suggested alternatives include:
  * Nystatin pessaries are the only licensed alternative to azole therapy and are therefore the first-line treatment for non-albicans infection.
  * Amphotericin B vaginal suppositories 50 mg OD for 14 days has a 70% success rate.
  * Limited evidence with boric acid vaginal suppositories 600 mg daily for 2–3 weeks. If mucosal irritation occurs, the dose can be reduced to 300 mg daily. There may be a teratogenic risk.
  * Intravaginal flucytosine either separately or with amphotericin to reduce the chances of resistance can be used for 2 weeks.

Pregnancy

- Asymptomatic (30–40%) and symptomatic colonization is more common in pregnancy.
- It is not associated with low birth weight or premature delivery.
- Treatment – topical imidazoles.
- Do not treat asymptomatic women.
- There is no evidence that any one topical imidazole is more effective than another.
- Longer courses are recommended; a 4-day course will cure just over 50% whereas a 7-day course cures over 90% of cases.
- Oral therapy is contraindicated.

What not to do

- Treatment of asymptomatic male sexual partners in either episodic or recurrent VVC.
- Recurrent VVC – use of tea tree oil, probiotics/Lactobacillus for prevention, or any dietary recommendations, including carbohydrate or yeast intake.
- Treatment of asymptomatic women in pregnancy.
- Oral antifungal therapy in pregnancy.

1. *The Management of Women of Reproductive Age Attending Non-genitourinary Medicine Settings Complaining of Vaginal Discharge.* FFPRHC and BASHH Guidance, January 2006.
2. *Management of Abnormal Vaginal Discharge in Women. Quick Reference Guide for Primary Care for Consultation and Adaptation.* HPA, 2007. www.hpa.org.uk.
3. *Clinical Knowledge Summaries – Vaginal Discharge.* http://www.cks.nhs.uk/vaginal_discharge.

CHAPTER 43 Trichomonas vaginalis

Background and prevalence

- A flagellated protozoan.
- Colonizes:
  * Women – vagina, urethra, and paraurethral glands. Urethral infection is present in 90% of episodes. The urinary tract is the sole site of infection in < 5% of cases.
  * Men – urethra, sub-preputial sac, and lesions of the penis.
- STI – Owing to site specificity, it inoculates only intravaginal or intraurethral sites.

History and examination

- Symptoms:
  * 10–50% are asymptomatic.
  * Vaginal discharge, vulval itching, dysuria, or offensive odour.
  * Occasionally low abdominal discomfort.
- Signs:
  * Vaginal discharge in up to 70% of women – varying in consistency from thin and scanty to profuse and thick; the classical discharge of frothy yellow occurs in 10–30% of cases.
  * Vu vitis and vaginitis.
  * Strawberry cervix appearance to the naked eye, in about 2%.
  * Higher rate on colposcopic examination.
  * 5–15% of women will have no abnormalities on examination.

Risks or complications

- Increasing evidence that TV infection may be associated with preterm delivery and low birth weight. Further research is needed to confirm these associations and to prove that the association is causal. However, studies reported that treatment in pregnancy does not improve pregnancy outcome.
- Screening of asymptomatic individuals for TV infection is not currently recommended.
- TV infection may enhance HIV transmission.

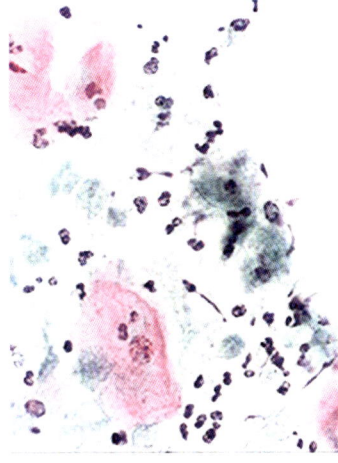

PAP smear, showing infestation by Trichomonas vaginalis

Investigations

- Wet mount or acridine orange staining is approximately 70% sensitive.
- Perform microscopy as soon as possible after the sample is taken as motility diminishes with time.
- Culture is the 'gold standard'.
- PCR-based diagnostic tests have been developed with sensitivities and specificities approaching 100%.
- If Trichomonads seen on cervical cytology, confirm by culture of vaginal secretions.
- Site to sample – posterior fornix. Self-taken vaginal swabs are likely to give equivalent results.

Management

• Metronidazole and related drugs (95% cure rate).
• There is a spontaneous cure rate of 20–25%.
• **Recommended regimens:**
  * Metronidazole 2 g orally single dose.
  * OR metronidazole 400–500 mg BD for 5–7 days.
• Single dose is cheaper with better compliance; however, failure rate is higher, especially if partners are not treated.
• **Alternative regimens** – tinidazole 2 g orally, single dose. Similar activity to metronidazole but is more expensive.

General advice

• Screen for other STIs.
• Treat sexual partner(s) simultaneously.
• Advise patients to avoid sexual intercourse (including oral sex) until they and their partner(s) have completed treatment and follow-up.

Management of sexual partners

• Screen current partners for STIs and treat for TV irrespective of the results of investigations.
• If a male contact is found to have NGU, it is reasonable to treat initially for TV and repeat the urethral smear before treating additionally for NGU.

Treatment failure

• Check compliance and exclude vomiting with metronidazole.
• Check possibility of re-infection.
• Check partner(s) has been treated.

Repeat course of standard treatment

Metronidazole-refractory TV

• A major therapeutic challenge, treatment options are extremely limited.
• Sensitivity testing is currently unavailable.
• Use of a broad-spectrum antibiotic such as erythromycin or amoxicillin before re-treating with metronidazole may improve the chances of a cure.
• Higher doses of metronidazole:
  * Metronidazole 400 mg TDS with metronidazole 1 g PR daily for 7 days or longer.
  * Metronidazole 2 g OD for 3–5 days.
  * High-dose intravenous metronidazole.
• High doses of oral tinidazole, e.g., 2 g BD for 2 weeks, with or without intravaginal tinidazole with a cure rate of 92%.

Test of cure is only recommended if the patient remains symptomatic following treatment, or if symptoms recur.

What not to do

• Screening of asymptomatic individuals for TV.

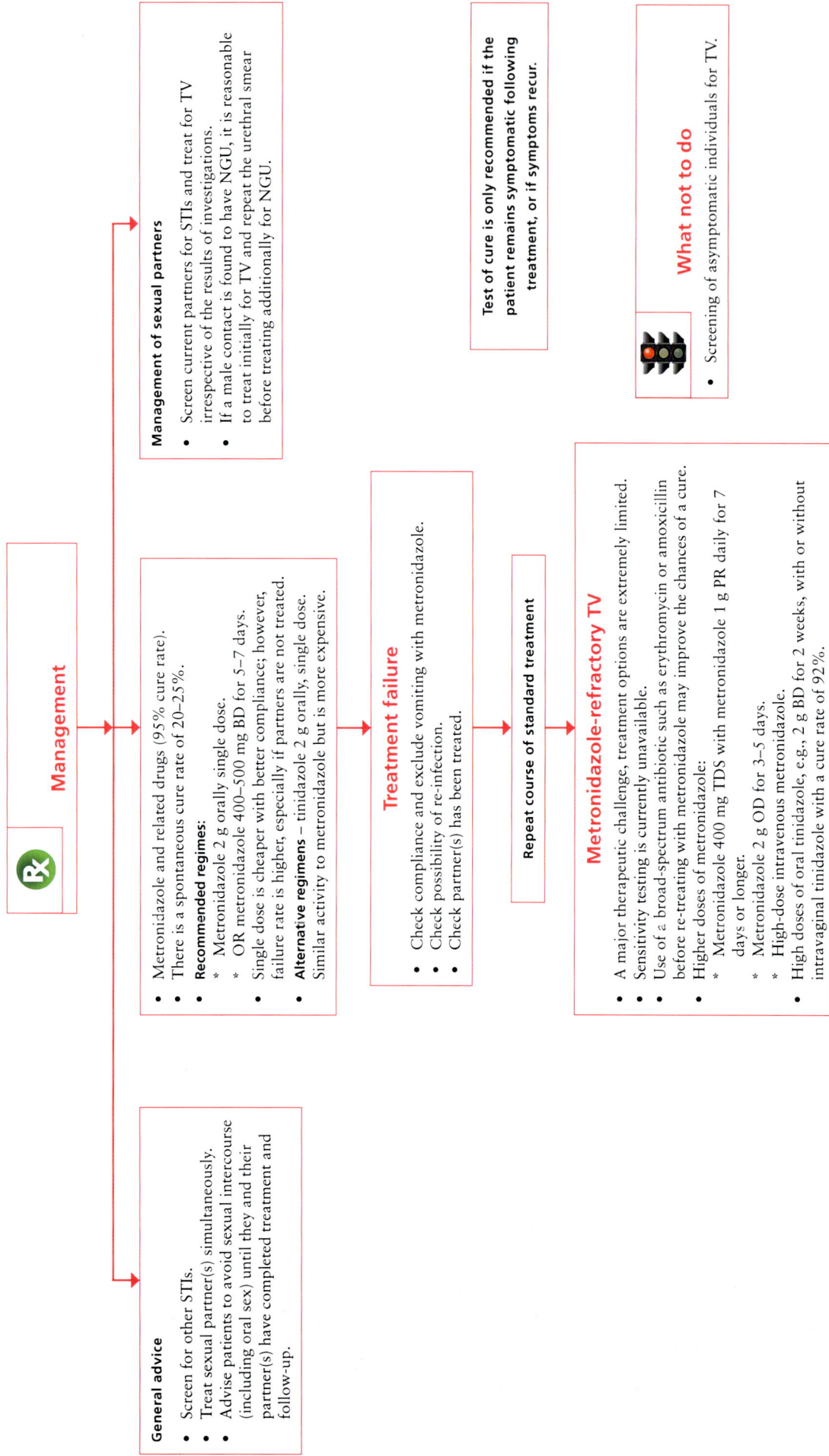

1. *The Management of Women of Reproductive Age Attending Non-Genitourinary Medicine Settings Complaining of Vaginal Discharge. FFPRHC and BASHH Guidance, January 2006.*
2. *Management of Abnormal Vaginal Discharge in Women. Quick Reference Guide for Primary Care for Consultation and Adaptation. Health Protection Agency, 2007.* http://www.hpa.org.uk.
3. http://www.cks.nhs.uk/vaginal_discharge.
4. http://en.wikipedia.org/wiki/Trichomonas_vaginalis.

STIs

- **Bacterial**
  * Gonorrhea – *Neisseria gonorrheae*.
  * Chlamydia – *Chlamydia trachomatis*.
  * Non-gonococcal urethritis – *C. trachomatis* or *Mycoplasma genitalium*.
  * Chancroid – *Haemophilus ducreyi*.
  * Granuloma inguinale – *Calymmatobacterium granulomatis*.
  * Lymphogranuloma venereum – *Chlamydia trachomatis*.
  * Syphilis – *Treponema pallidum*.
  * Mycoplasma – *Mycoplasma hominis*.
- **Viral**
  * Genital herpes – *herpes simplex virus*.
  * Genital warts – *human papillomavirus*.
  * Hepatitis B, D, A, C, E – *hepatitis viruses, types A–E*.
  * HIV/AIDS – *human immunodeficiency virus*.
  * Molluscum contagiosum – *poxvirus*.
- **Protozoal**
  * Trichomoniasis – *Trichomonas vaginalis*.
- **Fungal**
  * Yeast infections – *Candida albicans*.
- **Parasites**
  * Pubic lice or crabs – *Pediculosis pubis*.
  * Scabies – *Sarcoptes scabiei*.

Genital ulcer

- **Painful**
  * Herpes – *herpes simplex virus type 1, 2*.
  * Chancroid – *Haemophilus ducreyi*.
  * Systemic conditions – Behcet's syndrome.
- **Painless**
  * Syphilis – primary chancre, condylomata lata.
  * Condylomata accuminata – *human papillomavirus virus*.
  * Granuloma inguinale – *Calymmatobacterium granulomatis*.
  * Lymphogranuloma venerum (LGV) – *Chlamydia trachomatis*.

Guidance on screening and testing for STIs in patients attending GUM clinics

Asymptomatic women

- Cervix.
  * Gonorrhoea – culture.
  * Chlamydia – NAAT.
- Vagina (self-taken swabs; vulval-introital and posterior fornix swabs).
- Urine.
  * Chlamydia – NAAT.
- Blood.
  * Syphilis – EIA or TPPA, or cardiolipin test plus TPHA.
  * HIV – EIA.

Women presenting with genital discharge

- Urethra.
  * Gonorrhoea – microscopy plus culture.
- Cervix.
  * Gonorrhoea – microscopy plus culture.
  * Chlamydia – NAAT.
- Vagina (self-taken swabs; vulval-introital, wall smear, posterior fornix swabs).
  * Gonorrhoea – NAAT (not validated).
  * Chlamydia – NAAT (not validated).
  * Candida – microscopy plus culture.
  * Trichomonas – culture or latex agglutination +/– microscopy.
  * Bacterial vaginosis – microscopy.
- Rectum and oropharynx.
  * Gonorrhoea – culture.
  * Chlamydia – tissue culture.
- Urine.
  * Chlamydia – NAAT (if cervical/vaginal specimen is not available).

	Gonorrhoea	Chlamydia	Herpes
Aetiology	Neisseria gonorrhoeae.	Chlamydia trachomatis.	Herpes simplex virus 1 (orolabial herpes). Herpes simplex virus 2 (sexual transmission).
Organism	Gram-negative diplococcus.	Gram-negative obligate intracellular organism.	DNA virus.
Primary sites of infection	Mucous membranes of the urethra, endocervix, rectum, pharynx, and conjunctiva.	Mucous membranes of the urethra, endocervix, rectum, pharynx, and conjunctiva.	Genital. Oral.
Transmission	Direct inoculation of infected secretions from one mucous membrane to another.	Penetrative sexual intercourse.	Direct sexual contact. Orolabial contact.
Universal screening	Not advisable.	National Chlamydial Screening Programme.	Not available.
Diagnosis	Microscopy. NAAT. Culture.	NAAT. Cell culture. Enzyme immunoassays (EIAs).	Culture. Serology.
Specimen site	Women: vaginal or endocervical swab – NAAT; endocervical and urethral swab – culture. Men: first-pass urine – NAAT; urethral swab – microscopy and culture.	Women – cervical and vulvovaginal swabs; first-catch urine (FCU) specimen. Men – urine; urethral swab. Men and women – rectal, pharyngeal, and conjunctival specimens.	Ulcer base.
Treatment	Ceftriaxone and azithromycin.	Doxycycline, azithromycin, erythromycin, ofloxacin.	Aciclovir, valaciclovir, and famciclovir.
Test of cure	Recommended.	Not necessary.	Not applicable.

Tropical genital ulcers

	Chancroid	LGV	Donovanosis
Aetiology	*Haemophilus ducreyi.*	*Chlamydia trachomatis.*	*Klebsiella granulomatis.*
Organism	Gram-negative coccobacilli.	Gram-negative obligate intracellular organism.	Gram-negative.
Primary sites of infection	Anogenital ulceration and lymphadenitis.	Mucous membranes of the urethra, endocervix, rectum, pharynx, and conjunctiva.	Anogenital area, inguinal nodes, cevix, vagina, mouth.
Transmission	Penetrative sexual intercourse.	Penetrative sexual intercourse.	Penetrative sexual intercourse.
Diagnosis	Culture. PCR. Microscopy of a Gram-stained smear.	NAAT. Cell culture. Enzyme immunoassays (EIAs).	Demonstration of Donovan bodies.
Specimen site	Ulcer base or the undermined edges of the ulcer or from pus aspirated from the bubo.	Women – cervical and vulvovaginal swabs; first-catch urine (FCU) specimen. Men – urine, urethral swab. Men and women – rectal, pharyngeal, and conjunctival specimens.	Cellular material (scraping/smear/swab/crushing of pinched-off tissue fragment) or biopsy from the ulcers.
Treatment	Azithromycin, ceftriaxone, erythromycin.	Doxycycline, azithromycin, erythromycin, ofloxacin.	Azithromycin, ciprofloxacin, erythromycin.
Test of cure	Not necessary.	Not necessary.	Not necessary.

In general, the prevalence of chancroid has decreased from 40–50% to 15% or less, while HSV-2 has risen from 5–10% to 40%. The prevalence of LGV, however, has remained stable and has not exceeded 5% of GUD.

1. Screening Guideline Steering Group. *Sexually Transmitted Infections.* UK National Screening and Testing Guidelines, August 2006.
2. *UK National Guideline on the Management of Vulval Conditions.* CEG/BASHH, 2007.

CHAPTER 44 Sexually transmitted infections

CHAPTER 45 Gonorrhoea

Prevalence and incidence

- Second most common bacterial STI in the UK.
- Most common in young people under the age of 25 years, in men who have sex with men.
- Incidence of gonorrhoea has decreased in all age groups since 2002 in the UK. In 2005, 18,665 gonorrhoea infections were diagnosed in the UK in GUM clinics.
- Affects the mucous membranes of the urethra, endocervix, rectum, pharynx, and conjunctiva.

Symptoms

Women – symptoms usually develop within 10 days.

- Asymptomatic in up to 50% of cases.
- Increased or altered vaginal discharge (up to 50%).
- Lower abdominal pain (up to 25%).
- Urethral infection – dysuria (12%).
- IMB or HMB – rarely.
- Pharyngeal infection – asymptomatic in > 90% of cases.
- Rectal infection is by transmucosal spread rather than from anal intercourse and is usually asymptomatic.

Men – symptoms develop 2–5 days after infection.

- Urethral infection – urethral discharge (> 80%), dysuria (> 50%), asymptomatic (< 10%).
- Rectal infection – usually asymptomatic but may cause anal discharge (12%) or perianal/anal pain or discomfort (7%).
- Pharyngeal infection – asymptomatic in > 90% of cases.

Signs

Women:

- Mucopurulent endocervical discharge, easily induced bleeding (< 50%).
- Pelvic/lower abdominal tenderness (< 5%).
- No abnormal findings is common.

Men:

- Mucopurulent or purulent urethral discharge.
- Epididymal tenderness/swelling or balanitis is rare.

Risks or complications

- PID in women.
- Epididymo-orchitis or prostatitis in men.
- Disseminated gonococcal infection (<1%) – (haematogenous dissemination) skin lesions, arthralgia, arthritis, and tenosynovitis (uncommon).

There is no evidence to support widespread unselected testing for gonorrhoea in the community.

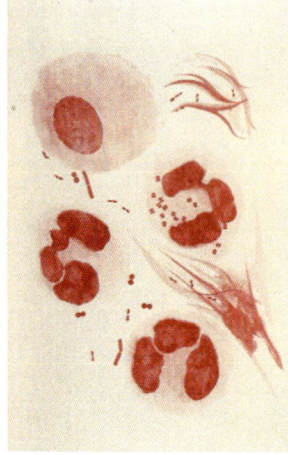

Gram-negative diplococci shown within polymorphonuclear leucocytes

Specimen site

- **Women:**
  - * Vaginal or endocervical swab – NAAT.
  - * Endocervical and urethral swab – culture.
  - * Urine is a suboptimal sample in women.
- **Men:**
  - * First-pass urine for NAAT.
  - * Urethral swab – microscopy and culture.
  - **Rectal and pharyngeal swab.**

Investigations – no test for gonorrhoea offers 100% sensitivity and specificity.

Microscopy

- Gram stain of genital specimens – Gram-negative diplococci within polymorphonuclear leucocytes.
- Poor sensitivity in women – 37–50% for endocervical smears and 20% for urethral smears; therefore, not recommended for urethral smears.
- Sensitivity of 90–95% in men with urethral discharge and is recommended to facilitate immediate diagnosis in symptomatic men. Staining of urethral smears in asymptomatic men is less sensitive (50–75%).
- Microscopy is not appropriate for pharyngeal specimens and asymptomatic rectal infections.

NAATs

- NAATs –more sensitive than culture and can test wider range of specimen types. **High sensitivity (> 9 6%) in both symptomatic and asymptomatic infection.**
- Equivalent sensitivity to culture in urine and urethral swab from men and in vaginal and endocervical swabs from women. Superior sensitivity to culture in extra-genital (anogenital and pharyngeal) specimens.
- **Sensitivity in female urine is significantly lower and urine is not the optimal specimen in women.**
- A dual NAAT for both pathogens (chlamydia and gonorrhoea) maximizes sensitivity and ease of specimen collection, transport, and processing.
- Positive NAATs require supplementary testing to confirm the diagnosis.

Culture

- Specific and sensitive diagnostic test.
- Allows confirmatory identification and antimicrobial susceptibility testing.
- Both direct plating of genital samples and use of transport media with prompt laboratory plating give acceptable results.
- Culture is necessary in patients with signs and symptoms compatible with gonorrhoea and/or with a confirmed NAAT result, prior to antibiotics being given, so that susceptibility testing can be performed and resistant strains identified.

Management

Indications for treatment

- Identification of intracellular Gram-negative diplococci on microscopy of a smear from the genital tract.
- A positive culture for N. gonorrhoeae from any site.
- A positive NAAT for N. gonorrhoeae from any site.
- Recent sexual partner(s) of confirmed cases of gonococcal infection.
- Following sexual assault.

General advice

- To abstain from UPSI until the patient and partner(s) have completed treatment; if azithromycin is used, this will be 7 days after treatment was given.
- Screen for other STIs. Test for C. trachomatis routinely on all adults with gonorrhoea or treat to eradicate possible co-infection.

Partner notification

- Male patients with symptomatic urethral infection should notify all partners with whom they had sexual contact within the preceding 2 weeks or their last partner if longer ago.
- Patients with infection at other sites or asymptomatic infection should notify all partners within the preceding 3 months.
- Offer sexual partners testing and treat epidemiologically for gonorrhoea.
- To confidently exclude infection in patients who attend within 3 days of sexual contact, consider a second set of tests if effective antimicrobial therapy is not given. Conventionally this would be 14 days after contact.

Uncomplicated anogenital infection in adults: treatment

- Ceftriaxone 500 mg IM as a single dose with azithromycin 1g oral as a single dose.
- Azithromycin is recommended as co-treatment irrespective of the results of chlamydia testing.
- There is a risk of resistance.
- Alternative regimens – cefixime, spectinomycin.

Follow-up and test of cure (TOC)

- Assess after treatment to confirm compliance with treatment, ensure resolution of symptoms, enquire about adverse reactions, take a sexual history to explore the possibility of re-infection, pursue partner notification and health promotion.
- TOC is recommended in all cases to identify emerging resistance.
- If TOC needs to be selective, prioritize the following patients – persisting symptoms or signs, pharyngeal infection (all treatments are less effective at eradicating pharyngeal infection), treatment with anything other than the first-line recommendations.
- **Method and timing of TOC:**
  * Persisting symptoms or signs – culture, at least 72 hours after completion of therapy.
  * If asymptomatic – NAATs followed by culture if positive. Test 2 weeks after completion of antibiotic therapy.
- Infection identified after treatment may well be due to re-infection.

1. *UK National Guideline for the Management of Gonorrhoea in Adults.* CEG/BASHH, 2011.
2. *Guidance for Gonorrhoea Testing in England and Wales.* HPA/BASHH, http://www.gyuk.org.uk.
3. http://fr.wikipedia.org/wiki/Gonorrhée.

CHAPTER 46 Chlamydia

Prevalence and incidence

- Most common STI in the UK.
- About 5–10% of sexually active women aged < 24 years and men between 20 and 24 years may be infected.
- Risk factors – age < 25 years, new sexual partner, > 1 sexual partner in the past year, and lack of consistent use of condoms.
- Site of infection – men: urethra; women: endocervix, urethra. It also infects the conjunctiva, rectum, and pharynx.
- Transmission – primarily by penetrative sexual intercourse; however, infection can be detected at the conjunctiva and nasopharynx without concomitant genital tract infection.
- Two thirds of sexual partners of chlamydia-positive individuals are also chlamydia positive.

Risks or complications

- PID in 10–40% cases; can result in tubal factor infertility, ectopic pregnancy, and chronic pelvic pain. Risk of PID and subfertility increases with each recurrence of infection.
- Other complications:
  * Fitz–Hugh–Curtis syndrome (peri-hepatitis).
  * Vertical transmission – neonatal conjunctivitis, pneumonia.
  * Epididymo-orchitis.
  * Adult conjunctivitis.
  * Reactive arthritis/Reiter's syndrome (more common in men).

Clinical features

- Asymptomatic in up to 70% of women and 50% of men with ongoing transmission in the community. If untreated, infection may persist or resolve spontaneously.
- Women – PCB, IMB; purulent vaginal discharge; mucopurulent cervical discharge; contact bleeding; dysuria, deep dyspareunia, pelvic pain and tenderness; inflamed or friable cervix.
- Men – urethral discharge, urethral discomfort, dysuria.
- Rectal infections – usually asymptomatic, but may cause anal discharge and anorectal discomfort (proctitis).
- Pharyngeal infections – asymptomatic and are uncommon.

Investigations

No test is 100% sensitive or specific.

Sites to be sampled

Women:
  * Cervical or vulvovaginal swab. Vulvovaginal swab has sensitivity of 90–95%.
  * If a speculum examination is not possible, then a self-taken vulvovaginal swab or urine sample can be used. Variable sensitivities (65–100%) with the first-catch urine specimen.

Men:
  * First-voided urine sample or urethral swab.
  * Rectal, pharyngeal, and conjunctival specimens – currently none of the NAATs have FDA approval for these sites.

NAAT

- NAATs are more sensitive and specific than enzyme immunoassays (EIAs).
- Confirm reactive tests using the same NAAT platform, but if possible with a second platform. However, offer treatment to all patients with unconfirmed reactive NAAT results.
- In general, NAATs are 90–95% sensitive. As the number of sites sampled or the number of different NAATs used increases, the detection rate increases.

Cell culture

- Sensitivity 60–80%; 100% specificity.
- Expensive, limited availability.
- Can be used on all specimen types.
- **Routine use is not recommended owing to high cost and low sensitivity.**

Enzyme immunoassays (EIAs)

- Labour intensive, requires skilled personnel.
- Unsuitable for large numbers of specimens.
- Can use all specimen types including rectal and pharyngeal.
- **Sensitivity is 40–70%, and their use is not recommended.**

Owing to the evidence of high and increasing rates of infection, the National Chlamydial Screening Programme (NCSP) has been introduced in the UK. All sexually active under 25-year-olds are to be tested for chlamydia annually or when there is a change of sexual partner.

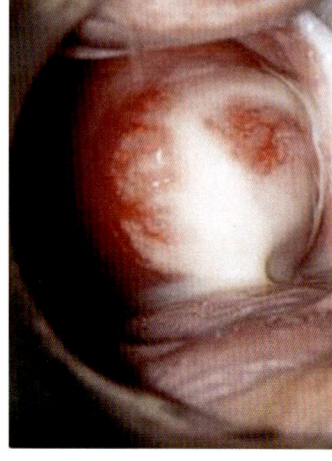

Inflamed cervix with mucopurulent discharge

Management Rx

General acvice

- To avoid UPSI (including oral sex) until patients and their partner(s) have completed treatment (or wait 7 days if treated with azithromycin).
- Explain long-term implications.
- Screen for other STIs. If the patient is within the window period for HIV and syphilis, repeat at an appropriate time interval.
- Uncomplicated infection is not an indication for removal of an IUS or IUD.

Pregnancy and breastfeeding

- Doxycycline and ofloxacin are contraindicated.
- Erythromycin 500 mg QDS for 7 days/500 mg BD for 14 days.
- Or amoxicillin 500 mg TDS for 7 days.
- Or azithromycin 1 g stat.
- Owing to higher positive chlamydia tests after treatment in pregnancy (possibly due to less efficacious treatment regimen, non-compliance or re-infection) – pregnant woman must have a test of cure 5 weeks after completing therapy, 6 weeks later if given azithromycin.
- Azithromycin is probably < 95% effective. Azithromycin 1 g stat is recommended by WHO; unlicensed in the UK. BNF recommends use only if no other alternative is available.

Treatment

- Recommended regimens:
  * Doxycycline 100 mg BD for 7 days.
  * Or azithromycin 1 g orally stat.
- Doxycycline and azithromycin have > 95% cure. There is no difference in the re-infection rates between the two.
- Alternative regimens: if either of the above treatments are contraindicated.
  * Erythromycin 500 mg BD for 10–14 days.
  * Or ofloxacin 200 mg BD or 400 mg OD for 7 days.
- Ofloxacin has similar efficacy to doxycycline and a better side-effect profile, but is more expensive so is not recommended as first-line treatment.
- Erythromycin – less efficacious than azithromycin or doxycycline; 20–25% of patients experience side effects that are sufficient to discontinue treatment.

Management of sexual partners

- Partner notification – offer all sexual partners a full STI screen. Offer epidemiological treatment.
- If declined, advise patients to abstain from sex until they have received a negative result. If found to be positive, screen and offer epidemiological treatment to any other potentially exposed partner(s).
- A cut-off of 4 weeks is used to identify those sexual partner(s) potentially at risk if the index patient is symptomatic. If the index case is asymptomatic, a cut-off of 6 months, or until the last previous sexual partner (whichever is the longer time period), is used.
- Re-testing positive can result from either suboptimal antimicrobial therapy or re-infection. Re-infection may result from having sexual intercourse with either an untreated, suboptimally treated, or a new partner who is C. trachomatis positive.

Test of cure

- Not routinely recommended.
- It should be performed in pregnancy or if non-compliance or re-exposure is suspected at 5 weeks (6 weeks if azithromycin given) after treatment is completed.

1. UK National Guideline for the Management of Genital Tract Infection with Chlamydia trachomatis. BASHH, 2006.
2. http//www.stdinfo.org.

Background

- HSV-1 or HSV-2.
- Primary infection: first infection with either HSV-1 or HSV-2 in an individual with no pre-existing antibodies.
- Recurrent episode: recurrence of clinical symptoms owing to reactivation of pre-existent HSV-1 or HSV-2 infection after a period of latency.

Natural history

- Majority of infections are asymptomatic (80%).
- Primary genital herpes – equally likely to be caused by HSV-1 or HSV-2.
- Following primary infection, the virus becomes latent in local sensory ganglia, periodically reactivating to cause symptomatic lesions or asymptomatic, but infectious, viral shedding.
- Virus can be shed asymptomatically from the external genitalia, anus, rectum, cervix, and urethra.
- Recurrence rate after a symptomatic first episode is 0.34 recurrences/month for HSV-2 and is four times more frequent than the recurrence rate for HSV-1. Recurrence rates decline over time.
- In HIV-positive HSV-2 seropositive individuals, both symptomatic and asymptomatic shedding are increased, especially in those with low CD4 counts and those who are also seropositive for HSV-16.

Clinical features

Symptoms

- Asymptomatic.
- Local symptoms – painful ulceration, dysuria, vaginal or urethral discharge.
- Systemic symptoms – fever and myalgia. Much more common in primary.

Signs

- Blistering and ulceration of the external genitalia (+/– cervix/rectum).
- Tender inguinal lymphadenitis, usually bilateral.
- First episodes – lesions and lymphadenitis are usually bilateral. In recurrent disease, it is usual for lesions to affect favoured sites. They may alternate between sides but are usually unilateral for each episode.

Risks or complications

- Autonomic neuropathy, resulting in urinary retention.
- Autoinoculation to fingers and adjacent skin, e.g., on thighs.
- Aseptic meningitis.

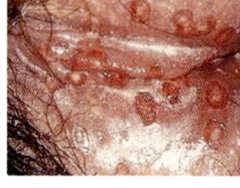

Female external genitalia showing severe blistering

Investigations

Virus detection and characterization

- HSV isolation in cell culture in swabs taken from the base of the genital lesion for confirmation of the infection and its type. Current routine diagnostic method in the UK.
- Virus typing to differentiate between HSV-1 and HSV-2.
- Virus culture – slow, labour-intensive, and expensive. Specificity is virtually 100%, but levels of virus shedding, quality of specimens, sample storage and transport conditions influence sensitivity.
- HSV DNA detection by PCR increases HSV detection rates compared with virus culture. It allows less stringent conditions for sample storage and transport than virus culture and new real-time PCR assays are rapid and highly specific. **Real-time PCR is recommended as the preferred diagnostic method for genital herpes.**

Serology

- HSV type-specific antibodies – HSV-1 or HSV-2 IgG represents HSV infection at some time. It is difficult to say whether the infection is recent as IgM detection is unreliable. Collection of serum samples a few weeks apart can be used to show seroconversion and, hence, recent primary infection. HSV-2 antibodies are indicative of genital herpes. HSV-1 antibodies do not differentiate between genital and oropharyngeal infection.
- Serology may be helpful in recurrent genital disease of unknown cause; counselling patients with initial episodes of disease, including pregnant women; investigating asymptomatic partners of patients with genital herpes.

Management

Counselling

- Most people with recurrences adjust over time but antiviral treatment can improve quality of life.
- Everyday stress does not affect recurrences.
- Use of antiviral drugs for symptom control.
- Abstinence from sexual contact during recurrences or prodromes.
- Reassure regarding transmission by fomites and autoinoculation after the first infection is over.
- Transmission may occur as a result of asymptomatic viral shedding.
- Condoms may help in reducing transmission; however, their use cannot completely prevent transmission.

First-episode genital herpes

- General advice – saline bathing; analgesia; topical anaesthetic agents, e.g., 5% lignocaine ointment may be useful but use with caution because of the risk of potential sensitization.
- Antiviral drugs reduce the severity and duration of episodes.
  * Oral antiviral drugs within 5 days of the start of the episode and while new lesions are still forming.
  * Aciclovir, valaciclovir, and famciclovir.
  * Antiviral therapy does not alter the natural history of the disease.
  * Topical agents are less effective than oral agents.
  * Combined oral and topical treatment is of no benefit.
  * IV therapy only when the patient cannot swallow or tolerate oral medication because of vomiting.
  * There is no evidence for benefit from courses longer than 5 days.
- Review the patient after 5 days and continue therapy if new lesions are still appearing at this time.
- Management of complications:
  * Hospitalize if urinary retention, meningism, and severe constitutional symptoms.
  * If catheterization is required, suprapubic catheterization is preferred to prevent theoretical risk of ascending infection, to reduce the pain associated with the procedure, and to allow normal micturition to be restored without multiple removals and recatheterizations.

Recurrent genital herpes

- Recurrences are self-limiting and generally cause minor symptoms.
- Manage according to recurrence frequency, symptom severity, and relationship status.
- General advice – saline bathing, analgesia, 5% lignocaine ointment.
- Episodic antiviral treatment:
  * Oral aciclovir, valaciclovir, and famciclovir reduce the duration (by 1–2 days) and severity of recurrence.
  * Patient-initiated treatment started early in an episode is most likely to be effective.
- Suppressive antiviral therapy – patients who have at least six recurrences per annum have fewer or no episodes on suppressive therapy. Patients with lower rates of recurrence will probably also have fewer recurrences with treatment. Balance the frequency of recurrence with the cost and inconvenience of treatment.

Asymptomatic viral shedding

- Most common in patients with genital HSV-2 infection in the first year after infection. In individuals with frequent symptomatic recurrences, it is an important cause of transmission. May be reduced by aciclovir 400 mg twice daily.
- Prevention of transmission:
  * Condoms may be partially effective.
  * Aciclovir, famciclovir, and valaciclovir all suppress symptomatic and asymptomatic viral shedding by about 80–90%.
- Suppressive antiviral therapy with valaciclovir reduces the rate of acquisition of HSV-2 infection and clinically symptomatic genital herpes in sero-discordant couples. Although valaciclovir reduces the risk of acquiring symptomatic infection by 75%, approximately 60 people need to be treated to prevent one transmission.

Partner notification

- May clarify whether a partner is infected or not.
- Is an effective way of detecting individuals with unrecognized disease.
- May help to relieve anxiety about transmission or reinforce the need to reduce the risk of transmission.
- Awareness of the diagnosis in a partner or ex-partner may prevent further onward transmission.
  - Herpes vaccines – there are no vaccines currently approved for prevention of genital herpes although trials are ongoing.

Genital herpes in pregnancy
See Obstetrics: evidence-based algorithms.

1. *National Guideline for the Management of Genital Herpes.* CEG/BASHH, 2007.

2. http://www.hardinmd.lib.uiowa.edu.

3. "<a href="http://commons.wikimedia.org/wiki/File:SOA-Herpes-genitalis-female.jpg#mediaviewer/File:SOA-Herpes-genitalis-female.jpg">SOA-Herpes-genitalis-female</a>" by SOA-AIDS Amsterdam - <a rel="nofollow" class="external text" href="http://www.aidsfonds.nl/">SOA-AIDS Amsterdam</a>. Licensed under <a href="http://creativecommons.org/licenses/by-sa/3.0/" title="Creative Commons Attribution-Share Alike 3.0">CC BY-SA 3.0</a> via <a href="//commons.wikimedia.org/wiki/">Wikimedia Commons</a>.

Background

- Systemic disease caused by Chlamydia trachomatis. • Rare in developed countries with 65 reported cases of 'tropical genital ulcers' (chancroid, LGV, and donovanosis) in England in 1998. Since 2003, there has been a series of LGV outbreaks in European cities, mostly among HIV-positive men who have sex with men (MSM); more than 75% are HIV positive, and many have concomitant STIs (e.g., gonorrhoea) or infection with hepatitis C virus.

Clinical features – three stages.

- **Incubation period** – 3–30 days.
- **Primary lesion** – transient, painless papule or pustule, or shallow erosion. Found on coronal sulcus of males and on the posterior vaginal wall, fourchette, vulva, and occasionally on the cervix of females. Extra-genital lesions – oral cavity (tonsil) and extra-genital lymph nodes.
- **Secondary lesions** – lymphadenitis or lymphadenopathy or Bubo. Chlamydia serovars L1–L3 are lymphotropic, resulting in thrombolymphangitis and peri-lymphangitis resulting in inflammation and swelling of lymph nodes and surrounding tissue. Lymphadenopathy commonly follows the primary lesion by a period of a few days to weeks.
  * Most common clinical manifestation – unilateral (2/3 of cases) tender inguinal and/or femoral lymphadenopathy. It may involve one lymph node or the entire chain, which can become matted with multiple points, creating chronic fistulae.
  * When both inguinal and femoral lymph nodes are involved, they may be separated by the so-called 'groove sign', which consists of the separation of these two lymph node systems by the inguinal ligament which is pathognomonic of LGV (only seen in 15–20% of cases).
  * Systemic spread may be associated with fever, arthritis, pneumonitis and, rarely, peri-hepatitis (Fitz–Hugh–Curtis syndrome).
- **Tertiary stage** – the genitoanorectal syndrome:
  * Majority recover after the secondary stage without sequelae, but in a few patients the persistence or progressive spread of Chlamydia in anogenital tissues results in a chronic inflammatory response, and destruction of tissue resulting in proctitis, acute proctocolitis mimicking Crohn's disease, fistulae, strictures, and a chronic granulomatous disfiguring condition of the vulva (esthiomene).

Risks or complications

- Destruction of lymph nodes may result in lymphoedema of genitals (elephantiasis) with persistent suppuration and pyoderma.
- An association with rectal cancer has been reported.

- In recent outbreaks, all cases presented with proctitis resulting in severe rectal pain, mucoid and/or haemorrhagic rectal discharge, tenesmus, constipation and other signs of lower gastrointestinal inflammation, which can be very intense. Some patients reported systemic symptoms such as fever and malaise. Genital ulcers and inguinal symptoms are rare.

Differential diagnosis

- Other causes of genital ulcerations or inguinal lymphadenopathy.
- Anorectal syndrome – exclude other causes of rectal bleeding.
- Investigations for other potentially co-existing STIs, in particular for syphilis.

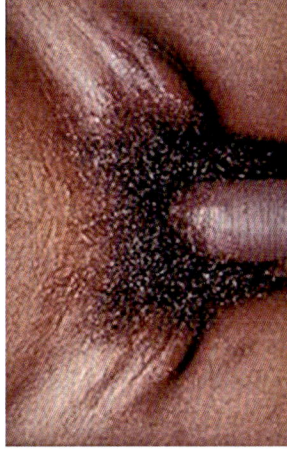

Sample sites

- Chlamydiae are intracellular organisms, thus samples must contain cellular material:
  * From the ulcer base exudate or from rectal tissue.
  * By aspiration from fluctuant lymph nodes.
  * Rectal swabs from MSM and women exposed rectally.
  * A urethral swab or first-catch urine sample when lymphadenopathy is present.

Investigations

- Original Frei test is abandoned owing to lack of sensitivity and specificity.
- Direct immunofluorescence of material from lesions to demonstrate Chlamydia trachomatis elementary and inclusion bodies is sensitive but requires expertise and is labour intensive.
- Enzyme immunoassay has lower sensitivity and it is no longer recommended.
- Histology of lymph nodes showing follicular hyperplasia and abscesses is nonspecific.
- Typing to distinguish LGV strains from other chlamydial serotypes with molecular diagnostic techniques are newer technologies becoming available.

- Detection of NAATs with PCR for urethral, cervical, or urine specimens is highly sensitive and specific. Confirm positive samples by real-time PCR for LGV-specific DNA.
- Culture from suspected LGV lesion is most specific, but its sensitivity is 75–85% and 30–50% in the case of bubo aspirate. It is labour intensive, expensive, and of restricted availability.
- Chlamydia trachomatis serology – a 4-fold rise of antibody (both IgM and IgG) in the course of suspected illness is diagnostic of active infection. Alternatively, single point titres of > 1/64 and > 1/256 are considered positive. The test may lack sensitivity for the earlier manifestations of LGV such as ulcers, and a high titre in the absence of symptoms cannot confirm LGV.

Management

General advice

- To avoid UPSI until the patient and partner(s) have completed treatment and follow-up.
- Screen for other possible causes of genital ulcerative disease – Haemophilus ducreyi, Treponema pallidum, herpes simplex, and Klebsiella/Calymmatobacterium granulomatis, and other STIs.
- Biopsy of lymph nodes may be required to exclude neoplasia.

Recommended regimens

- Treat early to reduce the chronic phase.
- Prolonged treatment (at least 3 weeks) is the norm.
- Recommended regimens:
  * 1st choice: doxycycline 100 mg BD orally for 21 days.
  * 2nd choice: erythromycin 500 mg QDS orally for 21 days.
- Alternative regimens – azithromycin may be effective in multiple doses over 2–3 weeks but clinical data are lacking.

- Consider surgical repair, including reconstructive genital surgery in patients with fibrotic lesions or fistulae.

Sexual partner(s)

- Examine persons who have had sexual contact with a patient with LGV within the 30 days before onset of the patient's symptoms; test for rectal, urethral, or cervical chlamydial infection and treat, or provide presumptive treatment (e.g., azithromycin 1.0 g orally or doxycycline 100 mg BD for 7 days).

Fluctuant buboes – aspirate fluctuant buboes through healthy adjacent skin. Surgical incision is usually contraindicated because of fear of complications.

Follow-up and test of cure (TOC)

- Follow clinically until signs and symptoms have resolved. This may occur within 3–6 weeks.
- Routine microbiological TOC depends on locally available resources. Specific NAAT tests can be used, although their use has not been rigorously evaluated and the optimum time for testing is not yet known.

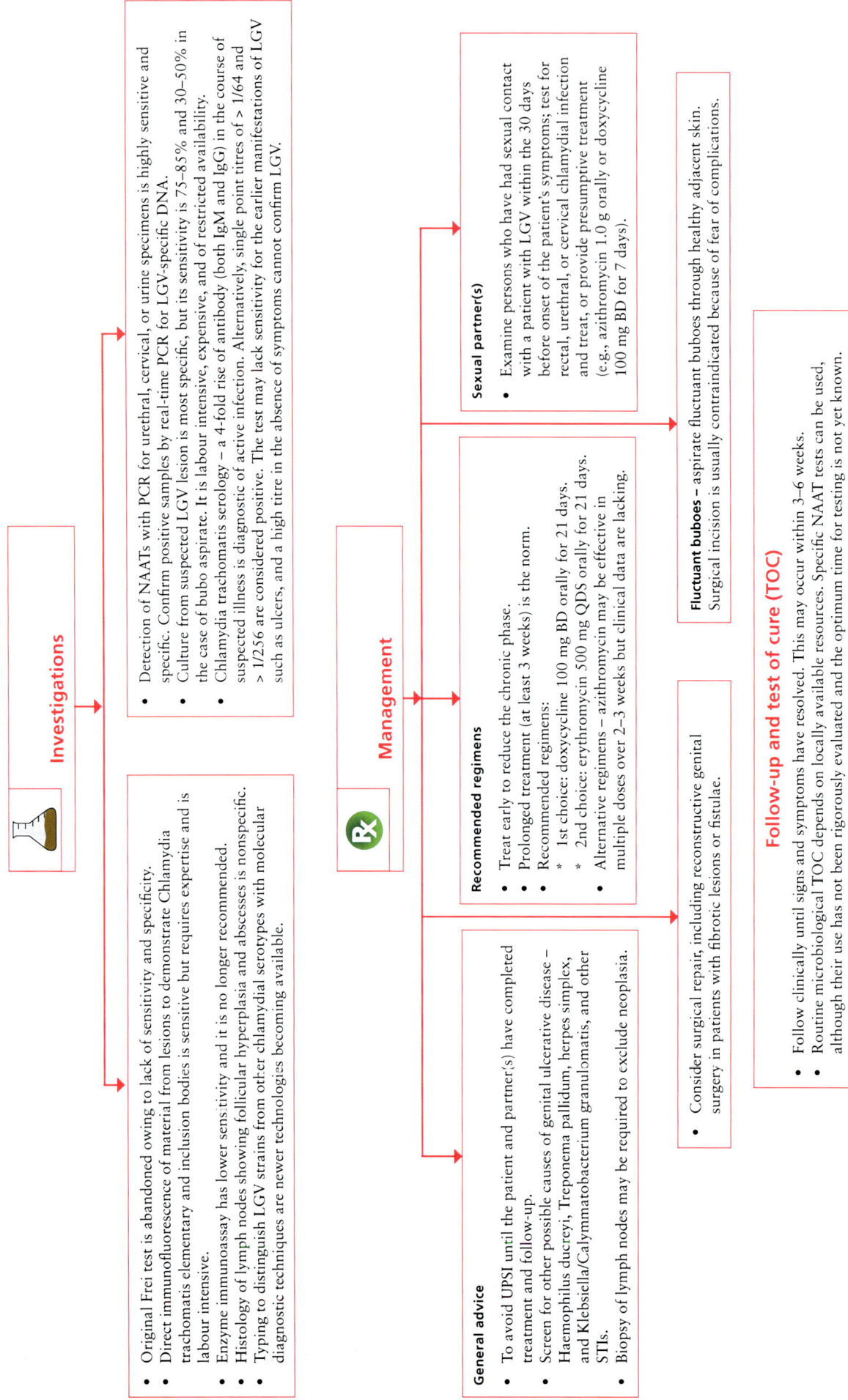

1. *National Guideline for the Management of Lymphogranuloma Venereum (LGV).* CEG/BASHH, 2006.
2. "<a href="http://commons.wikimedia.org/wiki/File:Lymphogranuloma_venerum_-_lymph_nodes.jpg#mediaviewer/File:Lymphogranuloma_venerum_-_lymph_nodes.jpg">Lymphogranuloma venerum - lymph nodes</a>" by Herbert L. Fred, MD and Hendrik A. van Dijk - <a rel="nofollow" class="external free" href="http://cnx.org/content/m14883/latest/">http://cnx.org/content/m14883/latest/</a>. Licensed under <a href="http://creativecommons.org/licenses/by/2.0" title="Creative Commons Attribution 2.0">CC BY 2.0</a> via <a href="//commons.wikimedia.org/wiki/">Wikimedia Commons</a>.

Background

- A benign viral skin infection most commonly seen in children. However, sexual contact in adults may lead to the appearance of lesions in the genital area.
- Caused by a poxvirus. The virus is probably passed on by direct skin-to-skin contact, and may affect any part of the body.

Complications

- Secondary bacterial infection may result if lesions are scratched.
- In the immunocompromised, e.g., in HIV infection, lesions may become large and exuberant, and secondary infection may be problematic.
- The main differential diagnosis is with genital warts, which are neither smooth nor umbilicated.

Clinical features

- Incubation period – 3–12 weeks.
- Discrete, pearly, papular, smooth or umbilicated lesions. In immunocompetent individuals the size of the lesions seldom exceeds 5 mm, and if untreated, there is usually spontaneous regression after several months.
- Facial lesions may be seen with HIV-related immunodeficiency.

Investigations

- Core of lesions can be examined by electron microscopy, under which typical poxvirus-like particles will be seen.
- HIV testing is recommended in patients presenting with facial lesions.

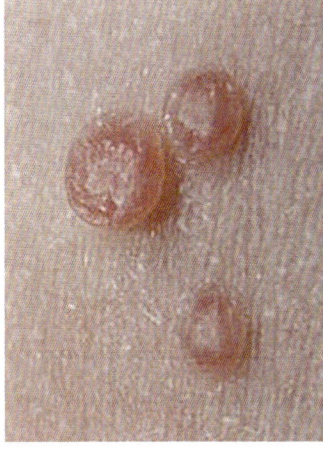

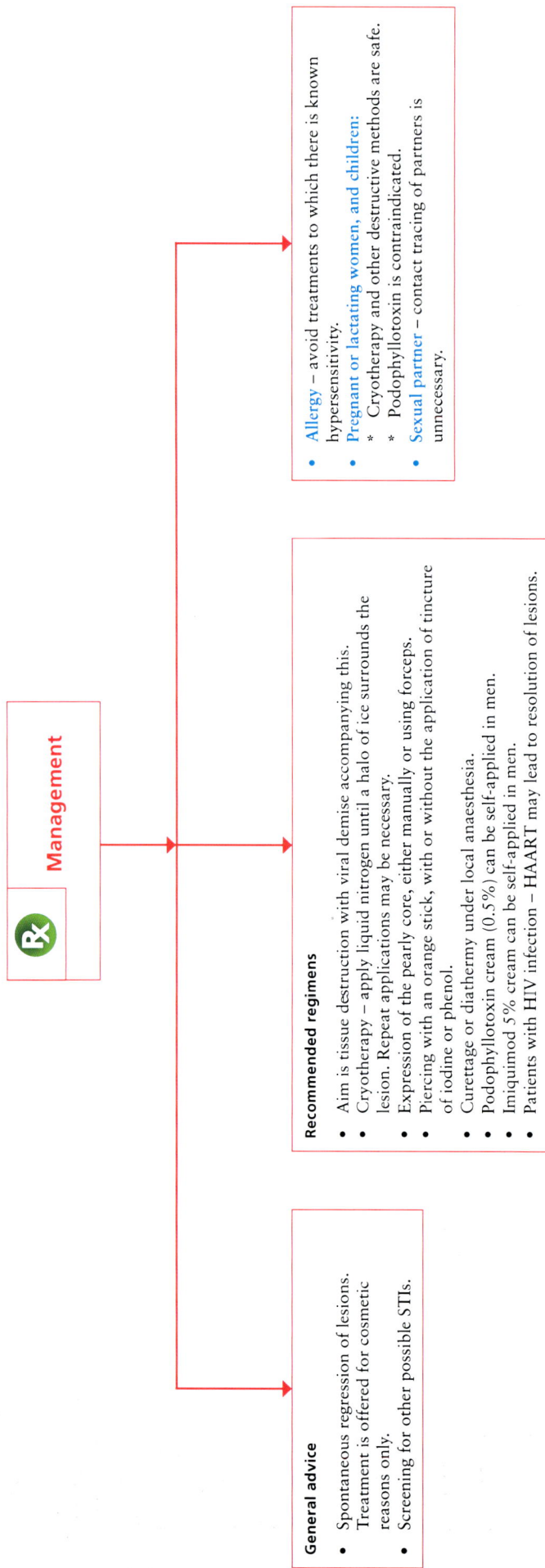

Management

General advice

- Spontaneous regression of lesions. Treatment is offered for cosmetic reasons only.
- Screening for other possible STIs.

Recommended regimens

- Aim is tissue destruction with viral demise accompanying this.
- Cryotherapy – apply liquid nitrogen until a halo of ice surrounds the lesion. Repeat applications may be necessary.
- Expression of the pearly core, either manually or using forceps.
- Piercing with an orange stick, with or without the application of tincture of iodine or phenol.
- Curettage or diathermy under local anaesthesia.
- Podophyllotoxin cream (0.5%) can be self-applied in men.
- Imiquimod 5% cream can be self-applied in men.
- Patients with HIV infection – HAART may lead to resolution of lesions.

- **Allergy** – avoid treatments to which there is known hypersensitivity.
- **Pregnant or lactating women, and children:**
  * Cryotherapy and other destructive methods are safe.
  * Podophyllotoxin is contraindicated.
- **Sexual partner** – contact tracing of partners is unnecessary.

1. http://www.cdc.gov.
2. *United Kingdom National Guideline on the Management of Molluscum Contagiosum.* CEG/BASHH, 2007.
3. "<a href="http://commons.wikimedia.org/wiki/File:Molluscaklein.jpg#mediaviewer/File:Molluscaklein.jpg">Molluscaklein</a>" by E van Herk - nl.wikipedia. Licensed under <a href="http://creativecommons
.org/licenses/by-sa/3.0/" title="Creative Commons Attribution-Share Alike 3.0">CC BY-SA 3.0</a> via <a href="//commons.wikimedia.org/wiki/">Wikimedia Commons</a>.

Background

- Previously the most common cause of genital ulcers in the developing world. Genital ulcers due to HSV-2 infection are increasing with decreasing H. ducreyi.
- H. ducreyi is an important co-factor in the transmission of HIV infection.
- Chancroid has been rare in developed countries. There had been 50–80 cases of 'tropical genital ulcers' (chancroid, LGV, and donovanosis) in England and Wales annually between 1996 and 2002; the recent increase to 300 cases is mainly due to the recent epidemic of LGV.
- Most cases are acquired abroad or with a partner who has been abroad.
- Co-infections of H. ducreyi with Treponema pallidum or HSV occur in over 10% of patients.

Clinical features

- Anogenital ulceration and lymphadenitis with progression to bubo formation.
- Incubation period is 3–10 days, and the initial lesion may progress rapidly to form an open sore. There are no prodromal symptoms.
- **The ulcer:** * Single or (often) multiple. * **Not indurated ('soft sore').** * With a necrotic base and purulent exudate. * Bordered by ragged undermined edges. * Bleeds easily on contact. * **Pain: a distinctive feature,** more common in men.
- Males – most ulcers are found on the prepuce near the frenulum or in the coronal sulcus.
- Females – most lesions are found at the entrance of the vagina, particularly the fourchette.
- Several lesions may merge to form gigantic ulcers.
- Painful inguinal adenitis is also a characteristic feature of chancroid and may be present in 50% of cases. The adenitis is unilateral in most patients. Buboes form and can become fluctuant and rupture, releasing thick pus, resulting sometimes in extensive ulceration.

Investigations

- Culture of material obtained from the ulcer base, or the undermined edges of the ulcer, or from pus aspirated from the bubo.
- Detection of DNA by amplification techniques such as PCR, using nested techniques.
- Microscopy of a Gram-stained smear (or other stains) of material from the ulcer base or of pus aspirated from the bubo: demonstration of characteristic Gram-negative coccobacilli, with occasional characteristic chaining. The test has low sensitivity and is not recommended as a diagnostic test.
- Serology – detection of antibody to H. ducreyi as a marker of chancroid using enzyme-linked immunoassays (EIAs). The method lacks sensitivity, specificity (cross-reaction with other Haemophilus species) and cannot distinguish between remote and recent infection; therefore, serology should not be used for management.

Risks or complications

- Mostly seen in men, these may include phimosis and partial loss of tissue, particularly on the glans penis (so called 'phagedenic' ulcers).
- H. ducreyi has not been shown to cause systemic infection or to spread to distant sites.

- Differential clinical diagnosis is often unreliable with an accuracy ranging from 33% to 80%. Two alternatives – (1) Combined: laboratory testing to rule out the presence of other genital ulcerative disease (GUD) pathogens such as syphilis and HSV-2; (2) Use of syndromic treatment, i.e., combined antimicrobials to cover all possible treatable aetiologies of GUD. WHO recommends it in places where diagnostic facilities are not readily available.
- The Centers for Disease Control and Prevention, 2007: a 'probable diagnosis' if the patient has one or more painful genital ulcers, and (a) no evidence of T. pallidum infection by dark field examination of ulcer exudate or by a serological test for syphilis performed at least 7 days after onset of ulcers, and (b) the clinical presentation, appearance of the genital ulcers, and regional lymphadenopathy, if present, are typical for chancroid, and a test for HSV is negative.

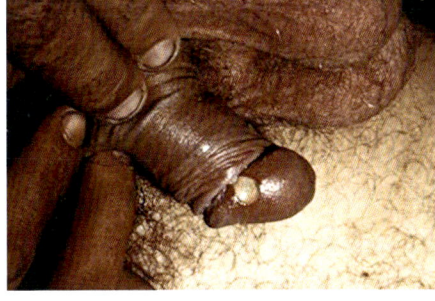

Rx

Management

General advice

- Avoid UPSI until patient and partner(s) have completed treatment and follow-up.
- Further investigations to screen for other possible causes of genital ulcerative disease such as T. pallidum and genital herpes, LGV, or donovanosis and HIV.
- Biopsy of lymph nodes may be required to exclude neoplasia.

Recommended regimens

* Azithromycin 1 g orally in a single dose.
* Or ceftriaxone 250 mg IM in a single dose.
* Or ciprofloxacin 500 mg orally in a single dose.
* Or ciprofloxacin 500 mg orally BD for 3 days.
* Or erythromycin base 500 mg orally QID for 7 days.

- Azithromycin and ceftriaxone offer the advantage of single-dose therapy. They have excellent in vitro activity against H. ducreyi with no reported resistance to date.
- Erythromycin given at high doses for 7 days is the WHO-recommended first line treatment for chancroid. Cure rates of 93% but associated with poor compliance and gastrointestinal intolerance.

Pregnant or lactating women, and children

- Safety of azithromycin for pregnant and lactating women has not been established.
- Ciprofloxacin is contraindicated for pregnant and lactating women, children, and adolescents younger than 18 years of age.
- Erythromycin or ceftriaxone regimens should be used.
- No adverse effects of chancroid on pregnancy outcome or on the fetus have been reported.

Patients co-infected with HIV

- Monitor closely, healing may be slower and treatment failures have been recorded with azithromycin, ceftriaxone or single dose fleroxacin, low dose erythromycin or ciprofloxacin.
- CDC – as data on therapeutic efficacy with ceftriaxone and azithromycin regimens among patients infected with HIV are limited, those regimens should be used among persons known to be infected with HIV, only if follow-up can be assured.
- Some experts suggest using the full-dose erythromycin 7-day regimen for treating HIV-infected persons.

Fluctuant buboes

- Needle-aspiration of fluctuant buboes from adjacent healthy skin. It is simpler and safer than incision, which is prone to complications (sinus formation).
- Careful incision and drainage under effective antibiotic cover is also reported to be an effective and safe method for treating fluctuant buboes, and avoids frequent needle re-aspirations.

Follow up and test of cure (TOC)

- Re-examine 3–7 days after initiation of therapy. If treatment is successful, ulcers improve symptomatically within 3 days and substantial re-epithelization occurs within 7 days after onset of therapy. The time required for complete healing is related to the size of the ulcer; large ulcers may require more than 2 weeks to heal.
- Clinical resolution of fluctuant lymphadenopathy is slower than that of ulcers and may require frequent needle aspiration (or drainage).
- **A test of cure is not recommended.**
- Treatment failures – investigate possible co-infections with T. pallidum or HSV; or determine possible resistance of H. ducreyi to antibiotics.
- Sexual partner – people who have had sexual contact with a patient who has chancroid within the 10 days before onset of the patient's symptoms should be examined, and treated even in the absence of symptoms, as asymptomatic carriage of H. ducreyi can occur. Screening is not recommended.

1. *National Guideline for the Management of Chancroid.* CEG/BASSH, 2007.
2. "<aref "http://commons.wikimedia.org/wiki/File:Chancroid_lesion_haemophilus_ducreyi_PHIL_3728_lores.jpg"> Chancroid lesion haemophilus ducreyi PHIL 3728 lores</a>" by CDC/Joe Miller - This media comes from the <a href="//en.wikipedia.org/ wiki/Centers_for_Disease_Control_and_Prevention" class="extiw" title="w:Centers for Disease Control and Prevention">Centers for Disease Control and Prevention</a>'s <a rel="nofollow" class= "external text" href="http://phil.cdc.gov/phil/home.asp">Public Health Image Library</a> (PHIL), with identification number <a rel="nofollow" class="external text" href="http://phil.cdc.gov/phil/ details.asp?pid=3728">#3728</a>.Note: Not all PHIL images are public domain; be sure to check copyright status and credit authors and content providers.<a class="external text" href="//commons.wikimedia.org/wiki/Template:CDC-PHIL/en">English </a> | <a class="external text" href="//commons.wikimedia.org/wiki/Template:CDC-PHIL/sl">Slovenščina</a> | <a class="external text" href="//commons.wikimedia.org/w/index. php?title= Template:CDC-PHIL/lang&action=edit">+/-</a>. Licensed under Public domain via <a href="//commons.wikimedia.org/wiki/">Wikimedia Commons</a>.

Background

- STI – usually manifests as genital ulceration.
- Seen chiefly in small endemic foci in tropical countries.
- Causative organism – Klebsiella granulomatis (Calymmatobacterium granulomatis).

Risks or complications

- Haemorrhage, genital lymphoedema, genital mutilation, and cicatrization.
- Development of squamous carcinoma.
- Haematogenous dissemination to bone and viscera (rare).
- Vertical transmission (rare) – lesions of the ears of infants.

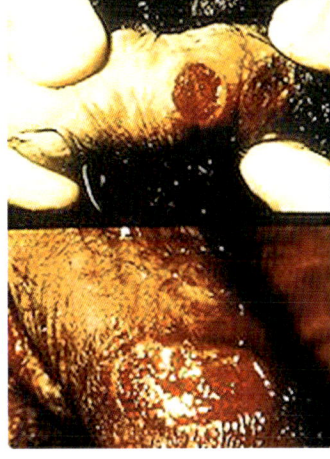

Clinical features

- At site of primary inoculation – painful papules/nodules whcih develop into friable ulcers or hypertrophic lesions, which gradually increase in size.
- Regional lymph nodes – swelling followed by spread of infection into overlying tissues, resulting in abscess (pseudobubo) or ulceration of overlying skin (mainly at inguinal nodes).
- Untreated infection may either resolve spontaneously or persist and slowly spread.
- Primary lesions of mouth and cervix can occur. Cervical lesions can be mistaken for malignant lesions.

Investigations

- **Donovan bodies** – demonstrated in:
  * Cellular material taken by scraping/smear/swab/crushing of pinched-off tissue fragment on to glass slide.
  * Tissue sample from biopsy.
- **Donovan bodies are characterized by:**
  * Location within large (20–90 μm) histiocytes.
  * Pleomorphic appearance 1–2 × 0.5–0.7 μm.
  * Bipolar densities and a capsule often visible.
  * Stain Gram negative.
  * Sensitivity is 60–80% in endemic areas.
- Culture of Klebsiella granulomatis has recently been reported.
- Both PCR methods and serological tests for donovanosis have been described but are not yet routinely available.

Rx Management

General advice

- To avoid UPSI until patient and partner(s) have completed treatment and follow-up.
- Further investigations – screen for other possible causes of genital ulcerative disease (syphilis, genital herpes, LGV), and HIV.
- Biopsy of lymph nodes may be required to exclude neoplasia.

Recommended regimens

- Azithromycin by the Australian Antibiotic Guidelines.
- CDC – ciprofloxacin is recommended, which has better bioavailability than norfloxacin. Gentamicin is recommended as an adjunct to therapy in patients whose lesions do not respond in the first few days to other agents.
- Duration of treatment is until lesions have healed. Healing times vary greatly between patients. CDC recommends a minimum of 3 weeks' treatment.

Pregnant or lactating women, and children

- Gentamicin, doxycycyline, co-trimoxazole, and norfloxacin are not recommended for pregnant or lactating women.
- Erythromycin has been used successfully in pregnant women.
- Children born to mothers with untreated genital lesions of donovanosis are at risk of infection; therefore, consider a course of prophylactic antibiotics.

Follow-up

- Follow patients until symptoms have resolved.
- Partner management – assess and offer treatment to any person with a history of UPSI with a patient with active donovanosis or within 40 days before the onset of lesions (incubation period of between 3 and 40 days in 92% of patients).

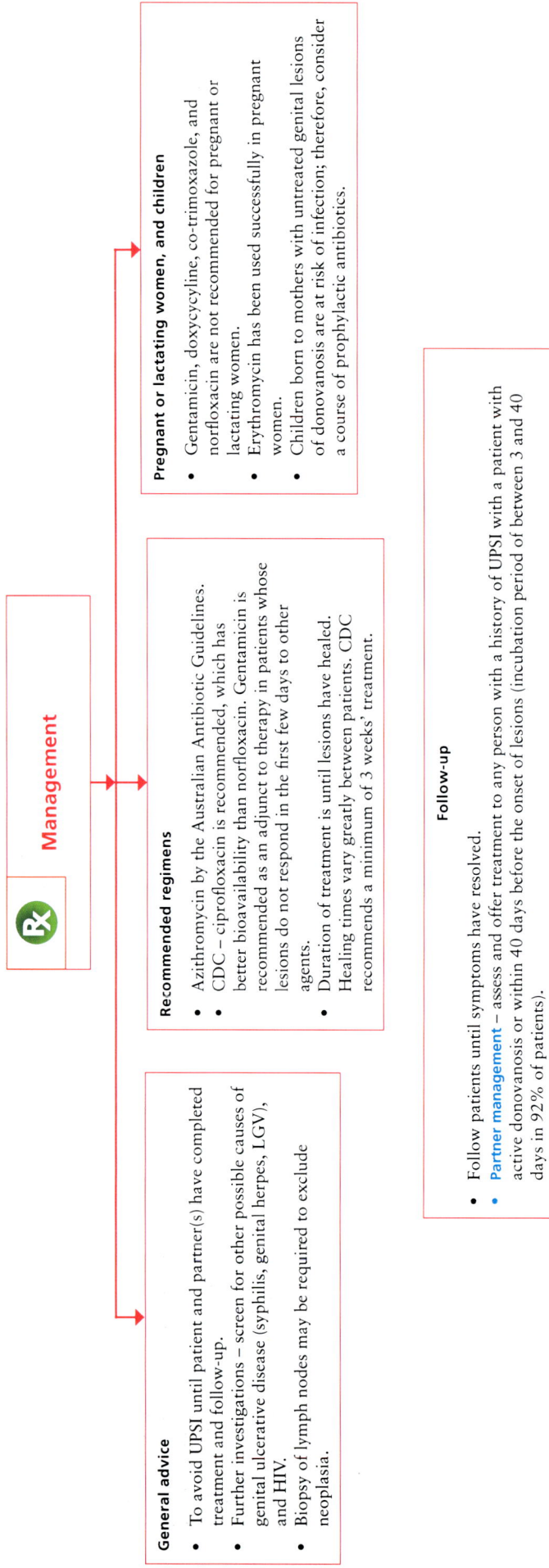

1. *United Kingdom National Guideline for the Management of Donovanosis (Granuloma inguinale)*. BASHH/CEG, 2011.
2. "<a href="http://commons.wikimedia.org/wiki/File:SOA-Donovanosis-male.jpg#mediaviewer/Archivo:SOA-Donovanosis-male.jpg">SOA-Donovanosis-male</a>". Disponible bajo la licencia <a href="http://creativecommons.org/licenses/by-sa/3.0/" title="Creative Commons Attribution-Share Alike 3.0">CC BY-SA 3.0</a> via <a href="//commons.wikimedia.org/wiki/">Wikimedia Commons</a>.

Background

- The crab louse Phthirus pubis is transmitted by close body contact.
- Incubation period is 5 days to several weeks.
- Occasionally individuals may have more prolonged, asymptomatic infestation.

Clinical features

- Adult lice infest coarse hairs of the pubic area, body hair, and, rarely, eyebrows and eyelashes.
- Eggs (nits) are laid, which adhere to the hairs.
- May be asymptomatic.
- Itching due to hypersensitivity to feeding lice.
- Blue macules (maculae caeruleae) may be visible at feeding sites.
- On examination – may see adult lice and/or eggs.

Investigations

- Examination under light microscopy can confirm the morphology if necessary.

℞ Management

General advice

- To avoid UPSI until the patient and partner(s) have completed treatment and follow-up.
- Screen for other possible STIs.
- Lotions are more effective than shampoos, and should be applied to all body hair including the beard and moustache if necessary. Advise a second application after 3–7 days.

Recommended regimens

- Malathion 0.5% – apply to dry hair and wash after at least 2 and, preferably, 12 hours, i.e., overnight.
- Permethrin 1% cream – apply to damp hair and wash after 10 minutes.
- Phenothrin 0.2% – apply to dry hair and wash after 2 hours.
- Carbaryl 0.5 and 1% – apply to dry hair and wash 12 hours later.
- Infestation of eyelashes – permethrin 1% lotion for 10 minutes.

- Allergy – avoid treatments to which there is known hypersensitivity.
- Pregnant or lactating women, and children – permethrin is safe during pregnancy and breastfeeding.
- Sexual partner – examine and treat current sexual partners. * Contact trace of partners from the previous 3 months.

Follow-up and test of cure

- Re-examine for absence of lice after 1 week.
- Provide an alternative from the above list for treatment failures.
- Dead nits may remain adherent to hairs and this does not imply treatment failure.

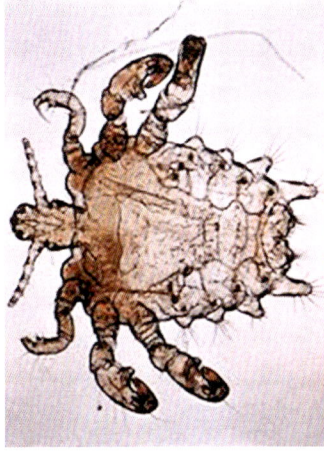

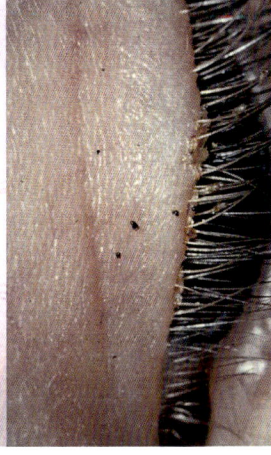

1. *United Kingdom National Guideline on the Management of Phthirus pubis Infestation.* BASHH/CEG, 2007.

2. http://commons.wikimedia.org/wiki/File:Pthius_pubis_-_crab_louse.jpg.

3. http://en.wikipedia.org/wiki/Crab_louse#mediaviewer/File:Pubic_lice_on_eye-lashes.jpg - "<a href="http://commons.wikimedia.org/wiki/File:Pubic_lice_on_eye-lashes.jpg#mediaviewer/File:Pubic_lice_on_eye-lashes.jpg">Pubic lice on eye-lashes</a>" by <a href="//en.wikipedia.org/wiki/User:KostaMumcuoglu" title="en:User:KostaMumcuoglu" class="extiw">KostaMumcuoglu</a> <a href="//en.wikipedia.org/wiki/User_talk:KostaMumcuoglu" class="extiw" title="en:User talk:KostaMumcuoglu">(Talk)</a> at <a class="external text" href="http://en.wikipedia.org">en.wikipedia.org"">en.wikipedia</a> - Transferred from <a class="external text" href="http://en.wikipedia.org">en.wikipedia.org"</a> to Commons by <a href="//commons.wikimedia.org/wiki/User:SMasters" title="User:SMasters">User:SMasters</a> using <a rel="nofollow" class="external text" href="http://tools.wikimedia.de/~magnus/commonshelper.php">CommonsHelper</a>. Licensed under <a href="http://creativecommons.org/licenses/by-sa/3.0/" title="Creative Commons Attribution-Share Alike 3.0">CC BY-SA 3.0</a> via <a href="//commons.wikimedia.org/wiki/">Wikimedia Commons</a>.

Complications

- Secondary infection of the skin lesions can occur following repeated scratching.
- The clinical appearance is usually typical, but there may be diagnostic confusion with other itching conditions such as eczema.

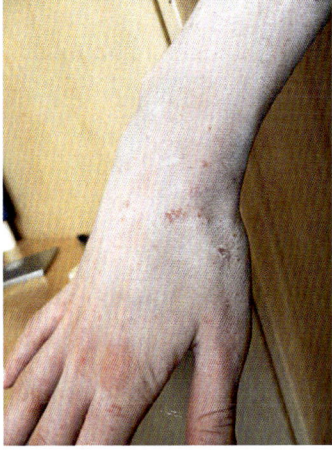

Background

- Caused by the mite Sarcoptes scabiei. • Mites burrow into the skin where they lay eggs. The resulting offspring crawl out onto the skin and make new burrows.
- The absorption of mite excrement into skin capillaries generates a hypersensitivity reaction.
- Any part of the body may be affected, and transmission is by skin-to-skin contact.

Clinical features

- Symptoms – generalized itch, especially at night. May take 4–6 weeks to develop.
- Signs: * Characteristic silvery lines may be seen in the skin, where mites have burrowed.
  * Classic sites – interdigital folds, wrists and elbows, and around breast nipples.
  * Papules or nodules that may result from itching often affect the genital area.
  * Norwegian scabies is seen in HIV infection; crusted lesions that teem with mites.

Investigations

- Scrapings taken from burrows may be examined under light microscopy to reveal mites.

Management

Recommended regimens

- Permethrin 5% cream.
- Malathion 0.5% aqueous lotion. Apply to the whole body from the neck downwards, and wash off after 12 hours, usually overnight.
- Norwegian scabies may be treated with oral ivermectin (200 µg/kg).

- Allergy – avoid treatments to which there is known hypersensitivity.
- Pregnant or lactating women, and children – permethrin is safe.
- Sexual partner – examine and treat current sexual partners as well as other members of the household.
  * Trace contacts with an arbitrary time span of the previous 2 months.

General advice

- To avoid close body contact until the patient and partner(s) have completed treatment.
- Screen for other possible STIs.
- Crotamiton cream and antihistamines may give symptomatic relief.
- To wash contaminated clothes and bedding at high temperature (> 50°C) if possible.

Follow-up

- There is no clear evidence as to optimal follow-up.
- Appearance of new burrows at any stage post-treatment is indicative of a need for further therapy, although in re-infection, symptoms of pruritus may recur before typical burrows have developed.
- Pruritus persisting > 2 weeks after treatment may reflect treatment failure, re-infection, or drug allergy.

1. *United Kingdom National Guideline on the Management of Scabies Infestation.* BASHH/CEG, 2007.
2. http://commons.wikimedia.org/wiki/File:ScabiesD04.jpg.

CHAPTER 54 Syphilis

Background

- Spirochaete – Treponema pallidum.
- Transmitted by direct contact with an infectious lesion (usually occurring during sexual contact), vertical transmission (may be passed trans-placentally from the 9th week of gestation onwards) or via infected blood products.
- In England, diagnoses of syphilis have increased substantially since 1997; 3762 cases were diagnosed in 2007.
- Epidemics of syphilis and LGV are continuing, especially among men who have sex with men (MSM) who are known to be HIV infected.
- MSM account for 73% of infectious syphilis and 99% of LGV cases.
- HIV co-infection is common in those diagnosed with LGV (74%) and syphilis (27%), reflecting the close relationships between the epidemics. (HPA, 2009)
- The increased number of syphilis cases in women of reproductive age has resulted in an increase in cases of congenital infection.

Clinical features

- Incubation period of 9–90 days.
- Primary syphilis – ulcer (the chancre) at the site of inoculation and regional lymphadenopathy. The chancre is classically in the anogenital region; single, painless and indurated, with a clean base discharging clear serum. However, it may be multiple, painful, purulent, destructive and on extra-genital (most frequently oral) sites.
- Secondary syphilis – incubation period of 6 weeks to 6 months; multisystem involvement within the first two years of infection. Rash (typically generalized macular, papular, or macular– papular, often affecting the palms and soles), condylomata lata, mucocutaneous lesions, generalized lymphadenopathy. Less commonly: patchy alopecia, anterior uveitis, meningitis, cranial nerve palsies, hepatitis, splenomegaly, periostitis, and glomerulonephritis.
- Latent syphilis – diagnosed on serological testing with no symptoms or signs. Early latent syphilis within the first 2 years of infection and late latent syphilis after 2 years of infection.
- Tertiary syphilis – used synonymously with late symptomatic syphilis; may develop in approximately one third of individuals. It is non-infectious; gummatous syphilis, neurosyphilis, and cardiovascular syphilis.

Screening is recommended for all asymptomatic patients attending a UK GUM clinic. Apart from the public health benefit of detecting infectious syphilis, it will detect non-infectious stages of syphilis, which will benefit the individual patient.

Congenital syphilis

- Early – diagnosed in the first two years of life; includes a rash, condylomata lata, vesiculobullous lesions, haemorrhagic rhinitis, osteochondritis, periostitis, pseudoparalysis, mucous patches, perioral fissures, hepatosplenomegaly, generalized lymphadenopathy, non-immune hydrops, glomerulonephritis, neurological or ocular involvement, haemolysis, and thrombocytopenia.
- Late – presenting after two years; includes stigmata: interstitial keratitis, Clutton's joints, Hutchinson's incisors, mulberry molars, high palatal arch, rhagades, deafness, frontal bossing, short maxilla, protuberance of mandible, saddle-nose deformity, sternoclavicular thickening, paroxysmal cold haemoglobinuria, neurological or gummatous involvement.

Recommended sites for testing

- Blood (all patients).
- Ulcer material (primary syphilis).
- Lesion material (secondary syphilis).

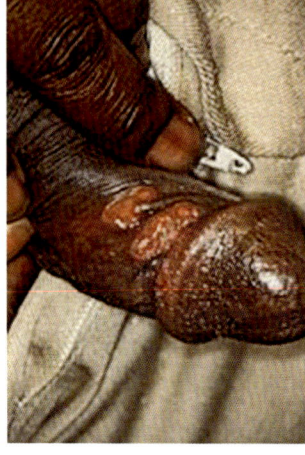

Risk groups

- MSM. • Sex workers. • 'Young' (under 25 years old) patients.
- Pregnant women.
- Patients who are known contacts of the infection need a request for an anti-treponemal IgM EIA on the blood specimen submitted for standard screening.

Investigations

Virus detection and serological tests

- **Dark-field microscopy** should be performed by experienced technicians. If the initial test is negative, repeat daily for 3 days. Less reliable in examining rectal and non-penile genital lesions and not suitable for examining oral lesions due to commensal treponemes.
- **PCR** may be used on oral or other lesions where contamination with commensal treponemes is likely. Owing to limited availability and the time taken to obtain a result, this is not a replacement for dark-field microscopy in the clinic setting. PCR may be helpful in diagnosis by demonstrating T. pallidum in tissue samples, vitreous fluid, and CSF.
- **Serological test – specific (treponemal) tests:**
  * Treponemal enzyme immunoassay (EIA) to detect IgG and IgM; T. pallidum chemiluminescent assay; T. pallidum haemagglutination assay (TPHA); T. pallidum particle agglutination assay (TPPA); fluorescent treponemal antibody absorbed test (FTA-abs); T. pallidum recombinant antigen line immunoassay.
  * EIA for anti-treponemal IgM if primary syphilis is suspected (tend to be more sensitive in primary infection). IgM becomes detectable in the serum 2–3 weeks after infection, therefore there will be a window of 1–2 weeks when routine screening tests may be negative.
  * All the specific tests are almost invariably positive in secondary and early latent syphilis.
  * T. pallidum particle assay (TPPA) is recommended in preference to the T. pallidum haemagglutination assay (TPHA).
- **Serological test – nonspecific cardiolipin tests:** VDRL carbon antigen test/RPR. A quantitative VDRL/RPR should be performed when treponemal; tests indicate syphilis as this helps stage the disease and indicates the need for treatment. A VDRL/RPR titre of > 16 and/or a positive IgM test indicates active disease and the need for treatment. A false-negative cardiolipin (reagin) test may occur in secondary or early latent syphilis. This may be more likely to occur in HIV-infected individuals.

Serological screening tests

- Treponemal EIA (both IgG and IgM) or TPPA or VDRL/RPR and TPHA.
- Screening with either EIA alone or the TPPA alone is recommended.
- The TPHA can be used in combination with a cardiolipin antigen/ reagin test such as VDRL or RPR to maximize the detection of primary infection on screening.

Additional and confirmatory serological tests

- Always repeat positive tests on a second specimen to confirm the result.
- Confirm a positive screening test with a different treponemal test.
- An immunoblot (T. pallidum recombinant antigen line immunoassay) is recommended when the standard confirmatory test does not confirm the positive treponemal screening test result. The FTA-abs is not recommended as a standard confirmatory test.
- A quantitative VDRL/RPR should be performed on a specimen taken on the day that treatment is started as this provides an accurate baseline for monitoring response to treatment.
- An EIA IgM test should be performed in addition to routine screening tests in all cases of genital ulceration as well as in those patients who are known contacts of syphilis.
- In patients who have previously been treated for syphilis a 4-fold increase in VDRL/RPR titre and/or a change in the EIA IgM from negative to positive (confirmed on a second specimen) suggests re-infection or relapse.

Management

General advice

- Offer screening for other STIs.
- Advise to refrain from sexual contact of any kind until the lesions of early syphilis (if they were present) are fully healed, or until after the results of the first follow-up serology are known.

- Penicillin is the treatment of choice. Clinical data are lacking on the optimal dose and duration of treatment and the long-term efficacy of antimicrobials other than penicillin.
- Parenteral treatment is the treatment of choice because therapy is supervised and bioavailability is guaranteed.
- 60% of untreated individuals do not develop late complications. The prevalence of late syphilis including neurosyphilis remains low, indicating that treatment is effective and suggests that host immune responses in early syphilis play an essential part.
- Cardiovascular lesions may progress despite adequate treatment. Steroids are recommended to prevent potential consequences of Jarisch–Herxheimer reaction.
- Neurosyphilis – procaine penicillin plus probenecid for 14 days. (CDC, 2006)

Non-penicillin antibiotics

- Erythromycin is least effective and does not penetrate the CSF or placental barrier well.
- Doxycycline 100 mg OD/BD for 14 days is effective; failure of OD dose has been reported.
- Single dose of 2 g of azithromycin has shown efficacy in early syphilis equivalent to that of benzathine penicillin; however, there are concerns regarding treatment failure.
- In small studies, a number of ceftriaxone regimens have been shown to be effective.

Syphilis in pregnancy

- Syphilis may be transmitted trans-placentally at any stage of pregnancy.
- May result in polyhydramnios, miscarriage, PTL, stillbirth, hydrops, and congenital syphilis.
- Maternal early stage syphilis and high titre RPR/VDRL are risk factors for congenital syphilis, although transmission rate in late latent disease could be up to 10%.
- Maternal co-infection with HIV may increase the transmission risk of syphilis.
- Treatment in the last trimester is also associated with poorer outcomes.

All pregnant women should be screened for syphilis at the initial antenatal visit.

- In pregnancy the rate of the Jarisch–Herxheimer reaction is the same as in the non-pregnant (40%).
- Woman may experience uterine contractions (40–65%) secondary to the fever, which resolve within 24 hours. FHR decelerations occur in 40%, concomitant with maternal fever, and resolve within 24 hours of maternal penicillin treatment.
- There is a theoretical increased risk of spontaneous and iatrogenic PTD and fetal demise associated with the Jarisch–Herxheimer reaction, though these complications are also associated with maternal and fetal syphilis infection.
- Management of the Jarisch–Herxheimer reaction in pregnancy is supportive with antipyretics. No evidence that high-dose oral prednisolone will reduce the occurrence of uterine contractions or FHR abnormalities.

Management

- MDT – obstetric, midwifery, paediatric, GUM physician teams.
- Referral to FMU for USS to evaluate fetal involvement showing non-immune hydrops or hepatospenomegaly.
- Fetal monitoring for fetal distress in the early stages of therapy is recommended after 26 weeks of gestation.

- A single dose of benzathine penicillin G 2.4 MU is effective in most cases, although failures have been reported; mainly in those at increased risk of transmission (higher RPR/VDRL titre, early stage maternal disease, and last trimester treatment).
- Physiological changes in pregnancy may result in reduced penicillin concentrations. Therefore, when maternal treatment is initiated in the third trimester, give a second dose of benzathine penicillin one week after the first. Assess the neonate carefully and consider treatment at birth.

- Consider re-treatment in those with a previous diagnosis of syphilis when:
  * There is uncertainty of efficacious past treatment.
  * A 4-fold drop in RPR/VDRL titre has not been achieved.
  * The RPR/VDRL titre is serofast at > 1:8.

- Non-penicillin alternatives are ceftriaxone (limited data), erythromycin, or azithromycin.
- There are no studies evaluating azithromycin in pregnancy and treatment failure has been reported with erythromycin and azithromycin. Treatment of the baby at birth with penicillin is recommended, following maternal treatment with macrolides.

Infants born to mothers with syphilis

Serological screening tests on infant's blood (not cord blood) and examination for signs of congenital syphilis.

If negative and no signs of congenital infection, no further testing is necessary.

If positive – perform treponemal IgM EIA, quantitative VDRL/RPR, and quantitative TPPA tests on the infant and mother in parallel.

A positive IgM EIA test and/or a sustained 4-fold or greater difference of VDRL/RPR titre or TPPA titre above that of the mother (confirmed on testing a second specimen from the infant) confirms **diagnosis of congenital infection.**

If IgM is negative, the other tests are reactive with titres < 4-fold higher than those of the mother, and there are no signs of congenital syphilis.

- Repeat reactive tests at 3, 6, and 12 months of age or until all tests become negative (usually by 6 months).
- Repeat IgM at 3 months in case the infant's response is delayed or suppressed.

- Screen older siblings for congenital syphilis.
- Manage congenital syphilis diagnosed in an older child or in adulthood as for late syphilis but screen the parents, all siblings, and any sexual partner(s) for syphilis.

Management

Monitor:
- Infants born to mothers treated for syphilis prior to pregnancy.
- Infants born to mothers treated with a penicillin-based regimen more than 4 weeks prior to delivery with no evidence of re-infection or relapse. CDC – a stat dose of benzathine penicillin G 50,000 units/kg.
- Treatment may be indicated particularly if follow-up is uncertain or if treatment was in the last trimester of pregnancy.

Treatment for congenital syphilis is indicated in:
- Infants with suspected congenital syphilis.
- Mothers
  * Treated < 4 weeks prior to delivery.
  * Treated with non-penicillin regimens.
  * Who were not treated.
  * Who were inadequately treated.
  * Who have no documentation of being treated.

Regimens:
- Benzyl penicillin sodium 100,000–150,000 units/kg daily IV (in divided doses) in the first 7 days of life and 8 hourly thereafter for 10 days.
- Procaine penicillin 50,000 units/kg daily IM for 10 days.
- In children, IV may be preferable due to the pain associated with IM injections.

1. *Sexually Transmitted Infections: UK National Screening and Testing Guidelines.* BASHH, August 2006.
2. Kingston M, French P, Goh B, et al. UK National Guidelines on the Management of Syphilis, 2008. *Int J STD AIDS* 2008;19:729–740.
3. *Update on Management of Syphilis in Pregnancy.* BASHH/CEG Statement, August 2011.
4. http://www.hpa.org.uk; www.webmd.com; drugline.org; www.cdc.gov.
5. "<aref="http://commons.wikimedia.org/wiki/File:Chancres_on_the_penile_shaft_due_to_a_primary_syphilitic_infection_caused_by_Treponema_pallidum_6803_lores.jpg#mediaviewer/File:Chancres_on_the_penile_shaft_due_to_a_primary_syphilitic_infection_caused_by_Treponema_pallidum_6803_lores.jpg">Chancres on the penile shaft due to a primary syphilitic infection caused by Treponema pallidum 6803 lores</a>" by CDC/M. Rein, VD - This media comes from the <a href="//en.wikipedia.org/wiki/Centers_for_Disease_Control_and_Prevention" class="extiw" title="w:Centers for Disease Control and Prevention">Centers for Disease Control and Prevention</a>'s <a rel="nofollow" class="external text" href="http://phil.cdc.gov/phil/home.asp">Public Health Image Library</a> (PHIL), with identification number <a rel="nofollow" class="external text" href="http://phil.cdc.gov/phil/details.asp?pid=6803">#6803</a>.Note: Not all PHIL images are public domain; be sure to check copyright status and credit authors and content providers.<a class="external text" href="//commons.wikimedia.org/wiki/Template:CDC-PHIL/en">English</a> <a class="external text" href="//commons.wikimedia.org/wiki/Template:CDC-PHIL/sl">Slovenščina</a> <a class="external text" href="//commons.wikimedia.org/wiki/Template:CDC-PHIL/lang&action=edit">+/-</a>. Licensed under Public domain via <a href="//commons.wikimedia.org/wiki/">Wikimedia Commons</a>.

Background

- Caused by the human papilloma virus (HPV), usually by HPV types 6 and 11.
- Over 100 genotypes have been identified.
- Most anogenital warts are benign proliferative growths; some may contain oncogenic types associated with genital tract dysplasia and cancers.
- Mode of transmission is mainly by sexual contact, but may be transmitted peri-natally.
- Genital lesions result from transfer of infection from hand warts in children.
- There is no good evidence of transmission from fomites.
- Incidence of new anogenital warts in the UK is about 100,000 cases/year.
- 55% of anogenital wart diagnoses were in those aged less than 25 years old.

Clinical features

Symptoms:
- Asymptomatic – majority cause little physical discomfort.
- May be associated with irritation and soreness, especially around the anus.
- May present with inflammation, fissuring, itching, bleeding, or dyspareunia.
- Vaginal discharge, IMB, PCB.
- Urinary symptoms – distortion of urine flow, bleeding from the urethra, urethral discharge, dysuria.
- Bleeding from anus.

Signs – benign epithelial skin tumours with clinical appearances of exophytic warts:
- * Single or multiple.
- * Warts on the warm, moist, non-hair-bearing skin are soft and non-keratinized; those on the dry hairy skin are firm and keratinized.
- * May be broad based or pedunculated or pigmented.

Assessment of lesions:
- Examine external anogenital and surrounding skin under good illumination.
- Females – vaginal speculum examination.
- Both sexes – proctoscopy may be indicated if history of anal receptive sex, or following clearance of perianal warts. Meatoscopy and proctoscopy if there is a history of distortion of urine flow or bleeding from the urethra or anus, respectively. Urethroscopy for more proximal warts.
- Classify warts as to morphology. Record lesions on genital maps at each visit; provides a visual record of approximate number, distribution, and response to treatment.
- Examine extra-genital sites (e.g., oral cavity) if clinically indicated.

Investigations

- Biopsy to rule out possible intra-epithelial neoplasia if in doubt, or if the lesion is atypical or pigmented (with or without a colposcope).

Site of the lesions

- Multifocal infection of the anogenital skin, most common at the site of trauma at sexual intercourse, but may occur at any site.
- Perianal lesions are common in both sexes, but are seen more commonly in homosexual men.
- Warts in the anal canal are associated with penetrative anal sex, and may indicate the need for samples to be taken from the anorectal region for other STIs.
- Occult lesions may be seen on the vagina, cervix, urethral meatus, and anal canal.
- Extra-genital lesions may be seen in the oral cavity, larynx, conjunctivae, and nasal cavity.

Risks or complications

- May be disfiguring, leading to psychological distress.
- Up to 20% of people with anogenital warts will also have another STI.

Differential diagnosis

- Molluscum contagiosum, skin tags, seborrhoeic keratoses.
- Secondary syphilis, which may present as anogenital condylomata lata (moist warty lesions at sites of skin friction such as perianal and vulval areas).
- Other STIs.
- Vulval, penile, or anal intra-epithelial neoplasia if the lesions are flat, only slightly raised, or pigmented.
- Malignancy if the lesions are ulcerated or bleeding.

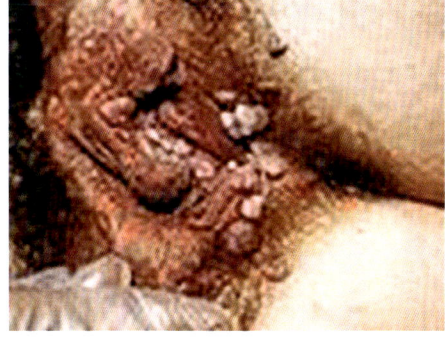

CHAPTER 55 Anogenital warts (condylomata acuminata)

Rx Management

Subclinical lesions

- Lesions not seen by the naked eye but detectable after applying 5% acetic acid (**aceto-white lesions**) and examining under colposcopic magnification.
- Usually asymptomatic, but may cause irritation and inflammation of the skin.
- **Issues:**
  - * Many aceto-white lesions are not caused by HPV.
  - * Histological changes are not specific for HPV infection.
  - * HPV detection is not routinely available.
  - * Treatment of these lesions has not been shown to affect the course of disease.
  - * Identification may cause unnecessary anxiety.
  - * **It is not recommended that these lesions are sought unless there is a clinical indication.**

General advice

- Condoms may protect against the HPV infection and genital warts, and may have a therapeutic effect when both partners are infected, possibly by preventing continued re-exposure to the virus.
- Latex condoms may be weakened if in contact with imiquimod.
- Psychological distress – refer for counselling.
- Smokers may not respond as well to treatment as non-smokers.
- Screen for other STIs.

Treatment options

- No treatment – as one third of warts disappear spontaneously within 6 months.
- Chemical applications – podophyllin, podophyllotoxin, trichloroacetic acid, 5-fluorouracil, interferons, imiquimod.
- Physical ablation – excision, cryotherapy, electrosurgery, laser.
- Imiquimod – an immune response modifier.
- Choice depends on the morphology, number, distribution of warts, and patient preference.
- All have significant failure and relapse rates; may cause discomfort and local skin reactions.
- Soft non-keratinized warts – podophyllin, podophyllotoxin, and trichloroatic acid.
- Keratinized lesions – cryotherapy, excision, or electrocautery.
- Imiquimod – for both keratinized and non-keratinized warts.
- Podophyllotoxin, for 4 week cycles, and imiquimod for up to 16 weeks can be used for home treatment by patients.

Sexual partners

- Assess current sexual partner(s) for any undetected genital warts and other STIs.
- Tracing of previous sexual partner(s) is not recommended.

Pregnancy

- Children may develop laryngeal papillomatosis and anogenital warts.
- Treatment aims to minimize the number of lesions present at delivery to reduce the neonatal exposure to the virus.
- Avoid podophyllin, podophyllotoxin, and 5-fluorouracil due to possible teratogenic effects; imiquimod is not approved for use in pregnancy.
- CS may be indicated due to the obstruction of vaginal outlet with warts or the presence of gross cervical warts. CS is not indicated to prevent laryngeal papillomatosis/anogenital warts in the neonate as both conditions are rare.

Consider the possibility of sexual abuse in any child with anogenital warts, particularly if younger than 13 years of age.

Follow-up

- Review at end of course to monitor response. Patients who respond well to treatment, but in whom new lesions develop, can continue with current regimen.
- Change of treatment is necessary if patient is not tolerating current treatment or there is < 50% response to current treatment by 6 weeks (8–12 weeks for imiquimod).
- Treat relapses according to the lesion types.

1. *United Kingdom National Guideline on the Management of Anogenital Warts.* BASHH/CEG, 2007.
2. http://en.wikipedia.org/wiki/Genital_wart - "<a href="http://commons.wikimedia.org/wiki/File:SOA-Condylomata-acuminata-female.jpg#mediaviewer/File:SOA-Condylomata-acuminata-female.jpg">SOA-Condylomata-acuminata-female</a>" by SOA-AIDS Amsterdam - <a rel="external text" href="http://www.aidsfonds.nl/">SOA-AIDS Amsterdam</a> - <a rel="nofollow" class="external text" href="http://creativecommons.org/licenses/by-sa/3.0/" title="Creative Commons Attribution-Share Alike 3.0">CC BY-SA 3.0</a> via <a href="//commons.wikimedia.org/wiki/">Wikimedia Commons</a>.

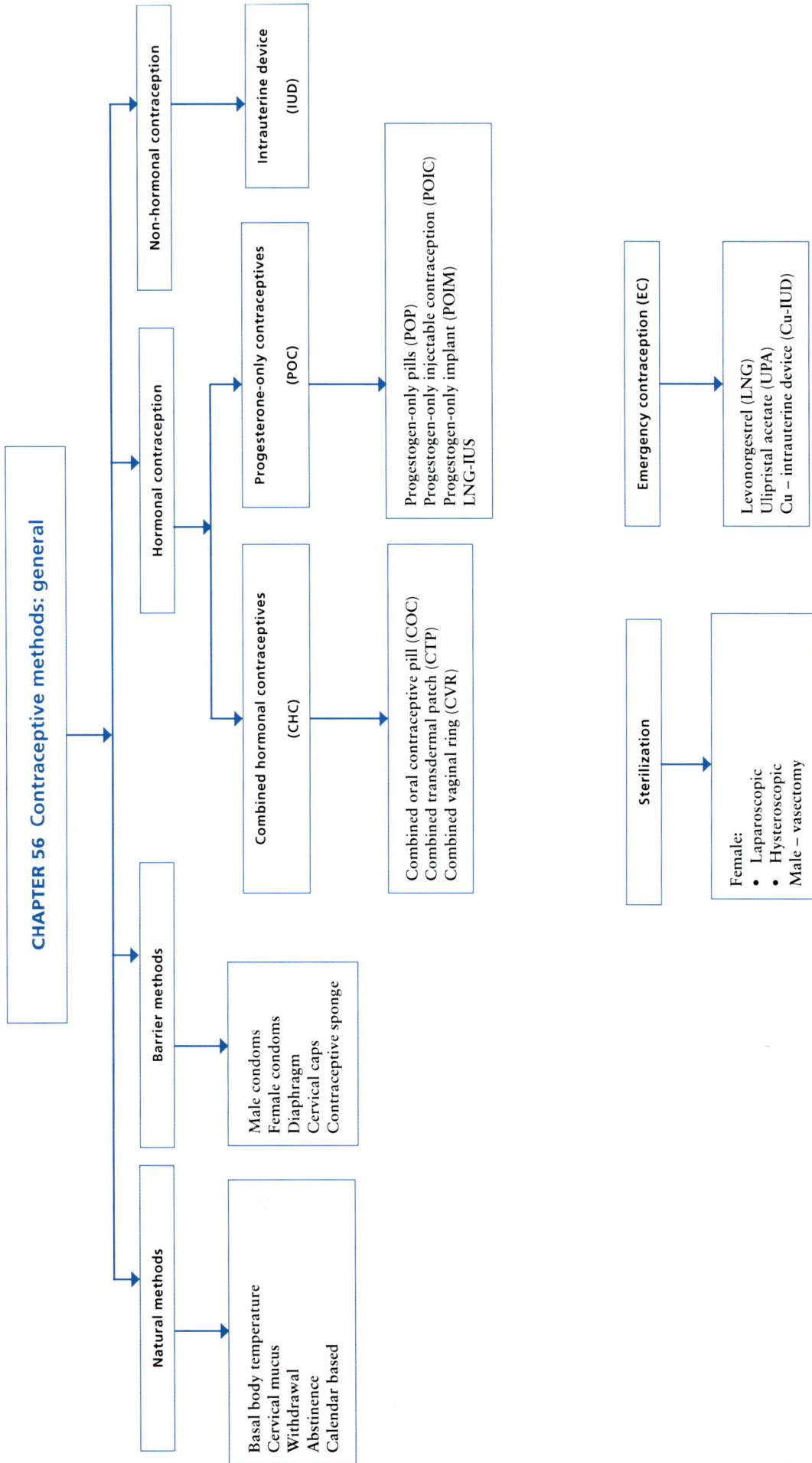

CHAPTER 56 Contraceptive methods: general

Natural methods

- Basal body temperature
- Cervical mucus
- Withdrawal
- Abstinence
- Calendar based

Barrier methods

- Male condoms
- Female condoms
- Diaphragm
- Cervical caps
- Contraceptive sponge

Hormonal contraception

Combined hormonal contraceptives (CHC)

- Combined oral contraceptive pill (COC)
- Combined transdermal patch (CTP)
- Combined vaginal ring (CVR)

Progesterone-only contraceptives (POC)

- Progestogen-only pills (POP)
- Progestogen-only injectable contraception (POIC)
- Progestogen-only implant (POIM)
- LNG-IUS

Non-hormonal contraception

Intrauterine device (IUD)

Sterilization

Female:
- Laparoscopic
- Hysteroscopic
Male – vasectomy

Emergency contraception (EC)

- Levonorgestrel (LNG)
- Ulipristal acetate (UPA)
- Cu – intrauterine device (Cu-IUD)

Male and female condoms

Correct use and caution – advice

- Counsel regarding correct use of condoms, appropriate use of lubricant, STI screening, and when EC may be required.
- To use polyurethane condoms or deproteinized latex condoms in case of latex sensitivity.
- If symptoms of local genital irritation associated with latex condom, take a clinical history to identify any cause. Consider further investigation and referral if necessary.
- Not to use condoms lubricated with spermicide.
- To use non-oil-based preparation if using lubricant with latex condoms.
- To use lubricant for anal sex to reduce the risk of condom breakage.
- Do not apply lubricant to the penis under a male condom as this is associated with slippage.
- Use of a thicker condom instead of standard condoms does not reduce the risk of breakage.

Effectiveness

- When used consistently and correctly:
  - * Male condoms are up to 98% effective at preventing pregnancy.
  - * Female condoms are up to 95% effective at preventing pregnancy.
- Pregnancy rates are similar for latex and non-latex condoms.

Condom failure

- Offer advance provision of POEC (progestogen-only emergency contraception) to women relying solely on condoms for contraception.
- Discuss post-exposure prophylaxis for HIV following sexual exposure (PEPSE) with condom failure.

Prevention of STIs

- Use of condoms reduces the risk of STIs. However, even with consistent and correct use, transmission may still occur.
- Consistent and correct use of:
  - * Condoms reduces the risk of C. trachomatis, N. gonorrhoeae, T. vaginalis, syphilis, HSV, and genital HPV transmission.
  - * Female condoms and non-latex male condoms may reduce the risk of HIV, HSV, syphilis, and genital HPV transmission.
- Male latex condoms may reduce the risk of transmission of hepatitis B. There is insufficient evidence to determine the efficacy of condoms in preventing transmission of hepatitis A and C.
- If condom failure – screen for STIs 2 weeks and 12 weeks later.

Female barrier methods

Female condoms: diaphragm, cervical caps, and contraceptive sponge

Assessment

- Take detailed history (including medical and sexual history). • Assess STI risk.
- Counsel about correct use of the method. Make sure woman can insert the diaphragm or cervical cap correctly to cover the cervix; method used is of correct size; woman is comfortable for the duration of its use, including during intercourse; and she can tolerate the use of spermicide.
- Offer vaginal examination at initial fitting to ensure the safe and effective use.
- Follow and review if she experiences any problems with the method and if she has lost or gained over 3 kg (7lb) in weight.

Effectiveness

- When used consistently and correctly, effectiveness at preventing pregnancy:
  * Diaphragm and cervical cap (used with spermicide) – 92–95%.
  * Female condoms – 95%.
  * Contraceptive sponge – 80–90%.

Emergency contraception

- Consider advance provision of POEC to women who use a diaphragm or cervical cap.
- Advice regarding EC (if a diaphragm or cervical cap is dislodged during sex or removed within 6 hours of sex).

STIs

- Female condoms reduce the risk of STIs including HIV. However, even with consistent and correct use, transmission may occur and male condoms provide better protection.
- There is little evidence to support the use of a diaphragm or cervical cap (with spermicide) or a contraceptive sponge to reduce the risk of STIs.
- There is limited evidence that a diaphragm may reduce the risk of CIN.

Correct use and caution

- Diaphragm and cervical cap:
  * Use with spermicide.
  * Must be left in place for at least 6 hours after the last episode of intercourse.
  * Can be inserted with spermicide any time before intercourse but additional spermicide should be applied if sex is to take place and the method has been *in situ* for ≥ 3 hours or if sex is repeated with the method in place.
  * Do not leave contraceptive sponge *in situ* longer than recommended by the manufacturer.
  * Sensitivity to latex proteins – use a silicone diaphragm/cervical cap or a polyurethane female condom.
- Check the diaphragm or cervical cap regularly for tears, holes, or cracks.
- Oil-based products can damage latex; therefore, avoid their use with latex diaphragms or cervical caps.
- There is no evidence that inserting the diaphragm dome up or dome down influences efficacy; however, woman should check that the diaphragm covers the cervix after insertion.
- Latex diaphragms and cervical caps can remain in place for a maximum of 30 hours.

(UKMEC 3) for use of female barrier methods

Conditions where the risks associated with use of contraceptive methods may outweigh the benefits (UKMEC 3)

- Condition

Condition	Diaphragms/cervical cap	Female condoms
* High risk of HIV/AIDS	UKMEC 3	UKMEC 1
* HIV infected	UKMEC 3	UKMEC 1
* AIDS and using HAART	UKMEC 3	UKMEC 1
* History of toxic shock syndrome	UKMEC 3	UKMEC 1
* Sensitivity to latex proteins	UKMEC 3	UKMEC 3*

- Evidence of repeated high-dose use of the spermicide nonoxynol-9 is associated with increased risk of genital lesions, which may increase the risk of HIV. The use of a diaphragm, cervical cap, or contraceptive sponge (all with nonoxynol-9) by women who have HIV or AIDS, or who are at high risk of HIV infection, is not recommended.
- Owing to a possible association between diaphragm use and non-menstrual toxic shock syndrome, for women with a history of toxic shock syndrome the use of a diaphragm, cervical cap, or contraceptive sponge is not recommended; they may use a female condom.
  * UKMEC 3 category is given but this refers to all condoms, which includes latex male condoms. For female polyurethane condoms, the benefits would outweigh the risks.

Combined hormonal contraception

Background

- CHCs contain oestrogen and progestogen:
  * Combined oral contraceptive pill (COC).
  * Combined transdermal patch (CTP).
  * Combined vaginal ring (CVR) – it is a flexible ring about 2 inches in diameter that is inserted into the vagina. It stays in the vagina for 3 weeks and is removed for 1 week, to allow menstruation.
- CHCs contain synthetic oestrogen (EE or mestranol), except Qlaira, which contains oestradiol valerate.
- Efficacy of all CHCs is generally similar.
- Use of extended or continuous regimens of CHC is off licence.

Assessment

- Take detailed history and recheck the history at least annually.
- History should include medical conditions such as migraine, drug use, family history, and lifestyle factors such as smoking.
- Record BP and BMI.
- Advice about expected bleeding patterns both initially and in the longer term.

Starting the pill

- Can start the pill at any time in the menstrual cycle if sure that the woman is not pregnant.
- If the pill is started on the first day or up to and including the 5th day of the period, woman will be protected from pregnancy immediately.
- If pill is started at any other time in the menstrual cycle, advise additional contraception such as condoms, for the first 7 days of pill taking.

Non-contraceptive health benefits

- CHC may help to improve acne.
- Can provide cycle regularity, improve primary dysmenorrhoea, and reduce HMB.
- May improve some of the symptoms associated with menopause.
- There is a reduction in the incidence of ovarian cysts and benign ovarian tumours.
- Benign breast disease – there may be a reduction in the incidence of benign breast disease (fibroadenoma and chronic cystic disease).
- Ovarian and endometrial cancer – CHC is protective against ovarian and endometrial cancer that continues for 15 years or more after stopping CHC.
- Colorectal cancer – there may be a reduction in the risk of colorectal cancer.
- CHC may be associated with mood changes but there is no evidence that it causes depression.
- Current evidence does not support a causal association between CHC and weight gain.

Drug interactions

- Lamotrigine (except in combination with sodium valproate) – owing to the risk of reduced seizure control while on CHC, and the potential for toxicity in the CHC-free week, the risks of using CHC may outweigh the benefits.
- Additional contraceptive precautions are not required when antibiotics that do not induce enzymes are used in conjunction with CHCs.
- Additional contraceptive precautions are required with drugs that are liver enzyme inducers.
- Women who do not wish to change from a CHC while on short-term treatment with an enzyme-inducing drug (and for 28 days after stopping treatment) may continue using a COC containing at least 30 µg EE, the patch, or ring along with additional contraception. An extended or tricycling regimen should be used and the hormone free interval (HFI) shortened to 4 days. Additional contraception should be continued for 28 days after stopping the enzyme-inducing drug.
- With the exception of the very potent enzyme inducers rifampicin and rifabutin, women who are taking an enzyme-inducing drug and who do not wish to change from COC or use additional precautions may increase the dose of COC to at least 50 µg EE (maximum 70 µg EE) and use an extended or tricycling regimen with an HFI of 4 days.

Risks and side effects with CHC

Risk of VTE

- Compared to non-users, the risk of VTE with use of CHC is approximately double but the absolute risk is still very low.
- There is continuing debate about the effects of the type of progestogen in CHCs on VTE risk, specifically whether CHCs containing desogestrel, gestodene, and cyproterone are associated with a higher risk than CHCs containing LNG and NET.
- Reducing the dose of oestrogen from 30 to 20 μg may reduce the risk of VTE.
- There is conflicting evidence in relation to COCs containing drospirenone.
- Transdermal patch has a similar or slightly increased risk compared with COCs.
- The RR of VTE with the CVR is unknown.
- A personal history of VTE or a known thrombogenic mutation is an unacceptable health risk for CHC use.
- For women with a family history of VTE, a negative thrombophilia screen does not necessarily exclude all thrombogenic mutations.
- A thrombophilia screen is not recommended routinely before prescribing CHC.

MI and stroke

- There may be a very small increased risk of ischaemic stroke, which may be influenced by smoking, HT, and migraine with aura.
- Smoking – as both smoking and age are independent risk factors, greater restrictions are placed on the use of CHC depending on the number of cigarettes smoked and age. After smoking cessation, risk of MI associated with smoking reduces with time (see Chapter 57). **CHC in women aged ≥ 35 years who smoke is not recommended.**
- HT – hypertensive individuals who use CHC are at higher risk of stroke and acute MI. The risks of using CHC in women with consistently elevated BP outweigh the advantages. **SBP ≥ 160 mmHg or DBP ≥ 95 mmHg is an unacceptable health risk. Even for women with adequately controlled HT, alternative methods are preferable to CHC.** (UKMEC 3)
- Migraine – risk of stroke is increased in CHC users with migraine compared to CHC users without migraine. The risk of stroke associated with migraine appears to affect only those with migraine with aura, and CHC use further increases the risk of ischaemic stroke. **CHC methods represent an unacceptable health risk in presence of migraine with aura.** (UKMEC 4)

Breast cancer

- Risk of breast cancer increases with age. There is no clear evidence as to the risk of breast cancer with use of CHC. Any risk of breast cancer associated with CHC use is likely to be small, and will reduce with time after stopping.
- Early case–control studies and meta-analysis showed an increased risk of pre-menopausal breast cancer while using COCs. However, other well-conducted observational studies have found no increased risk or a very small increased incidence of breast cancer.
- Any increased risk associated with use decreases with time after stopping, reducing to no significant risk 10 years after cessation.
- Women with current breast cancer – CHC methods are an unacceptable health risk. (UKMEC 4)
- A family history of breast cancer – No increased risk of breast cancer with use of CHC methods. (UKMEC 1)
- Women who are carriers of BRCA1 or BRCA2 – Evidence is mixed. The theoretical or proven risks of using CHC generally outweigh the benefits. Expert clinical judgement and/or referral to a specialist contraceptive provider is advised, as use of the method is not usually recommended unless other more appropriate methods are not available or not acceptable. (UKMEC 3)

- **Cervical cancer** – CHC use may be associated with a small increase in the risk of cervical cancer that is related to duration of use. CHC use does not appear to have a negative effect on overall mortality. Reassure that the benefits generally outweigh the risks. The risk of invasive cancer has been shown to decline after use ceases and, by 10 years or more, return to that of never users.

Others:

- Risk of using CHC in women with a BMI ≥ 35kg/m² usually outweighs the benefits.
- Advise about reducing periods of immobility during flights of > 3 hours.
- Women trekking to altitudes of > 4500 m for periods of >1 week may be advised to consider switching to an alternative method.

Progestogen-only contraception – health benefits and risks associated with POC

Progestogen-only pills (POP)
Progestogen-only injectable contraception (POIC)
Progestogen-only implant (POIM)
LNG-IUS

Reproductive cancers

- Breast cancer – evidence on association between breast cancer and POCs is inconclusive.
- Cervical cancer – a small increase in the risk of cervical cancer associated with long duration of POCs injectable contraceptives (> 5 years) has been reported, but the risk is smaller than that for CHC methods and the finding is based on very few women.

Dysmenorrhoea and menopausal symptoms

- Idiopathic dysmenorrhoea and ovulatory pain may be alleviated by POCs that inhibit ovulation such as the desogestrel POP, POIM, and POICs.
- LNG-IUS and DMPA may have beneficial effects on endometriosis.
- DMPA may help to alleviate vasomotor symptoms.

Bone health

- The POIC DMPA is associated with a small loss of BMD, which usually recovers after discontinuation.
- Women aged > 40 years – there is some reassuring evidence from small studies to support their use in women approaching the menopause.
- Women aged > 45 years – use of DMPA is UKMEC Category 2.
- DMPA can be used until maximum recommended age of 50 years, provided a re-evaluation of the risks and benefits of treatment for all women is carried out every 2 years.
- For women with significant lifestyle and/or medical risk factors for osteoporosis, consider other methods of contraception.
- There is currently no evidence of a clinically significant effect of other POCs on BMD.

Cardiovascular and cerebrovascular disease

- Although the data are limited, POC does not appear to increase the risk of stroke or MI, and there is little or no increase in VTE risk.
- Because of the adverse effect of progestogens on lipid metabolism, there is a theoretical risk of vascular disease in women with additional risk factors. DMPA has a greater effect on lipid metabolism than other POCs, hence the more restrictive categories in UKMEC (see Chapter 57). Be cautious when prescribing DMPA to women with cardiovascular risk factors because of the effects of progestogens on lipids.

Progestogen-only pills

Background

- Traditional POPs work by altering cervical mucus to prevent sperm penetration and by inhibiting ovulation in some women.
- Primary mode of action of the desogestrel-only pill is inhibition of ovulation.
- No data to suggest that some POPs are better at preventing pregnancy than others.
- No delay in return of fertility following discontinuation of a POP.
- If used consistently and correctly, all POPs are > 99% effective.

Assessment

- Take history to identify conditions given a UKMEC Category 3 or 4.
- BP and an assessment of BMI.

Starting the pill

- POPs can be started to provide immediate contraceptive protection:
    * Up to and including day 5 of the normal menstrual cycle.
    * Up to and including day 21 postpartum.
    * At the time of miscarriage/termination (< 24 weeks' gestation) or within 5 days.
    * If started after this time, advise condoms or abstinence for 48 hours.

Instructions for the pill

- To take one POP at or around the same time every day, without a pill-free interval.
- The desogestrel-only pill has a 12-hour window therefore may improve compliance.
- If a traditional POP is > 3 hours late or a desogestrel-only pill is > 12 hours late, advise women to:
    * Take the late or missed pill now.
    * Continue pill taking as usual (this may mean taking two pills at the same time).
    * Use condoms or abstain from sex for 48 hours after the pill is taken.
- If a woman vomits within 2 hours of pill taking, advise to take another pill ASAP.

Follow-up

- Women may be given up to 12 months' supply of POPs at their first and follow-up visits.
- POP can be continued until the age of 55 years. Alternatively check FSH levels on 2 occasions 1–2 months apart. If both FSH levels are > 30 IU/L suggestive of ovarian failure, advise them to continue with a POP or barrier contraception for 1 further year (or 2 years if aged < 50 years).

Bleeding pattern

- Changes in bleeding pattern are common: 2 in 10 women have no bleeding, 4 in 10 women have regular bleeding, and 4 in 10 women have irregular bleeding.
- Women who have a change in bleeding pattern when using a POP – assess and consider for risk of STIs, pregnancy, or gynaecological pathology.
- No evidence that changing the type and dose of progestogen will improve bleeding but this may help some individuals. If, after exclusion of other causes, bleeding patterns are still unacceptable, consider an alternative contraceptive method.

Drug interactions

- Liver enzyme-inducing drugs with short-term use – advise condoms in addition to POPs and for at least 4 weeks after the liver enzyme-inducer is stopped.
- Liver enzyme-inducing drugs with long-term use – the efficacy of POPs is reduced, therefore consider an alternative contraceptive method.

UK Medical Eligibility Criteria (Refer to Chapter 57)

- UKMEC 4 – current breast cancer.
- UKMEC 3:
  - ◆ Initiation of a POP in women with: * A history of breast cancer (no evidence of disease in the last 5 years).   * GTN (abnormal serum hCG).   * Active viral hepatitis.   * Severe decompensated cirrhosis.   * Liver tumours (benign and malignant).   * Liver enzyme-inducing medication.
  - ◆ Continuation of a POP in women with: * Current ischaemic heart disease.   * Stroke (history of cerebrovascular accident).   * Headaches, migraine with aura.
- UKMEC 2 – can initiate POP in women with history of ectopic pregnancy, ovarian cyst, VTE, stroke, ischaemic heart disease, or migraine with aura.

Other medical issues

- No evidence that the efficacy of POPs is reduced in women weighing > 70 kg and, therefore, the licensed use of one pill per day is recommended.
- No evidence of a causal association between POP and weight change, cardiovascular disease (MI, VTE, stroke), breast cancer, or headache.
- Mood change can occur with POP use, but there is no evidence of a causal association for depression.
- Women of any age with a history of migraine (with or without aura) may safely use POP.
- Women who develop new symptoms of migraine with aura while using POPs – advise to seek medical advice, as investigation may be appropriate. Consider continued use. (UKMEC 3)

Progestogen-only injectable contraception

Background

- Primary mode of action is prevention of ovulation.
- Failure rate if given within every 12 weeks is < 4/1000 over 2 years.
- There can be a delay of up to 1 year in the return of fertility after discontinuation.
- Altered bleeding patterns usually occur. Up to 70% of DMPA users are amenorrhoeic at 1 year of use. Up to 50% of POIC users discontinue by 1 year; the most common reason for discontinuation is changes to bleeding pattern.
- Women who experience unacceptable bleeding – take history, assess risk of STIs, and consider possible gynaecological pathology. Consider a COC pill (if appropriate) as a short-term treatment for women who have unacceptable bleeding but wish to continue with this method.

Assessment and when to start

- A medical history (including sexual history) to assess the appropriateness of POIC.
- Women aged < 18 years – DMPA can be used as first-line contraception after consideration of other methods.
- Women using DMPA who wish to continue – review every 2 years to assess individual situations and discuss the benefits and potential risks.
- Use may continue to age 50 years.
- POIC can be safely used by women who are breastfeeding.
- Women can start a POIC up to day 21 postpartum to provide immediate contraceptive protection. If started after that time, advise another method of contraception or abstinence for 7 days.
- POIC may be given following miscarriage or termination. If started within 5 days after the miscarriage/termination, then additional contraceptive or abstinence is not required.

Injections and follow-up

- Repeat injection of DMPA every 12 weeks (or every 8 weeks for NET-EN). If necessary, a repeat POIC can be given up to 2 weeks early.
- A repeat injection of POIC can be given up to 2 weeks late (i.e., 14 weeks since the last DMPA and 10 weeks for NET-EN) without additional contraception (unlicensed).
- Review if any signs or symptoms of infection at the site of injection.

Medical issues

- There is an association between DMPA use and weight gain.
- No evidence of a causal association between the use of POICs and mood change, libido, or headache.
- POIC use is associated with a small loss of BMD, which is usually recovered after discontinuation.
- No evidence available on the effect of DMPA on long-term fracture risk.
- Efficacy of POIC is not reduced with concurrent use of medication (including antibiotics and liver enzyme-inducing drugs) and the injection intervals do not need to be reduced.
- UKMEC for POIC use – see Chapter 57.

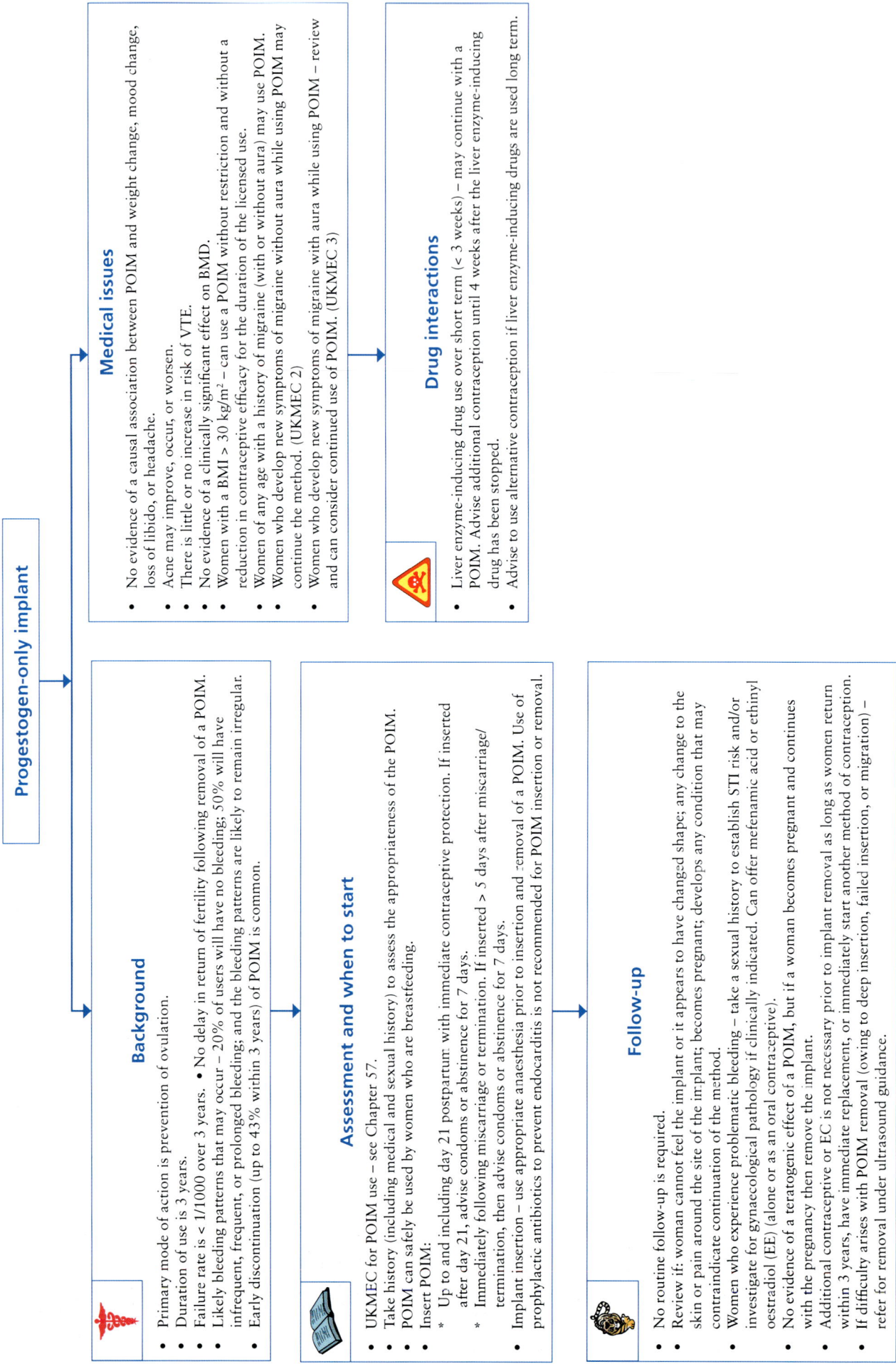

Progestogen-only implant

Background

- Primary mode of action is prevention of ovulation.
- Duration of use is 3 years.
- Failure rate is < 1/1000 over 3 years. • No delay in return of fertility following removal of a POIM.
- Likely bleeding patterns that may occur – 20% of users will have no bleeding; 50% will have infrequent, frequent, or prolonged bleeding; and the bleeding patterns are likely to remain irregular.
- Early discontinuation (up to 43% within 3 years) of POIM is common.

Assessment and when to start

- UKMEC for POIM use – see Chapter 57.
- Take history (including medical and sexual history) to assess the appropriateness of the POIM.
- POIM can safely be used by women who are breastfeeding.
- Insert POIM:
  * Up to and including day 21 postpartum with immediate contraceptive protection. If inserted after day 21, advise condoms or abstinence for 7 days.
  * Immediately following miscarriage or termination. If inserted > 5 days after miscarriage/termination, then advise condoms or abstinence for 7 days.
- Implant insertion – use appropriate anaesthesia prior to insertion and removal of a POIM. Use of prophylactic antibiotics to prevent endocarditis is not recommended for POIM insertion or removal.

Follow-up

- No routine follow-up is required.
- Review if: woman cannot feel the implant or it appears to have changed shape; any change to the skin or pain around the site of the implant; becomes pregnant; develops any condition that may contraindicate continuation of the method.
- Women who experience problematic bleeding – take a sexual history to establish STI risk and/or investigate for gynaecological pathology if clinically indicated. Can offer mefenamic acid or ethinyl oestradiol (EE) (alone or as an oral contraceptive).
- No evidence of a teratogenic effect of a POIM, but if a woman becomes pregnant and continues with the pregnancy then remove the implant.
- Additional contraceptive or EC is not necessary prior to implant removal as long as women return within 3 years, have immediate replacement, or immediately start another method of contraception.
- If difficulty arises with POIM removal (owing to deep insertion, failed insertion, or migration) – refer for removal under ultrasound guidance.

Medical issues

- No evidence of a causal association between POIM and weight change, mood change, loss of libido, or headache.
- Acne may improve, occur, or worsen.
- There is little or no increase in risk of VTE.
- No evidence of a clinically significant effect on BMD.
- Women with a BMI > 30 kg/m² – can use a POIM without restriction and without a reduction in contraceptive efficacy for the duration of the licensed use.
- Women of any age with a history of migraine (with or without aura) may use POIM.
- Women who develop new symptoms of migraine without aura while using POIM may continue the method. (UKMEC 2)
- Women who develop new symptoms of migraine with aura while using POIM – review and can consider continued use of POIM. (UKMEC 3)

Drug interactions

- Liver enzyme-inducing drug use over short term (< 3 weeks) – may continue with a POIM. Advise additional contraception until 4 weeks after the liver enzyme-inducing drug has been stopped.
- Advise to use alternative contraception if liver enzyme-inducing drugs are used long term.

Intrauterine contraception

Background

- Primary mode of action of Cu-IUD is prevention of fertilization.
- LNG-IUS works primarily by its effect on the endometrium preventing implantation; effects on cervical mucus reduce sperm penetration.
- Failure rates at 5 years' use: < 2% with TCu380A and TCu380S; <1% with the LNG-IUS. TCu380S and LNG-IUS are the most effective IUDs available.
- TCu380A and TCu380S can remain in place for 10 years and other Cu-IUDs for 5 years.
- TCu380S is the first-choice Cu-IUD to minimize the risks associated with reinsertion.
- LNG-IUS is licensed for 5 years of use as a contraceptive.
- No delay in return to fertility after removal of IUC.

Risk of STIs

- Take history (including sexual history), assess suitability for IUCs, and identify those at higher risk of STIs.
- Prior to insertion of IUC:
  * Women who are either at higher risk of STI or who request swabs – test for C. trachomatis and N. gonorrhoeae.
  * For women at higher risk of STIs, if results are unavailable before insertion – consider prophylactic antibiotics (at least to cover C. trachomatis).
  * In asymptomatic women, there is no indication to test or treat other lower genital tract organisms or delay insertion until the results of tests are available.
- Prophylactic antibiotics are NOT required for the insertion or removal of IUC in women with conditions where the risk of infective endocarditis may be increased.

Eligibility and when to insert

- Choose an IUC based on medical eligibility and the woman's preference.
- If women choose a Cu-IUD – TCu380S is recommended as it is the most effective and has the longest duration of use.
- A Cu-IUD and LNG-IUS can be inserted at any time in the menstrual cycle if it is reasonably certain that the woman is not pregnant.
- May be inserted any time after miscarriage if there is no suspicion that the pregnancy is ongoing.

Insertion of IUC

- Discuss and administer pain relief when appropriate.
- Perform a pelvic examination. • Assess pulse rate and BP.
- Use a 'no-touch' technique when sounding the uterine cavity and inserting IUC. If this technique is used then sterile gloves are not required.
- Stabilize the cervix with forceps and assess the length of the uterine cavity to facilitate fundal placement to reduce the risk of perforation.
- Document appropriate pre- and post-insertion counselling, the insertion procedure, and the type of device inserted.

Risks or side effects

- Uterine perforation – up to 2/1000 insertions.
- Risk of expulsion – 1/20; most common in the first year, particularly within 3 months of insertion. There are no differences in the rates of expulsion between different Cu-IUDs and between Cu-IUDs and LNG-IUS.
- Overall risk of ectopic pregnancy is reduced with use of IUC when compared to no contraception, and no particular device is associated with a lower rate of ectopic pregnancy.
- There may be an increased risk of pelvic infection in the 20 days following insertion of IUC, but the risk is the same as for the non-IUD-using population thereafter.
- Spotting, light bleeding, heavier or prolonged bleeding are common in first 3–6 months of Cu-IUD.
- Irregular bleeding and spotting are common in the first 6 months after insertion of the LNG-IUS, but by 1 year, amenorrhoea or light bleeding is usual.
- LNG-IUS – systemic absorption of progestogen occurs; however, rates of discontinuation due to side effects (such as acne and headache) are not significantly different from those of Cu-IUD users.
- Ovarian cysts may occur with LNG-IUS, but they are rarely a clinical problem.

Follow-up

- Give instructions on how to check for the coil threads and advise to seek help if they are unable to feel them (expulsion or perforation). Use alternative contraception until they seek medical advice.
- Advise to seek medical assistance at any time if they develop symptoms of pelvic infection, pain, persistent menstrual abnormalities, missed period, non-palpable threads, or they can feel the stem of the IUD.
- Follow-up routinely after the first menses following insertion of IUC or 3–6 weeks later.

- After counselling (about declining fertility, risks associated with insertion, and contraceptive efficacy), women who have a Cu-IUD inserted at the age of 40 years or over can retain the device for 1 year after the LMP if aged over 50 years (or 2 years if under 50 years), or until contraception is no longer required.
- Women who have the LNG-IUS inserted at the age of 45 years or over, for contraception, can retain the device until the menopause is confirmed or until contraception is no longer required.

Contraceptive methods available in the UK

(1) Hormonal methods

Method	Progestogen	Brand names
Combined oral contraception (COC) – monophasic pills		
20 µg ethinyl oestradiol	Norethisterone Desogestrel Gestodene	Loestrin 20 Mercilon Femodette, Sunya 20/75
30 µg ethinyl oestradiol	Levonorgestrel Norethisterone Desogestrel Gestodene Drospirenone	Microgynon 30*, Ovranette Loestrin 30 Marvelon Femodene*, Katya 30/75 Yasmin
35 µg ethinyl oestradiol	Norethisterone Norgestimate Cyproterone acetate	Brevinor, Norimin, Ovysmen Cilest Dianette, Clairette (co-cyprindiol)
50 µg mestranol (35 µg ethinyl oestradiol)	Norethisterone	Norinyl-1
(COC) – phasic pills		
Ethinyl oestradiol	Levonorgestrel Norethisterone Gestodene Dienogest	Logynon* BiNovum, Synphase, TriNovum Triadene Qlaira
Oestradiol valerate		
Combined patch Ethinyl oestradiol	Norelgestromin	Evra
Combined vaginal ring Ethinyl oestradiol	Etonogestrel	NuvaRing
Progestogen-only pill (POP)		
Desogestrel POP Traditional POPs	Desogestrel Levonorgestrel Norethisterone Etynodiol	Cerazette Norgeston Noriday, Micronor Femulen
Progestogen-only injectable	Medroxyprogesterone acetate Norethisterone enantate	Depo-Provera Noristerat
POIM	Etonogestrel	Implanon
Intrauterine system	Levonorgestrel	Mirena
Hormonal emergency contraception	Levonorgestrel Ulipristal acetate	Levonelle One Step, Levonelle 1500 ellaOne

(2) Non-hormonal methods

Method	Examples
Intrauterine	Copper-bearing intrauterine device
Barrier	Male condom, female condom, diaphragm, cap
Fertility awareness	Lactational amenorrhoea method, Persona™ device, calendar basal body temperature, cervical mucus (Billings), cervical palpation, symptothermal (combination of natural methods)

Failure rates of contraceptive methods

Method	Percentage of women experiencing an unintended pregnancy within the first year of use (%)	
	Typical use	Perfect use
No method	85	85
Withdrawal	29	18
Diaphragm	16	6
Condoms		
• Female	21	5
• Male	15	2
COC and POP	8	0.3
Evra patch	8	0.3
NuvaRing	8	0.3
Depo-Provera	3	0.3
Copper-IUD	0.8	0.6
LNG – IUS	0.2	0.2
Implanon	0.05	0.05
Female sterilization	0.5	0.5
Male sterilization	0.15	0.10

1. *Intrauterine Contraception*. Faculty of Sexual and Reproductive Healthcare Clinical Guidance, CEU, November 2007.
2. *Recommendation from the CEU: Antibiotic Prophylaxis for Intrauterine Contraceptive Use in Women at Risk of Bacterial Endocarditis*. Faculty of Sexual and Reproductive Healthcare Clinical Guidance, July 2008.
3. *Combined Hormonal Contraception*. Faculty of Sexual and Reproductive Healthcare Clinical Guidance, CEU, October 2011.
4. *Male and Female Condoms*. Faculty of Sexual and Reproductive Healthcare Clinical Guidance, CEU, January 2007.
5. *Female Barrier Methods*. Faculty of Sexual and Reproductive Healthcare Clinical Guidance, CEU, June 2007.
6. *Progestogen-only Implants*. Faculty of Sexual and Reproductive Healthcare Clinical Guidance, CEU, April 2008 (updated January 2009).
7. *Progestogen-only Injectable Contraception*. Faculty of Sexual and Reproductive Healthcare Clinical Guidance, CEU, November 2008 (updated June 2009).
8. *Progestogen-only Pills*. Faculty of Sexual and Reproductive Healthcare Clinical Guidance, CEU, November 2008 (updated June 2009).

CHAPTER 56 Contraceptive methods: general

CHAPTER 57　UKMEC category and definition for the use of the contraceptive method

- UKMEC category and definition for the use of the contraceptive method

1 – No restriction.
2 – Advantages of using the method generally outweigh the risks.
3 – Theoretical or proven risks usually outweigh the advantages. The provision of a method requires expert clinical judgement and/or referral to a specialist contraceptive provider, as use of the method is not usually recommended unless other more appropriate methods are not available or acceptable.
4 – An unacceptable health risk.

Condition	CHC	POP	DMPA/NET-EN	IMP	Cu-IUD	LNG-IUD	Sterilization
Age							
• Menarche to < 40 years.	1						
• ≥ 40 years.	2						
Age							
• Menarche to < 18 years.		1	2	1			
• 18–45 years.		1	1	1			
• > 45 years.		1	2	1			
Age							
• Menarche to < 20 years.					2	2	
• ≥ 20 years.					1	1	
Young age							C
Parity							
• Nullipara.		1	1	1	1	1	C
• Multipara.		1	1	1	1	1	A
Breastfeeding							
• < 6 weeks.	4	1	2	1			A
• ≥ 6 weeks to < 6 months (fully or almost fully BF).	3	1	1	1			
• ≥ 6 weeks to < 6 months (partial BF).	2	1	1	1			
• > 6 months.	1	1	1	1			
Postpartum (non-BF)							
• < 21 days.	3	1	1	1			
• ≥ 21 days.	1	1	1	1			
Postpartum							
(BF or non-BF, including post-Caesarean section)							
• 48 hours to < 4 weeks.					3	3	
• ≥ 4 weeks.					1	1	
• Puerperal sepsis.					4	4	
Postpartum							
• Following vaginal delivery or emergency CS.							D
• At the time of CS.							C

Condition	CHC	POP	DMPA/NET-EN	IMP	Cu-IUD	LNG-IUD	Sterilization
Post-abortion							
• First trimester.	1	1	1	1	1	1	D
• Second trimester (< 24 weeks).	1	1	1	1	2	2	
• Immediate post-septic abortion.	1	1	1	1	4	4	
Past ectopic pregnancy	1	1	1	1	1	1	A
Hx of pelvic surgery	1	1	1	1	1	1	
Smoking							
• Age < 35 years.	2	1	1	1	1	1	A
• Age ≥ 35 years.							
* < 15 cigarettes/day.	3	1	1	1	1	1	A
* ≥ 15 cigarettes/day.	4	1	1	1	1	1	A
* stopped smoking < 1 year.	3	1	1	1	1	1	A
* stopped smoking ≥ 1 year.	2	1	1	1	1	1	A
Obesity							
• BMI ≥ 30.	2	1	1	1	1	1	C
• BMI ≥ 35.	3	1	1	1	1	1	C
Cardiovascular disease – multiple risk factors (such as older age, smoking, diabetes, hypertension, obesity).	3/4	2	3	2	1	2	S
Hypertension							
• Adequately controlled.	3	1	2	1	1	1	C
• Consistently elevated BP.							
* SBP > 140–159; DBP > 90–94.	3	1	1	1	1	1	C
* SBP ≥ 160; DBP ≥ 95.	4	1	2	1	1	1	S
• Vascular disease.	4	2	3	2	1	2	S
• Hx of high BP during pregnancy (current BP – N).	2	1	1	1	1	1	A
Venous thromboembolism							
• Hx of VTE.	4	2	2	2	1	2	A
• Current VTE (on anticoagulants).	4	2	2	2	1	2	D
• Family Hx of VTE.							
* First-degree relative, age < 45 years.	3	1	1	1	1	1	A
* First-degree relative, age ≥ 45 years.	2	1	1	1	1	1	A
• Major surgery.							
* With prolonged immobilization.	4	2	2	2	1	2	A
* Without prolonged immobilization.	2	1	1	1	1	1	D
• Minor surgery without prolonged immobilization.	1	1	1	1	1	1	A
• Immobility unrelated to surgery.	3	1	1	1	1	1	D
Known thrombogenic mutations (e.g., Factor V Leiden, prothrombin mutation, protein S, protein C, and anti-thrombin deficiencies.)	4	2	2	2	1	2	A

CHAPTER 57 UKMEC category and definition for the use of the contraceptive method

Superficial venous thrombosis							
• Varicose veins.	1	1	1	1	1	1	A
• Superficial thrombophlebitis.	2	1	1	1	1	1	A
Current and history of ischaemic heart disease	4	I-2; C-3	3	I-2; C-3	1	I-2; C-3	D/C
Stroke							
(Hx of cerebrovascular accident, including TIA.)	4	I-2; C-3	3	I-2; C-3	1	I-2; C-3	C
Known hyperlipidaemias	2/3	2	2	2	2	2	A
Vascular and congenital heart disease							
• Uncomplicated.	2	1	1	1	1	1	C
• Complicated (pulmonary HT).	4	1	1	1	2	2	S
Headaches							
• Non-migrainous (mild or severe).	I-1; C-2	1	1	1	1	1	A
• Migraine without aura, any age.	I-2; C-3	2	2	2	1	2	A
• Migraine with aura, any age.	I-4; C-4	2	2	2	1	2	A
• Past Hx of migraine with aura (≥ 5 years ago), any age.	3	2	2	2	1	2	A
Epilepsy	1	1	1	1	1	1	C
Depressive disorders	1	1	1	1	1	1	C
Vaginal bleeding patterns							
• Irregular pattern without heavy bleeding.	1	2	2	2	1	I-1; C-1	A
• Heavy or prolonged bleeding (regular and irregular patterns).	1	2	2	2	2	I-1; C-2	A
Unexplained vaginal bleeding – (suspicious for serious underlying condition) before evaluation.	2	2	3	3	I-4; C-2	I-4; C-2	D
Endometriosis	1	1	1	1	2	1	S
Benign ovarian tumours including cysts	1	1	1	1	1	1	A
Severe dysmenorrhoea	1	1	1	2	1	1	A
Gestational trophoblastic disease							
• Decreasing or undetectable hCG levels.	1	1	1	1	3	3	A
• Pesistently elevated hCG levels or malignant disease	1	1	1	1	4	4	D
Cervical ectropion	1	1	1	1	1	1	A
CIN	2	1	2	2	1	2	A
Cervical cancer awaiting treatment	2	1	2	2	I-4; C-2	I-4; C-2	D

(contd.)

Condition	CHC	POP	DMPA/NET-EN	IMP	Cu-IUD	LNG-IUD	Sterilization
Breast disease							
• Undiagnosed mass.	I-3; C-2	2	2	2	1	2	A
• Benign breast disease.	1	1	1	1	1	1	A
• Family Hx of cancer.	1	1	1	1	1	1	A
• Carriers mutations associated with breast cancer (BRCA1).	3	2	2	2	1	2	A
• Breast cancer:							
* Current.	4	4	4	4	1	4	C
* Past and no evidence of current disease for 5 years.	3	3	3	3	1	3	A
Endometrial cancer	1	1	1	1	I-4; C-2	I-4; C-2	D
Ovarian cancer	1	1	1	1	I-3; C-2	I-3; C-2	D
Uterine fibroids							
• Without distortion of the uterine cavity.	1	1	1	1	1	1	C
• With distortion of the uterine cavity.	1	1	1	1	3	3	C
Anatomical abnormalities							
• Distorting the uterine cavity.					3	3	
• Other abnormalities (Cx stenosis) not distorting the uterine cavity.					2	2	
PID							
• Past PID (no current risk factors for STI).	1	1	1	1	I-1; C-1	I-1; C-1	A
• Current PID.	1	1	1	1	I-4; C-2	I-4; C-2	D
STIs							
• Chlamydia infection.							
* Symptomatic.	1	1	1	1	I-4; C-2	I-4; C-2	D
* Asymptomatic.	1	1	1	1	I-4; C-2	I-4; C-2	D
• Current purulent cervicitis or gonorrhoea.	1	1	1	1	I-4; C-2	I-4; C-2	D
• Other STIs (excluding HIV and hepatitis).	1	1	1	1	I-2; C-2	I-2; C-2	A
• Vaginitis (including Trichomonas vaginalis and BV).	1	1	1	1	I-2; C-2	I-2; C-2	A
• Increased risk of STIs.	1	1	1	1	I-2/3; C-2	I-2/3; C-2	A
HIV/AIDS							
• High risk of HIV.	1	1	1	1	2	2	A
• HIV-infected:							
* Not using anti-retroviral therapy.	1	2	2	2	2	2	A
* Using anti-retroviral therapy.	1–3	1–3	1–2	1–2	2–3	2–3	A
• AIDS (using retroviral).	2	2	2	2	2	2	S

Condition							
Other infections							
• Schistisomiasis:							
* Uncomplicated.	1	1	1	1	1	1	A
* Fibrosis of liver.	1	1	1	1	1	1	C
• Tuberculosis:							
* Non-pelvic.	I-1; C-1	I-1; C-1	1	1	1	1	A
* Known pelvic.	I-4; C-3	I-4; C-3	1	1	1	1	S
• Malaria.	1	1	1	1	1	1	A
Diabetes							
• Hx of gestational diabetes	1	1	1	1	1	1	A
• Non-vascular disease:							
* Non-insulin dependent.	1	2	2	2	2	2	C
* Insulin dependent.	1	2	2	2	2	2	C
• Nephropathy/retinopathy/neuropathy.	1	2	2	3	2	3/4	S
• Other vascular disease.	1	2	2	3	2	3/4	S
Thyroid disorder							
• Simple goitre.	1	1	1	1	1	1	A
• Hyperthyroid.	1	1	1	1	1	1	S
• Hypothyroid.	1	1	1	1	1	1	C
Gall-bladder disease							
• Symptomatic:							
* Treated by cholecystectomy.	1	2	2	2	2	2	A
* Medical treatment.	1	2	2	2	2	3	A
* Currently treated.	1	2	2	2	2	3	D
• Asymptomatic.	1	2	2	2	2	2	A
History of cholestasis							
• Pregnancy-related.	1	1	1	1	1	2	A
• Past COC-related.	1	2	2	2	2	3	A
Viral hepatitis							
• Acute or flare.	1	1	1	1	1	I-3/4; C-2	D
• Carrier.	1	1	1	1	1	1	A
• Chronic.	1	1	1	1	1	1	A
Cirrhosis							
• Mild – compensated without complications.	1	1	1	1	1	1	C
• Severe – decompensated.	1	3	3	3	3	4	S
Liver tumours							
• Benign:							
* Focal nodular hyperplasia.	1	2	2	2	2	2	C
* Hepatocellular (adenoma).	1	3	3	3	3	4	C
• Malignant (hepatoma).	1	3	3	3	3	4	C

Condition	CHC	POP	DMPA/NET-EN	IMP	Cu-IUD	LNG-IUD	Sterilization
IBD (Crohn's and ulcerative colitis)	2	2	1	1	1	1	S
Anaemia							
• Thalassaemia.	1		1	1	2	1	C
• Sickle cell disease.	2	1	1	1	2	1	C
• Iron deficiency anaemia.	1	1	1	1	2	1	
* Hb < 7 g/dl.							D
* Hb ≥ 7 to < 10g/dl.							C
Raynaud's disease							
• Primary.	1	1	1	1	1	1	A
• Secondary.							
* Without LAC.	2	1	1	1	1	1	A
* With LAC.	4	2	2	2	1	2	A
Systemic lupus erythematosus							
• Positive (or unknown) anti-phospholipid antibodies.	4	3	I-3; C-3	3	I-1; C-1	3	S
• Severe thrombocytopenia.	2	2	I-3; C-2	2	I-3; C-2	2	S
• Immunosuppressive.	2	2	I-2; C-2	2	I-2; C-1	2	C
• None of the above.	2	2	I-2; C-2	2	I-1; C-1	2	C
Local infection							D
Coagulation disorder							S
Respiratory disease							
• Acute.							D
• Chronic:							
* Asthma.							S
* Bronchitis.							S
* Emphysema.							S
* Lung infection.							S
Systemic infection or gastroenteritis							D
Fixed uterus due to previous surgery or infection							S
Umbilical wall or abdominal wall hernia							S
Diaphragmatic hernia							C
Kidney disease							C
Severe nutritional deficiency							C

Previous abdominal or pelvic surgery	S
Sterilization concurrent with abdominal surgery	
• Elective.	C
• Emergency (without previous counselling).	D
• Infectious condition.	D

A – accept, C – caution, D – delay, S – special.

Drug interactions	CHC	POP	DMPA/ NET-EN	IMP	Cu-IUD	LNG-IUD
Anti-retroviral therapy – effectiveness may be reduced and pregnancy itself may have a negative impact on health for some women with certain medical conditions.						
• Nucleoside reverse transcriptase inhibitors.	1	1	DMPA-1 NET-EN-2	1	I-2/3; C-2	I-2/3; C-2
• Non-nucleoside reverse transcriptase inhibitors.	2	2	DMPA-1 NET-EN-2	2	I-2/3; C-2	I-2/3; C-2
• Ritonavir-boosted protease inhibitors.	3	3	DMPA-1 NET-EN-2	2	I-2/3; C-2	I-2/3; C-2

Anticonvulsants – effectiveness may be reduced and pregnancy itself may have a negative impact on health for some women with certain medical conditions.
When a COC is chosen, a preparation containing a minimum of 30 μg EE should be used. Use of other contraceptives should be encouraged for women who are long-term users of any of these anticonvulsant drugs. Use of DMPA is a Category 1 because its effectiveness is NOT decreased by the use of certain anticonvulsants.
Lamotrigine – when a COC is chosen, a preparation containing a minimum of 30 μg EE should be used. Anticonvulsant treatment regimens that combine lamotrigine and non-enzyme inducing antiepileptic drugs (such as sodium valproate) do not interact with COCs.

Drug interactions	CHC	POP	DMPA/ NET-EN	IMP	Cu-IUD	LNG-IUD
• Certain anticonvulsants (phenytoin, carbamazepine, barbiturates, primidone, topiramate, oxcarbazepine).	3	3	DMPA-1 NET-EN-2	2	1	1
• Lamotrigine.	3	1	1	1	1	1

Antimicrobial therapy – effectiveness may be reduced and pregnancy itself may have a negative impact on health for some women with certain medical conditions.
The contraceptive effectiveness of COC is not affected by co-administration of most broad spectrum antibiotics.
Rifampicin or rifabutin therapy and COC – when a COC is chosen, a preparation containing a minimum of 30 μg EE should be used. If a woman on rifampicin or rifabutin decides to use CHC, the consistent use of condoms is recommended. Use of other contraceptives should be encouraged for women who are long-term users of rifampicin or rifabutin. Use of DMPA is a Category 1 because its effectiveness is unlikely to be decreased by the use of rifampicin or rifabutin.

Drug interactions	CHC	POP	DMPA/ NET-EN	IMP	Cu-IUD	LNG-IUD
• Broad spectrum antibiotics.	1	1	1	1	1	1
• Antifungals.	1	1	1	1	1	1
• Antiparasitics.	3	1	1	1	1	1
• Rifampicin or rifabutin therapy.	3	3	DMPA-1 NET-EN-2	2	1	1

Background

- Traditionally, initiation of contraception was delayed until the onset of the next menstrual period in order to avoid inadvertent use during pregnancy. Starting early in the cycle also avoids the need for additional contraception. Some methods may be started up to day 5 or day 7 (LNG-IUS) of the menstrual cycle without the need for additional contraception.
- 'Quick starting' – starting contraception at the time a woman requests contraception, rather than waiting for the next menstrual cycle.
- May also mean starting a method immediately after the use of EC. In this situation, there is a possibility of EC failure and pregnancy. Such practice is outside the licence. Consider it on an individual basis.

- Quick starting contraceptive methods can be started at any point in the menstrual cycle if reasonably certain that the woman is not currently pregnant or at risk of pregnancy.
- As sperm may be viable in the female reproductive tract for up to 7 days, consider if a woman is at risk of becoming pregnant as a result of UPSI within the last 7 days.
- The probability of pregnancy from a single act of UPSI in the first 3 days of the cycle is negligible. There is a theoretical concern that women with a short menstrual cycle may ovulate very early in their cycle, putting them at risk of pregnancy if contraception is started as late as day 5 or day 7 (LNG-IUS). FPA advises additional contraception for women in this situation, if they have a cycle shorter than 23 days.

Potential benefits

- Quick starting may reduce the time a woman is at risk of pregnancy; prevent her forgetting information on correct use of the method; prevent waning enthusiasm for the method and use of a less reliable alternative method; avoid patient costs and barriers to return for contraception, and reduce healthcare costs by reducing the number of appointments.
- Women who have taken EC or who have irregular cycles may have a longer wait for their next menses. There is a 2–3-fold higher risk of pregnancy in women who have other episodes of UPSI in the same cycle that EC has been given compared to those who abstain. Quick starting is expected to reduce unintended pregnancy rates by improving initiation and continuation of contraceptives compared to conventional start methods.
- **While there is currently a paucity of evidence demonstrating effectiveness, there are data to suggest women find quick starting acceptable.**

Potential disadvantages

- A small risk of woman being already pregnant or failure of EC.
- Diagnosis of pregnancy may be delayed if amenorrhoea is assumed to be a result of the contraceptive method or if bleeding is mistaken for a period.
- Effects of fetal exposure to steroid hormones – theoretical concerns that HC may be harmful to the fetus. There have been no consistent findings of specific fetal abnormalities.
- Animal studies – very high doses of progestogens may cause masculinization of female fetuses. A very small number of cases of clitoral enlargement have been reported in humans but there have been no reports of serious abnormalities.
- Dianette after the 45th day of pregnancy could cause feminization of male fetuses (phase of embryogenesis at which differentiation of the external genitalia occurs).
- Pregnancies conceived with a Cu-IUD in situ are not associated with congenital abnormalities but may be associated with an increased risk of miscarriage.
- Risks with the LNG-IUS may be higher owing to direct in utero exposure to progestogen. Teratogenicity (especially virilization) cannot be completely excluded, but in cases where pregnancies have continued with the LNG-IUS, there is no evidence of birth defects.
- Bleeding pattern – may be associated with more disruption to a woman's usual bleeding pattern than when initiating contraception at the beginning of the menstrual cycle.
- Insertion of IUCs – no evidence that the cervix dilates during menses or that insertion of an IUD is easier at this time.

- Quick starting contraception is likely to be an acceptable option for women requesting contraception, and may offer some benefits, with no strong evidence of adverse effects. Where appropriate, offer an immediate start of the method of choice or a bridging method as an alternative to waiting until the next menstrual period.
- Quick starting method may be continued as an ongoing method of contraception or it may be used as a temporary 'bridging' method until pregnancy can be excluded and a longer-acting method initiated.
- If a woman prefers to delay starting contraception or if she is concerned about potential risks, she may wait until her next period or until risk of pregnancy has been excluded.

Assessment – woman attending for contraception or EC

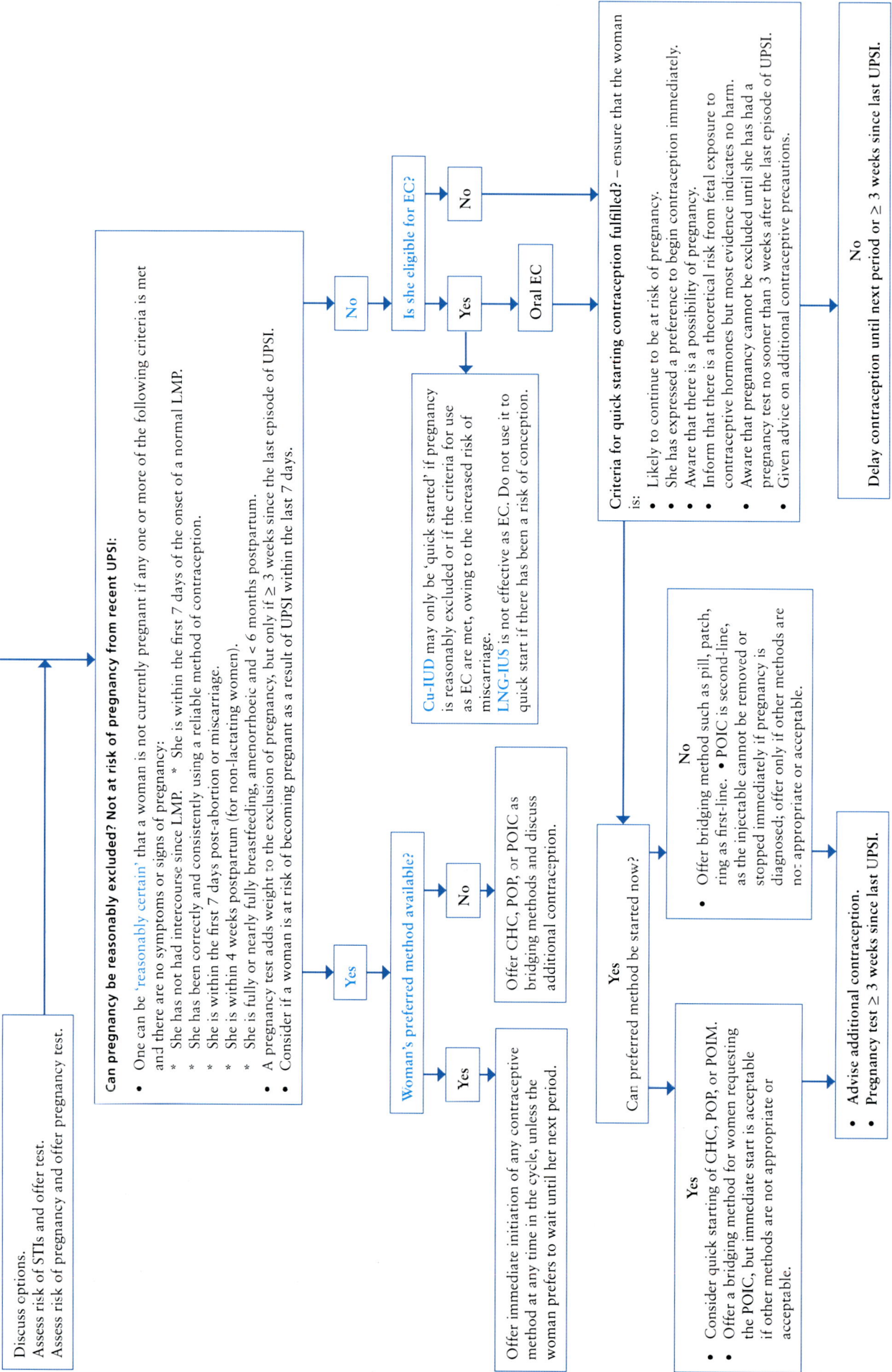

Discuss options.
Assess risk of STIs and offer test.
Assess risk of pregnancy and offer pregnancy test.

Can pregnancy be reasonably excluded? Not at risk of pregnancy from recent UPSI:

- One can be 'reasonably certain' that a woman is not currently pregnant if any one or more of the following criteria is met and there are no symptoms or signs of pregnancy:
  * She has not had intercourse since LMP.   * She is within the first 7 days of the onset of a normal LMP.
  * She has been correctly and consistently using a reliable method of contraception.
  * She is within the first 7 days post-abortion or miscarriage.
  * She is within 4 weeks postpartum (for non-lactating women).
  * She is fully or nearly fully breastfeeding, amenorrhoeic and < 6 months postpartum.
- A pregnancy test adds weight to the exclusion of pregnancy, but only if ≥ 3 weeks since the last episode of UPSI.
- Consider if a woman is at risk of becoming pregnant as a result of UPSI within the last 7 days.

Yes → **Woman's preferred method available?**

- **No** → Offer CHC, POP, or POIC as bridging methods and discuss additional contraception.

- **Yes** → Offer immediate initiation of any contraceptive method at any time in the cycle, unless the woman prefers to wait until her next period.

No → **Is she eligible for EC?**

- **Yes** → Oral EC

  Cu-IUD may only be 'quick started' if pregnancy is reasonably excluded or if the criteria for use as EC are met, owing to the increased risk of miscarriage.
  LNG-IUS is not effective as EC. Do not use it to quick start if there has been a risk of conception.

- **No** →

Criteria for quick starting contraception fulfilled? – ensure that the woman is:

- Likely to continue to be at risk of pregnancy.
- She has expressed a preference to begin contraception immediately.
- Aware that there is a possibility of pregnancy.
- Inform that there is a theoretical risk from fetal exposure to contraceptive hormones but most evidence indicates no harm.
- Aware that pregnancy cannot be excluded until she has had a pregnancy test no sooner than 3 weeks after the last episode of UPSI.
- Given advice on additional contraceptive precautions.

Yes → **Can preferred method be started now?**

- **Yes**
  - Consider quick starting of CHC, POP, or POIM.
  - Offer a bridging method for women requesting the POIC, but immediate start is acceptable if other methods are not appropriate or acceptable.

  - Advise additional contraception.
  - Pregnancy test ≥ 3 weeks since last UPSI.

- **No**
  - Offer bridging method such as pill, patch, ring as first-line. • POIC is second-line, as the injectable cannot be removed or stopped immediately if pregnancy is diagnosed; offer only if other methods are not appropriate or acceptable.

No → Delay contraception until next period or ≥ 3 weeks since last UPSI.

Additional contraceptive requirements when starting contraception

Method	Circumstances (day of menstrual cycle/method of EC)	Requirements for additional contraception (condoms/avoidance of sex)
COC pills except	Days 1–5. Day 6 onwards/'Quick starting' after POEC. Quick starting after UPA EC.	Not required. 7 days. 14 days.
Qlaira COC pill	Days 1. Day 2 onwards/'Quick starting' after POEC. Quick starting after UPA EC.	Not required. 9 days. 16 days.
Combined vaginal ring Transdermal patch	Days 1. Day 2 onwards/'Quick starting' after POEC. Quick starting after UPA EC.	Not required. 7 days. 14 days.
POP (traditional/desogestrel)	Days 1–5. Day 6 onwards/'Quick starting' after POEC. Quick starting after UPA EC.	Not required. 2 days. 9 days.
POIM/POIC	Days 1–5. Day 6 onwards/'Quick starting' after POEC. Quick starting after UPA EC.	Not required. 7 days. 14 days.
LNG-IUS	Days 1–7. Day 8 onwards.	Not required. 7 days.
Cu-IUD	Any start day.	Not required.

Follow-up

- Inform women of the need for additional contraceptive precautions and pregnancy testing. The timing of the pregnancy test should be no sooner than 3 weeks after the woman's last episode of UPSI.
- Inform women that bleeding during or soon after stopping HC is not the same as a natural period and even regular withdrawal bleeds on CHC may not be a reliable indicator that a woman is not pregnant.

Pregnancy diagnosed after starting contraception

- If the woman wishes to continue the pregnancy, stop or remove the method.
- Contraceptive hormones are not thought to cause harm to the fetus and do not advise to terminate the pregnancy for this reason.
- If a woman is using the POIM and she opts to abort the pregnancy, the implant can be left *in situ* for ongoing contraception.
- IUD *in situ* is associated with increased risks of second-trimester miscarriage, preterm delivery, and infection if left *in situ*. Removal in the first trimester is thought to reduce the overall risk of adverse outcomes but is associated with a small risk of miscarriage. If the threads are visible, or can easily be retrieved from the endocervical canal, remove the IUC up to 12 weeks' gestation. Do not remove IUDs if pregnancy is diagnosed after 12 weeks' gestation.

1. *Quick Starting Contraception*. Faculty of Sexual & Reproductive Healthcare Clinical Guidance, CEU, September 2010.

CHAPTER 59 Unscheduled bleeding with hormonal contraception (HC)

Background and definition

- Unscheduled bleeding – breakthrough bleeding, spotting, prolonged or frequent bleeding.
- Exact mechanism of unscheduled bleeding associated with HC is unknown.
- Oestradiol exposure during the follicular phase is responsible for endometrial proliferation. Exposure to progesterone in the luteal phase results in secretory differentiation. Progesterone is anti-oestrogenic and inhibits endometrial growth and glandular differentiation. It is the withdrawal of oestrogen and progesterone that triggers the onset of menstrual bleeding.
- Endometrial response to HC reflects circulating sex hormone concentration, dose, route, formulation of steroid delivery, and the timing and duration of administration.
- **Before starting HC, advise women about the expected bleeding patterns, both initially and in the longer term.**
- See Chapter 57 categories for use of HC by women with vaginal bleeding.
- POC are more likely to present with unscheduled bleeding than CHCs. Bleeding with POP is less likely to settle than bleeding with the POIC.

Expected bleeding patterns after commencing HC

CHC (pill, patch, or ring)–
- Up to 20% of COC users have irregular bleeding.
- No significant differences between pill or patch.
- Ovarian activity is effectively suppressed.

POP:
- One third of women have a change in bleeding and 1/10 have frequent bleeding. Bleeding may not settle with time and ovarian activity is incompletely suppressed.
- Long term: 10–15% are amenorrhoeic; up to 50% have a regular bleed; 30–40% have irregular bleeding.

POIC:
- Bleeding disturbances (spotting, light, heavy, or prolonged bleeding) are common.
- Up to 35% are amenorrhoeic at 3 months.
- Up to 70% are amenorrhoeic at 1 year.

POIM:
- Bleeding disturbances are common.
- After 6 months' use, 30% have infrequent bleeding; 10–20% have prolonged bleeding.
- Long term: 20% are amenorrhoeic; 50% have infrequent, frequent, or prolonged bleeding, which may not settle with time.

IUS:
- Irregular, light, or heavy bleeding is common (in the first 6 months).
- 65% have amenorrhoea or reduced bleeding at 1 year, with a 90% reduction in menstrual blood loss over 12 months of use.

History

To identify or exclude the possible causes of unscheduled bleeding:
- Assess compliance, current contraception, and the duration of use.
- Bleeding pattern before starting HC, since starting, and current pattern.
- Need for examination and investigation depends on the presence of any other symptoms suggestive of an underlying cause such as abdominal or pelvic pain, PCB, dyspareunia, or heavy bleeding.
- Identify risk of STIs – abnormal bleeding may be a presenting symptom of C. trachomatis.
- Cervical screening history. • Rule out the possibility of pregnancy.
- Use of medications that may interact with the contraceptive method, or any illness that may affect the absorption of orally administered hormones.

Examination

- **Speculum examination** can identify cervical conditions (polyps or ectopy) and the very occasional case of cervical cancer. Indicated if:
  * Persistent bleeding beyond the first 3 months' use.
  * New symptoms or a change in bleeding after at least 3 months' use of a method. * Requested by the woman.
  * Woman has not participated in a cervical screening programme.
  * After a failed trial of the medical management.
  * There are other symptoms such as pair, dyspareunia, or PCB.
- The 3-month cut-off is a guide only, as some methods such as the IUS or POIM may commonly cause bleeding even after the first 3 months of use.
- **Bimanual examination** if there are symptoms such as IMB or PCB, pelvic pain, or pressure symptoms suggestive of a structural or histological abnormality.

Examination is not necessary

- Unscheduled bleeding in the first 3 months after starting a new HC is common.
- Ensure there are no risk factors for STIs, no concurrent symptoms suggestive of underlying causes, and the woman is participating in the National Cervical Screening Programme (NCSP).
- Some women may be happy to continue with the method after this initial assessment but plan follow-up as bleeding may persist.

Investigations

- Women who are at risk of STIs – test for C. trachomatis as a minimum. Testing for N. gonorrhoeae will depend on sexual risk and local prevalence. A self-obtained low vaginal swab or a first-void urine if a speculum examination is not being performed can be done.
- Cervical smear in women who are not participating in an NCSP.
- Pregnancy test if there is a possibility of incorrect use (missed pills, late injection, or expelled IUS), drug interactions, or illness which may lead to malabsorption of oral hormones.
- Endometrial biopsy – perform in women aged ≥ 45 years or in women aged < 45 years with risk factors for endometrial cancer (e.g., obesity or PCOS), who have persistent unscheduled bleeding after the first 3 months of starting a method or who present with a change in bleeding pattern.
- The role of uterine polyps, fibroids, or ovarian cysts as a cause of unscheduled bleeding is limited. Nevertheless, if such a structural abnormality is suspected, a TVS and/or hysteroscopy may be indicated.

Management

Rx

- Bleeding with HC is common in the first few months of use and delay treatment until after the first 3 months.
- No evidence to suggest that bleeding patterns with one POC will predict the likely bleeding patterns with another POC.

CHC

- Unscheduled bleeding is less common with CHC than with POCs.
- Do not change a COC pill within the first 3 months of use as bleeding disturbances often settle in this time.
- For women using a COC pill, use the lowest dose of EE to provide good cycle control. The dose of EE can be increased to a maximum of 35 μg to provide good cycle control.
- Although some studies suggest bleeding may be better with COCs containing certain progestogens, it is not evident in systematic reviews.
- No evidence to support the use of a continuous regimen over the cyclical regimens to improve bleeding.
- Insufficient evidence to recommend the use of a biphasic and triphasic COC to improve bleeding patterns.

POP

- There is lack of evidence on the effective treatment of bleeding in women using POPs.
- No evidence to suggest that one POP is associated with less bleeding than any other (including the desogestrel-only pill).
- Although bleeding may settle with time, there is no definite time frame in which women can expect bleeding to stop or improve.
- There is no evidence that bleeding improves with two POPs per day, although this has been used in clinical practice.
- There is no evidence that changing the type and dose of POPs will improve bleeding, but this may help some.

POIM

- Women using an LNG implant (Norplant) – some evidence of a beneficial effect of mefenamic acid or EE (alone or as a COC) on bleeding patterns.
- Mifepristone may be beneficial but there is limited evidence to support its use in routine clinical practice.

POIC

- No evidence on the use of a low-dose (< 50 μg) COC to treat unscheduled bleeding with POIC. Despite this, use of EE (given as a COC) is advised as a *short-term treatment* option up to 3 months, if there are no contraindications to use of oestrogen. The COC can be taken in the usual cyclic manner or continuously without a pill-free interval.
- For women who have a contraindication to COC, consider mefenamic acid for 5 days. It can reduce the length of a bleeding episode but has little effect on bleeding in the longer term.
- Mifepristone – one RCT reported a significant reduction in breakthrough bleeding compared to placebo.
- There is some evidence that a COX-2 inhibitor (valdecoxib) is effective in the treatment of uterine bleeding with DMPA; however, the use of COX-2 inhibitors for this purpose is unlicensed in the UK.

LNG-IUS

- No evidence on treatment options for women with unscheduled bleeding with the LNG-IUS.
- Provide information about bleeding patterns likely to be experienced.

For women with unscheduled bleeding using a POIC, POIM, or IUS who wish to continue with the method and are medically eligible, a COC may be used for up to 3 months (cyclically or continuously).

1. *Management of Unscheduled Bleeding in Women Using Hormonal Contraception.* Faculty of Sexual and Reproductive Healthcare Clinical Guidance, May 2009.

CHAPTER 59 Unscheduled bleeding with hormonal contraception

CHAPTER 60 Missed pill

Definition – a missed pill is defined as one that is more than 24 hours late.
If >1 pill is missed, the rule applies to consecutive pills.
The rule applies to active pills.

Key elements

- If it is reasonably certain that the woman is not pregnant, COCs can be initiated on any day of the menstrual cycle. Additional contraception is required for the first 7 days if the pill is started after day 5 of the cycle.
- If one active pill is missed, there is no need to take additional precautions.
- If two active pills are missed, advise additional precautions for the next 7 days.

CHC

If one pill has been missed (> 24–48 hours late)

- **To continue contraceptive cover** – advise to:
  * Take the missed pill as soon as it is remembered.
  * Continue the remaining pills at the usual time.
- **To minimize the risk of pregnancy** – EC is not usually required, but consider EC if pills have been missed earlier in the packet or in the last week of the previous packet.

If ≥ 2 pills have been missed (> 48 hours late)

- **To continue contraceptive cover** – advise to:
  * Take the most recently missed pill ASAP.
  * Continue the remaining pills at the usual time.
  * Use condoms or abstain from sex until 7 consecutive active pills have been taken. This advice may be overcautious in the second and third weeks, but the advice is a backup in the event that further pills are missed.

- **If pills are missed in the first week (pills 1–7)** – consider EC if UPSI occurred in the pill-free interval or in the first week of pill-taking.
- **If pills are missed in the second week (pills 8–14)** – no indication for EC if the pills in the preceding 7 days have been taken consistently and correctly (assuming the pills thereafter are taken correctly and additional contraceptive precautions are used).
- **If pills are missed in the third week (pills 15–21)** – advise to omit the pill-free interval by finishing the pills in the current pack (or discarding any placebo tablets) and starting a new pack the next day.

Progestogen-only pill

Traditional POPs (Micronor, Noriday, Norgeston, Femulen): **> 3 hours late** (> 27 hours since the last pill was taken).
Desogestrel-only (Cerazette): **> 12 hours late** (> 36 hours since the last pill was taken).

Advice:
- To take a pill as soon as remembered.
- If >1 pill has been missed – just take one pill. Take the next pill at the usual time. This may mean taking two pills in one day.
- An additional method of contraception (condoms or abstinence) for the next 2 days (48 hours after the POP has been taken) is required.

1. *Missed Pill Recommendations*. Faculty of Sexual and Reproductive Healthcare, CEU Statement, May 2011.
2. *Progestogen-only Pills*. Faculty of Sexual and Reproductive Healthcare, CEU, November 2008 (updated June 2009).

Prevalence and background

- Choice of contraception is influenced by effectiveness, discretion, safety, side effect profile, invasiveness, ease of use, or how difficult it is to forget.
- Among women aged 16–29 years who are at risk of pregnancy, about 78% use the contraceptive pill and/or the condom.
- LARC is used by a minority of women; there is a trend towards increasing use.
- Use of POICs and POIMs is greater in young women compared with older women.

History for medical eligibility

- Young people have specific risks relating to pubertal development and risk of STIs.
- Take into account factors such as ability to adhere with contraception, eating disorders, family situation, obesity, and recreational drug/alcohol use.
- General health – prescription medications, drug use, smoking, alcohol use, non-prescription drugs, diet, and physical activity levels; HPV vaccination.
- Sexual and reproductive health – age at menarche, regularity of menstrual cycles, LMP, history of any pregnancy and its outcome.
Current and previous partners in last 6 months; relationship with the partner(s) – casual/regular/long-term; gender of partner(s); age of partner(s); type of sex practised – vaginal, oral, or anal sex; STI information and any past history of STI.
- Family history of any significant medical problems (e.g., heart disease, diabetes, VTE).
- Social history – do they go to school or work? Who lives at home? Any problems at home? Whether the partner or parents know about her visit. Any problems at school/college/work? Preferences for contraception. How well can she remember pills? Any problems in the past with using a particular contraceptive? How to access condoms and use them, etc.

Consultation – to improve compliance

- In women aged < 20 years – contraceptive failure rate is 16% in the first 12 months of use, compared with a rate of 8% in married women aged ≥ 30 years.
- LARC methods are less user-dependent, have lower failure rates with typical use, and are more cost-effective than COC or condoms if used for 1 year or longer.
- Discontinuation of methods may also be a factor in unintended pregnancies. Side effects (perceived or experienced) are often cited as the reason for method discontinuation.

Aim to maximize a young person's compliance:

- Provide a wide and appropriate choice of methods, dealing with specific health concerns, discussing specific health benefits, and providing appropriate follow-up.
- Develop rapport and create a safe and comfortable environment during the consultation.
- Be friendly and non-judgemental. • Allow as much time in the consultation as they need.
- Maintain confidentiality.
- Avoid making assumptions about reason for visit; sexual behaviour, sexual orientation, risk or capacity based on age, gender, or disability.
- Avoid appearing to moralize about sex, sexuality, and contraceptive choice, and be aware of cultural and sexual diversity.
- When accompanied by an adult, see the young person alone if possible.

Starting HC in young people

- Do not use regular HC prior to menarche. Advise condoms in young people requiring contraception before this time.
- POEC can be given to pre-menarchal women if required.
- 'Quick starting' may be appropriate as waiting may result in the individual never starting the method, because of waning enthusiasm or the inconvenience of rescheduling an appointment.
- Categories for each method in relation to age – see Chapter 57.
- There are no restrictions on using any of the methods based on nulliparity alone.
- Age alone should not limit contraceptive choices, including intrauterine methods.

Emergency contraception

- Use of EC is common in those aged < 30 years. EC may be influenced by factors such as perceived pregnancy risk, personal and perceived attitudes towards EC, and confidence in asking for it.
- POEC can be given if there is likely to be a delay between the initial consultation and IUD insertion.
- Offer all women Cu-IUD even if they present for EC within 72 hours of UPSI.

STIs

- Young people account for 65% of chlamydia, 55% of genital warts, and 50% of gonorrhoea cases diagnosed in UK GUM clinics.
- Advise on correct and consistent use of condoms to reduce the risk of STIs.
- Offer chlamydia testing for sexually active young people aged < 25 years. Encourage them to have regular STI testing, particularly when there has been a new sexual partner.
- UPSI – offer STI screening and repeat screening 12 weeks later to detect any recently acquired infection, as antibodies to HIV and syphilis may take up to 12 weeks to be detected.
- High-risk sexual exposure or assault – consider HIV post-exposure prophylaxis.

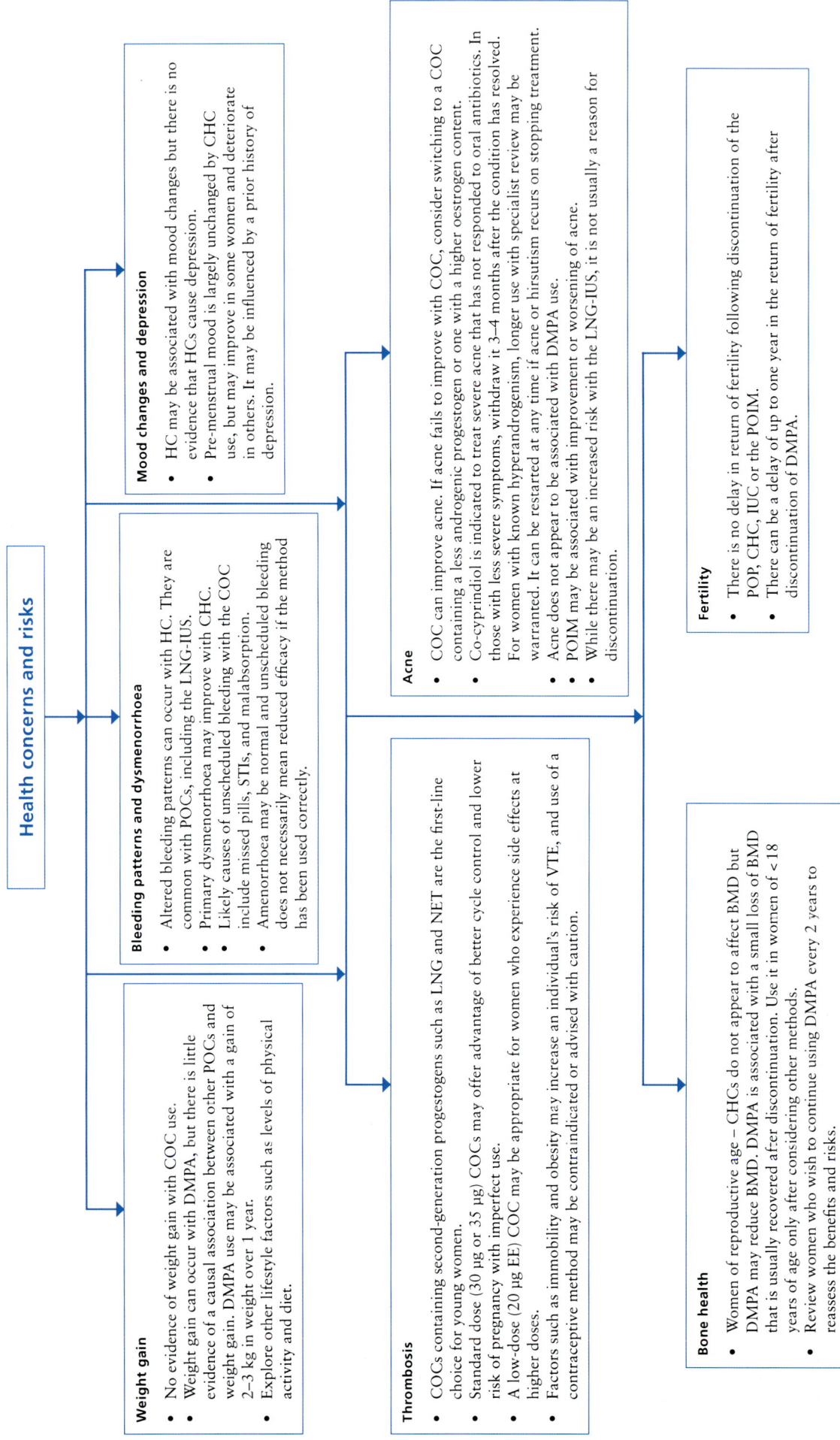

Health concerns and risks

Weight gain

- No evidence of weight gain with COC use.
- Weight gain can occur with DMPA, but there is little evidence of a causal association between other POCs and weight gain. DMPA use may be associated with a gain of 2–3 kg in weight over 1 year.
- Explore other lifestyle factors such as levels of physical activity and diet.

Bleeding patterns and dysmenorrhoea

- Altered bleeding patterns can occur with HC. They are common with POCs, including the LNG-IUS.
- Primary dysmenorrhoea may improve with CHC.
- Likely causes of unscheduled bleeding with the COC include missed pills, STIs, and malabsorption.
- Amenorrhoea may be normal and unscheduled bleeding does not necessarily mean reduced efficacy if the method has been used correctly.

Mood changes and depression

- HC may be associated with mood changes but there is no evidence that HCs cause depression.
- Pre-menstrual mood is largely unchanged by CHC use, but may improve in some women and deteriorate in others. It may be influenced by a prior history of depression.

Thrombosis

- COGs containing second-generation progestogens such as LNG and NET are the first-line choice for young women.
- Standard dose (30 μg or 35 μg) COCs may offer advantage of better cycle control and lower risk of pregnancy with imperfect use.
- A low-dose (20 μg EE) COC may be appropriate for women who experience side effects at higher doses.
- Factors such as immobility and obesity may increase an individual's risk of VTE, and use of a contraceptive method may be contraindicated or advised with caution.

Acne

- COC can improve acne. If acne fails to improve with COC, consider switching to a COC containing a less androgenic progestogen or one with a higher oestrogen content.
- Co-cyprindiol is indicated to treat severe acne that has not responded to oral antibiotics. In those with less severe symptoms, withdraw it 3–4 months after the condition has resolved. For women with known hyperandrogenism, longer use with specialist review may be warranted. It can be restarted at any time if acne or hirsutism recurs on stopping treatment.
- Acne does not appear to be associated with DMPA use.
- POIM may be associated with improvement or worsening of acne.
- While there may be an increased risk with the LNG-IUS, it is not usually a reason for discontinuation.

Bone health

- Women of reproductive age – CHCs do not appear to affect BMD but DMPA may reduce BMD. DMPA is associated with a small loss of BMD that is usually recovered after discontinuation. Use it in women of <18 years of age only after considering other methods.
- Review women who wish to continue using DMPA every 2 years to reassess the benefits and risks.

Fertility

- There is no delay in return of fertility following discontinuation of the POP, CHC, IUC or the POIM.
- There can be a delay of up to one year in the return of fertility after discontinuation of DMPA.

1. *Contraceptive Choices for Young People.* Faculty of Sexual and Reproductive Healthcare CEU, March 2010.

History and assessment

- Take sexual and reproductive history to assess the risk of STIs and sexual function.
- Take medical history as medical conditions are more common in this age group and could impact on contraceptive choice.
- Assess social factors such as frequency of intercourse, natural decline in fertility, sexual problems, wish for non-contraceptive benefits, menstrual dysfunction, etc.
- Smoking and BMI.
- Age – see Chapter 57 and table below.

Background – sexual and reproductive health in women aged over 40 years

- Fertility – although a natural decline in fertility occurs from the mid-30s, effective contraception is required to prevent an unintended pregnancy.
- Change of partner – average age for men and women to get divorced in the UK is 44 and 41 years, respectively. Many individuals in their 40s may therefore enter new relationships. There has also been a rise in the number of STIs diagnosed in > 40 year olds.
- Pregnancy – there is an increasing trend in the UK for women to have children later in life. The greatest increase in birth rate is seen in women aged ≥ 40 years, with the numbers nearly doubled from 1998 to 2008. At the same time, women in their 40s also experience unintended pregnancies. The rate of TOP in women aged 40–44 years is 4/1000 in the UK, which is almost equivalent to the rates for young women aged <16 years.
- Risks of pregnancy – see Obstetrics: evidence-based algorithms.
- Transition to menopause – women in their 40s and 50s move from normal ovulatory menstrual cycles to the cessation of ovulation and menstruation. During this time, intermittent ovulation occurs, resulting in irregular menstrual cycles.

Options

- None of the contraceptive options is contraindicated based on age alone.
- 4 most commonly used methods are sterilization (male or female), the pill, male condoms, and intrauterine methods.

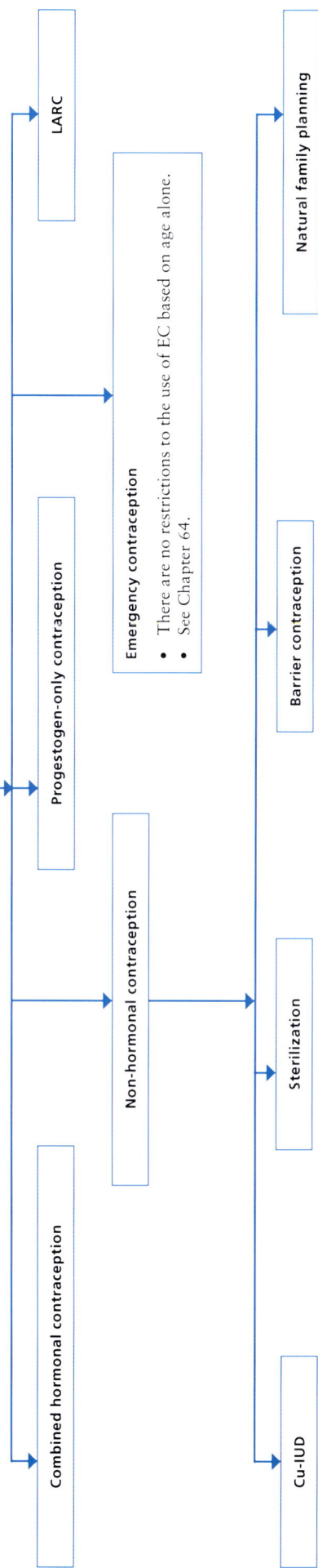

Combined hormonal contraception

Progestogen-only contraception

LARC

Non-hormonal contraception

Emergency contraception

- There are no restrictions to the use of EC based on age alone.
- See Chapter 64.

Barrier contraception

Natural family planning

Sterilization

Cu-IUD

Options: CHC – health benefits and risks associated with CHC use

Bone health – CHC in the peri-menopause may help to maintain BMD.

Dysmenorrhoea and cycle control, menopausal symptoms:

- CHC can provide cycle regularity, improve primary dysmenorrhoea, or reduce menstrual blood loss.
- CHC may improve some of the symptoms associated with menopause. Women experiencing menopausal symptoms while using CHC may try an extended regimen.

Ovarian cancer and endometrial cancer:

- CHC provides protection against ovarian cyst, ovarian cancer, and endometrial cancer.
- Risk of breast cancer increases with increasing age. There is no clear evidence as to the risk of breast cancer with use of CHC.

Cardiovascular and cerebrovascular disease:

- Morbidity and mortality from VTE, MI, or stroke are rare but the risk increases with age. Overall the absolute risks are small and women who have used oral contraceptives have no higher risk of mortality than those who have never used them.

  MI and stroke – risk is influenced by smoking, HT, and migraine with aura.
  Smoking – a very small increase in the risk of MI in smokers.

- As both smoking and age are independent risk factors, greater restrictions are placed on the use of CHC methods depending on the number of cigarettes smoked and age (see Chapter 57).

- After smoking cessation, risk of MI associated with smoking reduces with time, and therefore for former smokers aged > 35 years, the use of CHC becomes less restrictive. (UKMEC 2)

  HT – hypertensive individuals who use CHC are at higher risk of stroke and acute MI but not VTE compared to hypertensive non-CHC users. **Even for women with adequately controlled HT, alternative methods are preferable to CHC. (UKMEC 3)**

  Migraine – risk of stroke is increased in CHC users with migraine compared to CHC users without migraine. Risk of stroke affects those with migraine with aura and CHC use further increases the risk of ischaemic stroke. **CHC methods represent an unacceptable health risk in presence of migraine with aura.** (UKMEC 4)

VTE:

- The relative risk of VTE is increased with use of CHC. Reducing the dose of oestrogen from 30 μg to 20 μg may reduce the risk of VTE.

Prescribing CHC methods to women aged over 40 years:

- First choice of pill is the one containing the lowest dose of EE that provides adequate cycle control, i.e., pill with < 30 μg EE.
- In women who are aged ≥ 35 years and smoke, risks outweigh benefits.
- There may be a very small increased risk of ischaemic stroke with CHC.
- Advise women with cardiovascular disease, stroke, or migraine with aura against the use of CHC.
- HT may increase the risk of stroke and MI. Check BP before and at least 6 months and monitor at least annually thereafter.

Options (contd.)

LARCs

- Failure rates are lower than shorter-acting methods and are more cost effective.
- There is no delay in return of fertility with LARCs other than with the POICs, which can be delayed for up to 1 year after discontinuation. This may be unacceptable to those women who still wish to conceive, given the rapid decline in background fertility in this age group.
- LARC (POIM and the IUS) can be as effective as sterilization and offer a reliable, reversible alternative for women who do not want to be sterilized or for whom sterilization is not advised.

POCs – health benefits and risks associated with POC

HMB:

- POCs may be useful in the management of HMB and irregular bleeding because of the associated amenorrhoea.
- LNG-IUS is an option for HMB, which is particularly common in women aged > 40 years.

Bone health:

- The POIC DMPA is associated with a small loss of BMD, which usually recovers after discontinuation. For women aged > 40 years, there is some reassuring evidence from small studies to support DMPA use in women approaching menopause.
- Women aged > 45 years – DMPA is UKMEC Category 2. DMPA can be used until maximum recommended age of 50 years, provided a re-evaluation of the risks and benefits of treatment for all women is carried out every 2 years in those who wish to continue use.
- Consider alternative methods of contraception for women with significant lifestyle and/or medical risk factors for osteoporosis.
- There is no evidence of a clinically significant effect of other POCs on BMD.

Cardiovascular and cerebrovascular disease – be cautious when prescribing DMPA to women with cardiovascular risk factors because of the effects of progestogens on lipids.

Non-hormonal methods

Cu-IUD – menstrual bleeding problems are common in women aged > 40 years and also common in users of intrauterine methods. Spotting, heavier or longer periods, and pain are common in the first 3–6 months following Cu-IUD insertion. These bleeding patterns are not harmful and usually settle with time; however, advise women to seek medical help to exclude gynaecological pathology and infection if the bleeding problems persist or occur as new events.

Sterilization – inform about the lower failure rate and lower risk of major complications associated with vasectomy compared to laparoscopic tubal occlusion.

Barrier contraception – there is no restriction on the use of barrier methods based on age alone.

Natural family planning – when approaching the menopause, natural family planning may become more difficult owing to menstrual cycle irregularity and the increase of anovulatory cycles making it difficult to interpret ovulatory mucus.

Withdrawal – although not promoted as a method of contraception, coitus interruptus is reported by approximately 6–8% of women aged 40–49 years. Withdrawal, if used correctly (i.e., withdrawal before ejaculation every time), may work for some couples, particularly as a backup to other methods. However, it may be less effective than other methods of contraception.

Stopping contraception

Non-hormonal methods

- Can stop non-HC 1 year after the LMP in those aged > 50 years, and 2 years after the LMP in those aged < 50 years. The probability of menstruation (and ovulation) after a year of amenorrhoea for women aged > 45 years is estimated to be 2–10%.
- Women who have a Cu-IUD containing ≥ 300 mm² Cu, inserted at ≥ 40 years, can retain the device until the menopause or until contraception is no longer required.
- Remove IUD once contraception is no longer required.

LNG-IUS

- > 75% of women will have amenorrhoea or light bleeding in spite of ovulation.
- Women with LNG-IUS inserted at the age of ≥ 45 years and who are using the LNG-IUS solely for HMB can continue until the menopause.
- Women with LNG-IUS inserted for contraception at the age of ≥ 45 years can use the device for 7 years (off licence) or if amenorrhoeic until the menopause, after which remove the device.
- Discuss the risks of pregnancy over the age of 50 years, and the risks of removal and replacement. If bleeding/spotting occurs, this indicates ovarian follicular activity, in which case remove and replace the device or provide alternative contraception.

Hormonal methods

- In women using exogenous hormones, amenorrhoea is not a reliable indicator of ovarian failure. FSH is not a reliable indicator of ovarian failure in women using combined hormones, even if measured during the HFI. FSH levels may be used to help diagnose menopause, in women > 50 years using POCs. Women > 50 years who are amenorrhoeic and wish to stop POC – check FSH levels. If the level is ≥ 30 IU/L, repeat FSH after 6 weeks. If the second FSH level is ≥ 30 IU/L, contraception can be stopped after 1 year.

- In general, contraception may be stopped at the age of 55 years; however, tailor to the individual woman. Advise women who are not using HC and continue to have regular menstrual bleeding at the age of 55 years to continue with some form of contraception.
- Women > 50 years – do not use CHC or the POIC beyond the age of 50 years. Switch to an alternative method such as the POP, POIM, LNG-IUS, or barrier method until the age of 55 years or until the menopause can be confirmed.

Method	Age < 50 years	Age ≥ 50 years
CHC	Can continue up to age 50 years.	Stop at age 50 years and switch to a non-hormonal method or POCs (except DMPA).
Non-hormonal	After 2 years of amenorrhoea.	After 1 year of amenorrhoea.
DMPA	Can continue up to age 50 years.	Stop DMPA at age 50 years and switch to: • A non-hormonal method and stop after 2 years of amenorrhoea. • Or the POP, implant, or LNG-IUS.

POP, implant, or LNG-IUS	Can continue to age 50 years or longer.	Continue method:
		 • If amenorrhoeic.
		   * Check FSH levels and stop method after 1 year if serum FSH is ≥ 30 IU/L on two occasions, 6 weeks apart.
		   * Or stop at age 55 years when natural loss of fertility can be assumed for most women.
		 • If not amenorrhoeic, consider investigating any abnormal bleeding or changes in bleeding pattern, and continue contraception beyond age 55 years until amenorrhoeic for 1 year.

Follow-up

- Advise women to seek medical help:
  - * If any problems with their contraception.
  - * Or change in medical history that may influence contraceptive choice.
  - * Or when they reach 50 years of age.
  - * If new symptoms of pain, irregular or heavy bleeding.
  - * If bleeding problems do not settle within 3–6 months of IUD/IUS insertion.
- After the menopause, remove the intrauterine methods as cases of actinomyces-like organisms and pyometra have very occasionally been reported in postmenopausal women with IUDs.

HRT and contraception

- Advise women using HRT not to rely on this as contraception.
- POP can be used with HRT to provide effective contraception, but the HRT must include progestogen in addition to oestrogen.
- Women using oestrogen replacement therapy may use the LNG-IUS to provide endometrial protection. When used as the progestogen component of HRT, change the LNG-IUS no later than 5 years after insertion (the licence states 4 years), irrespective of age at insertion.

1. *Contraception for Women Aged Over 40 Years.* Faculty of Sexual and Reproductive Healthcare CEU Guidance, July 2010.

CHAPTER 63 Postnatal contraception

Background – postnatal fertility

- There is a wide variation in the time from delivery to resumption of sexual activity.
- Although return of menstruation is often the first sign of fertility, waiting for the first menstrual period before starting contraception may put some women at risk of pregnancy.
- Within 30 days of delivery, placental sex steroid levels decrease and gonadotrophins increase, stimulating ovarian activity.
- Breastfeeding women:
  - * Suckling disrupts the frequency and amplitude of gonadotrophin pulses and despite ovarian follicular activity, ovulation is suppressed.
  - * Ovulation returns when the frequency and duration of suckling episodes decrease.
  - * Menstruation occurs on average 28 weeks and ovulation 34 weeks after delivery.
- Prior to day 21 postpartum, no contraception is required.
- Non-breastfeeding women – ovulation may occur as early as day 28. As sperm can survive for up to 7 days in the female genital tract, contraception is required from day 21 onwards.
- Women who are fully breastfeeding may wish to rely on the lactational amenorrhoea method (LAM) alone. Women who are breastfeeding and wish to avoid pregnancy should use contraception. As fertility is reduced, any contraceptive method will be more effective.

- **See Chapter 57**: categories for methods that are applicable to breastfeeding and non-breastfeeding women.
- If starting an HC on or before day 21, there is no need for additional contraception.
- If starting an HC after day 21, make sure that the woman is not pregnant or at risk of pregnancy, and advise to avoid sex or use additional contraception for the first 7 days of use (2 days for POP), unless fully meeting LAM criteria.
- LARC methods are less user-dependent, provide the best protection against pregnancy, and may be more cost-effective.
- With regard to contraceptive choices for obese women, only CHC and sterilization are associated with potential risks.

Emergency contraception

- Both the Cu-IUD and POEC can be used. POEC can be used from day 21 onwards and the emergency Cu-IUD from day 28 onwards.
- As the earliest date of ovulation is predicted to be day 28, if UPSI occurs on days 21–27, the Cu-IUD can be used from day 28 until day 33 (i.e., 5 days after the earliest expected ovulation). Cu-IUD inserted for EC can be retained until the next menstrual period or it can be retained for ongoing contraception.
- UPSI or contraceptive failure before day 21 postpartum is not an indication for EC.

Starting contraception – assess

- Contraceptive needs (e.g., degree of efficacy required); sexual activity and function; woman's own beliefs, attitudes, and personal preferences; cultural practices that may impact on choice of method; whether a woman is breastfeeding; whether ovulation is likely to have resumed; whether there is any possibility of pregnancy.
- Social factors (e.g., return to work, ability to access services).
- Medical history (e.g., HT, migraine, VTE, obesity, HIV, cholestasis, GTN).
- Risk of STIs.

Provision of contraceptive advice

- Delaying future pregnancies may be beneficial as short inter-pregnancy intervals are associated with increased risk of poor perinatal outcome and risks to maternal health.
- Discuss contraception within the first week of delivery. (NICE)
- Postpartum contraception advice may be better delivered antenatally.
- Women who have required fertility treatment in the past are not necessarily infertile and may now require contraception.
- Risk of STIs – offer condoms to reduce STI either alone or as backup to other contraceptive methods.

Natural methods

- Fertility awareness-based methods – in breastfeeding women, delay the use of fertility awareness-based methods if the woman is < 6 weeks postpartum. From 6 weeks onwards, advise caution even if menses have begun.
- Lactational amenorrhoea method (LAM) – breastfeeding provides protection against unintended pregnancy. It can be started straight away.
- LAM is > 98% effective if: woman is amenorrhoeic, < 6 months postpartum, fully breastfeeding with no long intervals between feeds day or night (e.g., > 4 hours during day and > 6 hours at night).
- Risk of pregnancy is increased if the frequency of breastfeeding decreases (stopping night feeds, supplementary feeding, use of pacifiers), when menstruation returns or when > 6 months postpartum.

Contraceptive options – hormonal

CHC

- Not recommended before day 21 owing to the increased risk of VTE.
- Non-breastfeeding women may start CHC from day 21 postpartum.
- Breastfeeding women – avoid CHC in the first 6 weeks postpartum as there is insufficient evidence on safety of CHC while establishing breastfeeding.
- Contraceptive hormones are excreted in breast milk in very small amounts, and there is concern about their potential impact on infant growth and development. However, HC including COC do not appear to affect infant development adversely.
- Insufficient evidence on whether CHC affects breast milk volume.
- CHC between 6 weeks and 6 months is not recommended unless other methods are not acceptable or available. In partially breastfeeding women, the benefits of CHC may outweigh the risks.

POCs

No adverse effects on breastfeeding, infant growth, or development have been shown with POP, DMPA, Implanon, LNG-IUS, or the Cu-IUD.

POP

- Postpartum women (breastfeeding and non-breastfeeding) can start the POP at any time postpartum.
- If starting POP after day 21, advise additional contraception for the first 48 hours.
- Women wishing to move from LAM to an HC – no additional contraception is required in the first week of starting a POC as long as the conditions for LAM are still being met during this first week.

POIC

- Non-breastfeeding women – can start a POIC at any time postpartum.
- Breastfeeding women – do not start a POIC before day 21 unless the risk of subsequent pregnancy is high.
- Breastfeeding women – use of DMPA < 6 weeks postpartum is outside the product licence.
- Troublesome bleeding can occur with use of DMPA in the early puerperium.

POIM

- Implanon – insert between 21 and 28 days after delivery; it can be used during lactation.
- Women can choose POIM before day 21, although this is outside the product licence. There is no evidence to suggest that Implanon is more likely to cause bleeding when inserted at this time, but advise women to report bleeding problems so that other causes can be excluded.

LNG-IUS

- LNG-IUS – insert from day 28 postpartum.
- Advise women to avoid sex or use additional contraception for 7 days after insertion unless fully meeting LAM criteria.
- See intrauterine methods below.

Contraceptive options – non-hormonal

Intrauterine methods: Cu-IUD

- Immediate postpartum insertion is safe and effective, although expulsion rate may be higher.
- UKMEC – owing to increased risk of perforation, delay insertion until 4 weeks postpartum.
- Unless a Cu-IUD can be inserted within the first 48 hours postpartum, delay insertion until day 28 onwards.
- No additional contraception is required.

Barrier methods

- Condoms (male and female) can be used at any time postpartum. Even in the presence of another contraceptive method, advise correct and consistent use of condoms to protect against STIs.
- Diaphragms and caps are not recommended until 6 weeks postpartum when changes to the genital tract anatomy are complete and discomfort has usually resolved. A different size of diaphragm or cervical cap may be required. Another method of contraception should be used from day 21 until the woman is able to insert and remove a correctly fitted diaphragm or cap.

Sterilization

- Permanent method: inform about risks, benefits, failure rates, and other methods of contraception including LARC. Some LARC methods have failure rates comparable with female sterilization.
- There is no medical condition that would absolutely contraindicate sterilization, although precautions may be necessary in some cases.
- Vasectomy is associated with lower failure rate and lower risk of major complications compared to tubal occlusion.

1. *Postnatal Sexual and Reproductive Health*. Faculty of Sexual and Reproductive Healthcare, CEU, September 2009.

CHAPTER 64   Emergency contraception

Background and definition

- EC is a means of preventing unintended pregnancy following any UPSI. It is commonly supplied for 'off license' indications.
- Three methods available in the UK as EC:
  * Copper-bearing intrauterine device (Cu-IUD).
  * Levonorgestrel; progestogen-only emergency contraception (POEC).
  * Ulipristal acetate (UPA).
- 2002 judicial review concluded that pregnancy begins at implantation and not at fertilization. Explain the possible mechanisms of action to the patients as some methods may not be acceptable, depending on individual beliefs about the onset of pregnancy and abortion.
- Although EC has been shown to reduce the risk of pregnancy at an individual level, it has not shown to impact on overall unintended pregnancy or TOP rates in women with increased access (including advance provision) or at a population level. This may be because even with advance provision, women do not use EC on every occasion of UPSI and EC is used too infrequently by those women most at risk of pregnancy.

Determining a woman's precise risk of pregnancy

- This is complex as it depends on a number of factors including when ovulation is likely to have occurred, the fertility of both partners, and whether contraception has not been used or has been used incorrectly.
- In clinical practice, it is difficult to determine the precise timing of ovulation. The length of the luteal phase is relatively constant at 14 days. The follicular phase is more variable.
- Conception is most likely to occur following UPSI on the day of ovulation or in the preceding 24 hours. Owing to the natural variation in timing of ovulation, the timing of the 'fertile period' is highly variable, particularly among women with irregular cycles, and there are only a few days in the menstrual cycle when women are not theoretically at risk of pregnancy. The probability of pregnancy from a single act of UPSI in the first 3 days of the cycle appears to be negligible.

History for medical eligibility

- Consider the following factors when assessing a woman's need for EC:
  * Medical eligibility.
  * The most likely date of ovulation based on the date of the LMP and the usual cycle length.
  * Number and timing of all episodes of UPSI in the current cycle.
  * Previous EC use within current cycle.
  * Drug interactions – use of medications that may affect contraceptive efficacy.
  * Details of potential contraceptive failure (e.g., how many pills were missed and when).
  * Need for additional precautions/ongoing contraception.
  * Efficacy of method.
  * Individual choice.
- BMI: obese women (BMI > 30) using LNG are at greater risk of pregnancy compared with those with a normal or low BMI. While an increased risk is also noticed amongst UPA users, the difference is not statistically significant. More evidence is needed before specific recommendations can be made. Currently, all EC methods are recommended in obese women and it is not recommended to increase the dose of oral EC.

Investigations

- Pregnancy test – if a woman has been at risk earlier in the cycle, consider pregnancy test. A pregnancy test cannot reliably exclude pregnancy if there has been an episode of UPSI < 3 weeks previously.
- Prevalence of Chlamydia infection among women presenting for EC is up to 9% in women aged < 25 years. Offer STI testing including HIV. For women at risk of STIs, if test results are unavailable before IUD insertion, consider prophylactic antibiotics, at least to cover Chlamydia.

Indications for EC

UPSI or barrier failure during the time that additional contraceptive precaution is required

- When starting the hormonal methods of contraception.
- POIC – late injection (> 14 weeks since last injection of DMPA or > 10 weeks since NET-EN).

Missed pills – if UPSI or barrier failure

- COCs (other than Qlaira):
  - If ≥ 2 active pills are missed.
  - If the pills are missed in week 1.
- If the pill-free interval is extended – consider an emergency IUD up to 15 days after taking the 21st pill in the last packet, providing the preceding pills have been taken correctly.

POP – if UPSI or barrier failure

- Before efficacy has been re-established (i.e., 48 hours after restarting).
- Late or missed pill (> 27 hours since last traditional POP or > 36 hours since last desogestrel-only pill).
- Timing of ovulation after missed pills cannot be predicted accurately. An emergency IUD is therefore only recommended up to 5 days after UPSI.

Liver enzyme-inducing drugs

While on CHC, POP, and POIM:-

- UPSI, barrier failure, or failure to use additional contraception while using liver enzyme-inducing drugs or in the 28 days after use.
- EC – Cu-IUD or a double dose (3 mg) of LNG is recommended.
- UPA is not recommended.

Cu-IUD and LNG-IUS

- If UPSI has occurred in the 5 days prior to:
  - Removal without immediate replacement.
  - Partial or complete expulsion.
  - Threads missing, perforation, and IUD/IUS location unknown.
- Depending on the timing of UPSI and time since IUD known to be correctly placed, it may be appropriate to fit another IUD for EC.

Recommendations

- Cu-IUD can be inserted up to 120 hours after the first episode of UPSI or up to 5 days after the earliest expected date of ovulation, because of the low failure rate.
- UPA is effective up to 120 hours and can be offered to all eligible women during this period. It is the only oral EC licensed for use between 72 and 120 hours.
- The efficacy of LNG has been demonstrated up to 96 hours; its efficacy between 96 and 120 hours is unknown. Use of LNG beyond 72 hours is outside the product licence.
- Ideally, insert an emergency IUD at first presentation, but where this is not possible, provide oral EC in the interim.
- Consider advance supply of EC, but there is no evidence to support routine provision.

Method	Cu-IUD	LNG (POEC)	UPA
Class	Intrauterine contraceptive method	Progestogen hormone	Progesterone receptor modulator
Products	Various types licensed.	Levonelle One; Levonelle 1500 (prescription only).	ellaOne (prescription only).
Recommended dose/use	IUD retained until pregnancy excluded or for licensed duration (5–10 years).	1.5 mg single oral dose.	30 mg single oral dose.
Indications	Within the first 5 days (120 hours) following first UPSI in a cycle or within 5 days from the earliest estimated date of ovulation.	**Within 72 hours of UPSI or contraceptive failure:** • Efficacy of LNG has been demonstrated up to 72 hours after UPSI. There is uncertainty about its effectiveness thereafter. Risk of pregnancy on days 2, 3, and 4 after UPSI was not significantly different from that on day 1, suggesting that LNG is effective for up to 96 hours. • However, compared to day 1, LNG administered on day 5 increases the risk of pregnancy nearly 6-fold.	**Within 120 hours of UPSI or contraceptive failure:** • The efficacy of UPA has been demonstrated up to 120 hours after UPSI, with no apparent decline in efficacy within that period.
Effectiveness	Failure rate is < 1%.	Failure rate is 1.1%.	
Mechanism	**Primarily by inhibiting fertilization, but there is an anti-implantation effect as well.** • Copper is toxic to the ovum and sperm and the Cu-IUD is effective immediately after insertion and works primarily by inhibiting fertilization. If fertilization has already occurred, it may have an anti-implantation effect. • The mean time from ovulation to implantation is 9 (range 6–18) days. Therefore, to ensure that an IUD is inserted before the process of implantation begins, the Cu-IUD should be fitted within the first 5 days (120 hours) following first UPSI in a cycle or within 5 days from the earliest estimated date of ovulation.	**Precise mode of action is incompletely understood but it is thought to work primarily by inhibition of ovulation.** • It prevents follicular rupture or causes luteal dysfunction. LNG taken prior to the LH surge results in ovulatory dysfunction in the subsequent 5 days. It can thus inhibit ovulation for 5–7 days, by which time any sperm in the reproductive tract will have become non-viable. • LNG is no better than placebo at suppressing ovulation when given immediately prior to ovulation and is not effective once the process of fertilization has occurred. • LNG does not affect embryo–endometrial attachment.	**Primary mechanism of action is inhibition or delay of ovulation.** • If administered immediately before ovulation, UPA suppresses growth of lead follicles. • The contribution of the endometrial changes to the efficacy of UPA (e.g., by inhibiting implantation) is, as yet, unknown.

	Cu-IUD	LNG	UPA

Drug interactions	**No drug interactions.**
	• The efficacy of Cu-IUDs is unaffected by concomitant drug use.
		Double the dose with liver enzyme inducers.
		• Drugs that induce enzymes decrease the contraceptive efficacy of LNG, while using them and for 28 days afterwards. Women on liver enzyme-inducing drugs or who have stopped using them (≤ 28 days ago) who require EC – offer a Cu-IUD as the efficacy is not affected by drugs.
		• Women taking liver enzyme-inducing drugs (or who have stopped within the last 28 days), and who decline or are not eligible for a Cu-IUD – give a dose of 3 mg LNG (two Levonelle tablets) ASAP within 120 hours of UPSI. The efficacy of LNG after 96 hours is uncertain.
		• HIV – post-exposure prophylaxis after sexual exposure (PEPSE) and EC may be required simultaneously. It is recommended to use 3 mg LNG (two tablets) if a Cu-IUD is not available or not acceptable.
			Not recommended with liver enzyme inducers.
			• No interaction studies have been carried out to date. Not to use with liver enzyme-inducing drugs and for 28 days after these are stopped.
			• Not to be used concomitantly with drugs that increase gastric pH (e.g., antacids, histamine H2 antagonists, and proton pump inhibitors).
			• Do not double the dose of UPA.
			• As a progesterone receptor modulator, it blocks the action of progestogen and, therefore, could reduce the efficacy of contraceptives containing progestogen.
			• Additional precautions for 7 days in addition to:
			  * 7 days for starting HC (i.e., 14 days total).
			  * 2 days for the POP (i.e., 9 days if starting or continuing the POP).
			  * 9 days for Qlaira (i.e., 16 days for Qlaira).
			• Theoretically there is a risk that progestogen could also block the action of UPA but, to date, there is no evidence to support or refute this.

Side effects	• Pain – pain relief may facilitate insertion. Analgesics commonly used are NSAIDSs, topical lidocaine (Instillagel), and cervical local anaesthetic block.	• Nausea in 20% of women using LNG EC and vomiting in 1%. If a woman vomits within 2 hours of taking LNG, or within 3 hours of UPA – offer a repeat dose of the same method or a Cu-IUD. • Altered bleeding patterns – advise regarding menstrual disturbances after oral EC use. If there is any doubt about whether menstruation has occurred, perform a pregnancy test ≥ 3 weeks after UPSI. • It does not increase the chance of ectopic pregnancy. A previous ectopic pregnancy is not a contraindication. • Other side effects – headaches, abdominal pain, dysmenorrhoea, and dizziness.	
More than once in a cycle	NA	**Can be used.** • Giving repeated doses of LNG may be effective and further UPSI may be an indication for repeat LNG use. • Cochrane review – LNG used on a regular basis for pre- and post-coital contraception seemed reasonably efficacious and safe. • As there is no evidence to indicate that LNG is not safe in pregnancy, LNG can be used more than once in the same cycle or can be used for a recent episode of UPSI, even if there has been an earlier episode of UPSI outside the treatment window (> 120 hours). • No data regarding a minimum time interval between successive LNG treatments. However, if further UPSI occurs within 12 hours of a dose of LNG, further EC treatment is not required.	**Not recommended.** • It is not advised to use UPA more than once per cycle, or if there has been another episode of UPSI, outside the treatment window (> 120 hours). • There are limited data on its safety in pregnancy; therefore, where multiple episodes of UPSI have occurred and there is a risk that a woman may already be pregnant, its use is not advised. • If a Cu-IUD is declined or is inappropriate, LNG can be given for another episode of UPSI after administration of UPA. It is not known if UPA reduces the efficacy of LNG or how long after UPA administration any such interaction has an effect.

Future contraception	• May continue using the Cu-IUD for ongoing contraception. • If the woman does not require contraception or prefers another method, the Cu-IUD can be removed after pregnancy has been excluded, providing there has been no UPSI in the 7 days prior to removal, and guidance for switching methods is followed.	• These methods do not provide contraceptive cover for subsequent UPSI and women will need to use contraception or refrain from sex to avoid further risk of pregnancy. For options and additional contraceptive precautions, see Chapter 58.
Failure of EC	Should be managed as EC.	If a woman chooses to continue her pregnancy after exposure to UPA, this should be reported to the manufacturer of ellaOne for inclusion in the European register to monitor outcomes of exposure during pregnancy.

FOLLOW-UP

• Offer follow-up if women want a pregnancy test, STI screening, Cu-IUD removal, or they have any concerns or difficulties with their contraception.
• If a Cu-IUD is to be used as an ongoing contraceptive method, advise women to return for a follow-up visit after the first menses (or 3–6 weeks) after insertion.

Guideline comparator – SOGC recommendations

- Hormonal EC can be offered up to 5 days after UPSI.
- Two types of hormonal EC are available in Canada:
  * A regimen of 2 oral doses of 750 µg LNG taken 12 hours apart.
  * Yuzpe method – 2 doses of 100 µg of EE and 500 µg of LNG taken orally 12 hours apart. Ovral is the most commonly used product, with 2 tablets of Ovral being equivalent to 1 dose of the Yuzpe regimen.
- WHO – pregnancy rate of 1.1% with the LNG-only regimen, compared to 3.2% for the Yuzpe regimen.
- Hormonal EC – although they have generally been used only up to 72 hours after UPSI, the Yuzpe and LNG regimens have been shown to be effective when taken between 72 and 120 hours. The range of effectiveness seems to be slightly lower than before 72 hours.
- LNG prevented 95% of pregnancies for up to 24 hours, 85% for 25–48 hours, and 58% for 49–72 hours. Corresponding figures for the Yuzpe regimen were 77%, 36%, and 31%, respectively.
- The Yuzpe and LNG-only regimens reduce the risk of pregnancy by about 2.5% and 11%, respectively, but this does not mean that 2.5% of women using the Yuzpe regimen will become pregnant. Theoretically, if 100 women had UPSI once during the second or third week of their cycle, about 8 would become pregnant; following treatment with the Yuzpe regimen, only 2 would become pregnant, a reduction of 75%.
- A Cu-IUD can be used up to 7 days after UPSI.
- A meta-analysis – IUDs inserted within 5 days of UPSI are significantly more effective than hormonal EC, with an effectiveness rate of 98.7%.
- Use of a post-coital Cu-IUD between 5 and 7 days is less well studied; extending insertion of an IUD up to 7 days after UPSI may be acceptable if it falls within 5 days of the ovulation day.
- LNG EC regimen is more effective and causes fewer side effects than the Yuzpe regimen.
- Either 1 double dose of the LNG EC regimen (1.5 mg) or the regular 2-dose LNG regimen (0.75 mg each dose) may be used, as they have similar efficacy with no difference in side effects.
- The anti-progestin mifepristone (RU 486) has been shown to be a highly effective post-coital contraceptive, but this product is not currently available.
- Women of reproductive age should be provided with a prescription for hormonal EC in advance of need.

What not to do

- No need to increase the dose of oral EC in women with high BMI.
- UPA is contraindicated in:
  * Women with hypersensitivity to UPA or any of the other components and pregnancy.
  * Women with severe asthma insufficiently controlled by oral glucocorticoids.
- UPA – caution in women with hepatic dysfunction, hereditary problems of galactose intolerance, the Lapp lactase deficiency, or glucose–galactose malabsorption.
- UPA – breastfeeding is not recommended for up to 36 hours.
- UPA – current recommendations:
  * Not to use with liver enzyme-inducing drugs and for 28 days after these are stopped.
  * Not to be used concomitantly with drugs that increase gastric pH (e.g., antacids, histamine H2 antagonists, and proton pump inhibitors).
- Do not double the dose of UPA.
- POEC – if further UPSI occurs within 12 hours of a dose of LNG, further EC treatment is not required.
- Do not use UPA more than once in a cycle or concomitantly with LNG.
- Do not use UPA more than once per cycle or if there has been another episode of UPSI outside the treatment window (> 120 hours).
- Do not insert the LNG-IUS following administration of EC, and offer an alternative 'bridging' method until pregnancy can be excluded.

1. *Emergency Contraception (EC)*. Faculty of Sexual and Reproductive Healthcare Guidance, August 2011.
2. *Emergency Contraception*. SOGC Clinical Practice Guidelines No. 131, August 2003.

CHAPTER 65   Long-acting reversible contraception (LARC)

History and assessment

- Take history on menstrual, contraceptive, sexual, medical, and family history.
- Exclude pregnancy. • Assess risk for STIs.
- Provide information on: * Contraceptive efficacy.   * Duration of use.   * Risks and possible side effects.   * Non-contraceptive benefits.   * Procedure for initiation and removal/discontinuation.   * When to seek help while using the method.

Prevalence and background

- Contraceptive methods that require administration less than once per cycle or month.
  * Cu-IUD and progestogen-only methods (IUS, injectables, and the implants).
- About 8% of women aged 16–49 years in UK use LARC as a method of contraception.
- LARC's effectiveness does not depend on daily compliance.
- LARC methods are more cost effective than the COCs.
- IUDs, IUS, and implants are more cost effective than the injectable contraceptives.

Progestogen-only injectable contraceptives DMPA, NET-EN

Contraceptive efficacy and effect on periods

- POICs act primarily by preventing ovulation. Pregnancy rate is < 4/1000.
- Pregnancy rate with DMPA is lower than that with NET-EN.
- Repeat DMPA every 12 weeks and NET-EN every 8 weeks.
- There could be a delay of up to 1 year in the return of fertility after stopping POICs.
- Amenorrhoea is likely; this is more likely with DMPA than NET-EN; is more likely as time goes by, and is not harmful.
- Up to 50% of women stop using DMPA by 1 year. The most common reason for discontinuation being altered bleeding pattern, including persistent bleeding.

Practical details of giving POICs

- Give POICs by deep IM injection into the gluteal or deltoid muscle or the lateral thigh.
- Start POICs (provided that it is reasonably certain that the woman is not pregnant):
  * Up to and including 5th day of the menstrual cycle (no need for additional contraception).
  * At any other time in the menstrual cycle with an additional barrier contraception for the first 7 days after the injection.
  * Immediately after first or second-trimester abortion, or at any time thereafter.
  * At any time postpartum.

Follow-up and managing problems

- Repeat injection can be given to women attending up to 2 weeks late for repeat injection, without the need for additional contraceptives.
- Persistent bleeding associated with DMPA – treat with mefenamic acid or ethinyl oestradiol.
- Women who wish to continue DMPA use beyond 2 years – review and discuss the balance between the benefits and potential risks.
- Pregnancy during DMPA use – there is no evidence of congenital malformation to the fetus.

Risks and possible side effects

- DMPA may be associated with an increase of up to 2–3 kg in weight over 1 year.
- DMPA is not associated with acne, depression, or headaches.
- DMPA is associated with a small loss of BMD, which is largely recovered on discontinuation. There is no evidence that DMPA increases the risk of fracture.

Specific groups, medical conditions, and contraindications for POICs

- Owing to the possible effect on BMD, be cautious with the use of DMPA in:
  * Adolescents.
  * Women > 40 years.
  * However, the benefits outweigh the risks in the above groups, and it may be given if other methods are not suitable or acceptable.
- Women with a BMI > 30 can safely use DMPA and NET-EN.
- Women who are breastfeeding can use POICs.
- All progestogen-only methods may be used by women who have migraine with or without aura.
- DMPA is safe for women if oestrogen is contraindicated.
- Not contraindicated in women with diabetes.
- DMPA may be associated with a reduction in the frequency of seizures in women with epilepsy.
- DMPA is safe and effective in women with STIs, including HIV/AIDS.
- Women taking liver enzyme-inducing medication may use DMPA and the dose interval does not need to be reduced.

Progestogen-only subdermal implants

Implanon

Contraceptive efficacy and effect on periods

- Implanon acts by preventing ovulation.
- Pregnancy rate with Implanon is < 1/1000 over 3 years.
- Implanon has UK Marketing Authorisation for use for 3 years.
- No evidence of a delay in the return of fertility following removal of implants.
- Bleeding patterns – 20% of women will have no bleeding, while 50% will have infrequent, frequent, or prolonged bleeding. Bleeding patterns are likely to remain irregular over time.
- Dysmenorrhoea may be reduced with the use of Implanon.

Practical details of giving POIMs

- Insert Implanon (provided that it is reasonably certain that the woman is not pregnant):
  * At any time (but if the woman is amenorrhoeic or it has been more than 5 days since menstrual bleeding started, advise additional barrier contraception for first 7 days after insertion).
  * Immediately after abortion in any trimester.
  * At any time postpartum.
- Implanon insertion and removal both cause some discomfort and bruising but technical problems are unusual (< 1/100).

Follow-up and managing problems

- No routine follow-up is needed after implant insertion.
- Irregular bleeding associated with implant – treat with mefenamic acid or ethinyl oestradiol.
- There is no evidence of a teratogenic effect of Implanon use but if a woman becomes pregnant and continues with the pregnancy, remove the implant.
- If an Implanon implant cannot be palpated (due to deep insertion, failed insertion, or migration) – localize by ultrasound scan for removal. Refer to an expert for deeply inserted implants.

Risks and possible side effects

- Up to 43% of women stop using Implanon within 3 years; 33% of women stop because of irregular bleeding and < 10% of women stop for other reasons including hormonal (non-bleeding) problems.
- Implanon use is not associated with changes in weight, mood, libido, or headaches.
- Implanon use may be associated with acne.

Specific groups, medical conditions, and contraindications for POIMs

- No evidence that the effectiveness or adverse effects of implants vary with age.
- Women > 70 kg can use Implanon as an effective method of contraception.
- Contraceptive implants can safely be used by women who are breastfeeding.
- Implanon use is not contraindicated in women with diabetes.
- Implanon is safe and effective in women with STI, including HIV/AIDS.
- All progestogen-only methods, including contraceptive implants, may be used by women who have migraine with or without aura.
- Implants are medically safe for women to use if oestrogen is contraindicated.
- There is no evidence of an effect of Implanon use on BMD.
- Implanon is not recommended as a contraceptive method for women taking liver enzyme-inducing drugs.

IUD and IUS

Contraceptive efficacy

- IUDs – act by preventing fertilization and inhibiting implantation. Licensed duration of use for IUDs (380 mm^2 Cu) is 5–10 years, depending on the type of device. Pregnancy rate with IUDs (380 mm^2 Cu) is < 20/1000 over 5 years. Up to 50% of women stop using IUDs within 5 years; the most common reasons being unacceptable vaginal bleeding and pain.
- IUS – acts mainly by preventing implantation and sometimes by preventing fertilization. Licensed duration of use for IUS is 5 years for contraception. Pregnancy rate – < 10/1000 over 5 years. Up to 60% of women stop using the IUS within 5 years. The most common reasons are unacceptable vaginal bleeding and pain; a less common reason is hormonal problems.
- No evidence of a delay in the return of fertility following removal of IUDs/IUS.

Before fitting an IUD/IUS

- Test for:
  * Chlamydia trachomatis in women at risk of STIs.
  * Neisseria gonorrhoeae in women from areas where the disease is prevalent and who are at risk of STIs.
  * Any STIs in women who request it.
- If testing for STIs is not possible, or has not been completed, give prophylactic antibiotics to women at increased risks of STIs.
- Insert IUS/IUD (provided that it is reasonably certain that the woman is not pregnant):
  * At any time during the menstrual cycle.
  * IUS – if the woman is amenorrhoeic or it has been > 5 days since menstrual bleeding started; advise additional barrier contraception for the first 7 days after insertion.
  * Immediately after first or second-trimester abortion, or at any time thereafter.
  * From 4 weeks postpartum, irrespective of the mode of delivery.

Advice for women at time of fitting

- Inform women:
  * Symptoms of uterine perforation or infection that would warrant an early review.
  * Insertion may cause pain and discomfort for a few hours and light bleeding for a few days.
  * How to check for the presence of IUD/IUS threads and encourage to do this regularly with the aim of recognizing expulsion.
- Women who are aged ≥ 45 years at the time of IUS insertion and who are amenorrhoeic may retain the device until they no longer require contraception, even if this is beyond the duration of UK Marketing Authorisation.
- Women who are aged ≥ 40 years at the time of IUD insertion may retain the device until they no longer require contraception, even if this is beyond the duration of the UK Marketing Authorisation.

Risks and possible side effects

- IUD – heavier bleeding and/or dysmenorrhoea.
- IUS – irregular bleeding and spotting are common during the first 6 months. Oligomenorrhoea or amenorrhoea is likely by the end of the first year.
- There is no evidence that IUD/IUS use affects weight.
- Changes in mood and libido are small and similar with IUDs and IUS.
- Risks:
  * Uterine perforation at the time of insertion: < 1/1000.
  * PID following insertion: < 1/100 in women who are at low risk of STIs.
  * Expulsion: < 1/20 women in 5 years.
  * Ectopic pregnancy when using IUDs/IUS is lower than when using no contraception.
- Risk of ectopic pregnancy when using the IUD/IUS is 1/1000 in 5 years. If a woman becomes pregnant with the IUD/IUS *in situ*, the risk of ectopic pregnancy is 1/20.
- IUS – there may be an increased likelihood of developing acne as a result of absorption of progestogen, but only a few women discontinue IUS use for this reason.

Specific groups, medical conditions, and contraindications for IUD and IUS

- May be used by adolescents, but consider STI risk where relevant.
- Not contraindicated in nulliparous women of any age.
- Women of all ages can use them.
- Can be used by women who are breastfeeding and by women with a history of VTE.
- Not contraindicated in women with diabetes.
- Can be safely used in women who are HIV-positive or have AIDS. Effectiveness of the IUS is not reduced when taking any other medication.
- All progestogen-only methods, including the IUS, may be used by women who have migraine with or without aura.
- IUS is medically safe for women to use if oestrogen is contraindicated.

Follow-up and managing problems

- Follow-up the women after the first menses, or 3–6 weeks after insertion, to exclude infection, perforation, or expulsion.
- Heavier and/or prolonged bleeding associated with IUD – treat with NSAIDs and tranexamic acid. Consider changing to IUS in women who find heavy bleeding associated with IUD use unacceptable.
- Presence of actinomyces-like organisms on a cervical smear in a woman with a current IUD – assess to exclude pelvic infection. Do not remove IUD routinely, in women without signs of pelvic infection.
- Women who have an intrauterine pregnancy with an IUD *in situ* – remove IUD before 12 weeks of completed gestation, whether or not they intend to continue the pregnancy.

Continuous and extended hormonal contraception (SOGC)

Background and definition

- Extended use refers to the use of COCs with planned hormone-free intervals (HFI) (from two contiguous cycles), and continuous use refers to uninterrupted use without HFIs.
- A number of COCs have been studied using a range of continuous or extended (CECOC) regimens. The length of the CECOC regimen can be altered, depending on the side effects.
- All currently available 50 μg EE contraceptives (oral [monophasic or multiphasic], transdermal, vaginal) can be used in a CECOC regimen.
- A 3-day HFI can be considered. After a 3-day HFI, if the woman uses COCs, she must take the next pill of her pack; if the woman uses the patch or the ring, she must use a new patch or a new ring.
- CECOCs regimens are as effective as cyclic regimens in preventing pregnancy.
- In COCs users, frequent lack of compliance may lead to increased failure. Use of CECOCs may be more 'forgiving' about missed pills because of the absence of a cyclical HFI.

Medical/non-contraceptive usage

- A CECOC regimen compared with a cyclical regimen results in fewer total bleeding days.
- Endometriosis – CECOCs administered for 6 months are effective in reducing the frequency and the intensity of dysmenorrhoea, deep dyspareunia, and non-menstrual pelvic pain.
- Women with HMB, including bleeding related to uterine fibroids, may benefit from menstrual suppression with CECOC regimens.
- Women with haemorrhagic diatheses may consider CECOC regimens in order to decrease monthly withdrawal bleeding.
- Menstrual migraine and headaches may improve with CECOC regimens.
- Women experiencing hormonal withdrawal symptoms such as nausea, vomiting, breast tenderness, bloating, swelling, and mood changes during the HFIs while using cyclical COCs may benefit from CECOC regimens.
- Women in the peri-menopause with problematic bleeding and vasomotor symptoms may benefit from CECOC regimens rather than cyclical regimens because of the elimination of the HFIs. For women in the peri-menopausal transition who may be ovulating, CECOC is preferred to HRT for controlling problematic bleeding and vasomotor symptoms.
- **Cost effectiveness** – CECOC regimens are associated with significantly less menstrual hygiene product consumption than cyclical regimens. Provided that the total annual cost of HC remains lower than the total annual cost of menstrual-related products and medications, CECOC regimens are cost saving for the individual compared with cyclical regimens.

Side effects

- The frequency of unscheduled bleeding with a CECOC regimen is similar to that of a cyclical regimen and reduces over time.
- Evidence of lower frequency of side effects such as headaches, bloating, and menstrual pain than cyclical regimen. The side-effect profile with CECOC regimens is not worse than with cyclical regimens and may be better.
- If irregular bleeding and/or spotting persist with the use of CECOC regimen – rule out pregnancy, non-compliance, cervical infection, smoking, malabsorption, and use of concomitant medications.
- Short-term safety of CECOC regimens is similar to that of cyclical regimens.
- Evidence on long-term safety of CECOC regimens is currently unavailable.
- Greater exposure to EE over one year – although uncertain, studies do not indicate that side effects are made worse with CECOC regimens and, in fact, such regimens may decrease some of these side effects.

1. *Long-acting Reversible Contraception: the Effective and Appropriate Use of Long-Acting Reversible Contraception.* NICE, October 2005.
2. *Canadian Consensus Guideline on Continuous and Extended Hormonal Contraception.* SOGC Clinical Practice Guidelines No.195, 2007.

CHAPTER 66 Male and female sterilization

Background and indications for sterilization

- 47,268 tubal occlusions and 64,422 vasectomies were performed in England in 1999.
- There are no absolute contraindications to sterilization of men or women.

History and assessment

- Take history and examine to rule out any concurrent conditions, which may require an additional or alternative procedure or precaution.
- Provide advice, counselling, and access to other LARCs, including information on the advantages, disadvantages, and relative failure rates of each method.
- As a precaution against the risk of later regret, take additional care when counselling people under the age of 30 years or people without children.
- Take additional care in discussions with people taking decisions during pregnancy or in reaction to a loss of relationship, or who may be at risk of coercion by their partner or family, or health or social welfare professionals.
- Take into account cultural, religious, psychosocial, psychosexual, and other psychological issues, some of which may have implications beyond fertility.
- If there is any question of a person not having the mental capacity to consent to a procedure that will permanently remove his/her fertility – refer the case to court.

Specific consent issues

- Discuss both vasectomy and tubal occlusion. Vasectomy carries a lower failure rate and has fewer risks related to the procedure.
- Although the procedure is intended to be permanent, inform about the success rates associated with reversal, should this procedure be necessary.
- These are associated with failure rates and pregnancies can occur several years after the procedure.
  * The lifetime risk of failure for tubal occlusion: 1/200.
  * Filshie clips, after 10 years of use: 2–3/1000 procedures.
  * The failure rate for vasectomy is 1/2000 after clearance has been given.
- In a small minority of men, non-motile sperm persist after vasectomy. In such cases, 'special clearance' to stop contraception may be given when < 10,000 non-motile sperm/ml are found in a fresh specimen examined at least 7 months after vasectomy, as no pregnancies have been reported under these circumstances.
- Inform of risks of laparoscopy, particularly if they are at increased risk such as previous abdominal surgery or obesity.

- If tubal occlusion fails, the resulting pregnancy may be an ectopic pregnancy. After tubal occlusion, advise women to seek medical help if they think that they might be pregnant or if they have abnormal abdominal pain or vaginal bleeding.
- No precautions can be guaranteed to avoid early pre-existing pregnancy, which may be undetectable. Advise women to use effective contraception until the day of the operation and to continue to use it until their next menstrual period.
- Advise men to use effective contraception until azoospermia is confirmed.
- Tubal occlusion is not associated with an increased risk of heavier or irregular periods when performed after 30 years of age. There is an association with subsequent increased hysterectomy rates, although there is no evidence that tubal occlusion leads to problems that require a hysterectomy.
- Data are limited on the effect on menstruation when tubal occlusion is performed on women under 30 years of age.
- There is no increase in testicular cancer or heart disease associated with vasectomy.
- There is a possibility of chronic testicular pain after vasectomy.

Sterilization procedures

Tubal occlusion

- Can be performed at any time during the menstrual cycle provided that the woman has used effective contraception up until the day of the operation. Otherwise, defer the operation until the follicular phase of a subsequent cycle.
- Woman should use effective contraception until her next menstrual period.
- Wherever possible, perform tubal occlusion after an appropriate interval following pregnancy.
- Women who request tubal occlusion postpartum or following abortion are at increased risk of regret and the possible increased failure rate.
- If tubal occlusion is to be performed at the same time as a CS, counselling and agreement should have been given at least one week prior to the procedure.
- A pregnancy test must be performed before the operation to exclude a pre-existing pregnancy. However, a negative test does not exclude the possibility of a luteal phase pregnancy.
- Routine curettage at the time of tubal occlusion, in order to prevent a luteal phase pregnancy, is not recommended.

Vasectomy

- No-scalpel approach to identify the vas results in a lower rate of early complications.
- Division of the vas on its own is not an acceptable technique because of its failure rate. Division should be accompanied by fascial interposition or diathermy.
- Do not use clips for occluding the vas, as failure rates are unacceptably high.
- Irrigation of the vas during vasectomy does not reduce failure rates or reduce time to clearance.
- Perform vasectomy under local anaesthesia wherever possible.
- Send the excised portions of vas for histological examination only if there is any doubt about their identity.

Laparoscopic approach

- Quicker and associated with less minor morbidity compared with mini-laparotomy.
- Perform as a day case wherever possible.
- Local anaesthesia is an acceptable alternative.
- Topical application of local anaesthesia to the Fallopian tubes should be used whenever mechanical occlusive devices are being applied.
- Mechanical occlusion of the tubes by either Filshie clips or rings is the method of choice for laparoscopic tubal occlusion.
- Do not routinely use more than one Filshie clip.
- Do not use diathermy as the primary method of tubal occlusion because it increases the risk of subsequent ectopic pregnancies and is less easy to reverse than mechanical occlusive methods.
- It should only be performed at a site where there are facilities to perform a laparotomy safely.

Other approaches

- When a mini-laparotomy is used as the method of approach for an interval sterilization, any effective surgical or mechanical method of tubal occlusion can be used.
- A modified Pomeroy procedure rather than Filshie clip application may be preferable for postpartum sterilization using mini-laparotomy or at the time of CS, as it leads to lower failure rates.
- Hysteroscopic methods for tubal occlusion – see next section of chapter.
- Do not use Culdoscopy as a method of approach.

Hysteroscopic sterilization by tubal cannulation and placement of intra-Fallopian implants

Guidance

- Current evidence on its safety and efficacy is adequate to support its use provided that normal arrangements are in place for clinical governance and audit.
- Additional contraception must be used until appropriate imaging has been done. There is a small risk of pregnancy in the longer term after any form of tubal occlusion procedure.

Procedure

- Usually performed under local anaesthesia and/or intravenous sedation.
- A hysteroscope is inserted through the vagina and cervix. A flexible microinsert is passed through the hysteroscope using a guidewire, and placed into each of the Fallopian tubes. The microinserts induce scar tissue formation, which occludes the Fallopian tubes and prevents conception.
- An additional form of contraception should be used until imaging has confirmed satisfactory placement of the microinserts. Imaging may be by X-ray or ultrasound scanning initially, followed by HSG in selected patients, or by HSG as a routine test to confirm tubal blockage.

Efficacy

Seven case series reported:
- Successful bilateral placement of microinserts in 86–99%.
- Tubal occlusion was confirmed by HSG or the position of the microinserts confirmed by X-ray or ultrasound, 3 months after the procedure in 91–99% of women.
- In some cases (19/1477) women had tubal patency at 3 months, but a second HSG at 6 months confirmed occlusion.
- 1-year pregnancy prevention rate of up to 98.9%.

Adverse events

- Infection, vasovagal reaction.
- Risk of ectopic pregnancy.
- Microinsert expulsion and migration to the abdominal cavity: 1–4%.
- Uterine or tubal perforation caused by improper microinsert placement: 1–2%.
- Vaginal spotting and postoperative bleeding, postoperative pain, and cramping.
- Pelvic pain – 5 case reports of 8 women who required subsequent procedures 6 days to 3 years after hysteroscopic sterilization to remove the microinserts because of pain.

What not to do

- Routine curettage at the time of tubal occlusion.
- Vasectomy – do not use clips for occluding the vas.
- Irrigation of the vas during vasectomy.
- Routine use of more than one Filshie clip.
- Use of diathermy as the primary method of tubal occlusion.
- Use of culdoscopy as a method of approach.

1. *Male and Female Sterilisation.* RCOG Evidence-based Clinical Guideline Number 4, 2004.
2. *Hysteroscopic Sterilisation by Tubal Cannulation and Placement of Intrafallopian Implants.* NICE Interventional Procedure Guidance No. 315, September 2009.

Prevalence and background

- VTE includes DVT, PE, and cerebral venous sinus thrombosis (CVST).
- Background incidence of VTE in women of reproductive age is 50–100/100,000 woman-years. This is 10-fold higher than the widely quoted absolute risks for women of reproductive age who are not using contraception (5/100,000 woman-years).
- Non-RCTs suggest an increased risk of VTE with CHC use. The consistency of finding an increased risk among COC users in most of these studies (20 or more) strongly suggests that the effect is real.
- There is synergism between genetic factors associated with VTE (such as factor V Leiden mutation, prothrombin 20210A, protein C or protein S deficiency, antithrombin III deficiency) and acquired risk factors (such as APS, pregnancy, contraceptive use, surgery, trauma, immobilization, and malignancy).
- Hormonal contraception:
  * Combined hormonal contraceptive – pill (COCs), patch (CTP), and vaginal ring.
  * Progestogen-only contraceptive – pills (POPs), implant (POIM), injectable (POIC), and the LNG-IUS; progestogen-only emergency contraception (POEC).

History and risk assessment

- For the majority of women, the use of HC is safe; however, some medical conditions can contraindicate the use of particular methods. Take a detailed history to identify any conditions that fall within the categories 3 or 4 for use of HC.
- As POCs do not increase the risk of VTE, most of the risk assessment relates to CHC.

Screening for thrombophilia before prescribing HC

- Do not routinely screen general population for thrombophilia prior to HC use. Most episodes of VTE occur in women who do not have a thrombogenic mutation.
- Selective screening (based on the presence of personal or family history of VTE) is more cost-effective than universal screening. However, selective screening prevents fewer clinical adverse events (1/10,000) compared with universal screening (3/10,000) prior to HC use.

Contraceptive efficacy

- COC containing gestodene or desogestrel has a 2-fold increase in the risk of VTE compared with NET or LNG (second-generation pills). Progestogen norgestimate is metabolized to LNG and is considered to have a VTE risk similar to that of second-generation COCs.
- Data on VTE risk and CHC are based mainly on studies of oral methods; however, the risk is considered to be the same for all HC methods regardless of the mode of administration.
- COC users and the risk of VTE (Committee on Safety of Medicine data from 1999)

Population	VTE/100,000 woman-years	Relative risk
Non-pregnant non-users	5	
LNG or NET COC	15	3-fold increase
Gestodene/desogestrel COC	25	5-fold increase
Pregnant non-users	60	12-fold increase

- The RR of VTE increased with all CHCs. Nevertheless, the rarity of VTE in women of reproductive age means that the absolute risk remains small.
- The RR of VTE increases in the first 4 months after initiating CHC. This risk reduces with increasing duration of use but it remains above the background risk until the CHC is stopped.

COCs

- Recent Europe-wide surveillance study (EURAS):
  * A 2-fold increase in the RR of VTE with COC use compared with non-use.
  * No difference in risk was identified between any brands of COC, regardless of the progestogen (including those containing drospirenone).
  * The absolute risk of VTE associated with COC use was 10-fold higher than those quoted in the earlier CSM data, but this reflects the increase in the background risk.
- Intravaginal ring – the combined hormonal vaginal ring (2.7 mg EE and 11.7 mg etonorgestrel) provides a serum concentration of EE of around 15 μg/day. Insufficient data on the RRs of VTE compared with other combined methods.
- Cyproterone acetate-containing COC – COC containing cyproterone acetate with EE is not licensed to be used solely as a contraceptive but it can provide contraception. There is some evidence that it is associated with a 4-fold increase in the risk of VTE. Some of it may be due to inherent cardiovascular risks of women (PCOS).
- Transdermal patch – long-term data on VTE risk with the combined EE and norelgestromin transdermal patch are limited.
- EURAS – the incidence of VTE in patch users is 74/100,000 woman-years.
- The risk of VTE with patch use is slightly increased compared with that for a LNG contraceptive (OR 1.4), but this is not statistically significant.

POCs

- Limited data. POCs are not associated with an increased risk of VTE.
- Systematic review (2009) – 4 case–control studies. 3 reported an increased risk and 1 a decreased risk of VTE. The overall OR for POC-associated VTE was 1.45.
- No specific evidence was identified regarding the risk of VTE with the use of POIM, the LNG-IUS, POEC, or desogestrel-only pill; but data are limited.

Conditions predisposing to VTE

Current or previous VTE

- **CHC is contraindicated as this poses an unacceptable health risk (UKMEC 4).**
- POCs – benefits outweigh any risks (UKMEC 2).
- Women using anticoagulants – there is a small risk of haematoma with POIM or POICs, but the risk is small.
- The LNG-IUS can be used to manage menorrhagia associated with anticoagulant use.

Family history

- A family history of VTE may indicate an increased risk of VTE. Nevertheless, a family history alone cannot identify an underlying thrombophilia with any certainty.
- **CHC use by women with a family history of VTE in a first-degree relative of < 45 years of age is not recommended (UKMEC 3).**
- POCs may be used regardless of family history.

Known thrombogenic mutations

- Women with reduced levels of naturally occurring anticoagulant (anti-thrombin III, protein C, or protein S) or factor V Leiden who use COCs have up to a 5-fold increase in the risk of VTE compared with non-users without this deficiency.
- Women with factor V Leiden can have up to a 35-fold increase in the risk of VTE with COC use.
- **If a woman has an identified thrombogenic mutation, the use of CHC poses an unacceptable health risk (UKMEC 4).**
- POCs can be used without further increasing the risk of VTE.

Smoking

- **Do not use CHC in women aged > 35 years who are current smokers or who have stopped smoking less than 1 year previously.**
- Compared with non-smokers, light smokers (< 15 cigarettes/day) have a 2-fold increased risk of MI and heavy smokers (> 15 cigarettes/day) have a 4-fold increased risk. Use of CHC in heavy smokers appears to increase the risk 20-fold. VTE risk is increased with the increasing amount smoked.
- The risks of stroke, MI, and VTE increase with increasing age, and mortality from cigarette smoking increases from age 35 years. Advise smokers aged > 35 years against the use of CHC (UKMEC 3 for women who smoke <15 cigarettes/day and UKMEC 4 for women smoking ≥ 15 cigarettes/day).
- Can use POCs in women who smoke.

Obesity

- For women with a BMI ≥ of 35, the risks of CHC may outweigh the benefits.
- Obesity is an independent risk factor for cardiovascular disease and VTE.
- COC users who are obese have a 5–8-fold increased risk of VTE compared with non-users and up to a 10-fold increase in risk compared with that of non-users who are not obese. The absolute risk of VTE in women with increased BMI is still low.
- For women with obesity I (BMI 30.0–34.9), the benefits of using CHC generally outweigh the risks (UKMEC 2).
- For women with obesity II (BMI 35.0–39.9) and obesity III (BMI 40 or more) the risks of CHC may outweigh the benefits (UKMEC 3).
- Consider using CHCs with expert clinical judgement and/or referral if other methods are unavailable or unacceptable.
- POCs can be used safely regardless of weight.

Post-pregnancy use

- **For women who are postpartum and not breastfeeding, do not initiate CHC before day 21 postpartum.**
- In the first 3 weeks postpartum, coagulation and fibrinolytic factors have not returned to their pre-pregnancy state and therefore the risk of VTE is still greater then in non-pregnant women. In view of this, the risks of using CHC before day 21 postpartum outweigh the benefits (UKMEC 3).
- From day 21 postpartum, the benefits of CHC use for women who are not breastfeeding outweigh the risks (UKMEC 1).
- POCs can be started any time postpartum as they do not pose an increased risk.
- All HC can be safely initiated immediately following a first- or second-trimester TOP up to 24 weeks of gestation.

Surgery and other conditions leading to immobilization

- **Discontinue CHC and start an alternative oestrogen-free method at least 4 weeks before major elective surgery where immobilization is expected. CHC does not need to be discontinued before minor surgery without immobilization.**
- The benefits of using CHC outweigh the risks for women having minor surgery where immobilization is not expected or for major surgery without prolonged immobilization.
- For women undergoing major elective surgery with prolonged immobilization, the use of CHC poses an unacceptable health risk (UKMEC 4).
- POCs do not increase the risk of VTE and do not need to be discontinued before surgery.
- When the CHC has not been discontinued before surgery (e.g., in an emergency procedure), follow thromboprophylaxis guidelines.

Conditions predisposing to VTE (contd.)

Sickle-cell disease

- SCD is a chronic, inherited, haematological condition that can be complicated by vaso-occlusion by poorly deformable erythrocytes. An observational study comparing hormonal (combined and POCs) and barrier contraception in women with SCD showed no significant difference in haemostatic variables. A case–control study showed a reduction in painful sickle-cell crises with use of DMPA.
- Benefits of using any type of HC in SCD outweigh the risks.
- Women with SCD with pulmonary HT – CHC is not recommended.

Systemic lupus erythematosus

- Women with SLE are at an increased risk of heart disease, stroke, and VTE. Nevertheless, very few women with SLE will go on to develop VTE.
- Women with SLE and positive or unknown antiphospholipid antibodies – CHC poses an unacceptable health risk (UKMEC 4).
- POCs may be used in this situation based on individual risks and with liaison between contraceptive and SLE specialists (UKMEC 3).

Other medical conditions

- Women with IBS are not at increase risk of VTE. Offer the same contraceptive choices as other women. In women who are immobilized owing to disease exacerbation or major surgery, stop CHC and provide an alternative contraception.
- Women with varicose veins and superficial thrombophlebitis are not at an increased risk of VTE and can therefore use any hormonal methods (UKMEC 1).

Evidence round-up – individual VTE risk with COCs

- Systematic review of 25 studies (2012).
- The pooled RRs of VTE associated with the various CHCs, depending on their progestogen, were:
  * Gestodene vs LNG 1.3.
  * Desogestrel vs LNG 1.9.
  * Drospirenone vs LNG 1.7.
- The pooled OR for for:
  * Norgestimate vs LNG 1.1.
  * Cyproterone acetate vs LNG 1.7.
- **Safest CHCs in terms of VTE are those containing LNG or norgestimate.**
- Risk of VTE associated with desogestrel-, drospirenone-, or cyproterone acetate-containing CHCs is greater than that associated with CHCs containing LNG.
- Increased risk of VTE found for CHCs with gestodene compared with LNG seems smaller than in previous analyses.
- There were no differences in VTE risk between oral and transdermal CHCs containing norgestimate or norelgestromin, respectively.

What not to do

- Routine population screening for thrombophilia prior to HC.
- **CHC use in women with current VTE or previous VTE** (UKMEC 4).
- CHC use in woman with an identified thrombogenic mutation (UKMEC 4).
- CHC use in women with SCD with pulmonary HT.
- CHC use in women with SLE and positive or unknown APA antibodies (UKMEC 4).
- CHC use in smokers who are aged > 35 years (UKMEC 3 for women who smoke < 15 cigarettes/day and UKMEC 4 for women smoking ≥ 15 cigarettes/day).
- CHC use in women undergoing major elective surgery with prolonged immobilization (UKMEC 4).

1. *Venous Thromboembolism and Hormonal Contraception* RCOG Green-top Guideline No. 40, July 2010.
2. Bergendal A, Odlind V, Persson I, Kieler H. Limited knowledge on progestogen-only contraception and risk of VTE. *Acta Obstet Gynecol Scand* 2009;88(3):261–266.
3. Martinez F, Ramrez I, Perez-Campos E, Latorre K, Lete I. Venous and pulmonary thromboembolism and combined hormonal contraceptives. Systematic review and meta-analysis. *Eur J Contracept Reprod Health Care* 2012;17(1):7–29.